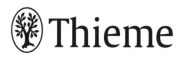

Pediatric Otolaryngology

Practical Clinical Management

R. W. Clarke, BA, BSc, DCH, FRCS, FRCS (ORL)
Consultant Pediatric Otolaryngologist
Alder Hey Children's Hospital
Senior Lecturer and Associate Dean
University of Liverpool
Liverpool, UK

454 illustrations

Thieme
Stuttgart • New York • Delhi • Rio de Janeiro

Library of Congress Cataloging-in-Publication Data is available from the publisher.

© 2017 by Georg Thieme Verlag KG

Thieme Publishers Stuttgart
Rüdigerstrasse 14, 70469 Stuttgart, Germany
+49 [0]711 8931 421, customerservice@thieme.de

Thieme Publishers New York
333 Seventh Avenue, New York, NY 10001 USA
+1 800 782 3488, customerservice@thieme.com

Thieme Publishers Delhi
A-12, Second Floor, Sector-2, Noida-201301
Uttar Pradesh, India
+91 120 45 566 00, customerservice@thieme.in

Thieme Publishers Rio, Thieme Publicações Ltda.
Edifício Rodolpho de Paoli, 25º andar
Av. Nilo Peçanha, 50 – Sala 2508,
Rio de Janeiro 20020-906 Brasil
Tel: +55 21 3172-2297 / +55 21 3172-1896

Cover design: Thieme Publishing Group
Typesetting by Thomson Digital, India

Printed in India by Replika Press Pvt. Ltd.   5 4 3 2 1

ISBN 978-3-13-169901-5

Also available as an e-book:
eISBN 978-3-13-169911-4

Important note: Medicine is an ever-changing science undergoing continual development. Research and clinical experience are continually expanding our knowledge, in particular our knowledge of proper treatment and drug therapy. Insofar as this book mentions any dosage or application, readers may rest assured that the authors, editors, and publishers have made every effort to ensure that such references are in accordance with **the state of knowledge at the time of production of the book.**

Nevertheless, this does not involve, imply, or express any guarantee or responsibility on the part of the publishers in respect to any dosage instructions and forms of applications stated in the book. **Every user is requested to examine carefully** the manufacturers' leaflets accompanying each drug and to check, if necessary in consultation with a physician or specialist, whether the dosage schedules mentioned therein or the contraindications stated by the manufacturers differ from the statements made in the present book. Such examination is particularly important with drugs that are either rarely used or have been newly released on the market. Every dosage schedule or every form of application used is entirely at the user's own risk and responsibility. The authors and publishers request every user to report to the publishers any discrepancies or inaccuracies noticed. If errors in this work are found after publication, errata will be posted at www.thieme.com on the product description page.

Some of the product names, patents, and registered designs referred to in this book are in fact registered trademarks or proprietary names even though specific reference to this fact is not always made in the text. Therefore, the appearance of a name without designation as proprietary is not to be construed as a representation by the publisher that it is in the public domain.

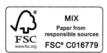

For Doreen and Emmet Clarke

"Nanny and Emmet"

Contents

Part II: The Ear

19. Obstructive Sleep Apnea 258
Ari DeRowe

20. Airway Obstruction in Children 272
Adam J. Donne and Michael P. Rothera

Foreword

It gives me great pleasure to write the foreword to this new textbook of pediatric otolaryngology, which seeks to encompass the essentials of the subspecialty within a single volume.

Pediatric otolaryngology has only become a subspecialty in relatively recent times. The first children's hospitals were founded during early 19th century, and by the end of the century, the first pediatric ENT ward was in existence in the Children's Hospital of Warsaw. But it was not until the middle of the 20th century that pioneering surgeons began to establish pediatric otolaryngology as a distinct subspecialty. Pediatric intensive care developed in the 1960s, and initially, this produced an epidemic of subglottic stenosis secondary to the intubation and long-term ventilation of premature infants who in earlier years would have perished. This, in turn, stimulated the development of open surgical techniques for laryngotracheal reconstruction in the early 1970s, and for many years thereafter, development of the subspecialty in Europe and North America largely ran in parallel with the evolution of pediatric airway surgery. Today, there is a network of children's hospitals in major cities across the developed world, each with a thriving department of pediatric otolaryngology, where multidisciplinary teamwork has increasingly become the normal practice for managing children with complex, often multisystem medical and surgical problems.

As the subspecialty became established, pediatric otolaryngology societies came into being at both national and international levels. In 1973, the Society for Ear Nose and Throat Advances in Children (SENTAC) was founded in the United States. In 1977, the European Working Group on Pediatric Otorhinolaryngology held its first meeting, and this was the precursor of the European Society of Pediatric Otorhinolaryngology (ESPO), which is now the umbrella organization for all the national European pediatric ENT societies and holds a large biennial congress attracting speakers and delegates from around the world.

As the subspecialty has become more important in clinical practice, postgraduate training and examinations in otolaryngology have been modified to incorporate it. A separate section in the British Intercollegiate FRCS examination was introduced in 1999, and in 2014, agreement was reached to add a pediatric section to the European Board Examination in ORL-HNS.

Since the middle of the 20th century, a number of textbooks on pediatric otolaryngology have been published, ranging from short handbooks to comprehensive multivolume reference works. There are now also various online resources, but nevertheless, the appeal of a printed book endures! There is, however, the need for a readable, single-volume book that is sufficiently comprehensive to prepare candidates for their higher surgical examinations, to act as a ready source of information for general otolaryngologists, and to serve as a quick point of reference for specialist pediatric otolaryngologists. Such a text sometimes derives from a successful course, and many of the authors of this book have taught on the annual British Paediatric Otolaryngology Course. Ray Clarke's dedication to teaching has inspired him to compile and edit this book, and in doing so, he has assembled an eminent group of authors to address all aspects of pediatric otolaryngology from a practical point of view, which will inform everyday clinical practice. I congratulate them upon their efforts and highly recommend their book to you.

Martin Bailey, BSc, FRCS, FRCSEd
Secretary-General
European Society of Pediatric Otorhinolaryngology

Preface and Acknowledgments

A small but increasing number of otolaryngologists devote the greater part of their professional time to children, usually in the specialist children's hospitals or the pediatric departments of large general hospitals. Pediatric otorhinolaryngology (ORL) is in the ascendancy and has changed out of all recognition during the professional lifetimes of the contributors to this book. Advances in endoscopy, in techniques to unravel the etiology of hearing loss, in the recognition and rehabilitation of the hearing-impaired child, in anesthesia and perioperative care, in diagnostic imaging, and in our understanding of the very different pathophysiological responses of children to disease have all made for an exciting, rewarding, and growing subspecialty. We are increasingly cognizant of the impact of disease on families and of the need for multidisciplinary teams to communicate with and to support children and their families often over a period of several years and, in some cases, over the lifetime of the child.

For the foreseeable future, it seems likely that ORL generalists with a mixed adult and pediatric workload will continue to manage many, probably most, ORL interventions in children; I hope this book will fulfil a need for them not easily met by the standard ORL texts. While the dedicated pediatric ORL will want to supplement his/her reading with recourse to the larger reference tomes, I hope this small book will be a useful working text covering most of the clinical scenarios he/she will come across. I am aware of the increasingly important place of pediatric ORL in the formal examinations and assessment of aspiring ORL specialists, and the chapters ahead will more than adequately cover their needs.

Putting this book together has been, much like pediatric ORL, a collaborative effort. I have been greatly helped by many friends and colleagues. I am indebted to the chapter authors, who patiently stuck to their brief of focussing on practical advice in the day-to-day management of children and their families and who showed great forbearance in accepting delays, indulging my many requests for changes, updates, and rewrites, and in putting up with my sometimes ruthless and seemingly quirky editorial changes to ensure consistency and harmony between chapters. Vicki Gregory supported me and the chapter authors throughout with her almost saintly patience, courtesy, and charm. She made many substantial contributions to the text and suggestions to help with clarity of some difficult concepts. The book truly would not have happened without her. My former "Chief" and mentor, Peter Bull, FRCS, emeritus consultant at Sheffield Children's Hospital, who has always been a source of inspiration to me, generously put at my disposal some of his excellent collection of clinical images. Dr. Shiv Avula, pediatric radiologist in Liverpool, supplied many of the radiological images, and the team at the Medical Photography Department at Alder Hey were ever helpful and supportive.

I have been privileged to supervise, teach, and examine numerous young ORL specialists over the years and have taken great joy from seeing them progress. Much that I have learned from them, and from what they tell me are their learning needs, has found its way into this book in the "nuggets of wisdom" that I have incorporated in most chapters as "key points" and as highlighted text boxes.

Like all pediatric ORL specialists in the United Kingdom and throughout Europe. I am indebted to Martin Bailey, FRCS, Secretary-General of the European Society of Pediatric Otorhinolaryngology (ESPO) and thank him for his generous foreword.

Lastly, I thank my wife Mary for her support throughout and for putting up with my many hours on the computer when I should have been attending to more mundane domestic duties!

I am most of all grateful to the children and families I have known in a long career in pediatric ORL. The poet Seamus Heaney evokes the sense of wonder and magic that a child feels during his first contact with the world of medicine and healing when he describes his local doctor visiting the Heaney farmhouse in the 1940s, *like a hypnotist unwinding us.** That sense of wonder transcends all of the technological and scientific advances and remains a constant source of joy to those of us who work with children. Few of our patients will go on to be Nobel prize–winning authors, but they may vividly remember their first encounter with us. What a privilege we enjoy in looking after them!

R. W. Clarke, BA, BSc, DCH, FRCS, FRCS (ORL)

---

* The phrase is from Seamus Heaney's "Out of the Bag" in the collection "Electric Light," Faber and Faber, London, 2002.

Contributors

Marcus K. H. Auth, MD, PD, FRCPCH
Consultant Pediatric Gastroenterologist
Alder Hey Children's Hospital
Liverpool, UK

Fuad M. Baroody, MD, FACS
Professor of Surgery (Otolaryngology-Head and Neck
 Surgery) and Pediatrics
The University of Chicago Medicine and Biological
 Sciences
Chicago, Illinois, USA

An N. Boudewyns, MD, PhD
Pediatric ENT Surgeon
University Hospital Antwerp
Edegem, Belgium

R. W. Clarke, BA, BSc, DCH, FRCS, FRCS (ORL)
Consultant Pediatric Otolaryngologist
Alder Hey Children's Hospital
Senior Lecturer and Associate Dean
University of Liverpool
Liverpool, UK

Sujata De, FRCS (ORL-HNS)
Consultant Pediatric ENT Surgeon
Alder Hey Children's Hospital
Liverpool, UK

Frank Declau, MD, PhD
Chair of ENT Department
Sint-Vincentiusziekenhuis
Antwerpen, Belgium

Ari DeRowe, MD
Director, Pediatric Otolaryngology Unit
Dana Children's Hospital
Tel-Aviv, Israel

Adam J. Donne, PhD, FRCS (ORL-HNS)
Consultant in Pediatric Otolaryngology
Alder Hey Children's Hospital
Liverpool, UK

**Simon van Eeden, BSc, BDS, MBCHB (Hons),
 MChD (Hons), FRCS (Ed), FRCS (OMS)**
Consultant Maxillofacial and Cleft surgeon
Alder Hey Children's Hospital
Liverpool, UK

**Adel Y. Fattah, BSc (Hons), Bchir, PhD, FRCS (Plast),
 PGDipAesthSurg**
Consultant Plastic Surgeon
Alder Hey Children's Hospital
Liverpool, UK

Wytske J. Fokkens, MD, PhD
Professor of Otorhinolaryngology
Academic Medical Center
Amsterdam, The Netherlands

Michael Gleeson, MD, FRCS, FRACS, FDS
Professor of Skull Base Surgery
The National Hospital for Neurology and
 Neurosurgery
Honorary Consultant Skull Base Surgeon
Great Ormond Street Hospital for Sick Children
Emeritus Professor of Otolaryngology
Guy's, Kings and St Thomas' Hospitals
London, UK

**Benjamin Hartley, BSc (Hons), MBBS, FRCS
 (ORL-HNS)**
Consultant ENT and Head and Neck Surgeon
Great Ormond Street Hospital for Children
London, UK

William P. L. Hellier, MB ChB, FRCS (ORL-HNS)
Consultant ENT Surgeon
Southampton University Hospital
Southampton, UK

Balaji Krishnamurthy, MBBS, FRCPH
Consultant Pediatric Gastroenterologist
Alder Hey Children's Hospital
Liverpool, UK

Haytham Kubba, MBBS, Mphil, MD, FRCS (ORL-HNS)
Consultant Pediatric Otolaryngologist
Royal Children's Hospital
Melbourne, Australia

Fiona B. MacGregor, MB ChB (Ed), FRCS, FRCS (ORL-HNS)
Consultant Otolaryngologist
Royal Hospital for Sick Children
Glasgow, UK

Josephine Marriage, BSc, MSc, PhD
Senior Lecturer Pediatric Audiology
University College London Ear Institute
London, UK

Jane M. Martin, Cert Ed, NCTD, BEd, MEd
Head of Service/Specialist Advisory Teacher
   of the Deaf
The Listening for Life Centre
Bradford Royal Infirmary
Bradford, UK

Ann-Louise McDermott, BDS, FDS RCS, MBChB, FRCS, FRCS (ORL-HNS), PhD
Consultant Pediatric ENT Surgeon
Birmingham Children's Hospital
Birmingham, UK

Gavin A. J. Morrison, MA, FRCS
Consultant Pediatric Otolaryngologist
The Evelina Children's Hospital
Guy's and St Thomas' NHS Foundation Trust
London, UK

Frank A. Potter, MBChB, FRCA, FFICM
Consultant Pediatric Anesthetist
Alder Hey Children's Hospital
Liverpool, UK

Christopher H. Raine, BSc (Hons), MBBS, FRCS (Otol), ChM, MBE
Consultant Otorhinolaryngologist
Bradford Royal Infirmary
Bradford, UK

Michael P. Rothera, FRCS
ENT Consultant
Spire Manchester Hospital
Manchester, UK

Amir Sadri, BSc, MSc, MBChB, MRCS
Registrar in Plastic Surgery
Great Ormond Street Hospital for Children
London, UK

Michael Saunders, MD, FRCS
Consultant Pediatric ENT Surgeon
Bristol Royal Hospital for Children
Bristol, UK

Ravi K. Sharma, MBBS, FRCS (ORL-HNS), FRCS (Ed), DLO, MPhil, PGCERT Medical Education
Consultant Pediatric Otolaryngologist
Alder Hey Children's Hospital
Liverpool, UK

Patrick Sheehan, MB BCh MPhil, FRCSI, FRCSEd, FRCS (ORL-NHS)
Consultant Pediatric Otolaryngologist
Sidra Medical and Research Center
Doha, Qatar

Priya Singh, AuD
Director of Education
University College London Ear Institute
London, UK

Marie Gisselsson Solén, MD, PhD, MSc
Department of Otorhinolaryngology, Head and Neck
   Surgery
Lund University Hospital
Lund, Sweden

Gundula Thiel, MD, FRCSEd (ORL-HNS)
Consultant ENT Surgeon
Royal Hospital for Sick Children
Edinburgh, UK

Daniel Tweedie, MA (Cantab), FRCS (ORL-HNS), DCH
Consultant Pediatric ENT Surgeon
Great Ormond Street Hospital for Children
London, UK

Hilko Weerda, MD, DMD
Professor and Former Head
Department of Otorhinolaryngology and Plastic
   Surgery
University Hospital Schleswig-Holstein
Lübeck, Germany

Michelle Wyatt, MA (Cantab) FRCS (ORL-HNS)
Consultant Pediatric Otorhinolaryngologist
Great Ormond Hospital for Sick Children
London, UK

Part I

General Considerations in Children's ENT

1 Introduction to Pediatric Otolaryngology

R. W. Clarke

1.1 Introduction

The majority of ear, nose, and throat (ENT) specialists have experience in both pediatric and adult practice; many work in hospital or clinic settings where both adults and children are cared for. A growing number of clinicians in recent years have focused their practice exclusively on children and work in a specialized children's hospital or in the children's section of a larger general hospital.

This specialization and streamlining of expertise has made for great advances in the management of children with otorhinolaryngology (ORL) disorders.

1.2 Training and Accreditation

The diagnosis and management of ORL conditions in children forms an integral part of the syllabus for all ENT surgeons in training. Examinations in ORL, including the European Board Examination,[1] put much emphasis on this, and in general, otolaryngologists are well trained in the principles of looking after children with common disorders of the upper respiratory tract. Although subspecialization in ORL is largely based on "system" (otology, head and neck surgery, rhinology) rather than on age, a growing number of otolaryngologists now choose to undertake advanced training in a fellowship program in one of the major children's hospitals with a view to taking a special clinical interest in the care of children. In addition to basic and fellowship training, it is essential that all of us who care for children have up-to-date knowledge and skills in topics such as child protection, prescribing for children, analgesia, and pediatric resuscitation, and that we continue to maintain and refresh this knowledge and skill.

1.3 History of Pediatric Otorhinolaryngology

Doctors have treated ENT disorders in children from the beginnings of medicine, centuries before otology or laryngology emerged as discrete specialties. There are references to tonsillectomy in some of the earliest clinical texts, for example, Celsus's "De Medicina" dating from the first century. Tracheostomy for the relief of airway obstruction has been known since ancient times.[2,3] Congenital deafness, craniofacial dysmorphia, infective disorders of the head and neck, and perinatal airway obstruction were recognized and described long before otorhinolaryngology developed. As the age of enlightenment and scientific discovery progressed throughout the 18th and 19th centuries, clinicians began not only to bring the principles of

science to bear on their work, but also to focus their attention on particular body systems and, in some cases, specific diseases (medical specialization). Otology grew largely from the early endeavors of the clinics of Adam Politzer (1835–1920) and Josef Gruber (1827–1900), who treated both adults and children at the Allgemeines Krankenhaus in Vienna, Austria, where they hosted hundreds of pupils from all over Europe and North America. These pupils included Sir William Wilde (1815–1876) and Joseph Toynbee (1815–1866) in Britain, each of whom published what were to become definitive English language textbooks of the new specialty.[4,5] Toynbee's avowed aim was "to rescue aural surgery from the hands of quacks." Wilde's book includes a substantial section cataloguing and recording the etiology of deafness in children, and an impassioned essay championing the cause of improved education for "deaf mutes." Wilde also described an early form of myringotomy (▶ Fig. 1.1,

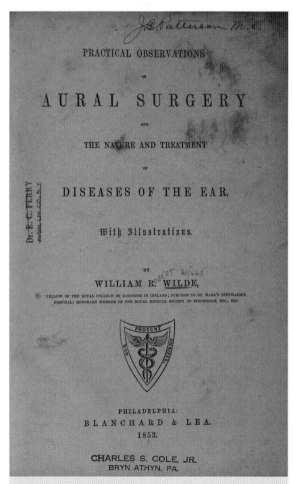

Fig. 1.1 Frontispiece of Wilde's textbook (1853).

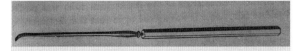

Fig. 1.2 Wilde's myringotomy knife, as illustrated in Wilde WR. Practical Observations on Aural Surgery and the Nature and Treatment of Diseases of the Ear. Philadelphia; Blanchard and Lea: 1853.

▶ Fig. 1.2) and tympanocentesis for "strumous otitis" (otitis media with effusion), myringoplasty, and a surgical approach to drain the mastoid for suppurative mastoiditis in children.

Laryngology advanced in parallel, and it was well into the 20th century before the two disciplines combined as "otorhinolaryngology." The early laryngologists—Morell Mackenzie and Sir Felix Semon, both in London—had substantial pediatric practices. Mackenzie described recurrent respiratory papillomatosis in a postmortem specimen of the larynx of a child who had died in a "home for the friendless." Semon did much to popularize tonsillectomy; he was a laryngologist to the British Royal family and undertook the procedure on the grandchildren of Queen Victoria, making it a fashionable intervention in the drawing rooms of the aristocracy.[6] Laryngeal tuberculosis and congenital syphilis were common causes of laryngotracheal stenosis, and by the early 20th century, there were well-established techniques for tracheotomy and for airway dilatation in children. Diphtheria was an important and often fatal cause of airway obstruction, and acute epiglottitis became a common indication for tracheostomy.

Gustav Killian in Freiburg pioneered suspension laryngoscopy and tracheabronchoscopy, and the technique was soon extended to children. Chevalier Jackson in Philadelphia became a celebrated teacher of pediatric airway endoscopy throughout Europe and the United States.

Children's hospitals were established in Paris (1802), Berlin (1830), St Petersburg (1834), Vienna (1837), and Great Ormond Street, London (1852). As these hospitals expanded, otologists and laryngologists joined the staff, particularly in Eastern Europe. Dr Jan Gabriel Danielewicz opened the first pediatric ENT ward in Warsaw shortly after the end of the second world war.[7] By the 1950s, designated children's ENT wards were becoming commonplace in the larger children's hospitals. Children's health in general improved greatly after the Second World War due to improved sanitation, availability of antibiotics, and widespread adoption of vaccination programs (see Chapter 2).

Pediatric ENT surgeons are acutely aware of the debt they owe to pioneers in other scientific disciplines. Endoscopy was greatly advanced by the discovery of the rod lens optical system by physicist Harold Hopkins in the United Kingdom[8] and developed and refined by the Storz company in Germany. Advances in anesthesia, intensive care, and neonatology are such that many chil-

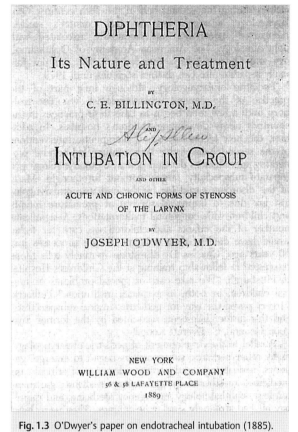

Fig. 1.3 O'Dwyer's paper on endotracheal intubation (1885).

dren who now come under our care are graduates of special care baby units, neonatal intensive care units, or the pediatric intensive care unit (PICU). They often have complex perinatal histories including congenital anomalies, extreme prematurity, and cardiorespiratory diseases that would have been fatal in an earlier generation.

Joseph O'Dwyer of New York (▶ Fig. 1.3) is credited with the first successful endotracheal intubation in a child, but the technique was not widely taken up until the 20th century when it was popularized for the management of diphtheria and croup. Modern pediatric anesthesia owes much to the early endotracheal tubes of Magill.[9] As anesthesia progressed, so did the new subspecialties of pediatric anesthesia and intensive care. Prolonged endotracheal intubation and management on a PICU only became commonplace from the 1960s onward. As recently as 1955, Wilson,[10] in the first English language textbook of pediatric ENT, wrote of tracheostomy in children: "these are desperate cases at best, and it may be a comfort to remember that the worst thing that will happen is that the patient will die. This is a likely event in any case."

Pediatric airway endoscopy even in the very young is now a safe day-case undertaking, and the fear and trepidation that surrounded tracheostomy in children is happily a distant memory.

Audiology has its own history. Physicians, pediatricians, otologists, and teachers took a keen interest in the hearing impaired child from the earliest times, but the profession of audiology began in the 1920s when the first audiometers became commercially available. Early devices for measuring hearing—known as "sonometers" or "acoumeters"—were produced in the late 19th century, and a variety of trumpet devices were used as primitive "hearing aids." Electronic hearing aids became available in the early 20th century, gradually becoming smaller and more efficient. The modern-day digital aids are highly sophisticated programmable devices. The term "audiology," and with it a more effective organization and regulation of the specialty, came after the Second World War. Education and teaching of the deaf child progressed hugely in the 20th century. Edith Whetnall in London was a pioneer in this area. She established a network of clinics, which became a model for the assessment and treatment of hearing impaired children, and her textbook, "The Deaf Child" (1964), was the standard work for many years.[4] Cochlear implantation, developed in the 1970s and, refined and improved upon throughout the next 30 years, transformed the lives of hearing impaired children and their families (see Chapter 15) in the developed world.

The assessment and rehabilitation of the hearing impaired child has advanced greatly in recent years (see Chapter 13 and Chapter 15), and pediatric audiology is an important and growing medical specialty.

1.4 Ear, Nose, and Throat Societies

As subspecialties develop, practitioners need to meet to exchange ideas, foster education and learning, and to advocate for their specialty interests. Ad hoc meetings of otolaryngologists with an interest in pediatric work took place at various venues particularly in Eastern Europe from the early 20th century. The European Working Group in Pediatric ENT was formed in 1973 and later became the European Society of Pediatric Otorhinolaryngology (ESPO).[11] The Society for Ear Nose and Throat Advances in Children (SENTAC) was formed in 1977 and the American Society of Pediatric Otolaryngology (ASPO) first met in 1985.[12] Most national ENT societies have a group focusing on pediatric practice, and there are now many national pediatric ORL societies.

1.5 Organizing Otorhinolaryngology Services for Children

The philosophy and thinking that influences how we care for children has undergone a radical transformation in recent years. Doctors are no longer seen as infallible.

Parents are well informed and expect full participation in decision-making. They expect that their child will be treated in an environment that serves the needs of the child and family, and that carers and other staff are fully trained not only in delivering health care, but also in the principles of looking after children and families. There is growing expectation that service organization should be driven not by the needs of professionals but by the needs of children and families. These legitimate expectations put an onus on us as doctors and planners when setting up services for children.

ORL is the specialty with the biggest pediatric surgical workload. It is important that we as ORL clinicians are to the fore in driving service changes forward to best serve children, families, and the next generation of specialists.

> Children should be treated safely, as close to home as possible, in an environment that is suitable to their needs, with their parents' involvement in decisions, and with the optimal quality of care.[13]

Despite the desirability of treating children close to home, children with unusual or complex conditions or who are in need of highly specialized intervention will have their care best delivered in one of a small number of more specialized settings, where resources and skills are concentrated.

Political priorities, cultural preferences, resources, and governance arrangements inevitably differ across jurisdictions and in different health care models and settings. It is impossible to be too proscriptive about how pediatric ORL services should be managed in any one system, but the fundamental principles and aspirations are the same.

1.5.1 Hospitals and Clinics

Clinicians caring for children and young people should undertake a level of pediatric clinical activity that is enough to maintain minimum competencies. This is rarely a problem in ORL due to the mixed adult and pediatric nature of the specialty. Most ENT interventions in children—both out-patient consultations and surgery—are delivered by ENT surgeons with a mixed adult and pediatric workload and in a hospital or clinic setting that caters for both adults and children.

Hospitals that undertake the care of children should be committed to exemplary standards of care, with the involvement of senior staff in ensuring that the specific requirements of children are met. In a hospital with several otolaryngologists on staff, one should ideally be designated as lead for pediatrics so that he/she can advocate for children at the highest level and can coordinate management, transfer, and referral of children with complex needs who may need treatment in a specialized center.

Well-established liaison networks and good communication with specialist centers, pediatricians, community pediatric services, social services, parents, and advocacy groups are a cornerstone of good pediatric practice.

> **i**
>
> It is best practice that children are seen at a designated children's clinic.

Ideally, a registered children's nurse should be available to supervise this clinic. It should be "child-friendly" with suitable toys, papers and pens, and facilities for parents and siblings (see Chapter 2).

> **i**
>
> Ideally, and where operating room scheduling permits, children scheduled for surgery should have that surgery performed on a dedicated children's operating list.

The operating room staff will need to be suitably trained, and in particular the anesthesiologist should be competent in pediatric anesthesia with a sufficient workload and throughput to maintain his/her skills in the perioperative care of children. Children under the age of 3 years will usually require more specialized anesthetic care, and the professional associations that govern anesthesia in different jurisdictions have their own recommendations with which anesthesiologists will generally be familiar. If at all possible and provided it is safe, children should be admitted and discharged on the same day ("day" surgery or "ambulatory care").

Children are best looked after in a children's ward rather than in a mixed ward with adults, again with appropriately trained and accredited nursing staff. Parents will usually wish to stay with the child overnight, and provision should be made for them.

If children require overnight nursing care, for example, following adenotonsillectomy for obstructive sleep apnea, experienced pediatric ENT nurses are usually best placed to look after them. A small number of children will need more thorough monitoring and supervision perhaps with one-to-one nursing care, admission to a high dependency unit, or exceptionally a PICU.

1.5.2 Emergencies and Transport

> **i**
>
> Hospitals that admit children must be prepared to deal with emergency presentations. Making provision for such emergencies well in advance is an integral part of a pediatric service.

ORL emergencies best dealt with locally include post-tonsillectomy hemorrhage, foreign bodies in the aerodigestive tract that require immediate removal, quinsy, and neck abscesses, provided the emergency team, particularly the surgeon and anesthetist, are appropriately trained and skilled to deal with the scenario. Many of these emergencies can be safely dealt with in a general hospital setting, but some children will need to be transferred to a specialist center, including on occasion a center with a PICU that may be some distance away. The nature of the emergency will determine the need for transfer, but there are occasions when a child with a relatively straightforward condition that would usually be easily dealt with locally may need to be transferred. This may be due to the availability of staff and facilities, but factors unique to the child can also be important. A child with significant cardiorespiratory comorbidity (e.g., congenital heart disease) may be best looked after in a tertiary center where anesthesia and medical pediatric facilities are more suitable. There is an acknowledged higher morbidity related to anesthesia and perioperative care in children with developmental delay or multiple disabilities, and consideration should be given prior to surgery whether surgical care should be undertaken in a specialist center.

It is important that senior clinicians engage with hospital management to make sure that policies and protocols are in place, including networked arrangements with a tertiary receiving center and defined mechanisms for speedy liaison with a transport or "retrieval" team of which there are now several, each serving different areas.[14,15] The initial priority is resuscitation of the child followed by stabilization so that he/she can be safely transported. This may involve a senior ENT surgeon, not only for ENT emergencies but also to ensure that the child has a safe and stable airway. If the child needs an alternative airway, endotracheal intubation is usually preferable and is nowadays safely undertaken by skilled and trained anesthesiologists, pediatricians, or intensive care physicians. In exceptional circumstances, a tracheotomy may be considered, but this is nowadays a very rare occurrence indeed. If the child is to be transported, a senior clinician, in liaison with the senior clinical staff at the receiving center, needs to decide on the best mode of travel, and the skill mix and seniority of the staff that accompany the transport team. Analgesia is an important component of the care of the sick child at all times, but can be easily neglected in a fraught emergency situation. Assessment and treatment of pain must start at first presentation and should be regularly reassessed.

"Retrieval" teams are an increasingly important part of networked care for children. These teams may include pediatricians, anesthesiologists, intensive care physicians, nurses, paramedics, and a pediatric otolaryngologist. These teams have particular training needs, including ongoing attention to maintaining their skills, and the otolaryngologist will often have a key role in the team.

1.6 Key Points

- Pediatric ORL is not new; ENT surgeons have always looked after sick children.
- Developments in medicine, anesthesia, and intensive care have brought about a need for increasingly specialist care for children with ORL disorders.
- Dedicated children's ENT wards were established in Eastern Europe from mid-20th century.
- The improvements in endoscopy brought about by the discoveries of Harold Hopkins transformed pediatric airway care.
- ENT surgeons with a substantial involvement in the care of children need to take a strong advocacy role to make for better services for children.
- Children frequently need to be transferred to specialist centers. Arrangements for safe transfer often involve the local ENT surgeon.

References

[1] Website of the European Board Examination in Otolaryngology – Head and Neck Surgery. Available at http://ebeorl-hns.org. Accessed February 8, 2016

[2] Porter R. The Greatest Benefit to Mankind: A Medical History of Humanity. London: Fontana Press; 1999

[3] Weir N, Mudry A. Otorhinolaryngology: An Illustrated History. 2nd ed. Ashford, UK: Headleys of Ashford; 2013

[4] Toynbee J. Diseases of the Ear: Their Nature Diagnosis and Treatment. London: Churchill; 1860

[5] Wilde WR. Practical Observations on Aural Surgery and the Nature and Treatment of Diseases of the Ear. Philadelphia, PA: Blanchard and Lea; 1853

[6] Harrison D. Eponymists in Medicine: Felix Semon 1849–1921: A Victorian Laryngologist. London: Royal Society of Medicine Press; 2000

[7] Allen GC, Stool SE. History of pediatric airway management. Otolaryngol Clin North Am. 2000; 33(1):1–14

[8] Bhatt J, Jones A, Foley S, et al. Harold Horace Hopkins: a short biography. BJU Int. 2010; 106(10):1425–1428

[9] Magill IW. Endotracheal anaesthesia. Proc RSM 1928;22(2):85–8

[10] Wilson TG. Diseases of the Ear Nose and Throat in Children. London: William Heinemann; 1955

[11] Website of the European Society of Pediatric Otorhinolaryngology. Available at www.espo.eu.com. Accessed February 8, 2016

[12] Website of the American Society of Pediatric Otolaryngology. Available at www.aspo.us. Accessed February 22, 2016

[13] Children's Surgical Forum of the Royal College of Surgeons of England. Standards for Children's Surgery. London: RCSENG; 2013. Available at www.rcseng.ac.uk/publications/docs/standards-in-childrens-surgery. Accessed February 8, 2016

[14] Website of North West & North Wales Paediatric Transport Service. Available at www.nwts.nhs.uk. Accessed February 22, 2016

[15] Website of Children's Acute Transport Service. Available at site.cats.nhs.uk. Accessed February 22, 2016

2 The Pediatric Consultation

R. W. Clarke

2.1 Introduction

A good pediatric first consultation is far more than a forum for making a diagnosis and planning management. It is an opportunity to establish a rapport with a family who may need to see you many times over the ensuing years. It can be used to familiarize the child and family with the hospital, the clinic, and the members of the team who may be looking after them during one or more admissions and outpatient visits.

Otolaryngologists are well trained in the general principles of history taking, examination, and consultation in both adults and children, but there are aspects of the pediatric consultation that set it apart. Children and their parents will often vividly remember their earliest encounters with a doctor. For many, this will be the child's first contact with clinics and hospitals, and may set the scene for subsequent visits. Attention to a few details can make for a far better experience. It is worth putting time, effort, and preparation into making the exchange as pleasant as possible for the child and family and as productive as possible for the doctor and the other health care professionals who will look after the child.

It goes without saying that the health and welfare of the child are paramount and must be at the forefront of any decisions made, but the decision to see you will have typically come from the parents (often the mother) who may be extremely anxious, perplexed, and wondering if they are "doing the right thing."

This makes for one of the important differences between the adult and pediatric consultation: the diagnosis, the discussion of management options, and the decision-making are essentially "by proxy" and will usually involve the parents or carers rather than the child. The older child may be able to express her views, but with babies and young children, you need to look after essentially two patients, the child and the parent or parents.

2.2 Setting Up

2.2.1 The Waiting Area

The clinic experience for the family starts well before they see you. Easy road access, car parking, a bright and friendly environment with adequate facilities for food and drinks, baby-feeding facilities, wheelchair-friendly access, and an environment where children and parents feel safe and welcome not only contribute greatly to parental and child satisfaction with their visit but also probably influence outcomes. Planning modern children's hospitals is a highly skilled endeavor and ideally will involve close liaison between the building architects and

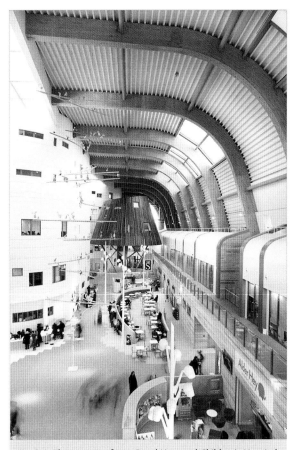

Fig. 2.1 The entrance foyer, Royal Liverpool Children's Hospital, Alder Hey.

their design team, clinicians, hospital staff, children and their advocates, and planning authorities (▶ Fig. 2.1).

A bright, spacious waiting room well stocked with toys, pens, paper, crayons, and computer games and able to withstand the rough and tumble that is inevitable in a group of children will make for a far happier experience than a cramped shared facility (▶ Fig. 2.2). Play therapists are invaluable, and if the hospital authorities can be persuaded to hire a professional clown, better still.

It goes without saying that easy access to bathrooms, baby-change facilities, and adequate space for breast-feeding mothers is essential.

2.2.2 The Clinic Room

One of the paradoxes of caring for children is that despite their small size they need far more space than adults. A clinic room needs to accommodate two parents, the

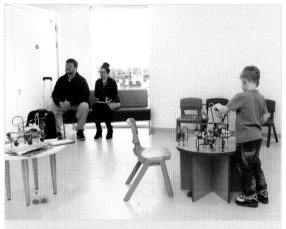

Fig. 2.2 The ENT waiting area.

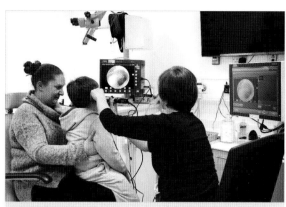

Fig. 2.3 Examining a child's ear using the otoendoscope. The parent can see the screen image, which can be recorded and kept.

child—sometimes in a Moses basket or a pushchair—one or more siblings, equipment such as oxygen cylinders or a ventilator, the doctor, a nurse, and often one or more medical students or trainee surgeons. This is in addition to the equipment required for ear, nose, and throat (ENT) examination and treatment. Ideally, each clinic room will have a microscope, suction apparatus, a camera, a light source and stacker system with a monitor for nasal and airway endoscopy, image capture facilities, and a range of flexible and rigid endoscopes (► Fig. 2.3). Discreetly put away as many sharp instruments, such as hooks, picks, and needles, as you can so they are not on display. They are better stored on a shelf out of view as they can be extremely intimidating to young children. Hand-washing facilities are, of course, mandatory. The physical environment needs to be safe with no sharp or pointed corners, spirit lamps, or loose cables.

> Audiological testing rooms are an integral part of an ENT consultation and should be adjacent to the clinic so that the child can easily move from one room to the other.

The preceding represents an ideal state of affairs and many ENT surgeons have to see children in less than optimum circumstances, but it is important that we as clinicians advocate as robustly as we can for the best facilities for our pediatric patients.

2.2.3 Support Staff

Reception staff and care assistants who have had training and experience in dealing with parents and children help to make for a better clinic experience. Best practice is that a registered children's nurse should ideally be available "to assist, supervise, support, and chaperone children,"[1,2] but clearly arrangements will vary in different jurisdictions and in different health care settings.

> Audiological professionals are an integral part of pediatric ENT practice, and as a minimum, a fully registered audiology technician with appropriate facilities for audiometry and tympanometry should be available for all children's ENT clinics.

Other professionals may be needed depending on the nature of the clinic, for example, a speech and language therapist for voice disorders or cleft palate, or specialist audiological personnel for children with bone-anchored hearing aids or cochlear implants.

Trained specialist nurses who liaise with families outwith the clinic, for example, in supporting home tracheostomy care, greatly enhance the clinical experience for parent and child. Some units arrange a "preadmission" clinic so that when a child is scheduled for surgery, he/she can have preoperative checks in advance of the day of admission. A dedicated nurse usually runs these clinics, and it can be useful for the family to meet her/him at the first clinic visit so that they can plan ahead. If the family does not speak the same language as the doctor and clinic staff, an interpreter may be needed, and this should, of course, be arranged well in advance of the visit.

Many ENT surgeons run "specialist" clinics with a focus on multidisciplinary care, for example, an allergy clinic will require an ENT surgeon and a specialist in pediatric allergy. It is important to strike a good balance between involving the required staff and overwhelming the child with a surfeit of adults in a single room.

2.2.4 Preparing for the Consultation

The parents may have had to book time off work, child care for siblings, a day off school for the child, and transport for the trip. Ideally, the children's clinic must be separate from the adult clinic. If it is not possible to have a clinical area and a set of consulting rooms that are used exclusively for children throughout the working week, they should be scheduled for a dedicated pediatric session; children should no longer be seen in a "mixed" adult and pediatric setting. It can be very uncomfortable for children and their parents—and for adult patients and their relatives—if they are allocated the same clinic and have to share a waiting area. Parents or children must not feel rushed in clinic; if you have to hurry them along, the clinic has not been properly planned.

Take time to read the case notes, including the results of investigations, if applicable, before the child enters the room. If the child has a chronic medical condition or a syndrome, read up on it in advance if you can. This should be relatively easy in most settings nowadays as so much information is available online. Parent and child will appreciate continuity, and if you are seeing a child for repeat visits, it is ideal if the same doctor sees them each time.

2.3 The Consultation

2.3.1 The History

Greet the child by name, make eye contact, and introduce yourself and any other staff in the room. Establish who is with the child—it may be a parent, a carer, or a grandparent. Be clear on who is going to give you the history and make sure the child gets an opportunity to speak if she is old enough. Doctors are taught to take very focused histories, but in a pediatric setting it is often better to ask an open question such as, "What are your worries about Kirsten?," rather than steering the parent down a particular set of symptoms. Many doctors regard themselves as good communicators because they can explain illnesses and procedures in easy-to-follow terms, but of course communication is a two-way street and listening without interruption can be more useful than talking. It is essential that the parent, usually the mother, feels that her account has been carefully listened to and understood before you probe with more direct questions. Watch the child, look at the mother's facial expressions, note how she interacts with the child, and pick up as much information as you can from both verbal and nonverbal clues.

If the parents offer to show you the child's growth chart, a record of their visits to the doctor, diary entries, photographs, or short video clips, do look at them. The parents will feel any record of their child's health is important and they may give you much information, for example, about the child's overall development or, in the case of video clips, the child's sleep pattern. The birth and perinatal history may be important, particularly with airway pathology, it is helpful to ask the mother about the delivery, whether the baby was term or premature, whether there were any concerns about breathing and feeding as a newborn, and in particular whether there was any airway intervention, for example, an endotracheal tube or a period on the special care baby unit.

Parents may be angry, upset, seeming not to listen, or challenging in a variety of ways, but unless they are overtly abusive or threatening, they should be carefully listened to and treated with the utmost courtesy.

2.3.2 Examination

The examination begins as soon as the child comes into the room. An astute clinician will note the child's gait, breathing pattern, and state of alertness as he/she is taking the history. Once they have had a chance to settle in the clinic room, most young children are happy to be examined. Smaller children are best examined sitting on their mother's knee.

It is not appropriate to restrain an older child for the purpose of an elective clinical examination, but the parent can gently but firmly hold a baby or toddler to facilitate otoscopy, examination of the nose, and examination of the neck.

I

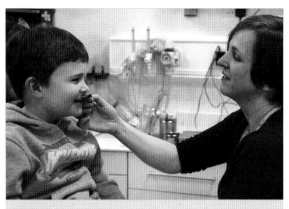

Fig. 2.4 Testing the nasal airway.

Most children will tolerate otoscopy, and if there is wax or debris, it is usually possible to remove it by suction to get a better view. Use the biggest speculum that will comfortably fit in the ear canal. If you need a better view, use the microscope, which should be as well tolerated as a standard otoscope. Thin otoendoscopes with high-quality cameras and viewing monitors are becoming more widely available and represent a good opportunity to record findings, to facilitate better explanations of pathology to parents, and as an aid to teaching.

A good way to start a nasal examination is to assess the nasal airway using a cold metal spatula to look for the pattern of condensation (▶ Fig. 2.4). Children do not like Thudicum's speculum; you can get a good view of the nasal cavities by simply elevating the tip of the nose and looking with a good light source, but again high-quality endoscopes have made rhinoscopy far easier and better tolerated. In a cooperative child, you should get a good view using a standard 0- or 30-degree telescope. Although some surgeons like to use a local anesthetic spray, the author has not found this useful, and, in general, if a child will not tolerate a nasendoscope, he/she will tolerate a spray even less so, and you are better getting the best view you can using a headlight.

To examine the pharynx, use a standard headlight. Children dislike tongue depressors; the author very rarely uses them. You can get a good view of the nasopharynx using a telescope with an angled lens gently placed between the tonsils.

Examining the larynx can be difficult in an older child, but flexible transnasal endoscopy will give you a very good view in a cooperative older child or in the case of a baby who is gently but firmly held by the mother. As with nasendoscopy, the author has not found local anesthesia very helpful as it can cause as much distress as the endoscope. Clearly, if a child is anxious or distressed, it is inappropriate to proceed, and if you have to get a view of the larynx, then you may need to arrange admission for a general anesthetic.

Neck examination should focus on observation for lumps, bumps, sinuses, and asymmetry, gently palpating to assess for lymph nodes. "Lymphadenopathy" is probably a misnomer in children as some degree of lymph node enlargement is physiological and should cause no alarm (see Chapter 25).

2.3.3 Investigations

> **i**
>
> Few, if any, investigations are needed for most common ENT presentations in children.

Pure-tone audiometry (provided the child is old enough) and tympanometry are essential components of a full ENT examination. Radiological imaging may be needed depending on the pathology, and ultrasonography is commonly used to quickly assess neck swellings. Some ENT surgeons are now skilled at getting good ultrasound images in clinic. If the child needs blood tests, then he/she should have local anesthetic cream (e.g., EMLA cream, an emulsion containing lidocaine and prilocaine) before being sent for phlebotomy. Photography can be useful, for example, for facial and neck lesions, and close liaison with a skilled medical photography department will make for a much better pediatric ENT service.

2.3.4 Management Plan

The parents have come to see you to hear your opinion on their child's condition and to discuss management options with you. In most cases, you should be able to make a plan having taken a history and conducted the examination.

> **i**
>
> This part of the consultation is vital and must not be rushed.

Very often there will be more than one option, including and perhaps most important avoiding any intervention, and it is essential that you present each of the options and get a feel for how the parents want to proceed. Diagrams, models, and wall charts can be very helpful in trying to explain pathologies and interventions, and it is good practice in writing to the referring clinician to copy in the parents, using this as an opportunity to reinforce and amplify any explanations you may have given. If a decision is made to admit the child for surgery, it is ideal if a date can be agreed with the parents, but this is not always possible and practice will vary in different settings. The more information parent and child have about the admission process the better. Many units run a "pre-admission" clinic when the child and family can visit the ward and meet the staff. Parents greatly appreciate information leaflets and some surgeons maintain good quality websites with video clips and explanations of common ENT conditions and interventions.

2.4 Normal Growth, Development, and Child Health Promotion

Otolaryngologists are not experts in assessing and monitoring child development, but all health care professionals who deal with children need to acquaint themselves with the major events in children's normal progression and to be alert to signs that all is not well. Some important milestones are shown in ▶ Table 2.1, but of course children develop at different rates, and it is the overall pattern of progress that is important.

The otolaryngologist may be the first specialist the parents see if a child is slow to speak, develops obstructive sleep apnea related to muscle hypotonia, or presents with suspected earache or hearing loss when a neurodevelopmental disorder is to blame. Parents who worry about their child's progress need to have their concerns taken seriously, and if you are in any doubt or have concerns about a child's overall growth and development, seek the opinion of a general pediatrician.

It is very reassuring for parents to record and plot their child's milestones so as to keep a permanent record. Arrangements for this vary in different jurisdictions and in different health care settings. Parents in the United Kingdom are given a "personal child health record" or "Red Book" in which they can plot their baby's progress (▶ Fig. 2.5 a, b) and record events such as hospital visits, developmental milestones, test results, and immunization history.

Table 2.1 Some milestones in normal child development

0–4 wk	Likes looking at faces
4–6 wk	Starts to smile
4–12 wk	Lifts her head
4–6 mo	Babbles and makes noise
6–8 mo	Sits up
10–18 mo	Walks
18 mo to 2 y	Uses two or more words together

Parents and health care visitors will usually plot a baby's weight and length on a graph such as the standard "growth charts" (▶ Fig. 2.6), which are included in the "Red Book." Poor weight gain or "failure to thrive" can be a feature of a number of ENT disorders such as severe laryngomalacia or obstructive sleep apnea. A good plot on the growth charts, while by no means excluding serious disease, is at least very reassuring for both doctor and parents. In the case of a baby, the author finds it very helpful to enquire how he/she is progressing in terms of weight gain and to ask for a look at the graph.

2.5 Promoting Child Health

ENT specialists, like all health care personnel, have a duty to promote good health. Breast-feeding should be encouraged, and in situations where ENT intervention can facilitate breast-feeding, for example, surgery for tongue-tie or correction of choanal atresia, it should be offered promptly, otherwise the momentum may be lost. Many ENT disorders in children, such as otitis media with effusion, rhinitis, and respiratory infections, are related to parental smoking; thus, parents may need advice and counseling. While vaccination regimes are generally the responsibility of family practitioners and community nurses, it is useful to be aware of the normal routines. ▶ Table 2.2 shows a typical immunization schedule for the United Kingdom.

2.6 Pediatric Medical Assessment

ENT surgeons are not medical pediatricians, but if you are seeing a significant number of children, you will inevitably come across conditions that are best diagnosed and dealt with by pediatrician colleagues. Some knowledge of these conditions can help early detection and referral so that parents and children are offered support as soon as is practicable. Attention deficit hyperactivity disorders (ADHDs), autistic spectrum disorders (ASDs), and "child protection" issues may well present first to the otolaryngologist.

2.6.1 Attention Deficit Hyperactivity Disorders

Every clinician will be familiar with the child who fidgets, will not sit still, and seems to have a poor attention span. Parents will often volunteer that the child is "hyperactive" or disruptive. In extreme cases, this may constitute a behavioral syndrome termed attention deficit hyperactivity disorder. This condition is now thought to affect 3–4% of children worldwide. They occasionally present with suspected hearing loss or poor sleep patterns.

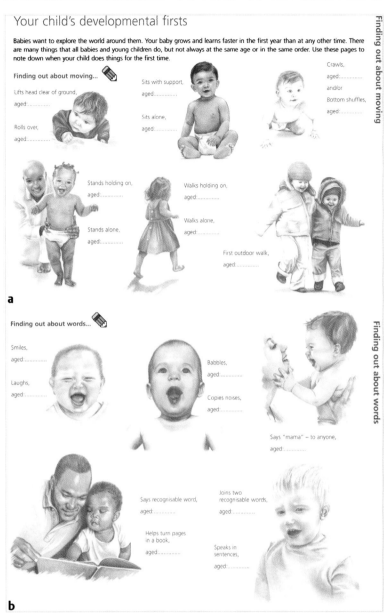

Your child's developmental firsts

Babies want to explore the world around them. Your baby grows and learns faster in the first year than at any other time. There are many things that all babies and young children do, but not always at the same age or in the same order. Use these pages to note down when your child does things for the first time.

Finding out about moving...

Lifts head clear of ground, aged:..............

Rolls over, aged:..............

Sits with support, aged:..............

Sits alone, aged:..............

Crawls, aged:..............

and/or

Bottom shuffles, aged:..............

Stands holding on, aged:..............

Walks holding on, aged:..............

Stands alone, aged:..............

Walks alone, aged:..............

First outdoor walk, aged:..............

a

Finding out about words...

Smiles, aged:..............

Laughs, aged:..............

Babbles, aged:..............

Copies noises, aged:..............

Says "mama" – to anyone, aged:..............

Says recognisable word, aged:..............

Joins two recognisable words, aged:..............

Helps turn pages in a book, aged:..............

Speaks in sentences, aged:..............

b

Finding out about moving

Finding out about words

Fig. 2.5 (a, b) Example pages from a Personal Child Health Record in the United Kingdom (the "Red Book"). (© Harlow Printing Limited. Reproduced with permission.)

> The defining features are hyperactivity, impulsivity, and inattention, but, of course, these characteristics are distributed in varying degrees throughout the population.

While ADHD diagnostic criteria vary somewhat, the core feature of the diagnosis is that these symptoms are associated with "at least a moderate degree of psychological, social, and/or educational or occupational impairment." ADHD is not a categorical diagnosis, and it should only be made with great care following a thorough assessment by a skilled and experienced pediatric team. A diagnosis of

ADHD has serious potential implications; it is generally a persisting disorder. Most affected children will go on to have significant difficulties in adulthood, which may include continuing ADHD, personality disorders, emotional and social difficulties, substance misuse, unemployment, and involvement in crime. Management may involve social and educational services, the family doctor and his/her team, specialist pediatricians, and, of course, the child's family, and can be very taxing.[3]

2.6.2 Autistic Spectrum Disorders

Autism was once thought to be an uncommon developmental disorder but is now estimated to occur in at least

2

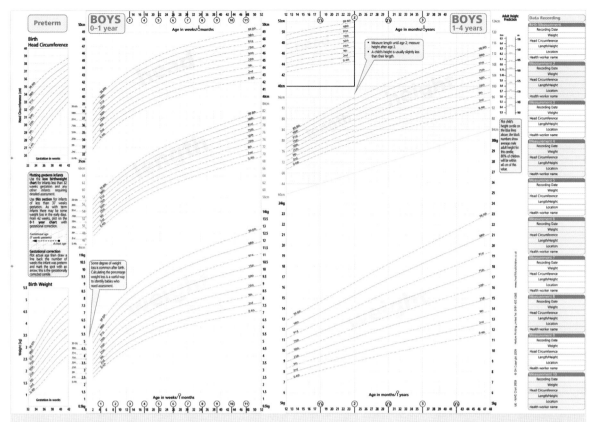

Fig. 2.6 UK-WHO growth charts for boys aged between 0 and 4 years. (© 2009. Royal College of Paediatrics and Child Health. Reproduced with permission.)

Table 2.2 Typical vaccination schedule in the United Kingdom

Age	Vaccine
2 mo	5-in-1 (DTaP/IPV/Hib) vaccine[a] Pneumococcal (PCV) vaccine Rotavirus vaccine Men B vaccine
3 mo	5-in-1 (DTaP/IPV/Hib) vaccine, second dose Men C vaccine Rotavirus vaccine, second dose
4 mo	5-in-1 (DTaP/IPV/Hib) vaccine, third dose Pneumococcal (PCV) vaccine, second dose Men B vaccine, second dose
12–13 mo	Hib/Men C booster, Hib, fourth dose MMR vaccine, given as a single jab Pneumococcal (PCV) vaccine, third dose Men B vaccine, third dose
2–4 y	Children's flu vaccine (annual)
From 3 y and 4 mo (up to starting school)	MMR vaccine, second dose 4-in-1 (DTaP/IPV) preschool booster, given as a single jab[b]
12–13 y (girls only)	HPV vaccine, two injections given between 6 mo and 2 y apart[c]

Abbreviations: DTaP, diphtheria, tetanus, acellular pertussis; Hib, Haemophilus influenzae type B; HPV, human papillomavirus; IPV, inactivated polio vaccine; MMR, measles, mumps, and rubella; PCV, pneumococcal conjugate vaccine.
[a]Protects against five separate diseases: diphtheria, tetanus, whooping cough (pertussis), polio, and Haemophilus influenzae type B.
[b]Protects against diphtheria, tetanus, whooping cough (pertussis), and polio.
[c]Protects against cervical cancer.

Table 2.3 Some features of autistic spectrum disorders in preschool children

Spoken language	Delayed speech development Frequent repetition of set words and phrases
Responding to others	Not responding to their name being called Rejecting cuddles
Interacting with others	Not aware of other people's personal space Intolerant of people entering their personal space Avoiding eye contact
Behavior	Repetitive movements Playing with toys in a repetitive way Getting upset if there are changes to normal routine

1% of children. Health care personnel need to be aware of some of the features so as to facilitate early diagnosis and intervention. The characteristic features are impairment in reciprocal social interaction and social communication, combined with restricted interests, and rigid and repetitive behaviors. In recognition of the great heterogeneity of autism, the term "autistic spectrum disorder" is now commonly used. The list of possible symptoms is very large indeed, but some key features are shown in ▶ Table 2.3. The diagnosis needs to be made with great care and warrants a full assessment by an experienced team. Families, carers, and the child or young person themselves can experience a variety of emotions, shock, and concern about the implications for the future. Some have a profound sense of relief that others agree with their concerns. Diagnosis and the assessment of needs can offer an understanding of why a child or young person is different from their peers and can open doors to support and services in education, health services and social care, and a route into voluntary organizations and contact with other children and families with similar experiences. All of these can improve the lives of the child or young person and his/her family.[4]

> **i**
>
> Children with ASD may present to the ENT clinic with language delay or suspected hearing loss.

Given the frequency of the condition, many children who present to the clinic will have a background history of ASD, and it is important to be aware of the condition because of its very common association with comorbidity. Autism is strongly associated with a number of coexisting conditions. Recent studies have shown that approximately 70% of people with autism also meet diagnostic criteria for at least one other (often unrecognized)

psychiatric disorder that is further impairing their psychosocial functioning. Intellectual disability (intelligence quotient below 70) occurs in approximately 50% of young people with autism. Deafness and other sensory impairments are more common and may be difficult to recognize.

> **i**
>
> Children with ASD need particular sensitive care and attention if they are admitted for surgery.

Many children with ASD find the company of other children distressing and are especially likely to become upset if they have to wait too long. In general, they should be assessed early by the anesthesiologist, considered for a sedative (premed), scheduled first on the operating list, and discharged as soon as they are fit. Day surgery is preferable unless there are very good medical reasons to keep the child overnight.

2.6.3 Functional Disorders

Just as in adult medicine, a significant number of children present to the ENT clinic with symptoms for which no organic pathophysiological explanation can be found despite a thorough examination and, in some cases, extensive investigation (▶ Fig. 2.7). The term "functional disorders" is often used to emphasize the notion that although there is no structural or anatomical abnormality that can be demonstrated, for example, on imaging, endoscopy, or microscopy, there may be physiological dysfunction. Terms such as "medically unexplained," "psychogenic," "stress-related," "psychosomatic," and "hysterical" were used in the past but have been abandoned as they were unhelpful, became derogatory, and implied a certain amount of "blame" on the part of the patient.

> **i**
>
> Functional disorders are emphatically not the same as factitious or feigned illness, and it is hugely counterproductive to make the child or parent feel that they are not believed.

The symptoms are very real to the patient and can cause great distress, which can be exacerbated if they are treated in an insensitive or judgmental way.

ENT symptoms include the following:
- Earache.
- Tinnitus.
- "Functional" or nonorganic hearing loss (see Chapter 14).

There is often a background history of environmental or psychological stress, but a certain amount of anxiety, uncertainty, and insecurity is a part of growing up. Children can consciously or unconsciously describe symptoms that bring about some "secondary gain" for them, for example, time off school, increased parental attention in the event of a new sibling, and the benefits associated with being perceived as "sick." Functional disorders are distinct from true malingering or feigned symptoms, although these do occasionally present. It is difficult to know on the basis of a single consultation whether there is any significant psychological morbidity, and too early referral to a psychological support service can be counterproductive.

> **i**
>
> Many functional disorders are short-lived and should not be "overmedicalized."

It is the author's practice in most circumstances to reassure the family that the majority of these symptoms are transient and rarely need intensive intervention. It is, of course, wise to bear in mind that depression, pathological anxiety, and rarely overt psychosis do occur in children and that skilled psychiatric help will be needed in some circumstances. Referral protocols vary, but most children's hospitals will have a child and adolescent mental health service team, who will see and assess children at short notice. Many hospitals and training programs will have specific policies covering this type of scenario, and again clinicians should ensure they have the appropriate training for the setting in which they work. Management must be tailored to the individual child and family and prognosis varies greatly.

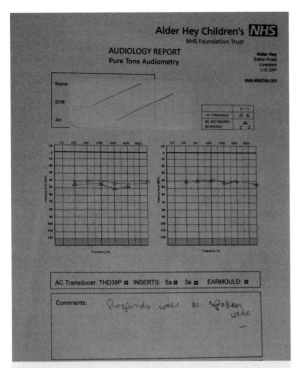

Fig. 2.7 Audiogram of a 13-year-old girl complaining of hearing loss. She responds well to normal conversation, and the audiology technician reports that her hearing seems better than the graph suggests. This is the typical pure-tone audiogram in "functional hearing loss." Auditory brainstem response is normal.

- Dysphagia.
- Neck pain.
- Balance disorders.
- Dysphonia.
- Very occasionally, stridor.

The clinician's role is to take a full history; examine the child thoroughly; arrange investigations including audiometry, imaging, and endoscopy, as needed; and formulate a diagnosis. If you suspect a functional basis for the symptoms, it is reasonable to enquire into issues such as school, relationships with siblings, friends, and family, and whether there has been any change in circumstances. Parental disharmony, bullying at school, and the trauma of the physiological and psychological changes of puberty and adolescence can all have an impact on health and well-being, with somatic symptoms not uncommonly coming to the fore. An experienced clinician will need to strike a balance between a thorough investigation to outrule an organic etiology and a more minimal approach focusing on history, examination, and reassurance that there is no worrying pathology. A sensitive and thoughtful explanation of the findings to parent and child will allay fears and make for a good rapport for follow-up visits.

2.7 Delivering Bad News

Parents, and older children, will remember with chilling clarity being told of their child's deafness, the need for a long-term tracheostomy, or a suspicion or confirmation of malignancy for many years after the event. Insensitive or even well-meaning but inexperienced handling of such situations can be very destructive.

> **i**
>
> If you have to impart such news, get the help and support of a senior clinician or, in the case of malignancy, of the oncology team.

Consider the setting, the availability of support staff, the need for further discussion, the need for detailed written information, and the time required. This type of consultation should not be delegated to a junior member of the team and above all must not be rushed. In the case of a child needing, for example, a tracheostomy, it may be best to introduce the subject on one occasion and have more detailed and focused discussions with the family on another occasion. Hospitals and training programs will have specific policies covering this type of scenario, and again clinicians should ensure they have the appropriate training for the setting in which they work.

2.8 Consent and Parental Responsibility

It goes without saying that every medical intervention requires the consent of the patient. What is different in the case of young children is that they may not have the capacity and understanding (competence) to weigh the benefits and risks of an intervention, and consent will usually need to be given on their behalf.[5,6,7,8,9] The interests of the child must, of course, take precedence over the wishes of others, even parents, but all clinicians will want to respect the legitimate concerns of parents, be they mothers, fathers, single, married, or divorced. It is wise to involve the child at all times if at all possible. The concept of "duty of candor" has recently been introduced in UK practice. The principle is that health care providers must be open and transparent with service users about their care and treatment, including when it goes wrong.[10] The legalities that govern these processes vary in different jurisdictions and health care settings but the principles are broadly similar.

> Once children reach the age of 16 years, they are deemed legally "competent" in the United Kingdom.

This means that they are responsible for decisions relating to consent themselves, but it is, of course, wise to involve parents if at all possible in major decisions in the young. If a young person up to the age of 18 years is not "competent," for example, due to learning disability, reduced consciousness, or severe illness, then a parent or person with "parental responsibility" (see below) can give consent for them, but over the age of 18 years in UK law, a parent cannot give consent on behalf of a young person. This causes difficulties in the case of young adults with learning disabilities, many of whom remain under the care of children's hospitals. In these instances, the clinician must make the decision on the young person's behalf, ideally with the written agreement of another senior clinician and with the full approval of the parent, albeit with uncertain legal standing.

A child under the age of 16 years may well be able to understand the implications of a treatment strategy. In UK law, such a child who has "sufficient understanding and intelligence to enable him or her to understand fully what is proposed" is deemed "Gillick competent" or as it sometimes known "Fraser competent." The decision as to whether a child fulfills the criteria for "Gillick competence" rests with the clinician; hence, teenagers undergoing tonsillectomy, for example, may give their own consent. The issues around consent in children can cause great sensitivity and are fraught with medicolegal pitfalls. If in any doubt, seek the advice of one or more senior clinicians.

The medico-legal framework governing consent in the UK was clarified in a recent judgment—the "Montgomery" case. This has placed even greater emphasis on the need for doctors discussing treatment options to consider whether a reasonable person in the patient's position would be likely to attach significance to the risk, or the doctor is or should reasonably be aware that the particular patient would be likely to attach significance to it." In other words, the consent discussion should be open, frank, and customized for individual patient or family. Some families will attach greater significance to a particular risk than others, and the clinician needs to be mindful of these differences.[11]

> In the case of a child who is not "competent," consent has to be sought from and given by a person with "parental responsibility."[5]

This is usually one or both of the parents. The situation varies in different jurisdictions, but in England and Wales, "parental responsibility" is automatically given to the mother and to most fathers. A father will have parental responsibility if he is married to the child's mother or listed on the child's birth certificate (after a certain date, which varies in different jurisdictions). Fathers who do not have parental responsibility can get it via an agreement with the mother or they can apply for it through the courts. Grandparents, foster parents, and others who look after children do not have parental responsibility unless special legal arrangements have been made. Consent from one parent is legally valid, but it is best practice to obtain consent where applicable from both. A written record of consent signed by the doctor and the parent is an important document, and although a written record of consent is not legally mandatory, in general, no invasive intervention should proceed without it. Verbal consent for surgery is possible and, in many circumstances, entirely reasonable. If, for example, a newborn baby needs urgent surgery, very often the mother will be recovering in the maternity unit. The surgeon should speak to her by telephone and explain the natural history of the condition, the implications of treatment, the consequences of not treating, and the timing of treatment. It is good practice to get another health care professional (e.g., a nurse) to confirm with the mother that she understands and agrees with what is being proposed and to record the exchanges in the case notes.

It may be necessary in emergency scenarios to proceed without consent, for example, when a child needs urgent intervention following an accident and the person with parental responsibility is not immediately available.

2.9 Child Protection

> **i**
>
> Every professional involved in the care of children needs to be aware of the potential for children to be subject to abuse or neglect.[12]

This can take the form of physical, emotional, or sexual abuse and may be perpetrated by family members, by friends and acquaintances, or by professionals who come in contact with the child. Professional regulatory bodies, for example, the General Medical Council in the United Kingdom, expect doctors working with children and young people to be especially conversant with the features of abuse and neglect and to act upon any concerns they have. Arrangements for raising such concerns vary in different health care settings and in different jurisdictions but the principles are essentially the same.

> **i**
>
> You should be familiar with the main presentations in your area of practice that can be caused by abuse and with the strategy for seeking appropriate advice and support.

Most children's hospitals will have a "child protection" team who can be contacted for advice in confidence. Anecdotal evidence would suggest that few ENT surgeons make a diagnosis of child abuse, but it is essential that they are aware of it as a possible explanation for some unusual presentations. Up to 75% of children who suffer physical abuse have injuries to the head and neck. Some ENT presentations that may be linked with child abuse are shown in Box 2.1. If you suspect that a child's symptoms may be due to abuse or neglect, you should seek advice from an experienced colleague. Most children's hospitals have a designated team headed up by a pediatrician "child protection lead," who has the expertise and sensitivity to give advice and support to you as a worried clinician and, where necessary, to explore the issue with the parents.

This is clearly an area where great sensitivity and delicacy is needed. An accusation of abuse or neglect can have devastating consequences for the child and family.

> **Box 2.1 Some Possible Nonaccidental Injuries in the Head and Neck**
>
> - Tears to the lingual frenulum.
> - Bruises to the cheeks, lips, gums.
> - Nasal injuries.
> - Injuries to the pinna, especially "pinch" marks.
> - Auricular hematomas.
> - Traumatic perforation of the eardrum.
> - Maxillofacial fractures.
> - Dental trauma.
> - Injuries to the palate, for example, due to forceful feeding.
> - Bruising to the neck.

A very small number of parents deliberately bring about symptoms and signs of disease in their child in an attempt to gain attention from health care personnel. ENT examples include ear injuries, blocked tracheostomy tubes, and deliberate smothering. This is a serious psychiatric condition (Munchausen's syndrome by proxy) and needs urgent and expert management.

A small number of children may, for various reasons, be best looked after outwith their family setting, for example, by social services or the local authority. They may be placed in a designated care setting or with an alternative family (foster family). Arrangements will vary in different health care settings, but, in general, these children ("looked-after children" or "children in care") need particularly vigilant medical attention. They will usually have a named social worker, and close liaison with her/him is important in ensuring continuity of medical management, especially if they require surgery, investigations, or repeat follow-up visits.

2.10 Key Points

- A visit to the hospital is a routine event for the doctor. It is a major episode in the life of the child and parent.
- Children should be seen in appropriately staffed "child-friendly" clinics dedicated only to children.
- Audiological professionals and audiological testing facilities are an integral part of children's ENT clinics.
- Children with suspected ASD are increasingly common and may present to the otolaryngologist.
- Make sure you are familiar with the procedures governing consent in children in your health care setting. Read the guidance and keep up to date with changes.
- Health promotion and child protection is everybody's business. Know what to do if you suspect a child is being maltreated.

References

[1] Royal College of Nursing. Defining Staffing Levels for Children and Young People's Services. London: Royal College of Nursing; 2013. Available at www.rcn.org.uk/-/media/royal-college-of-nursing/documents/publications/2013/august/pub-002172.pdf. Accessed February 9, 2016

[2] Children's Surgical Forum. Standards for Children's Surgery. London: Royal College of Surgeons of England; 2013. Available at www.rcseng.ac.uk/publications/docs/standards-in-childrens-surgery. Accessed February 9, 2016

[3] National Institute for Health and Care Excellence. Attention Deficit Hyperactivity Disorder: Diagnosis and Management. NICE guidelines [CG72]. London: NICE; September 2008

[4] Care Quality Commission. Brief guide: capacity and competence in under 18 s. Available at https://www.cqc.org.uk/sites/default/files/20151008%20Brief%20guide%20-%20Capacity%20and%20consent%20in%20under%2018s%20FINAL.pdf

[5] Department of Health. Consent – What You Have a Right to Expect: A Guide for Children and Young People. Department of Health Publications; 2001. Available at ethics.grad.ucl.ac.uk/forms/DH_Guide-ForChildrenAndYoungPeople.pdf. Accessed February 9, 2016

[6] General Medical Council. Consent Guidance: Involving Children and Young People in Making Decisions. GMC UK; 2016. Available at www.gmc-uk.org/guidance/ethical_guidance/consent_guidance_involving_children_and_young_people.asp. Accessed February 9, 2016

[7] General Medical Council. 0–18 years: Guidance for All Doctors. GMC UK; 2007. Available at www.gmc-uk.org/guidance/ethical_guidance/children_guidance_index.asp. Accessed February 22, 2016

[8] General Medical Council. Consent: Patients and Doctors Making Decisions Together. GMC UK; 2008. Available at www.gmc-uk.org/Consent___English_1015.pdf_48903482.pdf. Accessed February 22, 2016

[9] Department of Health. Reference Guide to Consent for Examination or Treatment. 2nd ed. Department of Health; 2009. Available at www.gov.uk/government/uploads/system/uploads/attachment_data/file/138296/dh_103653__1_.pdf. Accessed February 22, 2016

[10] General Medical Council and Nursing and Midwifery Council. Openness and Honesty When Things Go Wrong: The Professional Duty of Candour. GMC UK/NMC UK; 2015. Available at www.gmc-uk.org/DoC_guidance_englsih.pdf_61618688.pdf. Accessed February 22, 2016

[11] Coulter A, Hopkins A, Moulton B. Montgomery v Lanarkshire Health Board: transforming informed consent. Bulletin of Royal College Surgeons England 2017;99(1):3638

[12] National Institute for Health and Care Excellence. Child Maltreatment: When to Suspect Maltreatment in Under 16 s. NICE guidelines [CG89]. London: NICE; July 2009

3 Anesthesia and Perioperative Care

Frank A. Potter

3.1 Introduction

In nearly all branches of children's treatment, there is a tension between centralization and convenience, specialization and practicality, and this is particularly true of ear, nose, and throat (ENT) surgery. Outside of the neonatal period, most otherwise well children will undergo most of the common pediatric ENT procedures very satisfactorily in general hospitals. In recent years, there has been a general drift toward a degree of specialization within this setting, with cohorting of children onto pediatric lists and concentrating their care into the hands of fewer anesthetists. There are gray areas, and clearly both the nature of the patient and his/her particular surgery have to be borne in mind when deciding where a child is best treated. For example, a well child with Down's syndrome requiring routine glue ear surgery may have this safely and conveniently done in a nonspecialized center, whereas the same child presenting for a tonsillectomy for sleep-disordered breathing (SDB) is probably best cared for in a major pediatric center.

In all likelihood, much ENT surgery will continue to be delivered in a general hospital setting, and both surgeons and anesthetists who care for these children will have a mixed adult and pediatric practice.

3.2 Anesthesia

There are two basic methods of providing a general anesthetic for a child: simple anesthesia and balanced anesthesia (▶ Fig. 3.1).

3.2.1 Simple Anesthesia

In simple anesthesia, a single anesthetic agent is given in sufficient dosage to provide unconsciousness (sleep), lack of movement in response to surgical stimulation, and attenuation of the cardiovascular responses to such stimulation. Traditionally, the anesthetic agent was given in the form of a vapor. The patient would inhale this; it would take a minute or two for consciousness to be lost (induction of anesthesia). The vapor would continue to be inhaled for the duration of the surgical procedure (maintenance of anesthesia), and then the vapor would be discontinued and the patient would wake up.

Sometimes the process of inducing anesthesia could be speeded up so as to take only seconds by giving an intravenous (IV) anesthetic agent at the start and before continuing with the maintenance vapor. The idea of following the bolus of IV anesthetic with an IV infusion of the same drug, replacing the anesthetic vapor altogether, is relatively recent.

> **i**
>
> Today, simple anesthesia is used for short operations in patients who are well.

The child breathes for himself/herself throughout (spontaneous ventilation). If the child is breathing an anesthetic vapor and there is an unnoticed disconnection of the breathing circuit, then the child will continue to breathe, but will now be breathing room air and so start to awaken. Generally, this will produce some movement and thus alert both the surgeon and the mortified anesthetist before full consciousness returns.

3.2.2 Balanced Anesthesia

In the second method, balanced anesthesia, separate drugs are used to produce unconsciousness, paralysis, cardiovascular control and analgesia. These drugs are typically an anesthetic agent, a muscle relaxant, and an opiate, respectively. The patient is given sufficient anesthetic agent to induce unconsciousness, but not enough to stop muscle contraction or movement in response to surgical stimulation. Instead, lack of movement is now produced by the action of the muscle relaxant—a drug that directly but reversibly paralyzes all skeletal muscles. Thus, the patient can no longer breathe for himself/herself, so the anesthetist must ventilate the patient's lungs, either by hand or by using a mechanical ventilator. Unnoticed disconnection of the breathing tubing in this circumstance will now cause hypoxia with potentially disastrous consequences—neurologic damage or even death—rather than just causing the child to wake up and the surgeon to complain. More sophisticated monitoring to alert the anesthetist to the early signs of hypoxia is therefore essential. Balanced anesthesia also introduces the possibility of accidental awareness if insufficient anesthetic drug is given while the completely paralyzed patient cannot move to convey his/her wakefulness.

> **i**
>
> Given these risks, why would anyone choose to give (or receive) a balanced anesthetic? The answer is that by taking these risks in a controlled and carefully monitored fashion, anesthetists can safely use balanced anesthetics to allow frailer, sicker, younger, and older patients to undergo more invasive and longer procedures more conveniently and, more importantly, with less postoperative morbidity and better outcomes.

3

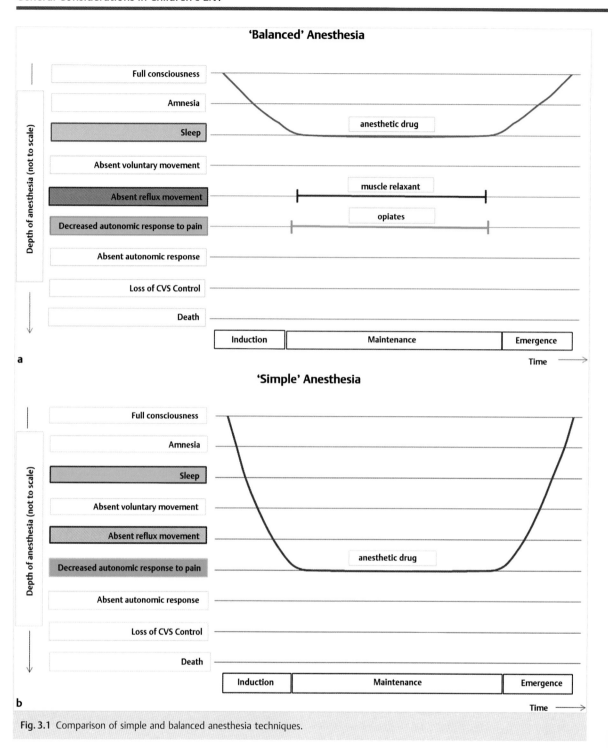

Fig. 3.1 Comparison of simple and balanced anesthesia techniques.

There are, of course, many refinements to this basic pattern of anesthesia and so we will examine how these apply to children's ENT surgery in more detail.

The decision as to the precise method of anesthesia used for children's ENT surgery takes many things into consideration. Important factors are as follows:

- How anesthesia is to be induced and maintained (using an inhaled and/or an IV agent).
- Duration of surgery.
- Surgical requirements.
- Patient comorbidity.
- Patient preference.
- Method of control of the airway.

3.3 Induction of Anesthesia

Inhalational induction continues to be widely used, but nowadays IV induction is more popular. This is because it is rapid and safe and avoids having to get the child to cooperate with the use of a face mask. Patient (or parental) preference, an obvious lack of easily cannulated veins, and poor patient tolerance of IV injection (despite use of effective topical anesthesia to the site of injection) are the usual indications for inhalational induction. However, many authorities would consider that the most important indication for inhalational induction in a child to be the presence of a partially obstructed or potentially difficult airway, and this is of obvious relevance to ENT surgery.

3.3.1 Intravenous Induction

IV anesthetic induction agents include *thiopentone* and *midazolam*, but *propofol* has become the ubiquitous agent of modern times because it gives a very rapid and reliable onset of unconsciousness and suppresses laryngeal and upper airway reflexes.

In children, IV induction is facilitated by applying local anesthetic cream (Ametop [Smith & Nephew], EMLA [AstraZeneca]) over a suitable vein beforehand, a small cannula (24 gauge), oral sedative premedication, some distraction for the child, and a good anesthetic assistant (usually in that order).

Who Needs a "Premedication?"

Basically, any child who one would predict will be too uncooperative to induce without undue upset to all concerned would need a premedication. Previous experience helps with prediction, particularly in spotting the child who masks his/her apprehension by maintaining an all-consuming interest in his/her book/electronic entertainment, but it remains more art than science.

- Oral midazolam is currently the most popular premedication, having a rapid onset of effect (15–20 minutes), giving good antegrade amnesia, and yet wearing off sufficiently quickly that it allows same-day discharge.
- Alternative drugs include other benzodiazepines (diazepam, temazepam) and oral clonidine.
- Clonidine has a slower, less predictable onset, which makes timings more difficult, but it has the merit of being virtually without taste.
- Some older patients with very severe behavioral difficulties may require very heavy premedication with both a benzodiazepine and oral ketamine (6 mg/kg).[1] While this is effective, it gives a significant "hangover" which may necessitate an overnight stay if given on an afternoon list.

IV induction takes seconds. One drawback of IV induction is that it usually produces a near-immediate 10 to 30 seconds of apnea. This acute severe reduction of respiratory drive may be used to advantage most of the time, allowing easier insertion of a laryngeal mask or even an endotracheal tube (ETT), but this may be severely disadvantageous in cases of partial airway obstruction where there may be loss of the airway.

3.3.2 Inhalational Induction

Unconsciousness can also be induced using an inhalational anesthetic agent. Worldwide, common inhaled vapors used for anesthesia include *halothane*, *isoflurane*, and *desflurane*, but the most popular agent for inhalational induction in children is *sevoflurane*. This gives a smooth, cough-free induction within a minute or so (often claimed to be faster still if nitrous oxide is used in the carrier gas, though there is little or no evidence for this[2]). After induction, a simple anesthetic may continue (maintenance anesthesia) with either sevoflurane or another inhalational agent, or an infusion of IV agent (propofol) may be used once IV access has been secured. Alternatively, a combination of drugs may be needed for a balanced anesthetic.

I

3.4 Methods of Control of the Airway

It is essential that the anesthetist has good control of the child's airway and that the child is protected from the risks of airway obstruction and aspiration. Anesthetists use a variety of methods for this purpose.

3.4.1 Face Mask

The simplest method of controlling the airway in an anesthetized child is to hold a face mask over the mouth and nose. The airway is held open by pulling the angle of the jaw forward, thus pulling the base of the tongue away from the posterior pharyngeal wall. A well-fitting face mask allows spontaneous ventilation to continue or intermittent positive pressure ventilation (IPPV) to be given ("bag-and-mask" ventilation), but it provides no separation of airway and gastrointestinal tract, so the stomach can be distended by gas during bag-and-mask ventilation and there is an ever-present risk of aspiration.

3.4.2 Oropharyngeal and Nasopharyngeal Airways

An oral Guedel airway or a nasopharyngeal airway (usually, in pediatrics, a cut-down ETT) may be inserted to help keep the airway patent.

3.4.3 The Laryngeal Mask Airway

The laryngeal mask airway (LMA; ▶ Fig. 3.2, ▶ Fig. 3.3) has revolutionized anesthesia in the past 20 years. It has all but replaced the use of the face mask for everything other than "bag-and-mask" ventilation prior to intubation and has greatly reduced the numbers of patients undergoing endotracheal intubation. It has popularized a return to "simple" (spontaneously breathing) anesthesia for short- and medium-duration surgery, and in pediatrics, the LMA may also be used as a conduit for flexible fiberoptic scopes, both in cases of difficult airway and for fiberoptic tracheobronchoscopy.

The LMA consists of a small (usually inflatable) collar, which is inserted into the mouth and pushed backward and downward until it comes to rest on the ridge of mucosa overlying cricopharyngeus muscle. In this position, the orifice of the mask should sit behind the inferior surface of the epiglottis, facing the glottic opening. The tubular part of the airway then passes up through the pharynx and mouth to connect up to the anesthetic breathing circuit.

This provides an excellent "anesthetist's hands-free" airway for spontaneous ventilation and also provides a good enough seal to allow IPPV in most circumstances.

> **i**
>
> The LMA provides protection of the airway from blood or secretions emanating from the nose, mouth, and pharynx, but it does not protect the airway from regurgitated liquid from the stomach, that is, aspiration.

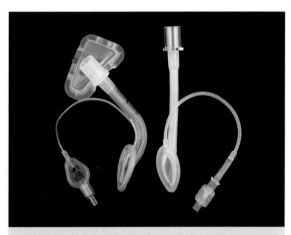

Fig. 3.2 Laryngeal masks; performed and straight versions. The inflatable cuff helps to keep the distal mask orifice opposite the glottic opening.

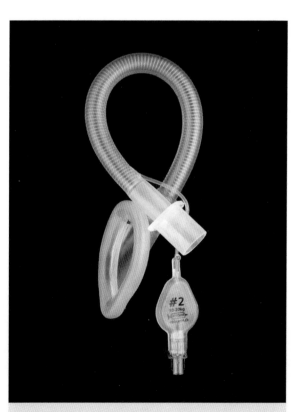

Fig. 3.3 Reinforced laryngeal mask (LM). Note how the wire helix within the wall of the tubular part of the mask resists kinking when the LM is distorted.

Indeed, it could be argued that by occupying the laryngopharynx, the LMA will direct such liquid into the airway. Newer variants of the laryngeal mask (ProSeal [Teleflex Health]) have a second channel to allow easy passage of a nasogastric tube to try to reduce this problem. The LMA can be readily inserted at a relatively light plane of anesthesia and is particularly easy to insert if propofol is used as an IV induction agent as propofol diminishes the gag and cough reflexes.[3]

3.4.4 Endotracheal Tubes

An ETT (▶ Fig. 3.4) not only provides a safe and easily accessible airway but also brings about definitive separation of the airway and gastrointestinal tract to reduce the risk of aspiration. In adults, the narrowest part of the airway is the inverted-**V**-shaped glottis, so in order to provide a leak-free connection between ETT and the airway, a thin cuff about the tube had to be inflated to form a seal.

3.4.5 Cuffed or Uncuffed Endotracheal Tube?

It was argued from cadaveric studies that since the narrowest part of the infant airway was the cricoid, and since this was all but circular in cross-section, then a well-chosen plain (uncuffed) ETT could provide an adequate seal both to allow inflation of the lungs and to protect the airway from overt aspiration of blood or regurgitated gastric contents.[4] Later, this view that a cuff was unnecessary developed into the idea that a cuff was positively contraindicated. This came about because there was recognition that following intubation, a proportion of patients suffered damage to the tracheal mucosa in the region of the subglottis, which could, on healing, form a constricting scar

which decreased the size of the tracheal lumen, subglottic stenosis. It is thought that the development of this subglottic stenosis relates to the degree of radial force exerted by either a "too large" tube being forced into the trachea or by an overinflated cuff pressing on the subglottic mucosa (see Chapter 21). Thus, cuffed ETTs fell out of use within pediatrics, and the smaller the child, the truer this was. This view has been challenged over recent years.[5]

There has been a marked increase in the use of cuffed ETTs in children and infants. Reasons for this center on the fact that cuffed tubes provide a better seal of the airway, which, in turn, allows use of low-flow anesthesia with inherently better humidification of gases, better use of mechanical ventilation, more accurate monitoring of end-tidal carbon dioxide, and less environmental pollution. "Sizing" of the tube is easier; if the tube chosen always errs on the side of being too small, then the leak can always be compensated for by inflating the cuff, avoiding the scenario of trying several tubes to get the best tracheal fit. The problem of the radial pressure of the cuff has been addressed in several ways. The cuffs themselves are of higher volume and more cylindrical than "olive shaped" (▶ Fig. 3.5) and

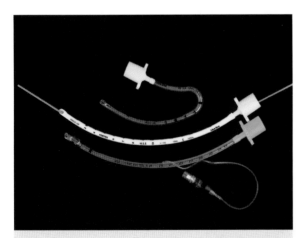

Fig. 3.4 Pediatric endotracheal tubes. Top: "south facing"; often used in ear, nose, and throat work as the circuit connector is kept clear of the immediate operating field. Middle: plain Ivory (Smiths Medical) tube (with introducing bougie). Bottom: Microcuff (Halyard Health) cuffed endotracheal tube.

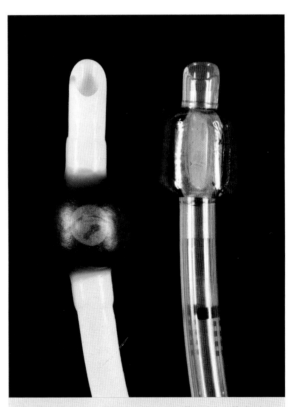

Fig. 3.5 Conventional (left) and Microcuff (right) cuffed tubes. The cuffs are filled with dye rather than air for clarity. Note that the cuff of the Microcuff tube is more cylindrical in shape and lies nearer to the distal end of the tube than the olive-shaped cuff of the conventional ETT.

there is greater emphasis on care with their use, for example, intermittent deflation and continuous monitoring of cuff pressure.

Oral or Nasal Intubation?

In the context of children's ENT surgery, endotracheal intubation is usually through the oral route, as this is quicker and easier to establish. Endotracheal intubation through the nose allows easier and more secure fixation and is more readily tolerated by lightly sedated patients, and for these reasons, nasal intubation is the preferred route for medium-term intubation (days to weeks) in the intensive care unit.

Tips and Tricks ☞

Insertion of an ETT is very stimulating to the patient. Potentially it will give rise to coughing, bucking, and laryngospasm and will produce a marked rise in blood pressure and heart rate. These features are undesirable in virtually all circumstances, particularly in the context of ENT surgery. There are several ways of avoiding this scenario.

- First, intubation can be performed under the effect of the induction agent at a deep plane of anesthesia. For example, if a child has anesthesia induced with sevoflurane, then it may be convenient to simply deepen the anesthetic until a degree of respiratory depression has been achieved, "bag-and-mask" ventilate for a short time, intubate, and then reduce the concentration of sevoflurane to allow spontaneous ventilation to resume.
- An additional refinement to this technique is to spray the larynx with local anesthetic (lignocaine 1–2 mg/kg) before passing the ETT so that afferent stimulation from the airway is decreased, allowing the ETT to be better tolerated at any given plane of anesthesia.

3.5 Muscle Relaxation (Paralysis) during Anesthesia and Reversal

3.5.1 Paralysis

All movement associated with intubation can be abolished by administering a muscle relaxant (paralyzing agent) before intubation. This gives the best possible conditions for intubation, but commits the anesthetist, first, to knowing that he/she will be able to intubate the patient and, second, to ventilating the patient for the duration of action of the muscle relaxant.

Suxamethonium is unique in that it is a depolarizing muscle relaxant, causing an initial contraction of muscle fibers before inducing paralysis. It is all but no longer used in elective surgery because of the problem of postoperative myalgia, though it retains a use in the emergency situation of the patient with a full stomach at risk of aspiration, where the rapid onset of paralysis is of overriding importance. All the other muscle relaxants are nondepolarizing agents. Some relevant properties of the commonly used muscle relaxants are given in ▶ Table 3.1.

The use of suxamethonium is usually reserved for patients with a full stomach at risk of aspiration.

3.5.2 Reversal

In balanced anesthesia for elective surgery, nondepolarizing neuromuscular blocking agents (NMBs) are used to paralyze the patient.

Table 3.1 Comparison of modern muscle relaxants in common use

	Depolarizing relaxants	Nondepolarizing relaxants			
		Hydroxyquinoline	Steroidal type		
	Suxamethonium	Atracurium	Vecuronium	Rocuronium	
				Normal dose	High dose
Dosage	1–1.5 mg/kg		100 micrograms/kg	600 µg/kg	1 mg/kg
Onset	20 s	90 s	60 s	60 s	20–25 s
Duration	5 min	40 min	50 min	40 min	60 min
Elimination	Serum cholinesterase	Hoffman elimination: pH and temperature-dependent hydrolysis	Hepatic metabolism		
Reversal	Spontaneous	Neostigmine	Neostigmine	Neostigmine	
Side effects	Hyperkalemia Muscle pains Idiosyncratic prolonged action	Pharmacological histamine release	Injection pain + +	Sugammadex Injection pain + + +	

+ +, very painful; + + +, extremely painful.

- Acetylcholine released into the neuromuscular cleft by the nerve impulse causes the muscle to contract. A nondepolarizer works by binding to an acetylcholine receptor on the muscle end plate, thereby blocking the effect of acetylcholine and inhibiting muscle contraction.
- The binding of NMB to acetylcholine receptors is not permanent and after 40 to 50 minutes there are sufficient "free" acetylcholine receptors for neuromuscular transmission to be reestablished.
- Thus, if a muscle relaxant is used to facilitate intubation, then the anesthetist is usually committed to giving at least 40 to 50 minutes of anesthesia if he/she wishes to allow paralysis to wear off spontaneously.
- This time may be reduced to 15 to 20 minutes if the anesthetist reverses the neuromuscular blockade using neostigmine. This neostigmine is an acetylcholinesterase enzyme inhibitor; it increases the amount of acetylcholine within the neuromuscular cleft, favoring acetylcholine in the competition with the NMB drug for binding with the muscle end plate acetylcholine receptors and so speeding up the restoration of neuromuscular transmission.

Reversal with neostigmine increases acetylcholine concentrations at nerve endings throughout the peripheral nervous system, producing unwanted muscarinic autonomic effects (bronchoconstriction, bradycardia, increased salivation, increased gastrointestinal peristalsis), and so neostigmine needs to be given with an antimuscarinic drug (atropine or glycopyrrolate) to attenuate these effects.

This is often inconvenient in, say, a list of tonsillectomies that may take on average 15 to 20 minutes. If the surgeon is quick, then this necessitates prolonging the anesthetic while the surgeon prowls about room and indulges in rhetorical requests to "send for the next." If the surgeon is slow and paralysis wears off, the anesthetist has to judge whether to give a second dose of muscle relaxant, risking a rapid conclusion of surgery and further demonstrating surgical impatience, or to eke out inadequate muscle relaxation with deeper anesthesia and loss of the "light plane of anesthesia" advantage of the balanced technique.

Newer Muscle Relaxants and Reversing Agents

There is now an elegant, if presently expensive, solution to the problem of using muscle relaxants with a surgeon of unpredictable speed: use *rocuronium* as the muscle relaxant and then reverse its action using *sugammadex* rather than neostigmine.

- In using neostigmine to restore neuromuscular transmission, there need to be sufficient free acetylcholine receptors on the muscle end plate with which

acetylcholine can interact. Immediately after a dose of nondepolarizing muscle relaxant is given, virtually all of the acetylcholine receptors are occupied with molecules of nondepolarizing drug, and so giving neostigmine will be entirely ineffective. It needs some time to elapse (usually at least 20 minutes) before sufficient acetylcholine receptors on the muscle end plate are free of their occupation by molecules of nondepolarizing agent.
- Sugammadex has an entirely different mechanism of action. It is a rocuronium-chelating drug that "removes" the muscle relaxant from the neuromuscular junction. Thus, it does not require any time to have elapsed before it can be used, allowing earlier and complete reversal of neuromuscular blockade.[6]

3.6 Duration of Surgery

Difficulty in predicting duration of surgery has given rise to another approach: trying to combine the good intubating conditions of the relaxant technique with the flexibility of duration of the simple anesthetic approach, avoiding the use of muscle relaxants completely.

- The patient is induced with a generous dose of propofol.
- Then the laryngeal and cough reflexes are further suppressed with a dose of short-acting opiate (fentanyl, alfentanil, or the ultrashort-acting remifentanil). This is usually sufficient to allow smooth intubation (by a smooth anesthetist).
- Following intubation, the patient's lungs are mechanically ventilated using deeper anesthesia rather than muscle relaxants to suppress coughing and bucking.

> Skilled exponents of this technique can combine tranquil operating conditions with a turnover sufficiently rapid as to leave the surgeon with several cold half-consumed cups of coffee at the end of a well-run list.

3.7 Analgesia

It is probably fair to say that postoperative pain and its control has not been uppermost in the minds of either surgeons or anesthetists thinking about the difficulties of pediatric ENT surgery. The usual strategy has been to use paracetamol for most minor procedures; give some intraoperative opiate (morphine or fentanyl) with one or, at most, two postoperative doses following tonsillectomy or mastoid type ear surgery; and to prescribe codeine and nonsteroidal anti-inflammatory drugs (NSAIDs) liberally to paper over the cracks for everything in between. Some thought has been given to trying to minimize the use of opiates to avoid postoperative nausea and vomiting

I

(PONV), so add "infiltration of local anesthetic wherever possible" to the recipe and one could reasonably claim to have the subject comprehensively covered and leave for home with a clear conscience.

Two recent developments have troubled this picture:

- The first is the inexorable pressure to minimize length of hospital stay. Inpatient ENT beds are becoming more scarce, day-beds or ambulatory services are the future, and even the hallowed overnight stay following tonsillectomy is buckling under economic pressure. Children must be rendered fit to go home quickly following surgery with pain-relief regimens that are simple, effective, and safe.
- The second event has been the abrupt demise of codeine.

Codeine

Codeine, a "weak" oral opiate, had been a mainstay of children's analgesia following minor-to-moderate surgery. In fact, its analgesic action was mainly the result of hepatic conversion to morphine by the enzyme cytochrome P4502D6 (CYP4502D6). This enzyme has several different forms, and the efficiency with which a subject converts codeine to active morphine varies according to which of the forms of the enzyme they have inherited. Most children, with the "EM" form of the enzyme, convert approximately 10% of their codeine to morphine. Some children, with the "PM" form, convert little or no codeine to morphine and so derive little or no analgesic effect from the drug—bad enough—but children with the "UM" form of the enzyme convert 15 to 20% of codeine to morphine and so can suffer opioid toxicity (central nervous system depression and apnea) even when given standard doses of codeine.

The frequency distribution of the enzyme forms varies between populations: overall, 1 to 10% of children are CYP2D6 UM type but this rises to nearly 30% in case of North African children.[7]

Following reports from the United States of deaths in toddlers having adenotonsillectomy for obstructive sleep apnea (OSA), regulatory authorities in the United States, United Kingdom, and Europe issued warnings against the use of codeine, which have effectively seen the end of its use in children's ENT surgery. However, there is as yet no single better drug to replace codeine. Thus, ENT anesthetists would seem to be facing a stark choice for their patients, particularly for those undergoing more painful procedures such as tonsillectomy:

- Stop using opiate drugs altogether as postoperative analgesics, thus avoiding the contribution of these drugs to PONV and respiratory depression. This approach calls for greater reliance on NSAIDs such as diclofenac and ibuprofen, but risks children having inadequate analgesia particularly 12 to 48 hours postoperatively when they are at home.
- Switch to using opiates such as oral morphine in the hope that its effects will be more predictable than those of codeine. The idea here would be that any occasional idiosyncratic sensitivity to morphine would become apparent while the child was still in hospital (in which case they could join children with severe OSA in being kept as inpatients), whereas the vast majority of patients, having demonstrated adequate respiratory drive in the face of morphine, could be safely treated as day-patients and allowed home with their "rescue" oral morphine. The rub here lies with early discharge; many anesthetists would be happy to adopt this approach of morphine "rescue" but would have misgivings about discharging patients home on respiratory depressants.

3.8 Anesthesia for Common Pediatric ENT Procedures

3.8.1 Myringotomy and Grommets

This is the obvious example for "simple anesthesia."

- Anesthesia may be induced intravenously (propofol) or using an inhalational agent (sevoflurane).
- Anesthesia is usually maintained with the patient breathing sevoflurane in an oxygen/air or oxygen/ nitrous oxide mixture through a laryngeal mask.

The "virtuous circle" of inhalational anesthesia may present a problem during an operation for insertion of grommets. All anesthetic agents are respiratory depressants. As anesthesia deepens, so too does the respiratory depression. With inhalational agents, increasing respiratory depression results in less anesthetic being inhaled, so anesthesia lightens. This negative feedback loop (virtuous circle) makes it difficult for the patient to become too deeply anesthetized (i.e., to reach such a depth of anesthesia where apnea is followed by cardiovascular collapse), but in this particular circumstance where surgical stimulation is minimal up to the point of the myringotomy, the patient may settle into a relatively light plane of anesthesia such that he/she rouse to produce some movement or cough at the very moment when the surgeon requires complete stillness.

Tips and Tricks

This problem may be overcome by giving several manually assisted breaths to deepen anesthesia just before the point of surgical stimulus.

Patients for "grommets" are usually otherwise well but frequently present with a "runny nose." Children who have or are recovering from an upper respiratory tract infection (URTI) have more irritable upper airways and are more likely to suffer "respiratory events" such as coughing, bronchospasm, laryngospasm, and transient arterial desaturation. Such events are readily dealt with by an experienced anesthetist and children rarely, if ever, suffer significant morbidity (e.g., longer hospital stay) in consequence.[8]

Common practice is to proceed with anesthesia in these circumstances, provided that the child does not have a temperature of more than 38°C and does not have any systemic upset.

If a child presenting for ENT surgery does have an active URTI requiring postponement of their operation, there is some controversy as to the optimal delay. Virally induced airway hyperreactivity (as assessed by aerosol challenge) persists for approximately 6 weeks and children typically suffer 6 to 8 upper URTIs each year. It may be that the best compromise is a 7- to 10-day postponement, allowing just enough time to get over the worst of the present infection but unlikely to coincide with the start of the next.

3.8.2 Adenoidectomy

This is the simplest example of the "shared airway." Surgical access precludes the use of a face mask to maintain anesthesia, and the larynx trachea and lungs must be protected from blood trickling (flowing) down from the nasopharynx.

- Reasonable surgical access may be provided by use of a "flexible" (wire helix) LMA. This will also provide good protection of the larynx and lower airway from blood. The LMA lends itself to maintaining spontaneous ventilation and the inherent flexibility of the "simple" anesthetic technique.
- Intraoperative autonomic control and postoperative analgesia may be provided by a combination of paracetamol (given orally preoperatively or intravenously intraoperatively), an NSAID, and a judicious (good analgesia balanced against respiratory depression) dose of IV opiate intraoperatively.

Alternatively, a well-sized plain or cuffed "south facing" oral ETT will allow excellent surgical access and very good protection of the airway against blood or inadvertently regurgitated gastric contents.

- Inserting the tube using a nondepolarizing muscle relaxant will probably commit us to 25 to 30 minutes of anesthesia, which may exactly match requirements for "adenoids by coblation and grommets" or may involve a quarter hour of "anesthesia, no useful surgical activity."
- Inserting the tube without muscle relaxant may require a greater depth of anesthesia to remain elegant, but it has the advantage of flexibility to accommodate both the quick and the slower operator.

3.8.3 Tonsillectomy

Pretty well every permutation of ETTs, LMAs, anesthetic agents (inhalational and IV), muscle relaxants, analgesics, and antiemetics has been used successfully by someone for this procedure.

No technique has ever been shown to be unequivocally better than the rest, and most anesthetists will tailor their favored technique to the particular patient (and operator) with whom they are faced.

That said, there are a number of particular considerations.

Patient Characteristics

The population of children presenting for adenotonsillectomy has changed over the past quarter of a century. Otherwise well children missing lots of secondary school because of recurrent tonsillitis have become rather less common, whereas younger children with coexisting medical problems and symptoms, which are, or may be, related to obstructive breathing patterns, have become much more common.

Well children who do not have any symptoms suggestive of OSA are usually presented as candidates for day-stay surgery. Their anesthetics are usually designed with this in mind. Common considerations are as follows:

- Using short-acting agents with little "hangover."
- Producing adequate analgesia but with a minimal sedative effect.
- Minimizing PONV.
- Minimizing postoperative bleeding and ensuring that it is recognized if it does occur.
- Predicting the need for postoperative respiratory monitoring and support.

Choice of Anesthetic Agent

- Propofol and sevoflurane are good agents for induction, whereas propofol, sevoflurane, and desflurane are excellent for maintenance of anesthesia.

I

- Most anesthetists consider that at least some intraoperative opiate, for example, fentanyl (0.5–1.5 µg/kg) or morphine (25–100 µg/kg), is needed to cover at least the pain of the immediate postoperative period. Some think that using morphine intraoperatively can help predict whether the patient will tolerate its use as a postoperative analgesic without suffering undue respiratory depression. Others consider fentanyl to give good immediate postoperative analgesia with less contribution to ongoing nausea and vomiting.

- Topical local anesthetic agents such as bupivacaine to the tonsil bed are thought to enhance analgesia (this has become very popular though the evidence indicates only modest efficacy[9]).

- Oral NSAIDs such as ibuprofen and diclofenac have become the mainstay of analgesia to allow "opiate sparing." Many people have been concerned that the use of NSAIDs might cause an increased incidence of postoperative hemorrhage,[10] but the present consensus is that the benefits of this group of drugs in this context outweighs their drawbacks.[11,12]

Postoperative Nausea and Vomiting and Tonsillectomy

In studies of vomiting following pediatric adenotonsillectomy, control groups have shown vomiting rates of 70%.[13] Thus, in addition to trying to avoid factors that may exacerbate this problem, such as excessive fasting and the overuse of nitrous oxide (its use appears to increase the risk of vomiting, as has been demonstrated in high-risk adult patients, and there is no reason to suppose that children should respond differently),[14] there is agreement that active pharmacological prophylaxis is justified.

> Serotonin antagonists, such as ondansetron or granisetron, and, more controversially, the steroid dexamethasone, are commonly used in this regard.

Trials have lessened though not abolished concerns about the effects of dexamethasone on infection and tissue healing (bleeding),[15] and as there seems to be little evidence of a significant dose–response relationship, there would seem to be no case for giving more than a very small dose, 0.0625 mg/kg.[16]

Post-tonsillectomy Bleeding

Most postoperative bleeding occurs in the first 6 hours after surgery. Many units only perform day-stay tonsillectomies as a morning procedure.

Respiratory Problems in Tonsillectomy

> SDB is a spectrum of disorders that affects approximately 10% of children. It encompasses everything, from simple snoring to the most severe form of OSA.

OSA is associated with episodes of hypopnea, apnea, and arterial desaturation. The "gold standard" for diagnosis of OSA is polysomnography (PSG), an investigation that is sufficiently expensive and time consuming, and seldom performed in ordinary clinical practice; the vast majority of children with a diagnosis of OSA achieve this status on clinical grounds, perhaps reinforced with an overnight oximetry reading.

A prospective trial looking at children with PSG-proven OSA undergoing adenotonsillectomy using a standard anesthetic technique demonstrated that compared to a group of children with recurrent tonsillitis operated on and anesthetized in the same way, children with OSA had a much higher incidence of perioperative airway complications (including breath-holding, desaturation, and supraglottic obstruction) and required more anesthetic interventions (use of oral airway, assisting ventilation, supplemental oxygen to maintain oxygen saturation), but the children with OSA did not require less opiate analgesia nor did they have longer hospital stays.[17]

The central problem in anesthetizing infants and children with preoperative airway obstructive symptoms for tonsillectomy is their postoperative care. The anatomical removal of the lymphoid tissue of Waldeyer's ring does not produce immediate physiological improvement in the degree of obstruction; in practice, it may appear to be at least as bad for some days after surgery, and the situation is worsened by any decreased level of consciousness and respiratory depression produced by residual anesthesia or sedative analgesia.

> The patient with preoperative airway obstruction may be more at risk of hypoxia and apnea on the first postoperative night than on the last preoperative night.[18]

Many of the anesthetic considerations for the day-stay patient are applicable to trying to decrease this risk for the obstructive patient—particularly choosing drugs with the least residual sedative and respiratory depressant effects and trying where possible to avoid the use of opiates for postoperative analgesia.[19]

Notwithstanding this, these patients must be monitored for significant respiratory depression, and there must be a means of taking effective action to treat impending hypoxia.

Monitoring Respiratory Depression

- The best monitors—experienced nurses with enough time to devote to the task—are also the scarcest.
- Other technological monitors alone, such as apnea mattresses and pulse oximeters, are much less good.
- Pulse oximetry gives little enough advance warning of the problem if the child is breathing air, and if the child is breathing a higher inspired oxygen concentration, then this problem is made worse as the pulse oximeter will continue to give a satisfactory reading long (many seconds) after the onset of severe respiratory depression or even complete loss of the airway.
- Continuous capnography at the nostril would be a more useful electrical adjunct, but it is seldom available in the ward setting.

The anesthetist has to insist that monitoring and staffing levels are of a sufficient standard so that children with obstructive symptoms can undergo adenotonsillectomies safely. In practice, this means that they should be in a ward environment or nursed in a high dependency unit (or even, on occasion, occupy a place in the pediatric intensive care unit [PICU]). This may impose limits on how many such children can safely undergo surgery on a particular list or involve increasing staffing allocations to allow several such children to be operated on at one particular time.

3.8.4 Anesthesia for Airway Problems in Infants

Surgical considerations usually dictate the method of anesthesia here. For diagnostic examination of the airway, the surgeon wants to make an unhurried, detailed inspection of the tracheobronchial tree with as little alteration of the dynamics of respiration as possible. Hence, it is nearly always a priority to maintain spontaneous ventilation.
- Traditional anesthetic management of such an infant would be to induce anesthesia with sevoflurane in oxygen.
- Then, having secured IV access, the larynx would be sprayed with topical local anesthetic, and a plain ETT would be passed either orally or nasally into the trachea.

- Having "sized" the subglottis in this manner and maintaining spontaneous ventilation through a Jackson Rees T-piece circuit (low resistance), a suspension laryngoscope is set up and the supraglottis can be examined microscopically and at leisure (▶ Fig. 3.6).
- Keeping the infant breathing spontaneously, the ETT is then withdrawn until its tip lies in the oropharynx, and passing the tube nasally helps to maintain the stability of the tube at this point. The sevoflurane concentration may have to be increased at this point as the infant's anesthetic gases are now diluted with air.
- The vocal cords, subglottis, and trachea can now be inspected with a rigid Hopkins Rod of appropriate size.
- If the surgeon wishes to perform a more extended rigid bronchoscopy, then the Jackson Rees circuit can be attached to the side arm of the bronchoscope (▶ Fig. 3.7).
- After completing inspection of the lower airway, the sevoflurane is switched off and the patient's level of consciousness is allowed to lighten until he/she reaches the point of spontaneous vocal cord movement. It is difficult to maintain elegance at this point in the procedure, as the surgeon has to assess the quality of cord adduction/abduction before the patient lightens to the point of coughing and bucking.
- Thereafter, inhalational anesthesia may be deepened once more and the patient's trachea can be reintubated, or, alternatively, the suspension laryngoscope can be removed and the patient's airway can be controlled with a face mask until full consciousness returns.

There are, of course, alternatives and refinements to this technique. Some anesthetists are concerned that what is seen as the great advantage of this technique—anesthesia being maintained through the airway, which must perforce be kept clear— is in fact its great disadvantage as it invites the possibility of awareness through inadequate anesthesia at times of maximal stimulation, particularly when the patient's anesthetic gases are diluted with air. They favor maintaining anesthesia by infusion of an IV agent or agents, for example, propofol or propofol/remifentanil, while the patient breathes oxygen-enriched air.

Modern anesthesia is extremely safe, but parents and health care professionals understandably worry about the potential effects of anesthetic agents on the developing brain and nervous system. This is of particular concern in the newborn.[20]

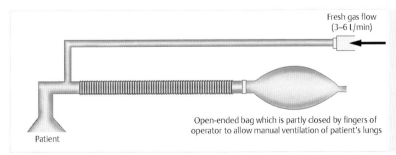

Fresh gas flow (3–6 L/min)

Open-ended bag which is partly closed by fingers of operator to allow manual ventilation of patient's lungs

Patient

Fig. 3.6 The Jackson Rees circuit (modified Ayre's T-piece).

I

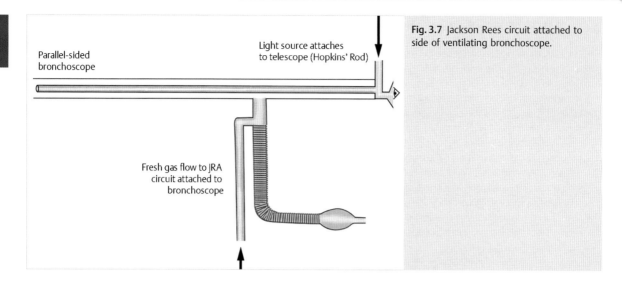

Parallel-sided
bronchoscope

Light source attaches
to telescope (Hopkins' Rod)

Fig. 3.7 Jackson Rees circuit attached to
side of ventilating bronchoscope.

Fresh gas flow to JRA
circuit attached to
bronchoscope

An international multicenter trial that compared infants
having awake-regional anesthesia with those having
short periods (less than 1 hour) of sevoflurane anesthesia found no evidence of an increased risk of adverse
neurodevelopmental outcomes at 2 years of age, but it
is wise to remain cautious about recommending surgery
or anesthesia in the very young.[21]

3.8.5 Tracheostomy in Infants

Speaking as a spectator, no matter how gifted the surgeon, the operator's hands and instruments always
appear to be oversized and cumbersome during this operation and so the anesthetist needs to do all he/she can to
facilitate matters in terms of positioning.

A roll under the child's neck helps to optimize neck extension, and a tape about the chin smooths the skin for
the incision (see Chapter 23).

Safety demands that the anesthetist has good access to
the patient's head and he/she should never be further
away than the length of the T-piece of a Jackson Rees
circuit from the airway.

I personally would caution against too elaborate head
draping ("turbanning" the head) and would recommend a
single "porthole" type drape with the porthole at the
neck allowing the anesthetist to rummage easily to
release the ETT fixation if all goes well and to facilitate

easy removal of the drape to allow reintubation if things
do not go well.

The crucial time in this procedure is the breaching of
the trachea and the exchange of tracheostomy for the ETT.

- The infant should be preoxygenated for a few minutes
  prior to this point.
- The surgeon opens the trachea between two "stay"
  sutures with a vertical incision at the level of the second
  and third tracheal rings, exposing the ETT.
- The anesthetist then withdraws the ETT under direct
  vision such that the surgeon can insert the tracheostomy tube or can guide the ETT back into the distal
  trachea if there is any problem such as the tracheal
  opening being too small or the tracheal tube slipping
  laterally off the trachea ("how unlikely!," I hear you say,
  but this does happen).
- When the tracheostomy tube is in situ, it is connected
  to a clean breathing circuit with a capnograph inline to
  confirm airway placement by the detection of carbon
  dioxide.
- The position of the end of the tracheostomy tube relative to the carina should then be checked with a flexible
  bronchoscope, in the position in which the infant will
  be lying in his cot rather than in the artificial, neck-
  extended position of the operating room, and any
  adjustments of the tube are made at this point. It is
  good to have at least 1 cm of trachea between the
  end of the tracheotomy tube and the bifurcation at the
  carina.
- Postoperatively, infants with a newly fashioned tracheostomy need to be nursed in an environment where
  the tube will be maintained and there are personnel
  and facilities to regain and maintain the airway if the
  tracheostomy tube blocks or becomes dislodged. In
  practice, this usually requires the infant to be kept in a
  PICU until it is clear that all is well.

3.9 Anesthesia in Children with Specific Syndromes or Disabilities

Some of the potential ENT and anesthetic problems associated with Down's syndrome are outlined in ▶ Table 3.2.

A child with a Fontan circulation or severe cerebral palsy should fall under the remit of a specialist center for even the most trivial of interventions. In general, age of less than 1 year, multisystem disease, severe learning difficulty, or airway problems of any sort should have a default position of referral to a specialist pediatric center.

3.10 Key Points

- Simple anesthesia, using a single anesthetic agent to provide unconsciousness, lack of movement in response to surgical stimulation, and attenuation of the cardiovascular responses to such stimulation, is used for short operations in patients who are well.

- Balanced anesthesia, using separate drugs (typically an anesthetic agent, a muscle relaxant, and an opiate) to produce unconsciousness, paralysis, cardiovascular control, and analgesia, allows frailer, sicker patients to undergo more invasive and longer procedures, with less postoperative morbidity.
- Induction can be inhalational (usually with sevoflurane) but is most commonly achieved using IV administration of propofol.
- In children, IV induction is facilitated by applying local anesthetic cream.
- Premedications may be necessary in children who would be too uncooperative to induce without undue upset to all concerned.
- Oral midazolam is currently the most popular premedication.
- The LMA has revolutionized anesthesia and has replaced the use of the face mask for everything other than "bag-and-mask" ventilation prior to intubation.
- The LMA provides protection of the airway from blood or secretions from the nose, mouth, and pharynx, but it does not completely protect the airway from aspiration.

Table 3.2 Clinical features of Down's syndrome and anesthetic considerations

Anatomy	Tendency to small midface, mandible, choanae, subglottis, trachea Relatively large tongue
Central nervous system	Severe learning difficulty Epilepsy Cervical spine abnormalities
Hematology	Poorer T and B cell function Reduced immunity More common URTIs Higher incidence leukemia
Cardiovascular system	>40% have congenital heart disease (60% endocardial cushion defect, CAVSD) PDA VSD Fallot's tetralogy Pulmonary hypertension Conduction defects following repair
Gastrointestinal system	Duodenal obstruction Gastroesophageal reflux Hirschsprung's disease
Endocrine	Hypothyroidism
ENT	Middle ear disease producing conductive deafness (up to 60%) Sleep-disordered breathing Rhinitis
Anesthetic implications	Poorer ability to cooperate Require smaller ETT than predicted[22] Generally increased incidence of complications specifically[23]: Severe bradycardia (3%) Natural airway obstruction (2%) Difficult intubation (0.5%) Postintubation stridor (2%) Cervical spine problems are difficult to assess, both clinically and radiologically, but potentially devastating. In practice, rarely a problem, but avoid hyperflexion and extention (extreme care or avoid suspension laryngoscopy)[24]

Abbreviations: CAVSD, complete atrioventricular septal defect; ENT, ear, nose, and throat; ETT, endotracheal tube; PDA, patent ductus arteriosus; URTIs, upper respiratory tract infections; VSD, ventricular septal defect.

- An ETT provides a safe and easily accessible airway and also reduces the risk of aspiration.
- In children's ENT surgery, endotracheal intubation is usually through the oral route following administration of a muscle relaxant.
- In balanced anesthesia, nondepolarizing NMBs are usually used to paralyze the patient.
- Postoperative pain is typically managed by intraoperative and, sometimes, postoperative opiates (morphine or fentanyl), infiltration of local anesthetic wherever possible, administration of paracetamol for most minor procedures, and postoperative codeine or NSAIDs, when necessary.
- Serotonin antagonists, such as ondansetron or granisetron, and, more controversially, the steroid dexamethasone, may be used to control PONV.
- The "shared airway" demands close cooperation between the anesthetist and surgeon.

References

[1] Rainey L, van der Walt JH. The anaesthetic management of autistic children. Anaesth Intensive Care. 1998; 26(6):682–686

[2] Sun X-G, Su F, Shi YQ, Lee C. The "second gas effect" is not a valid concept. Anesth Analg. 1999; 88(1):188–192

[3] McKeating K, Bali IM, Dundee JW. The effects of thiopentone and propofol on upper airway integrity. Anaesthesia. 1988; 43(8):638–640

[4] Eckenhoff JE. Some anatomic considerations of the infant larynx influencing endotracheal anesthesia. Anesthesiology. 1951; 12(4): 401–410

[5] Weber T, Salvi N, Orliaguet G, Wolf A. Cuffed vs non-cuffed endotracheal tubes for pediatric anesthesia. Paediatr Anaesth. 2009; 19 Suppl 1:46–54

[6] Hunter JM, Flockton EA. The doughnut and the hole: a new pharmacological concept for anaesthetists. Br J Anaesth. 2006; 97(2):123–126

[7] Yiannakopoulou E. Pharmacogenomics and Opioid Analgesics: Clinical Implications. International Journal of Genomics 2015. http://dx. doi.org/10.1155/2015/368979

[8] Tait AR, Malviya S. Anesthesia for the child with an upper respiratory tract infection: still a dilemma? Anesth Analg. 2005; 100(1):59–65

[9] Grainger J, Saravanappa N. Local anaesthetic for post-tonsillectomy pain: a systematic review and meta-analysis. Clin Otolaryngol. 2008; 33(5):411–419

[10] Marret E, Flahault A, Samama CM, Bonnet F. Effects of postoperative, nonsteroidal, antiinflammatory drugs on bleeding risk after tonsillectomy. Anesthesiol. 2003; 98(6):1497–1502

[11] Lewis SR, Nicholson A, Cardwell ME, Siviter G, Smith AF. Nonsteroidal anti-inflammatory drugs and perioperative bleeding in paediatric tonsillectomy. Cochrane Database Syst Rev. 2013; 18(7):CD003591

[12] Jeyakumar A, Brickman TM, Williamson ME, et al. Nonsteroidal anti-inflammatory drugs and postoperative bleeding following adenotonsillectomy in pediatric patients. Arch Otolaryngol Head Neck Surg. 2008; 134(1):24–27

[13] Bolton CM, Myles PS, Nolan T, Sterne JA. Prophylaxis of postoperative vomiting in children undergoing tonsillectomy: a systematic review and meta-analysis. Br J Anaesth. 2006; 97(5):593–604

[14] Leslie K, Myles PS, Chan MT, et al. ENIGMA Trial Group. Risk factors for severe postoperative nausea and vomiting in a randomized trial of nitrous oxide-based vs nitrous oxide-free anaesthesia. Br J Anaesth. 2008; 101(4):498–505

[15] Plante J, Turgeon AF, Zarychanski R, et al. Effect of systemic steroids on post-tonsillectomy bleeding and reinterventions: systematic review and meta-analysis of randomised controlled trials. BMJ. 2012; 345:e5389

[16] Kim MS, Coté CJ, Cristoloveanu C, et al. There is no dose-escalation response to dexamethasone (0.0625–1.0 mg/kg) in pediatric tonsillectomy or adenotonsillectomy patients for preventing vomiting, reducing pain, shortening time to first liquid intake, or the incidence of voice change. Anesth Analg. 2007; 104(5):1052–1058

[17] Sanders JC, King MA, Mitchell RB, Kelly JP. Perioperative complications of adenotonsillectomy in children with obstructive sleep apnea syndrome. Anesth Analg. 2006; 103(5):1115–1121

[18] Nixon GM, Kermack AS, McGregor CD, et al. Sleep and breathing on the first night after adenotonsillectomy for obstructive sleep apnea. Pediatr Pulmonol. 2005; 39(4):332–338

[19] Baijal RG, Bidani SA, Minard CG, Watcha MF. Perioperative respiratory complications following awake and deep extubation in children undergoing adenotonsillectomy. Paediatr Anaesth. 2015; 25(4):392–399

[20] Nasr VG, Davis JM. Anesthetic use in newborn infants: the urgent need for rigorous evaluation. Pediatr Res. 2015; 78(1):2–6

[21] Davidson AJ, Disma N, de Graaff JC, et al. GAS consortium. Neurodevelopmental outcome at 2 years of age after general anaesthesia and awake-regional anaesthesia in infancy (GAS): an international multicentre, randomised controlled trial. Lancet. 2016; 387(10015):239–250

[22] Shott SR. Down syndrome: analysis of airway size and a guide for appropriate intubation. Laryngoscope. 2000; 110(4):585–592

[23] Borland LM, Colligan J, Brandom BW. Frequency of anesthesia-related complications in children with Down syndrome under general anesthesia for noncardiac procedures. Paediatr Anaesth. 2004; 14(9):733–738

[24] Hata T, Todd MM. Cervical spine considerations when anesthetizing patients with Down syndrome. Anesthesiology. 2005; 102(3):680–685

4 Pediatric Ear, Nose, and Throat Emergencies

Ann-Louise McDermott

4.1 Introduction

A high percentage of illnesses affecting the head and neck in children present acutely, occasionally with airway obstruction or impending intracranial sepsis. Children are not "little adults" and often they are unable to provide a helpful history. Diagnosis can be difficult, delayed, and uncertain. Examination can be fraught, especially if the child is frightened and unwell. This can be very challenging for clinicians managing such pediatric ear, nose, and throat (ENT) emergencies. If you are responsible for the care of children, you need to be conversant with the main emergencies that present and with the principles of early management, especially pediatric resuscitation and life support.[1] The immediate priorities are to recognize those children at risk of significant and at times life-threatening complications if they are not treated immediately, to identify those who need early transfer to a specialized unit, and then to manage those who can be looked after in a local setting. Once a decision has been made that a child needs transfer to a specialist unit, the appropriate arrangements must be made to ensure the safety of the child throughout the transfer process. In some circumstances, a standard ambulance will be satisfactory but for very sick children or children with a precarious airway, you may need access to a specialized pediatric retrieval team, assuming one is available in your area (see Chapter 1).

> If a child needs to be transferred to a specialist unit, make sure he/she has a good airway, and you have commenced resuscitation–for example, fluid replacement–given analgesia, as needed, and arranged the appropriate staff to accompany him/her on the journey. Liaise closely with the receiving unit and with the specialized pediatric retrieval services, if available.

This chapter aims to highlight common nasal and aerodigestive tract emergencies in children and to guide the clinician in making these vital decisions. Otological emergencies such as acute mastoiditis and the suppurative complications of otitis media are dealt with in Chapter 7.

4.2 Foreign Bodies

Children are notoriously curious and enjoy experiments. Foreign bodies in the ear and upper aerodigestive tract are very common, particularly in young (preschool) children who, as their manual dexterity develops, are inclined to insert objects into the ear, nose, and mouth.

4.2.1 Foreign Bodies in the Ear

Foreign bodies in the ear are often fairly innocuous (▶ Fig. 4.1). The parent or carer may report their suspicions, or the child may have been seen inserting an object in the ear. Hearing loss and pain are reported in some cases. Many children are completely asymptomatic and the foreign body is an incidental finding by the carer or doctor.

The physical characteristics, size, and duration of the foreign body are very important. Inert objects such as beads, fragments of toys, crayons, and sponge are commonly found and may lead to impaction of wax and to otitis externa if not removed. Organic objects such as nuts, food particles, and occasionally insects tend to be more prone to infection.

> Batteries are not uncommon, may be very destructive, and should be promptly removed. "Button" batteries may look innocuous but modern technology has produced very powerful small electrochemical cells, and even if they do not leak, they can cause an electrochemical reaction when in contact with tissue. If left, they can give rise to desquamation of the skin and soft tissue, osteitis of the bones of the ear canal, and perforation of the drum.

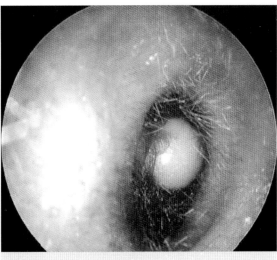

Fig. 4.1 Foreign body in the ear.

I

Removal of foreign bodies from the nose and ear should only be attempted if the clinician has the appropriate equipment and experience. An inert foreign body, such as a bead or piece of plastic, may be removed by gentle syringing. Otherwise, microsuction and instrumentation may be needed. Multiple failed attempts may result in further trauma and distress to the child making any further attempts impossible without general anesthesia.

> **Tips and Tricks**
>
> Check both ears; mischievous children may not always volunteer the whole truth.

4.2.2 Foreign Bodies in the Nose

Objects in the nose may present several days or weeks after they have been inserted with an offensive unilateral discharge and/or epistaxis. There may be crusting at the vestibule, and in prolonged cases, the skin of the vestibule and above the upper lip can become excoriated and inflamed. Sometimes the child may report self-insertion of such a foreign body but more often they present with symptoms.

Planning the timing for removal of nasal foreign bodies depends on the nature of the foreign body and the symptoms. As with ear foreign bodies, batteries can be notoriously destructive, even over a period of a few hours, and need to be removed as soon as possible. If they can be removed in the outpatient setting or the emergency department, this would be ideal, and if the child needs a general anesthetic, it should be arranged as soon as the child is starved and ready. The potential risk of inhalation of nasal foreign bodies is well recognized, but there is little evidence that this is a significant risk.[2] In a neurologically normal child, a nasal foreign body that slips back into the pharynx will almost certainly be swallowed rather than inhaled. If the child is neurologically compromised, for example, with a poor swallow and an absent gag reflex, it may be best to admit the child and arrange very early removal to avoid the risk of aspiration. It is recommended that a nasal foreign body should be removed at the earliest reasonable opportunity,[3] ideally on the next available operating list.

> **Tips and Tricks**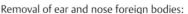
>
> Removal of ear and nose foreign bodies:
> - Nonorganic foreign bodies in the ear that are not completely occluding the ear canal may sometimes be removed by syringing with warm water.
> - Spherical bead-like objects can often be removed with suction.
> - Always use good lighting and appropriate instruments.
> - Grasping instruments, for example, "crocodile" forceps, are best for irregularly shaped objects, but for smooth or impacted material such as beads, use a hook-like instrument to gently dislodge the object from behind rather than letting it slip in further.
> - Live insects should be immobilized prior to removal. This is best achieved by filling the ear canal with fluid containing an anesthetic such as lidocaine.
>
> Button batteries in the ear and the nose can cause rapid and severe tissue destruction. Arrange for urgent removal.

Presentation and Early Management

Foreign bodies inhaled or ingested are a true medical emergency. A foreign body in the airway can cause rapid progressive airway obstruction, and a foreign body in the esophagus can compress the trachea and cause severe asphyxia. These children need prompt referral to the ENT department.

A clinical history of sudden coughing, choking, shortness of breath, and wheeze should alert the clinician to the possibility of inhalation, even if nobody has seen the child ingest or inhale an object. Similarly, drooling and a painful swallow would suggest an ingested foreign body. The nature of the foreign body is very important and again the clinician should be especially wary of very sharp objects and of batteries (▶ Fig. 4.2, ▶ Fig. 4.3).[4]

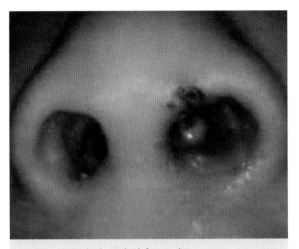

Fig. 4.2 Foreign body in the left nostril.

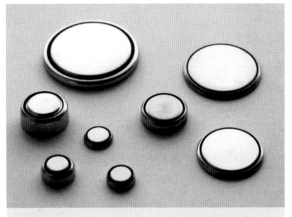

Fig. 4.3 Button batteries. (Courtesy of Gerhard H Wrodnigg.)

National Health Service (NHS) England Patient Safety Alert

In December 2014, NHS England issued the following Patient Safety Alert on the risk of death and serious harm from delays in recognizing and treating ingestion of button batteries[5]:

"Ingestion of button batteries can cause serious harm and death. Severe tissue damage results from a build up of sodium hydroxide (caustic soda) as a result of the electrical current discharged from the battery, and not, as commonly supposed, from leakage from the battery. The sodium hydroxide causes tissue burns, often in the oesophagus, which can then cause fistulisation into major blood vessels, resulting in catastrophic haemorrhage. Even apparently discharged ('flat') batteries can still have this effect, and button batteries pushed into ears or nostrils can also cause serious injuries.

"Button battery ingestion affects all age groups, although most cases involve children under the age of six who mistake the battery for a sweet, or older people with confusion or poor vision who mistake the battery for a pill. Older children and adults may ingest batteries as a means of self harming.

"Review of incident reports from a recent four year period identified five cases where severe tissue damage occurred after apparent delays in suspecting, diagnosing or treating button battery ingestion in small children; one child died.

"Incident reports suggested that when ingestion was reported, healthcare staff did not recognise the need for this to be **treated as a medical emergency**. Additionally, symptoms of tissue damage such as haematemesis, haemoptysis and respiratory difficulties can **manifest up to 28 days** after ingestion of the battery. Incident reports suggested that where such symptoms occur, staff did not always consider the possibility of prior button battery ingestion.

"Removal of the battery alone may be insufficient action to prevent further damage, with further symptoms manifesting later; patients need expert input, and careful monitoring and follow-up. One further incident described the death of a child from late complications after they had been treated and sent home.

"A further 241 incidents also described a range of battery types swallowed as self-harm by inpatients; whilst only one incident described severe tissue damage from delay in treatment, the incident reports suggested some nursing and medical staff believed battery ingestion would be harmless unless the battery was damaged or leaking, and therefore urgent advice was not always sought.

"Whilst the focus of this Alert is on prompt recognition and treatment of ingestion, healthcare providers caring for children, vulnerable adults or people who may self-harm should also consider if action to protect patients from button battery ingestion needs to be taken; the review of incidents above identified six occasions when older patients accidentally swallowed button batteries from hearing aids."

Reproduced with permission. Contains public sector information licensed under the Open Government License v3.0.

The size of the object and the site of the impaction and the timing of inhalation are important. A foreign body in the larynx or trachea may be quickly fatal. Immediately after ingestion/impaction or inhalation of a foreign body, the child is usually in considerable distress and needs prompt intervention. In children with potentially fatal impaction, first-aid measures at the scene can be lifesaving. These includes the Heimlich maneuver, positioning maneuvers and the removal of a foreign body obstructing the laryngeal inlet using a laryngoscope and Magill forceps if the attending physician is suitably trained and skilled. Suctioning may be needed as the child will often vomit.

In the case of a foreign body impacted in a bronchus, the child may have some degree of oxygen desaturation but will usually breathe well using the unaffected lung. Airway endoscopy need not be immediate and it is best to arrange safe transfer under supervision to a center where the child can have a laryngotracheobronchoscopy and removal of the foreign body under controlled conditions, with the support of a skilled pediatric anesthetist and ideally with access to a pediatric intensive care unit (PICU).

In some children, the inhalation may have occurred days or weeks previously and they may present with new features of unexplained cough or wheeze or even an unusual pneumonia. Retained foreign bodies, especially organic matter such as peanuts and food particles, can be an extreme irritant, and if treatment is delayed, the child may get bronchiectasis and chronic lung infection. In the case of a foreign body that is radiolucent (e.g., a peanut or a food particle), the only radiological evidence may be hyperinflation of the lung on the side where the object has lodged in the bronchus causing partial obstruction, that is, air enters the lung but is "trapped" beyond the foreign body ("obstructive emphysema"; ▶ Fig. 4.4).

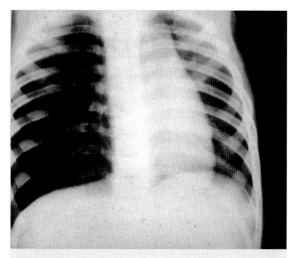

Fig. 4.4 Chest X-ray showing hyperinflation of the right lung. Foreign body in the right main-stem bronchus.

ⓘ

"All that Wheezes is not Asthma": Chevalier Jackson
- Think of an inhaled foreign body in the wheezy child.
- Be suspicious of a foreign body in a child with chronic laryngeal symptoms.
- Beware sudden onset of new persistent respiratory symptoms.
- Consider a chest (inspiration and expiration) and a lateral neck X-ray if it is safe to do so.
- Negative findings on X-ray do not exclude an inhaled or ingested foreign body.
- If in doubt, refer for diagnostic endoscopy.

Pharyngeal and upper esophageal foreign bodies need to be removed by pharyngoesophagoscopy. Be ready to undertake laryngotracheobronchoscopy as well if there is any suspicion of inhalation (▶ Fig. 4.5, ▶ Fig. 4.6).

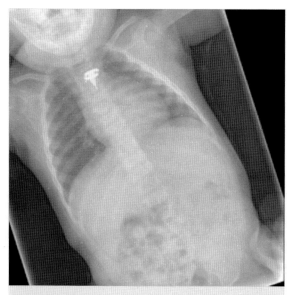

Fig. 4.5 Chest X-ray showing a "Coco Chanel" earring in the upper esophagus of a young girl.

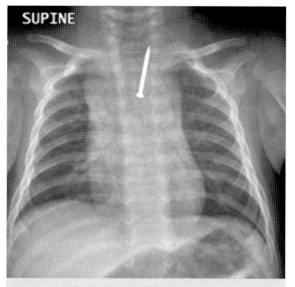

Fig. 4.6 Chest X-ray showing a nail in the upper esophagus of an infant boy. Urgent removal is necessary.

4.3 Epistaxis

4.3.1 Presentation

The nasal cavity has a very rich blood supply from both the internal and external carotid arteries. Epistaxis is a very common problem in childhood and is mostly mild and self-limiting. In a small number of cases, it may be severe and potentially life threatening.

The commonest cause of epistaxis in children is local trauma as a result of nose picking. Crusting within the nostrils is often identified in these children. Other causes must be considered especially if epistaxis is recurrent, severe, or fails to settle conservatively. Epistaxis may occasionally be the first sign of underlying hematological abnormalities and coagulopathies, as well as rarer pathology such as juvenile angiofibromas in young boys.

The site of the bleeding in children is typically a prominent retrocolumellar vein or the arterial plexus at Little's area (Kiesselbach's plexus) on the mucosa of the septum. Bleeds are typically slow and persistent, and stop quite quickly with pressure. The less common but more troublesome posterior epistaxis originates from the sphenopalatine artery and is a more profuse, prolonged, and severe bleed.

> **Tips and Tricks** 👉
>
> With severe bleeding in a young adolescent male, suspect juvenile angiofibroma until proven otherwise (▶ Fig. 4.7).

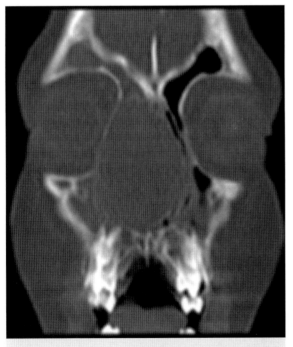

Fig. 4.7 Coronal computed tomography scan of the nose of a 10-year-old boy with a juvenile angiofibroma. He had presented with nasal obstruction and severe epistaxis.

4.3.2 Management

Adequate resuscitation is the first line of management for epistaxis but is rarely necessary in children.

Take a thorough history to identify any potential risk factors. Examine the child in a good light. An otoscope gives a good view of the anterior nose in a child.

For the majority of children, an emollient cream without other treatments has been shown to significantly reduce epistaxis when it is used twice daily for 4 weeks.[6] Naseptin (chlorhexidine hydrochloride and neomycin sulfate antiseptic cream) is a popular choice but many ENT surgeons recommend a simple petroleum jelly (Vaseline, Unilever).

The management of the acute bleed depends on the age of the child as outlined in Box 4.1 and Box 4.2.

4

> ### Box 4.1 Management of Acute Bleeds in Older Children Who Can Cooperate
>
> - Apply digital pressure to the nose. Sit the child upright with his/her chin down.
> - Apply cotton wool soaked in local anesthetic solution for 1 to 5 minutes.
> - Remove the cotton wool and dry the nose with tissue or cotton wool.
> - Use a 75% silver nitrate stick to outline the bleeding point and then follow with a second application of silver nitrate to the bleeding point itself.
> - Dry the inside of the nostril again with tissue or cotton wool.
>
> Follow with Naseptin cream* twice a day for 1 month.
>
> *Naseptin cream contains peanut oil. Check for peanut allergy before you use it.

> ### Box 4.2 Alternative Management for Younger Children
>
> - Use resorbable packs (e.g., Nasopore [Stryker], a fully synthetic biodegradable fragmented foam) to tamponade the bleeding.
> - Use Floseal (Baxter) hemostatic matrix (gelatin granules). This liquid can be syringed into the nostril, and hemostasis can be established within 2 minutes.
> - Surgiflo (Ethicon) hemostatic matrix (gelatin paste) can be applied to the nostril as above.
> - Give antibiotics to any child with a nasal pack to prevent infection and toxic shock syndrome.

4.4 Sinusitis and Its Complications

4.4.1 Presentation

In young children, the maxillary and ethmoid sinuses are the only sinuses present at birth. The bony boundary between the orbit and the ethmoids (lamina papyracea) is poorly developed. The sphenoid and frontal sinuses are not of any great size until at least the age of 5 to 6 years.

Acute rhinosinusitis is a common infection in the pediatric population. The classical symptoms of acute rhinosinusitis include coryzal symptoms, fever, nasal discharge, and cough. Headache is common.

The symptoms and presentation may vary greatly from those in adults, and infection can be more extensive. Although most cases resolve spontaneously, acute sinusitis can give rise to serious complications. Infection can spread into the orbit with a threat to vision, and intracranially to cause meningitis, extradural sepsis, or brain abscess, with a mortality rate quoted as high as 20 to 30% (▶ Fig. 4.8, ▶ Fig. 4.9, ▶ Fig. 4.10).

4.4.2 Management of Acute Sinusitis

Antibiotics are still recommended in pediatric practice. Amoxicillin or Co-amoxiclav is the first choice for uncomplicated sinusitis. The short-term use of topical nasal vasoconstrictors to reduce mucosal edema and improve sinus ventilation is vital and greatly speeds up the recovery period.[7]

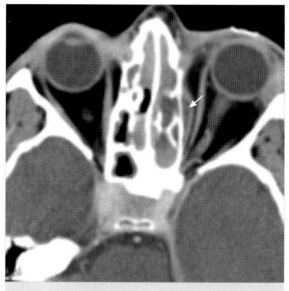

Fig. 4.8 Axial computed tomography scan showing a subperiosteal collection within the left orbit secondary to acute sinusitis of the ethmoid sinuses.

If there is any suspicion of orbital infection or of intracranial sepsis, commence high-dose antibiotics, prescribe nasal congestants, and arrange for urgent assessment including computed tomography (CT) imaging.

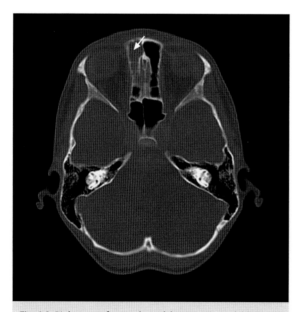

Fig. 4.9 Right acute frontoethmoidal sinusitis in a child presenting with a reduced Glasgow Coma Score.

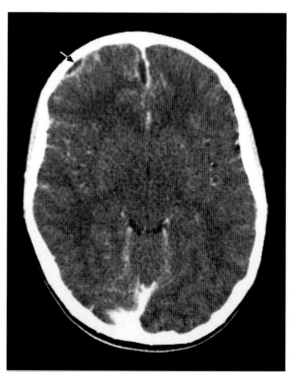

Fig. 4.10 Computed tomography scan showing a subdural empyema in the patient from ▶ Fig. 4.7.

4.4.3 Complications of Sinusitis

Spread of infection beyond the bony confines of the paranasal sinuses can give rise to the major complications of sinusitis: orbital cellulitis or abscess and/or intracranial sepsis.

> **i**
>
> "Red Flags" in Acute Sinusitis
> • Severe headache.
> • Neurologic dysfunction.
> • Eye signs.

Orbital Complications

The infection typically spreads from the ethmoid sinus through the lamina papyracea.

Chandler's classification[8] of orbital complications is widely accepted:
- Stage 1: preseptal cellulitis. Inflammation is confined to the eyelid.
- Stage 2: orbital cellulitis, that is, more extensive involvement of the soft tissues in the bony orbit but *no* abscess formation.
- Stage 3: orbital cellulitis with a subperiosteal abscess collection. There may be mild proptosis and some restrictions to eye movement (ophthalmoplegia).
- Stage 4: orbital cellulitis with intraperiosteal abscess collection; more severe proptosis and ophthalmoplegia. Risk to vision is high.
- Stage 5: cavernous sinus thrombosis; bilateral symptoms; high risk of blindness (50%) and mortality (10–27%).

> **i**
>
> Coronal CT scans with good bone window views are essential to localize any intraorbital collection prior to surgery (▶ Fig. 4.11).

Treatment depends on the staging of the orbital complications (▶ Fig. 4.12). Admit the child for careful monitoring, intravenous antibiotic therapy, and imaging, as dictated by clinical progress. Initial management is medical with broad-spectrum antibiotics pending the results of culture and sensitivity, analgesia, and nasal decongestions. A subperiosteal abscess with very minimal ophthalmoplegia and proptosis in a very young child may be managed in the first instance with aggressive medical therapy alone. If the child does not respond quickly, ideally within 24 hours, or if the infection is more advanced at presentation, then early surgical drainage is indicated.

Endoscopic nasal surgery to approach the ethmoid sinuses and the medial orbital wall is within the ability of most ENT surgeons, but bleeding due to the grossly

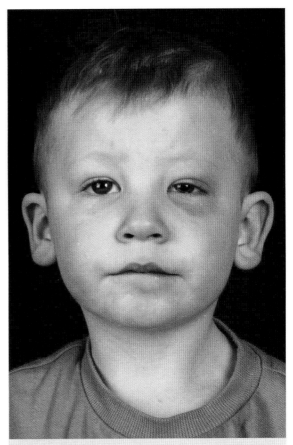

Fig. 4.12 Orbital cellulitis: preseptal. Chandler grade 1, usually responsive to medical treatment. Pupil has been dilated for fundoscopy.

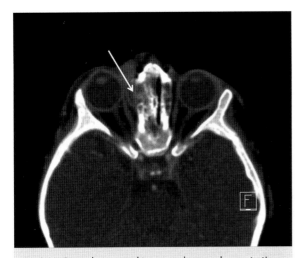

Fig. 4.11 Coronal computed tomography scan demonstrating a breach in the lamina papyracea and a subperiosteal collection (*arrow*) in the right orbit.

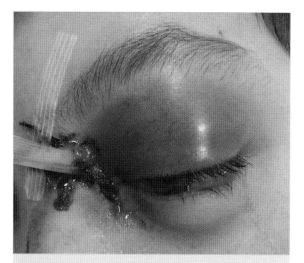

Fig. 4.13 Chandler grade 4 orbital cellulitis. Proptosis, chemosis, and ophthalmoplegia. The medial abscess has been opened but there is a more lateral abscess.

inflamed mucosa can make this very challenging in an emergency setting. It is also difficult to extend the endoscopic dissection beyond the medial orbital wall and into the orbit proper, where abscesses can collect (▶ Fig. 4.13, ▶ Fig. 4.14). An external approach through an incision at the medial canthus, carefully following the disease laterally until pus is found, achieves the prime aim of draining the abscess. Often there is a clear breach in the orbital lamina papyracea where the pus has entered the orbit from the adjacent sinuses (▶ Fig. 4.8). Lavage of the maxillary sinuses can be undertaken in addition if they are involved, or the maxillary antra can be opened by an endoscopic middle meatal antrostomy, but this must be in addition to rather than as a substitute for drainage of the sepsis within the orbit itself. A soft drain can be left in place for a day or two postoperatively while antibiotic therapy is continued and resolution occurs. An external trephine (directly accessing the frontal sinuses through a cosmetic incision in the eyebrow) is a well-established means of efficiently draining the frontal sinuses and may be needed if there is extensive involvement of the frontal sinuses, but this is not usually required in children.

---

i

Indications for Surgery in Orbital Cellulitis
- Proptosis.
- Chemosis (edema of the cornea).
- Ophthalmoplegia.
- Reduced visual acuity.

Poor color vision (as assessed by an ophthalmologist).

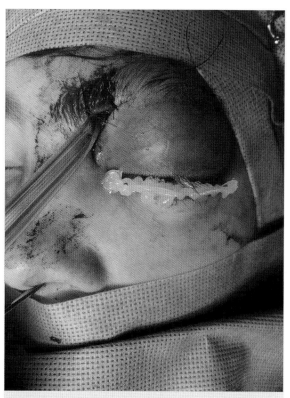

Fig. 4.14 Same patient as in ▶ Fig. 4.13. The lateral abscess has been drained through the incision at the medial canthus. The proptosis has now reduced.

Intracranial Complications

Maintain a high level of suspicion for a child with sinusitis who develops severe headaches or any neurologic symptoms. Commence intravenous antibiotics and arrange urgent imaging, ideally CT and magnetic resonance imaging (MRI) scan with contrast. These patients are often very unwell and will need neurosurgical care. Any one or more of a spectrum of complications can present, such as extradural abscess, subdural collections, meningitis, and cerebral abscess. Joint management with neurosurgical teams is vital for the best patient outcome.

Frontal and sphenoid sinuses are the more common causes of intracranial sepsis. Urgent medical antimicrobial therapy may need to be followed by craniotomy and surgical drainage. Surgical attention to the sinuses at the time of neurosurgery may be needed. The precise technique and approach is dictated by the condition and the experience of the ENT clinician. Endoscopic drainage of the ethmoids, lavage of the maxillary and sphenoidal sinuses, external frontal trephine using a cosmetic incision within the eyebrow, or a combination of these techniques may be needed.

4.5 Nasal Trauma

This is a common presentation to the accident and emergency department.

With any facial trauma it is important to examine the septum and the facial bones including the maxilla, the zygoma, and the orbit. A septal hematoma may be easily overlooked. The consequences of not treating such a hematoma are cartilage necrosis, abscess formation, and later an unsightly saddle deformity to the external nose. Both unilateral and bilateral septal hematomas require early evacuation to preserve the integrity of the nasal cartilage. Broad-spectrum antibiotics are recommended for 7 days (▶ Fig. 4.15).

Fractures of the nasal bones are fortunately uncommon in children. In young children, the nose is predominantly cartilaginous and the bones are small and flattened. In children over the age of 6 years, it is more common for bony displacement to occur following nasal trauma, but if so, simple manipulation is all that is usually required.

4.6 Neck Abscesses

4.6.1 Superficial Cervical Lymphadenopathy

Cervical lymphadenopathy is a frequent finding in children and a neck infection is a very common cause for acute admission. Typically there is a recent history of an upper respiratory tract infection and the child presents with a swollen and tender lymph node/nodes. The key clinical features are neck pain and swelling, fever, and dehydration. This is in contrast to the painless swelling associated with a chronic lymphadenitis such as that which occurs in nontuberculous mycobacteria, although sometimes an acute infection can supervene (▶ Fig. 4.16).

4.6.2 Deep Neck-Space Infections

Most children will have self-limiting respiratory infections but some will develop sepsis in a mass of lymph nodes or in the fascial spaces of the neck, for example, parapharyngeal and retropharyngeal abscesses (deep neck-space infections).

Thorough clinical assessment is important, and with the use of appropriate imaging, children requiring surgical intervention can be treated early. Since the airway is potentially at risk in these cases, a prompt referral to appropriately experienced clinicians is essential.[9]

Immediate management should focus on rehydration, analgesia, and broad-spectrum antibiotics, with baseline biochemical and hematological investigations including blood cultures.

For smaller abscesses, medical management may suffice. Children who fail to respond and those with large fluctuant abscesses should be treated with incision and drainage. The decision for surgical intervention can be helped by the use of ultrasound examination to identify those lymph nodes that have liquefied.

The concern with any deep neck-space infection is the risk of further extension. The possible spread of infection is dictated by the anatomical boundaries of each deep

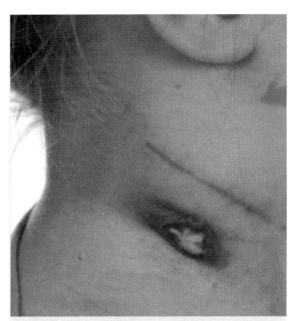

Fig. 4.16 Clinical photograph of a discharging sinus (nontuberculous mycobacteria) right aspect of the neck in an otherwise systemically well child.

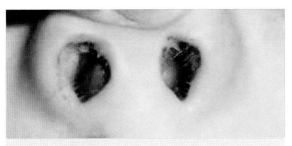

Fig. 4.15 Clinical photograph showing bilateral septal hematoma.

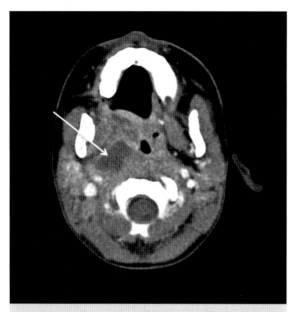

Fig. 4.17 An axial CT scan illustrating a right parapharyngeal collection (*arrow*) causing lateral displacement of the airway.

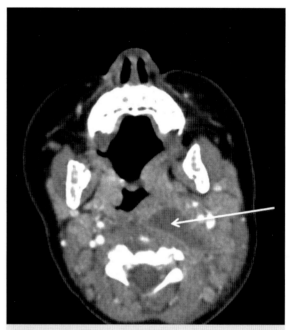

Fig. 4.18 Axial CT scan showing a left parapharyngeal abscess with anterolateral displacement of the carotid sheath.

neck space. The parapharyngeal space contains the carotid sheath and the internal jugular vein (IJV), so infection here can cause thrombophlebitis, pseudoaneurysm, and septic emboli. The retropharyngeal space extends from the skull base to the upper mediastinum, and the prevertebral space extends from skull base to the diaphragm, so infection here can track into the mediastinum.

> ℹ️
>
> Any infection in these spaces has the potential to cause septic mediastinitis with a significant mortality.

A *parapharyngeal abscess* typically presents with generalized lateral neck swelling and a systemically unwell child. They often have trismus and a reluctance to turn their head. The trismus is caused by pain and inflammation and not a true mechanical obstruction to mouth opening. Intraoral examination reveals a normal tonsil which may be displaced medially. Medial swelling from any deep neck-space infection may compromise the airway, so early senior anesthetic assessment is essential. A small abscess in an otherwise well child may respond to antimicrobial therapy, but if there is no early improvement, if there is a large abscess, or if the child is toxic, then arrange for incision and drainage. An enthusiastic interventional radiologist may be able to aspirate pus under ultrasound guided vision, but, in general, an external

drainage procedure through a transverse skin crease incision is best. Make sure the incision is at least 2 cm below the angle of the mandible to avoid damage to the marginal mandibular branch of the facial nerve. This approach is ideal when, as is usual, the vessels (IJV and carotid sheath) are displaced medially by the abscess (▶ Fig. 4.17).

Intraoral drainage has been advocated in some circumstances, mainly if the IJV and the carotid sheath are known to be displaced laterally by the abscess. This often involves excision of the tonsil so that the dissection can progress into the parapharyngeal space (▶ Fig. 4.18).

4.6.3 Lemierre's Syndrome

Spread of infection into the carotid sheath can cause thrombophlebitis of the IJV (Lemierre's syndrome). Particles of the infected thrombus may embolize to the lungs and cause shortness of breath, chest pain, and pneumonia. The most common organism nowadays is a fusobacterium, an otherwise normal organism in the oropharynx.

Management consists of intravenous antibiotics and drainage of any potential infective source. Antibiotic treatment may need to be prolonged for several weeks. The role of anticoagulants is controversial and uncertain, but warfarin is increasingly used in cases of thrombosis of the IJV for periods of 3 to 6 months in consultation with a hematologist.

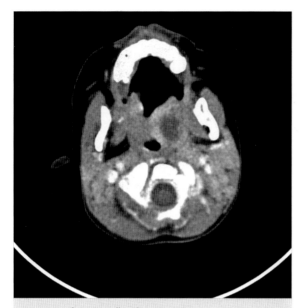

Fig. 4.19 Left peritonsillar abscess.

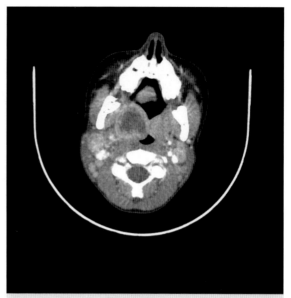

Fig. 4.20 Right peritonsillar abscess.

4.6.4 Peritonsillar Abscess (Quinsy)

This is very difficult to diagnosis in younger children since they may not permit examination of the oropharynx. An ultrasound examination may be helpful in some situations but it can be very difficult to get the child to tolerate a probe (▶ Fig. 4.19, ▶ Fig. 4.20). The child typically has an antecedent history of tonsillitis, with pyrexia, trismus, and an altered voice. Treatment is with intravenous antibiotics, rehydration, and analgesia. Incision and drainage may be needed, but if so, the child will rarely tolerate local anesthesia and a general anesthetic is needed. In this situation many otolaryngologists may recommend tonsillectomy (hot tonsillectomy) to avoid the risk of recurrence.

> **i**
>
> Treatment of Quinsy
> - Commence intravenous broad-spectrum antibiotics.
> - If there is no clinical sign of improvement, plan for surgery.
> - A young child will need general anesthesia.
> - Consider a "hot" tonsillectomy.

4.6.5 Retropharyngeal Abscess

In infants and in younger children up to the age of approximately 3 years, lymph nodes are prominent in the retropharyngeal space. Suppuration of these nodes and formation of a retropharyngeal abscess can cause a very serious airway problem.

The clinical features are given as follows.

> **Retropharyngeal Abscess**
>
> - Young child/infant typically less than 2 years of age.
> - Pyrexia.
> - Drooling.
> - Dysphonia/stertor.
> - Neck-flexed, head-extended position.

Imaging ,either MRI or CT, will confirm the diagnosis (▶ Fig. 4.21).

Commence intravenous antibiotics and monitor the airway carefully. Unless there is frank pus and a fluctuant abscess, surgery can be unrewarding, but if there is pus and the child needs drainage, then prepare for transoral incision and drainage (▶ Fig. 4.22). The airway is at risk, and a suitably experienced anesthetist is needed, ideally with PICU as a backup in case safe extubation proves difficult.

The retropharyngeal space extends from the skull base to the level of the first thoracic vertebra (T1), and mediastinitis is an ever-present risk. Consider a CT of the chest and an echocardiogram if there is any worry about mediastinal spread.

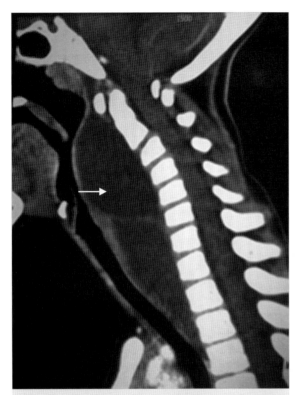

Fig. 4.21 Sagittal computed tomography scan showing a large retropharyngeal collection in an unwell child who presented with stridor and drooling.

4.7 Key Points

- Make sure you have arrangements in place for safe transfer of sick children to a specialist center.
- Beware the button battery foreign body, especially in the esophagus.
- Think of an inhaled foreign body in a wheezy child, especially if there is a poor response to the bronchodilators.
- Unilateral nasal discharge or vestibulitis is due to a nasal foreign body unless proved otherwise.
- Epistaxis in children is usually mild and self-limiting.
- Neck-space infections, particularly retropharyngeal abscess, can cause severe airway obstruction.
- Neck-space infections can track in to the carotid sheath or the mediastinum with potentially life-threatening results.
- Nasal fractures in young children rarely need reduction.
- Sinusitis can cause life-threatening complications.

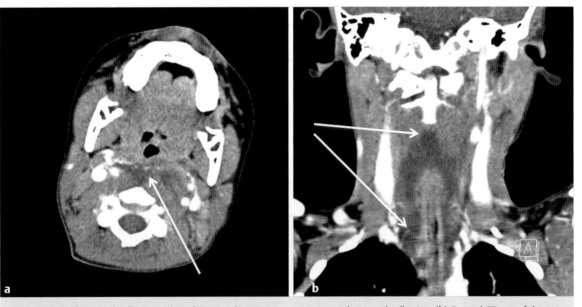

Fig. 4.22 Retropharyngeal collection. (a) Axial CT scan showing an extensive retropharyngeal collection. (b) Coronal CT scan of the same child showing the extensive downward spread of the collection into the superior mediastinum. An interesting bifurcation of the retropharyngeal collection is noted.

References

[1] Advanced Paediatric Life Support. Advanced Life Support Group. Available at www.alsg.org/uk. Accessed Feb 12, 2016

[2] Qureshi AA, Lowe DA, McKiernan DC. The origin of bronchial foreign bodies: a retrospective study and literature review. Eur Arch Otorhinolaryngol. 2009; 266(10):1645–1648

[3] Finkelstein JA. Oral Ambu-bag insufflation to remove unilateral nasal foreign bodies. Am J Emerg Med. 1996; 14(1):57–58

[4] Thomson M, Sharma S. The hazards of button battery ingestion. Arch Dis Child. 2015; 100(11):1010–1011

[5] England NHS. Patient Safety Alert. Stage One: Warning. Risk of death and serious harm from delays in recognising and treating ingestion of button batteries. NHS England December 2014. Available at http://www.england.nhs.uk/wp-content/uploads/2014/12/psa-button-batteries.pdf. Accessed September 15, 2015

[6] Kubba H, MacAndie C, Botma M, et al. A prospective, single-blind, randomized controlled trial of antiseptic cream for recurrent epistaxis in childhood. Clin Otolaryngol Allied Sci. 2001; 26(6):465–468

[7] Jones H, Trinidade A, Jaberoo MC, Lyons M. Periorbital cellulitis, subgaleal abscess and superior sagittal sinus thrombosis: a rare combination of complications arising from unilateral frontal sinusitis. J Laryngol Otol. 2012; 126(12):1281–1283

[8] Chandler JR, Langenbrunner DJ, Stevens ER. The pathogenesis of orbital complications in acute sinusitis. Laryngoscope. 1970; 80(9):1414–1428

[9] Adil E, Tarshish Y, Roberson D, Jang J, Licameli G, Kenna M. The public health impact of pediatric deep neck space infections. Otolaryngol Head Neck Surg. 2015; 153(6):1036–1041

4

5 The Child with Special Needs

Patrick Sheehan

5.1 Introduction

The best definition of a child with special needs is a child who, because of his/her unique medical or developmental difficulties, has needs in addition to those of his/her age-matched peers. This description may encompass an umbrella of diagnoses. It may include children who have mild learning disabilities or profound cognitive impairment; medical conditions or syndromes including neurologic impairment, severe allergies, and children with terminal illness; and a spectrum of disorders such as autism, attention deficit hyperactivity disorder (ADHD), and developmental delay (see Box 5.1).

Box 5.1 Child with Special Needs: One Term, Many Conditions

- Congenital anomaly or syndromes, for example, cystic fibrosis, cleft palate, choanal atresia, polysaccharidosis, dwarfism, Down's syndrome, Treacher Collins' syndrome, CHARGE syndrome (*coloboma, heart* defects, *atresia of the choanae, retardation of growth/development, genitourinary, and ear malformations*), craniofacial anomalies, fetal alcohol syndrome.
- Birth injury, for example, cerebral palsy.
- Extreme prematurity, respiratory failure, children on home ventilation.
- Developmental delay, epilepsy.
- Progressive conditions or degenerative disorders, for example, neuromuscular disorders, muscular dystrophy, malignant disease.
- Malignant disease, severe immune dysfunction, children on immunosuppressants.
- Behavioral disorders, for example, ADHD, Asperger's syndrome, disorders of the autistic spectrum, Tourette's syndrome.
- Learning disabilities.

Many of the common ear, nose, and throat (ENT) problems may be more frequent, more persistent, and more challenging in children and adults with special needs.[1] In this chapter, we discuss head and neck examinations in the clinic environment, common otological conditions, nasal and sinus diseases, throat and airway management, and complications in these children. Children who have special needs may require otolaryngological services beginning in the neonatal period, through their childhood, and lasting well into adult life.

ENT care in children has come a long way in recent years, and these advances have had a particular effect in improving outcomes for children with special needs and

their families. Children are now usually seen in dedicated pediatric clinics. Children with developmental delay are now managed in the same caring ethos as typically developing children. Diagnostic techniques have improved; the nasal cavity and the airways can be evaluated with pediatric endoscopes. Digital imaging with high-quality monitors in outpatient clinics allow parents and child to see his/her own conditions, for example, showing a child a screen image of their own eardrum can be of interest to the child as well as help the clinician explain the clinical findings to parents. Management of many conditions has also changed dramatically. Digital and programmable hearing aids, bone-anchored hearing aids (BAHAs), and cochlear implants have significantly improved access to sound for many people with permanent hearing loss, with resultant improvement in their speech and language development (see Chapter 15). This has led to better communication skills and ultimately greater integration into society for a large number of children who in an earlier era might have been marginalized and disadvantaged.[2,3] Head and neck malformations and tumors that would have required extensive and mutilating surgery can now often be managed by radiological interventional techniques or by chemotherapy. Advances in surgical techniques allow for safer and more effective resection of large head and neck tumors, and vascular or lymphatic malformations.[4,5]

5.2 The Ear, Nose, and Throat Consultation

5.2.1 General Considerations

Examining any child may be challenging but examining a child with developmental or learning difficulties may be even more difficult. The child may be frightened and have a limited ability to communicate or understand. Accompanying parents or carers will have additional concerns specific to the child's disability. The examination may need to be modified if the child is upset, is using a wheelchair, or is unable to stay still.

To provide the best care and environment for these children and their families, the consultation should be in an adequately staffed pediatric clinic. Pediatric trained nurses and play specialists that are accustomed to dealing with children and have a good knowledge of child development can make the hospital visit less intimidating and will greatly enhance the prospect of a good outcome. Clinic waiting areas need to be conducive to a playful environment for children, with appropriate toys, pictures, and suitable seating and flooring arrangements that are both comfortable and safe (see ▶ Fig. 2.2). Beware of excessively noisy toys that can make a conversation in the nearby consultation room difficult.

> **Tips and Tricks**
>
> Clinics should display helpful information or provide material for parents to read in their waiting areas. Information on hearing accessories from National Deaf Children's Societies can be displayed or leaflets on local services and local support groups can be provided.

Many clinicians set aside a specific clinic for children with special needs. This may not always be compatible with the demands of a busy service, but if these children are seen in a general clinic, some adjustments can greatly improve the experience for the clinician, child, and parent/carer alike. Consider allocating a first or last appointment slot to children with special needs; they may need an extended consultation session and will appreciate a quick passage into the consultation room as soon as possible after arrival. In most jurisdictions, health care providers now have a legal duty to ensure that children must not be discriminated against on the grounds of a medical condition or a disability and must make reasonable adjustments to ensure no such discrimination occurs.

Often families have to deal with multiple medical appointments, frequent crises, uncertainty about the child's future and prognosis, and constant worry. Clinicians need to acknowledge the parents' concerns and not appear condescending, rushed, dismissive, or unwilling to listen.

5.2.2 The History

Sometimes the child may be accompanied by carers rather than parents. The parents or carers may be sensitive but are often very knowledgeable about their child's condition and associated issues. Parents will not expect you to have a detailed and nuanced knowledge of often-rare disorders, which they may know a great deal about, but it can be tiresome to have to repeatedly tell a succession of new doctors about the child's previous medical history and treatment.

> **Tips and Tricks**
>
> The parents and carers will often be most knowledgeable about the underlying condition. They will frequently seek guidance from clinicians or clarification of advice they have read online. The clinician should not be suspicious of patients with Internet information at hand or feel intimidated by well-informed parents.

Gather as much information as possible about the child before beginning the consultation. Read the notes carefully before the child comes into the consultation room. Few parents appreciate seeing their doctor shuffling through notes to acquaint himself/herself with basic information during a consultation. As medical records are increasingly digitized and stored electronically, it can be even more difficult to glean important details about a child's previous history. Both parent and child will greatly appreciate seeing a doctor who knows them and with whom they have built a rapport on successive visits. Important aspects of the history include the social background of the child, for example, the number of siblings, if the child lives with parents or in a residential home, whether he/she goes to a special or a mainstream school, and what support he/she has at home and in school. Enquire on the parent's membership and knowledge of local parent support groups or national associations. Make open enquiries as to the general health of the child but importantly specifically to elucidate conditions that may be related to the syndrome or underlying condition (▶ Table 5.1), for example, thyroid status in Pendred's syndrome, cardiac status in Down's syndrome, or kidney function in Alport's syndrome. The associated conditions may have important implications when considering general anesthesia and perioperative care, such as cardiac status or neck stability in a child with Down's syndrome or airway access and ongoing oxygen dependency in a child with mucopolysaccharidosis.

The child will usually have a named lead pediatrician, and the otolaryngologist is only one of a number of clinicians looking after him/her. If the child has no lead pediatrician, consider enlisting one so that her overall

Table 5.1 Specific medical issues common in individuals with Down's syndrome

Cardiac	Congenital anomalies, cor pulmonale
Gastrointestinal	congenital malformations, feeding difficulties, gastroesophageal reflux, Coeliac's disease, Hirschsprung's disease
Vision	Refractive errors, nasolacrimal obstruction, cataracts, Keratoconus
Dental	Delayed eruption, bruxism
Hematological	Transient myeloproliferative disorder, leukemia
Endocrine	Hypothyroidism, diabetes
Immunological	Immune dysfunction, autoimmune disease, e.g., arthropathy, alopecia, vitiligo
Dermatological	Dry skin, folliculitis
Orthopaedic	Cervical spine instability, hip subluxation, patellar instability, Metatarsus varus, scoliosis
Neuropsychiatric	Infantile spasms and other myoclonic epilepsies, autistic spectrum disorders, dementia

medical care is under the surveillance of one team as far as possible. Always communicate the results of the consultation with the relevant clinicians, including the community nursing team, particularly if surgery is planned as there may be important considerations regarding perioperative care, for example, prophylactic antibiotics, perioperative steroids, etc.

Tips and Tricks

Clinicians can refresh their knowledge of a condition or access the latest information related to their patient's special needs by using the Internet in clinic. There are multiple Web sites including:
- www.patient.info
- www.intellectualdisability.info (good site for resources on intellectual disability)
- www.dsmig.org.uk (Down Syndrome Medical Interest Group)
- www.ndcs.org.uk (National Deaf Children's Society)
- www.emedicine.com (Medscape, a comprehensive resource)

There are parent/carer support groups for all of the common, and many uncommon, syndromes and conditions. National association Web sites can be very helpful for further information. Parents will often get a great deal of useful advice and support from the families of children with a similar condition.

In increasingly multiethnic societies, appropriate interpreters should be available throughout the entire care pathway so that an adequate history can be obtained, to explain the nature of the examination before it takes place, to explain the findings, and to explain the range of treatment options available. A "hospital passport booklet" (► Fig. 5.1) as used in the United Kingdom,[6] or its equivalent, ensures people with special needs are more involved in their care and that the care is provided in a personalized and dignified manner.

5.2.3 Examination

Note the child's general development including speech, comprehension, socialization, and motor skills. Much useful information can be gained just by watching the child's behavior during the consultation, for example, gait abnormalities and difficulties with fine motor skills may suggest spinal cord compression from atlantoaxial subluxation.

When examining, approach the child gently and cautiously, for example, by first using a polished metal spatula below the nostrils to give important information on the patency of the nasal passageway rather than by intro-

ducing a speculum (see ► Fig. 2.4). Examine the ears with the child in the parent's lap or in the wheelchair (► Fig. 5.2). Examining the mouth and oropharynx can often be more rewarding if a small child is placed into the examiner's lap. This permits a nonconfrontational view of the oropharynx from above rather than a more intimidating frontal examination.

In a teaching setting, junior doctors and medical students should appreciate that they may not get an opportunity to examine the child independently but may have to share the consultation and learning experience with the senior clinician as the time available to examine the child may be short.

---

i

The terminology used with parents is very important as it will set the scene for the consultation and the parent's attitude to the consultation. Remember that the child comes first and the underlying condition second, that is, *a child with Down's syndrome* not *a Down's syndrome child*. Take care in the language you use when comparing the child with a disability to a typically developing child (► Table 5.2). The term *normal* can be hurtful to the parents of a child with special needs if it is used to contrast a typically developing child with their child. Parents will often remember what they consider crass or insensitive phrases for many years after the event. This can make for a far less satisfactory rapport between parents and a clinician who may be completely unaware of the distress he/she has caused.

If special investigations are required, consider the associated issues for the parents, whether the child needs admission, sedation, or indeed general anesthesia to accomplish the investigation, and consider carefully the value of the information that will be derived. A home sleep study may be far easier for the parents to accommodate than a hospital inpatient sleep study and often provides better information as the child will be in his/her own bed and environment. Indeed, a couple video clips on a mobile device of the child asleep in his/her own bed may provide much of the information the clinician needs to confirm a diagnosis.

Occasionally, an adequate ENT examination is not possible in clinic, in which case a general anesthetic may be required to fully evaluate the child with special needs. In these cases or when arranging an admission, the clinician should consider the total care pathway. If the child has behavioral issues that other children on a ward would find upsetting, the child may require a single room. Some children on the autistic spectrum may become distressed on a general ward and may similarly require a single

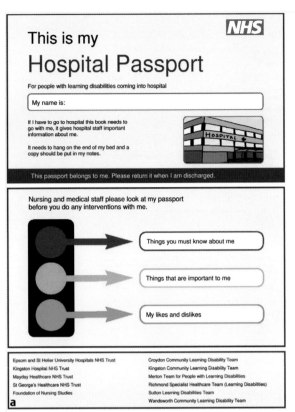

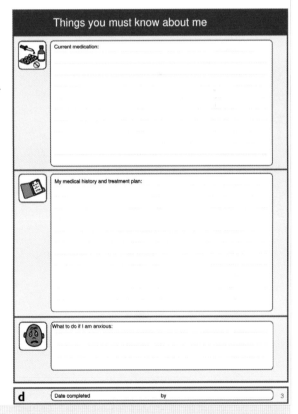

Fig. 5.1 Pages from a "hospital passport," as used in the United Kingdom for a child with a learning disability, developed by the South West London Access to Acute Group and based on original work by Gloucester Partnership NHS Trust.

5

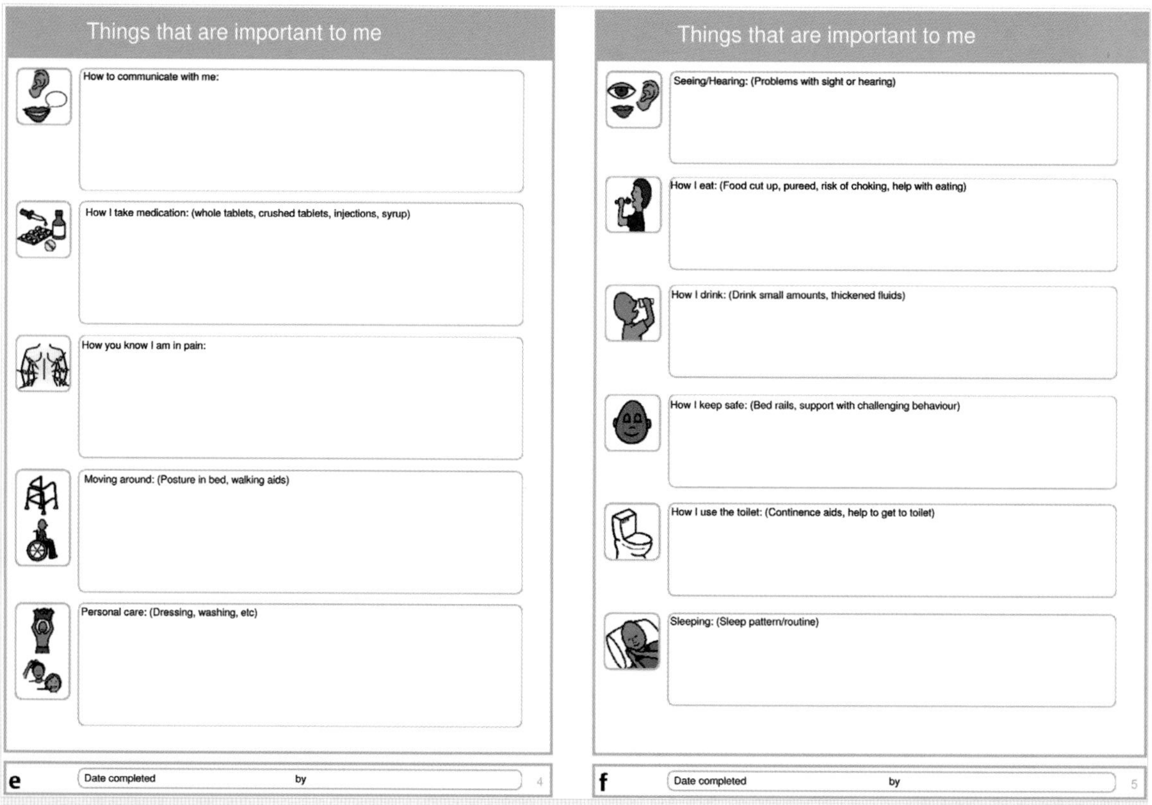

Things that are important to me

How to communicate with me:

How I take medication: (whole tablets, crushed tablets, injections, syrup)

How you know I am in pain:

Moving around: (Posture in bed, walking aids)

Personal care: (Dressing, washing, etc)

| e | Date completed | by | 4 |

Things that are important to me

Seeing/Hearing: (Problems with sight or hearing)

How I eat: (Food cut up, pureed, risk of choking, help with eating)

How I drink: (Drink small amounts, thickened fluids)

How I keep safe: (Bed rails, support with challenging behaviour)

How I use the toilet: (Continence aids, help to get to toilet)

Sleeping: (Sleep pattern/routine)

| f | Date completed | by | 5 |

Fig. 5.1 (*Continued*)

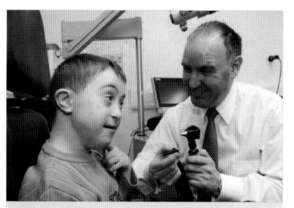

Fig. 5.2 Approach to otoscopic examination of a child with Down's syndrome.

room or an early morning admission with, for example, arrangements for recovery from anesthesia behind a screened area. Often children with special needs will need multiple interventions under the care of a variety of clinicians. Consideration should be given to coordinating with other specialties to include or combine evaluations and procedures, for example, venipuncture for thyroid function tests in Down's syndrome, feeding gastrostomies and changes of feeding tubes, dental examinations or procedures, evoked response audiometry, or the making of earmolds while the child is asleep.[7] This practice may save an extra general anesthetic in the future. Planning the postoperative care setting of the child is important as many children with special needs may require a high dependency bed or intensive care bed in the hours or days after a general anesthesia.[8]

Table 5.2 Terminology to improve patient–clinician relationship

Do not say	Do say
A Down's child or cerebral palsy child	Child has Down's syndrome or cerebral palsy
Suffers from or is a victim of Down's syndrome or cerebral palsy	Child with Down's syndrome or who has cerebral palsy
Mentally retarded/handicap	Child has learning difficulties
Compared with other "normal" children	Compared with another typically developing child

5.3 Otological Conditions

Managing the ears of children who cannot cooperate for otoscopic examination may be very difficult, especially if they have anatomical abnormalities of the ear canals and pinna. Occasionally, general anesthesia in the operating room is required to adequately examine the ears, remove wax, perform brainstem evoked response audiometry or otoacoustic emission testing, and make earmolds for hearing aids. If necessary, imaging studies of the temporal bones can also often be accomplished under general anesthesia.

5.3.1 Otitis Media

> Children with craniofacial anomalies or with mucociliary dyskinesias that predispose to Eustachian tube dysfunction (e.g., cleft palate, Down's or Alport's syndrome, CHARGE syndrome, Kartagener's syndrome) are more likely to develop otitis media with effusion (OME) and/or persistent middle ear problems well into their teens or indeed adulthood than their age-matched typically developing counterparts.

The management of the otitis media may involve hearing aids or ventilation tubes. These children often have frequent clinic visits for microsuction, hearing evaluations, and hearing- aid mold fittings. They may require frequent or long-term ventilation tubes to manage their OME and associated hearing loss. There is a high incidence of otitis media complications (e.g., tympanic perforation, chronic suppurative otitis media, and atelectasis of the tympanic membrane). Tympanic membrane perforations are often associated with conductive hearing loss, recurrent otorrhea, and the need for water precautions when bathing and swimming. Closing the perforation requires a general anesthetic but may prevent repeated ear infections especially if the child wears hearing aids. Frequent removal of wax can help lower the incidence of otitis externa and facilitate more comfortable and successful hearing aid usage. Chronic suppurative otitis media may be exacerbated by ongoing laryngopharyngeal reflux (LPR) or ciliary dysmotility.[9,10,11]

Even with close and careful management of otitis media, many of these children will have ear problems well into adulthood, and many develop chronic although relatively stable middle ear disease. A clinician's knowledge of a given child's ear status, hearing, and other developmental needs over many years or even decades can help formulate an approach that works for the individual and his/her family. In the United Kingdom, the majority of consultant ENT surgeons will be able to continue to follow these children into their adult practice.

5.3.2 Hearing Impairment

> Conductive hearing loss of even a mild form can be a significant disability to a child with learning difficulties, any other sensory impairment, or developmental delay, and should be managed appropriately.

Permanent conductive hearing loss associated with some conditions–for example, congenital atresia and microtia, or chronic ear disease–may not be amenable to surgical intervention, or intervention may improve but not completely resolve the hearing loss. In these instances, alternative solutions should be considered. Bone-conduction hearing aids, worn on a Softband (Cochlear Ltd.) or BAHAs, provide significant benefit and should always be considered if a conventional hearing aid is not feasible.[12] The same speech and language, and school peripatetic support services provided to children with sensorineural hearing loss children should be considered for children with special needs and concomitant significant conductive hearing loss.

> Sensorineural hearing loss is one of the most common birth defects, with a prevalence of permanent significant hearing loss present in 1 to 2 per 1,000 live births (see Chapter 13).

This number increases to approximately 13 per 1,000 by the age of 19 years if mild and unilateral hearing losses are included.[13,14] Hearing loss may occur alone or in association with other syndromes and medical conditions. Many of these children will require hearing aids and support accessories for the home and school environment. Surround-sound amplification systems and radiofrequency aids could benefit the child. The support of teachers of the hearing-impaired children is crucial. In profound hearing loss, referral to the local cochlear implant team for a full evaluation may be needed. Many children with severe comorbidity do well from surgery; their disability alone should not prevent them from obtaining appropriate medical care.

5.3.3 Sinuses and Nasal Diseases

> Sinus disease is more prevalent and more chronic in children with craniofacial anomalies and in certain other groups, including those with nasal and food allergies, cystic fibrosis, immunodeficiency, and ciliary dyskinesia.[15]

5

Table 5.3 ENT problems in individuals with Down's syndrome

Conductive hearing loss	Narrow external auditory canals, otitis media with effusion, ossicular abnormalities, hyperacusis
Sensorineural hearing loss	Hypoplastic cochlea, inner ear dysplasia
Sleep disordered breathing	Adenotonsiller hypertrophy, midfacial hypoplasia, relative glossoptosis, hypotonia
Chronic catarrh	Nasosinus hypoplasia, dairy food intolerance
Respiratory	Tracheobronchomalacia, subglottic stenosis, tracheoesophageal fistula, recurrent respiratory infections
Thyroid	Hypothyroidism, Hashimoto thyroiditis
Cervical spine	Atlantoaxial instability
Gastrointestinal	Laryngopharyngeal reflux

Children with Down's syndrome are especially susceptible to paranasal sinus disorders (▶ Table 5.3). Sinus disease may often follow these children into adulthood. These conditions may predispose to stagnation of secretions within the nasal cavities, reduced ciliary function, infection, and thus chronic nasal symptoms that may be very difficult to manage. Many children with developmental disabilities have other medical problems such as anatomical sinonasal anomalies and LPR that may exacerbate their sinus disease. Recognition and management of LPR can ensure that these children are more comfortable and greatly facilitate the management of their underlying sinusitis, otitis media, or laryngeal issues.[16]

There are several lines of outpatient treatment options available for those with nasal symptoms. These include regular nasal saline douches, encouraging nose blowing, mechanical decongestants, a dairy-free diet if appropriate, oral antihistamines, nasal or oral decongestants, and low-dose antibiotics. Symptoms of reflux can be managed with simple measures including advice regarding feeding (avoid overfeeding, increase frequency, and decrease the volume of feeds), posture, and if needed antacids (e.g., infant Gaviscon). In severe cases and with appropriate assessment and monitoring, H2-receptor antagonists may help.

Some children, for example, those with cystic fibrosis, develop chronic sinusitis and nasal polyps that require frequent removal under general anesthesia and repeated outpatient appointments.

Although sinus disease is probably the most common nasal disease requiring treatment, other problems include epistaxis, nasal polyps (especially in children with cystic fibrosis), allergic rhinitis, and foreign bodies.

- Epistaxis may result from nose picking or drying of the mucosa from nasal oxygen prongs, or may be a manifestation of an underlying bleeding disorder such as von Willebrand's disease or very rarely a neoplasm such as an angiofibroma or rhabdomyosarcoma.
- Nasal foreign bodies often present with a foul-smelling unilateral nasal discharge. Recurrent nasal foreign bodies are more common in patients with learning difficulties. Vigilance and a high index of suspicion are needed to diagnose and subsequently to prevent further episodes.

5.4 The Airway in the Child with Special Needs

5.4.1 Tonsils and Adenoids

> Adenotonsillar hypertrophy or frequent tonsillitis is common in all children but may be a more difficult management issue in children and young adults with special needs.

The removal of adenoid may be part of the management of recurrent otitis media or chronic middle ear effusions. In children with craniofacial anomalies, the tonsils and adenoids may not be enlarged but lie in a limited space leading to obstruction. Chronic adenotonsillar hypertrophy of any etiology may lead to disturbed sleep patterns, obstructive sleep symptoms, or indeed frank sleep apneas, and if medical therapies are unsuccessful in relieving symptoms, then adenotonsillectomy may be required (see Chapter 19).

Although the surgery may be relatively straightforward, intubation for general anesthesia in a child with severe micrognathia or a child with mucopolysaccharidosis having a tonsillectomy may be more challenging than the tonsillectomy itself, requiring special fiberoptic intubation techniques (see Chapter 3).[17] Anesthesia may be complicated by other airway abnormalities and beset by cardiac and pulmonary compromise.[18] In such a child, tonsillectomy may not resolve all the airway issues, which may be due, at least in part, to the size, shape, or location of the mandible or tongue. Many of these children will require a prolonged postoperative stay in a high dependency unit following surgery because their return to baseline pulmonary status may be delayed.

> Liaise closely preoperatively with the pediatric anesthetist, the medical team looking after the child, the nursing staff, and the family to avoid unpleasant surprises on the day of surgery.

Many of the airway issues will follow the child into adulthood, requiring an increased level of vigilance with every anesthetic experience.

> Obstructive sleep disorders are more common in children with disabilities.[19]

A sleep study may be required to make the diagnosis or to evaluate the severity of the obstructive sleep apnea. In many instances, a postoperative sleep study will be required to determine if improvements are sustained. Many may have improvement in their symptoms but may still have some degree of obstruction during sleep or during upper respiratory illnesses. Some will continue to require oxygen or indeed continuous positive airway pressure (CPAP) during sleep to completely alleviate their sleep apnea. The need for CPAP may be lifelong but often allows the child to avoid tracheostomy.[20] Tracheostomy may be needed in a very small number of children.

5.4.2 Other Airway Conditions

Airway compromise can be related to other conditions including choanal atresia, micrognathia, retrognathia, glossoptosis, cleft palate, laryngomalacia, vocal cord paralysis, subglottic stenosis, tracheomalacia, and tracheal stenosis. Benign and malignant tumors can involve any part of the airway. In addition, children and young adults with neuromuscular or musculoskeletal abnormalities (e.g., Duchenne muscular dystrophy) may have severe and progressive hypotonia and pharyngeal muscle dysfunction that directly or indirectly impacts on the airways.[21]

Choanal atresia—seen in more than half of children with CHARGE syndrome—may need to be recognized and bypassed in the newborn period. Although endoscopic techniques have improved the management of choanal atresia, repeat surgery may be required, and the child may have lifelong symptoms of nasal obstruction that become particularly apparent with viral upper respiratory tract or sinus infections. In infants with Pierre Robin sequence or similar associations, the airway may be abnormal and ongoing vigilance is required, especially at the time of sedation or general anesthesia.

5.4.3 Tracheostomy

Although anesthetic and surgical techniques for the assessment and management of the child's airways have significantly improved, some children with special needs will have airway problems that require a tracheostomy. The tracheostomy may be relatively short-term, but it may need to be long-term, depending on the underlying indication (see Chapter 23).

> The clinician and parents/carers should be aware of the problems associated with the ongoing management of a tracheostomy, particularly the impact on families, teachers, and other professionals involved with the individual's care.[22]

The family and careers will need to be instructed in daily care of the tracheostomy and in emergency procedures in case of blockage or dislodgement of the tube. Many institutions have a dedicated tracheostomy care team who will follow the child though the whole process of tracheostomy care and training and be a source of support during the time the child has a tracheostomy.

The presence of a tracheostomy will have social implications for the child, sometimes restricting the child's ability to travel on a school bus or go on holidays or school trips. Many will require intensive support at school or a placement in a new school that can cater to the needs of the child. Home support and school nursing support will be needed. Arrangements for home oxygen and the provision of humidifiers, suction machines, and replacement tubes will be needed. Therefore, although a tracheostomy may be absolutely necessary for the health and safety of the child, it can have a profound effect on the quality of life of the child and family.[23,24]

Many children with airway problems, with or without tracheostomies, may have difficulties that continue into their teens and adulthood. They may have intermittent long-term respiratory problems, for example, recurrent upper or lower tract infections and poor exercise tolerance. Airway problems may get worse as they get older. Young adults with cerebral palsy, neuromuscular disease, or severe kyphoscoliosis may have progressive worsening of their airways. These children may need to remain within the pediatric sector where specialist services tend to be better organized to a much older age or at least until they are transferred to appropriate specialists who look after adults with disabilities. Their care pathways need to be adjusted to ensure a safe and individualized solution to their special needs.

5.5 Key Points

- Children with special needs frequently live at home or in small residential settings within the community.
- They will receive much of their care from their family doctor and the local outpatient facilities.
- Coordination of their medical services can be challenging and many children with special needs will need ongoing care continued into their adult lives.

- Many have a lifelong need for care of their airway, hearing and middle ear problems, and paranasal sinus diseases.
- Appropriate liaison between the general practitioner, local hospital facilities, specialist services, and community teams is vital to allow for better patient care and quality of life for children with disabilities or special needs.[25]

References

[1] Venail F, Gardiner Q, Mondain M. ENT and speech disorders in children with Down's syndrome: an overview of pathophysiology, clinical features, treatments, and current management. Clin Pediatr (Phila). 2004; 43(9):783–791

[2] Doshi J, Sheehan P, McDermott AL. Bone anchored hearing aids in children: an update. Int J Pediatr Otorhinolaryngol. 2012; 76(5):618–622

[3] Hans PS, England R, Prowse S, Young E, Sheehan PZ. UK and Ireland experience of cochlear implants in children with Down syndrome. Int J Pediatr Otorhinolaryngol. 2010; 74(3):260–264

[4] Boardman SJ, Cochrane LA, Roebuck D, Elliott MJ, Hartley BE. Multimodality treatment of pediatric lymphatic malformations of the head and neck using surgery and sclerotherapy. Arch Otolaryngol Head Neck Surg. 2010; 136(3):270–276

[5] Van Aalst JA, Bhuller A, Sadove AM. Pediatric vascular lesions. J Craniofac Surg. 2003; 14(4):566–583

[6] EasyHealth 2010. Hospital Passports. Available at http://www.easyhealth.org.uk/listing/hospital-passports-(leaflets). Accessed April 28, 2015

[7] Stapleton M, Sheller B, Williams BJ, Mancl L. Combining procedures under general anesthesia. Pediatr Dent. 2007; 29(5):397–402

[8] Tweedie DJ, Bajaj Y, Ifeacho SN, et al. Peri-operative complications after adenotonsillectomy in a UK pediatric tertiary referral centre. Int J Pediatr Otorhinolaryngol. 2012; 76(6):809–815

[9] Campbell R. Managing upper respiratory tract complications of primary ciliary dyskinesia in children. Curr Opin Allergy Clin Immunol. 2012; 12(1):32–38

[10] Santos VJ, Comes GT, Gonçalves TM, Carvalho MdeA, Weber SA. Prevalence of broncopulmonary and otorhinolaryngologic symptoms in children under investigation for gastroesophageal reflux disease: retrospective analysis. Braz J Otorhinolaryngol. 2011; 77(3):328–333

[11] Prulière-Escabasse V, Coste A, Chauvin P, et al. Otologic features in children with primary ciliary dyskinesia. Arch Otolaryngol Head Neck Surg. 2010; 136(11):1121–1126

[12] Doshi J, McDermott AL, Reid A, Proops D. The use of a bone-anchored hearing aid (Baha) in children with severe behavioural problems—the Birmingham Baha programme experience. Int J Pediatr Otorhinolaryngol. 2010; 74(6):608–610

[13] Burke MJ, Shenton RC, Taylor MJ. The economics of screening infants at risk of hearing impairment: an international analysis. Int J Pediatr Otorhinolaryngol. 2012; 76(2):212–218

[14] Ohl C, Dornier L, Czajka C, Chobaut JC, Tavernier L. Newborn hearing screening on infants at risk. Int J Pediatr Otorhinolaryngol. 2009; 73(12):1691–1695

[15] Fokkens WJ, Lund VJ, Mullol J, et al. EPOS 2012: European position paper on rhinosinusitis and nasal polyps 2012. A summary for otorhinolaryngologists. Rhinology. 2012; 50(1):1–12

[16] Sullivan PB. Gastrointestinal disorders in children with neurodevelopmental disabilities. Dev Disabil Res Rev. 2008; 14(2):128–136

[17] Walker RW. The laryngeal mask airway in the difficult paediatric airway: an assessment of positioning and use in fibreoptic intubation. Paediatr Anaesth. 2000; 10(1):53–58

[18] Blum RH, McGowan FX, Jr. Chronic upper airway obstruction and cardiac dysfunction: anatomy, pathophysiology and anesthetic implications. Paediatr Anaesth. 2004; 14(1):75–83

[19] Lam DJ, Jensen CC, Mueller BA, Starr JR, Cunningham ML, Weaver EM. Pediatric sleep apnea and craniofacial anomalies: a population-based case-control study. Laryngoscope. 2010; 120(10):2098–2105

[20] Randhawa PS, Ahmed J, Nouraei SR, Wyatt ME. Impact of long-term nasopharyngeal airway on health-related quality of life of children with obstructive sleep apnea caused by syndromic craniosynostosis. J Craniofac Surg. 2011; 22(1):125–128

[21] Simons JP, Greenberg LL, Mehta DK, Fabio A, Maguire RC, Mandell DL. Laryngomalacia and swallowing function in children. Laryngoscope. 2016; 126(2):478–484

[22] Smith JC, Williams J, Gibbin KP. Children with a tracheostomy: experience of their carers in school. Child Care Health Dev. 2003; 29(4):291–296

[23] Patel MR, Zdanski CJ, Abode KA, et al. Experience of the school-aged child with tracheostomy. Int J Pediatr Otorhinolaryngol. 2009; 73(7):975–980

[24] Hopkins C, Whetstone S, Foster T, Blaney S, Morrison G. The impact of paediatric tracheostomy on both patient and parent. Int J Pediatr Otorhinolaryngol. 2009; 73(1):15–20

[25] Lewis-Gary MD. Transitioning to adult health care facilities for young adults with a chronic condition. Pediatr Nurs. 2001; 27(5):521–524

Part II

The Ear

6 Disorders of the External Ear

Hilko Weerda

6.1 Introduction

When I began my medical education in 1965 at the University-Hospital of Maxillo-Facial Surgery in Erlangen (Bavaria), the thalidomide disaster was just emerging and Erlangen was one of the centers for treating affected children. Because I had studied sculpture at an art academy earlier, I was asked to fashion auricular prostheses. The results were not satisfying.

My exposure to this group of children spurred a keen interest in this field during more than 40 years of my career in ear, nose, and throat and led to the book "Surgery of the Auricle: Tumors, Trauma, Defects, Abnormalities" in 2007.

This chapter considers the main causes of external ear conditions and their management. Additional information can be found in Chapter 1, Chapter 5, Chapter 7, Chapter 8, and Chapter 9.

6.2 Applied Clinical Anatomy and Development

The external ear includes the auricle and auditory canal (▶ Fig. 6.1 a). The *anterior and posterior surfaces* of the auricle are characterized by a typical relief (▶ Fig. 6.1 a, b) with a long axis of 62 to 64 mm (in the adult) and an inclination of 15 to 25 degrees. The distance between the anterior helical rim and the mastoid is less than 20 mm (▶ Fig. 6.19 c). The auricle consists of elastic cartilage (1.0–3.0 mm), enveloped within thick skin and firmly attached to the perichondrium, apart from the lobule which is free of cartilage. The posterior surface has an additional layer of fat between the skin and perichondrium. The auricle develops from the mesenchymal hillocks 1, 2, and 3, arising from the first "branchial arch" and the mesenchymal hillocks 4, 5, and 6 of the second "branchial arch." The auditory canal develops from the first branchial cleft (▶ Fig. 6.2).[1]

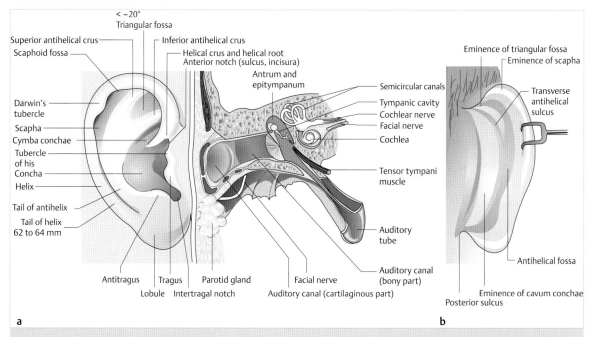

Fig. 6.1 External ear and adjacent structures. **(a)** Anterior auricular surface. **(b)** Posterior auricular surface. (Modified after Weerda H. Surgery of the Auricle: Tumors, Trauma, Defects, Abnormalities. Stuttgart/New York, NY: Thieme Publishing Group; 2007, with permission.)

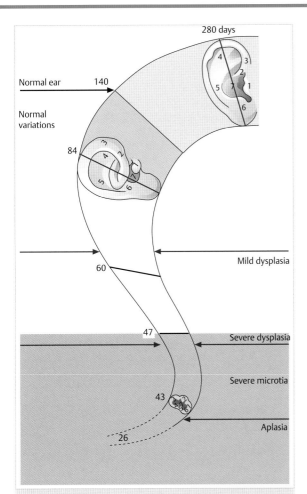

Fig. 6.2 Changes in the developing auricle as it migrates in the course of embryonic development, as described by Leiber,[1] and typical malformations associated with embryonic development. 1, 2, and 3: Hillocks from the first branchial arch. 4, 5, and 6: Hillocks from the second branchial arch. 7: first branchial cleft. (Modified after Weerda H. Surgery of the Auricle: Tumors, Trauma, Defects, Abnormalities. Stuttgart/New York, NY: Thieme Publishing Group; 2007, with permission.)

The auricle migrates from an anterocaudal position to a posterocranial position.

The auricle reaches 85% of its final length by the age of 6 years.

6.3 Acquired Disorders of the External Ear

> **Inflammatory Diseases of the External Meatal Skin and the Auricle** ℹ
>
> - Otitis externa circumscripta (furuncle).
> - Otitis externa diffusa (swimmer's ear).
> - Eczematous otitis.
> - Otitis bullosa hemorrhagica (bullous otitis).
> - Erysipelas (auricular cellulitis).
> - Chronic otitis externa.
> - Perichondritis.

6.3.1 Furuncle (Otitis Externa Circumscripta)

This is typically caused by a Staphylococcal infection of the hair follicle in the skin of the cartilaginous ear canal.

Diagnosis is made by finding a discrete red swelling of the ear canal with ear pain and tenderness, made worse by gently pulling or pressing the pinna or tragus.

Treatment is with antibiotic and steroid dressings changed daily. Incision and drainage under general anesthesia may be necessary, and in *recurrent cases*, it is wise to check the child for *diabetes mellitus* or immune dysfunction.

6.3.2 Swimmer's Ear (Otitis Externa Diffusa)

This may be caused by traumatization of macerated skin of the ear canal. Other factors include infection of cerumen after cleaning, use of hearing aids, and contamination of the ear canal with materials from water. Bacterial and/or fungal infection may supervene with *Pseudomonas aeruginosa* (54%), *Staphylococcus epidermidis* (9.1%), *S. aureus* (1.0%), *Proteus, Candida* species, or *Aspergillus*. The skin is red, edematous, and desquamated. The child may complain of itching, pain, and discharge. He/she may be mildly hearing impaired due to accumulated debris in the ear canal and, in severe cases, may be febrile and unwell. (See ▶ Fig. 6.3.)

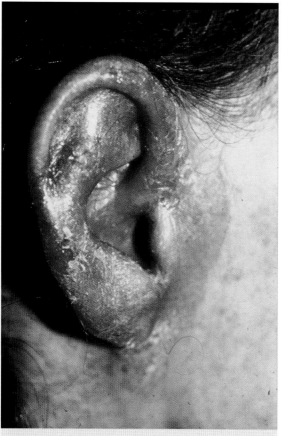

Fig. 6.3 Otitis externa.

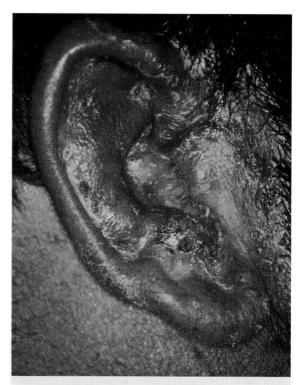

Fig. 6.4 Eczematous otitis.

Treatment is by meticulous cleaning of the ear (not always easy or possible in a child), adequate analgesia, and topical antimicrobial therapy, ideally with a local steroid, for up to a maximum of 2 weeks to avoid sensitization or mycosis. We recommend ciprofloxacin 0.3% and dexamethasone 0.1% as sterile otic suspension. A soft cotton or small pressed sponge, self-expanding[2] and soaked with antibiotic–steroid solution (based on culture results: Methicillin-resistant *S. aureus* 60%, clindamycin 33% resistance rate, increased resistance after long-time therapy), may be useful, with antimycotic therapy if necessary.[3]

6.3.3 Eczematous Otitis

This occurs with atopic eczema, seborrheic dermatitis, psoriasis, neurodermatitis, and purulent or chronic otitis externa (dermatological diagnoses) (▶ Fig. 6.4). Treatment is directed at the dermatological condition, with attention to aural toilet as needed. In susceptible children, it is important to avoid sprays and irritant shampoos.

6.3.4 Bullous Myringitis (Otitis Externa Bullosa Hemorrhagica)

This is caused by a viral infection (e.g., influenza). Pain is often severe.

Hemorrhagic bullae involve the tympanic membrane, skin, and medial canal, so the effects of otitis media and otitis externa are combined. The child may have a conductive deafness. Treatment is expectant with attention to pain control and draining the blebs.

6.3.5 Erysipelas (Auricular Cellulitis)

This is an acute infection with streptococcus in the ear region (▶ Fig. 6.5). It is characterized by a raised intensely red edematous eruption of the skin. The child complains of pain, high temperature, and increasingly bad general condition as the infection spreads into the skin of the face. It is distinguished from dermatitis as the child with erysipelas is usually systemically unwell, and from perichondritis, where the lobule is free of infection. Treatment is with antibiotics (penicillin), modified as needed by culture and sensitivity result, and analgesics.

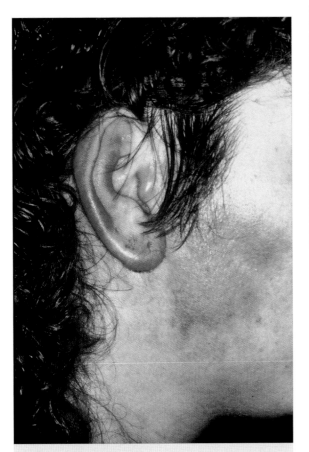

Fig. 6.5 Erysipelas of the pinna.

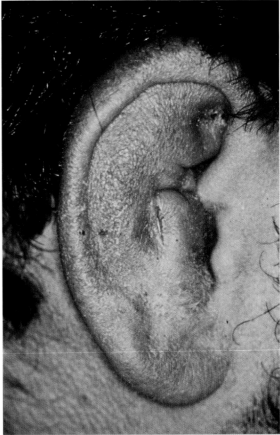

Fig. 6.6 Perichondritis.

6.3.6 Chronic External Otitis

This is characterized by debris and pus but seldom occurs in children.[4] There may be granulations on the tympanic membrane or the skin of the ear canal. Treatment is as for otitis externa diffusa, with management of acute exacerbations as they occur.

Chronic fungal infection may need antimycotic agents.

6.3.7 Perichondritis

This is covered later in the chapter (see section on Complications of Surgery to the Pinna; see also ▶ Table 6.3). See ▶ Fig. 6.6.

6.4 Trauma

The exposed position of the auricle predisposes it to a large number of different injuries. The cartilage is dependent upon nutrition from its surrounding tissues (a "bradytrophic" structure), so shearing forces can cause devascularization and necrosis.

Varieties of External Ear Trauma	ℹ

- Acute penetrating trauma (including piercing).
- Blunt trauma (hematoma and seroma auris).
- Chemical burns.
- Thermal burns.
- Avulsion injuries.

6.4.1 Penetrating Trauma

Some piercings even in the region of the helix cause inflammation associated with granulation tissue (▶ Fig. 6.7). This can lead to loss of the auricle by perichondritis.

6.4.2 Chemical Burns

Acid burns result in superficial coagulation necrosis, whereas alkali produces deeper more penetrating injuries.

The ear should be immediately cleaned with clear water with application of sterile, cool compresses, and steroid ointments. Later treatment may involve surgical removal of necrotic tissue and reconstruction at a later stage.[5,6]

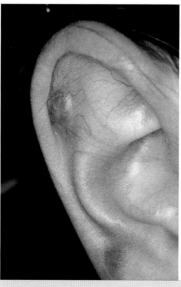

Fig. 6.7 Chronic inflammatory alterations after piercing, displaying in part scar hypertrophy and in part granulation tissue. (Reproduced from Weerda H. Surgery of the Auricle: Tumors, Trauma, Defects, Abnormalities. Stuttgart/New York, NY: Thieme Publishing Group; 2007, with permission.)

6.4.3 Thermal Injuries (Burns)

These are frequently caused by hot liquids (scalding) but are sometimes due to exposure to flames, for example, gas explosions or firework injuries.

- *First-degree burns* are caused by short exposure giving rise to painful erythema, tissue swelling, and superficial defects. Management is by cooling, local ointments, and analgesia. Complete recovery is usually observed within a few days.
- *Second-degree (partial-thickness) burns* involve the superficial layer of skin and the dermis. Therapy is as for first-degree burns, with spontaneous healing expected within 14 days.
- *Third-degree (full-thickness) burns* are caused by open fire or electrical burns, lead to tissue destruction and necrosis (even cartilage), and may be complicated by extensive tissue infection and deformity, requiring later reconstructive surgery.[6] Therefore, we need cartilage protection by a cooling sterile dressing. These children benefit from interdisciplinary cooperation (e.g., management on a burns unit) and tetanus prophylaxis.

6.4.4 Otohematoma and Otoseroma

Hematomas or seromas (▶ Fig. 6.8) develop between the cartilage and the nutrient skin–perichondrium layer. They are caused by tangential shearing movement due to *blunt trauma*, typically during sports without protective headgear. Approximately 80% of them are found on the superior aspect of the auricle.

Treatment involves drainage to remove the fluid, with secure apposition of the skin–perichondrium flap, otherwise the fluid will refill. This can be brought about by an *anterior* incision in the antihelical or conchal fold

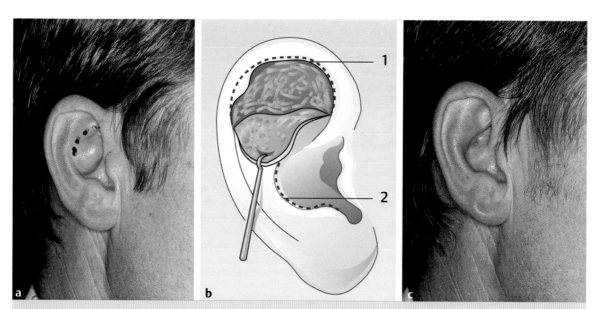

Fig. 6.8 Approaches of otohematoma otoseroma. **(a)** Concha hematoma (incision at the rim of antihelix). **(b)** Upper otohematoma; incision in the scapha (1) or beneath the antihelix for low conchal hematoma (2). **(c)** Result of **(a)**, 2 months after incision. (Reproduced from Weerda H. Surgery of the Auricle: Tumors, Trauma, Defects, Abnormalities. Stuttgart/New York, NY: Thieme Publishing Group; 2007, with permission.)

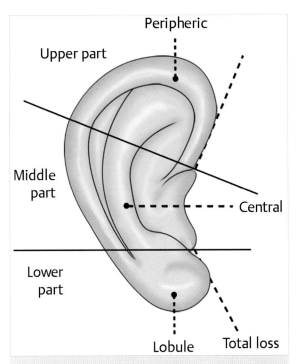

Fig. 6.9 Classification of defects: partial and total loss of the auricle (▶ Table 6.1). (Reproduced from Weerda H. Surgery of the Auricle: Tumors, Trauma, Defects, Abnormalities. Stuttgart/New York, NY: Thieme Publishing Group; 2007, with permission.)

(▶ Fig. 6.8), with removal of clotted blood and granulation tissue, and mild compression with mattress sutures for 1 week.

> **Hematoma of the Pinna**   i
>
> - Simple aspiration is not usually adequate.
> - If initial treatment is delayed or inadequate, the cartilage may undergo organization and fibrosis with thickened skin and cartilage (cauliflower ear). This may require surgical remolding but the damage may not be easily reversed.

6.4.5 Partial and Total Avulsion

Road traffic accidents are the cause in more than 40% of cases, and domestic accidents are the cause in over 30%. Although there will inevitably be overlaps when attempting to classify the defects, we still regard classification as worthwhile for didactic reasons (▶ Fig. 6.9, ▶ Table 6.1).

Partial defects and partial and total loss will be reconstructed with different methods in a one- or multistage technique, with cartilage of the contra-lateral auricle or rib cartilage. With modern surgical techniques, we are able to get satisfying results (▶ Fig. 6.10, ▶ Fig. 6.11).[5]

Reimplantation of the auricle as a composite graft only takes when small parts are amputated. Larger parts will

6

Table 6.1 Classification of auricular defects and their treatment (▶ Fig. 6.9)[5]	
Central defects	Concha Antihelix scapha Combined central defects
Peripheral defects (helix and helical crus)	Reconstruction with auricular reduction Reconstruction without auricular reduction
Partial reconstructions	Upper third of the auricle: • Reconstruction with auricular reduction • Reconstruction without auricular reduction Middle third of the auricle: • Reconstruction with auricular reduction • Reconstruction without auricular reduction (▶ Fig. 6.10) • Lower third of the auricle
Earlobe	Traumatic earlobe cleft Reduction of the earlobe (hyperplasia) Defects of the earlobe Loss of the earlobe (hypoplasia and aplasia) Hypertrophic scar formation Keloids (see ▶ Fig. 6.12)
Posterior defects	Postauricular defects (posterior surface of the ear) Retroauricular defects (mastoid region) Combined post- and retroauricular defects
Reconstruction after total auricular loss (▶ Fig. 6.11)	
Source note: Reproduced from Weerda H. Surgery of the Auricle: Tumors, Trauma, Defects, Abnormalities. Stuttgart/New York, NY: Thieme Publishing Group; 2007, with permission.	

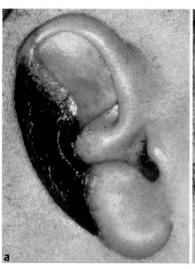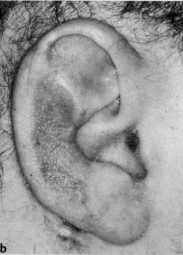

Fig. 6.10 Defect of the middle third of the auricle. **(a)** Necrosis after reimplantation. **(b)** Reconstruction of the middle part of the auricle with rib cartilage and skin of the mastoid region. (Reproduced from Weerda H. Reconstructive Facial Plastic Surgery. 2nd ed. New York, Stuttgart: Thieme; 2015, with permission.)

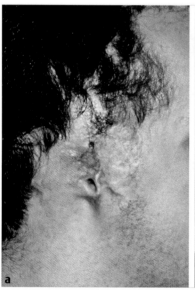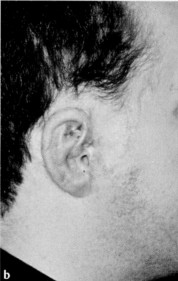

Fig. 6.11 Reconstruction of the auricle after total loss with rib cartilage and skin of the surrounding area in three stages. **(a)** Defect. **(b)** Reconstructed auricle. (Reproduced from Weerda H. Surgery of the Auricle: Tumors, Trauma, Defects, Abnormalities. Stuttgart/New York, NY: Thieme Publishing Group; 2007, with permission.)

become necrotic and must be reconstructed with cartilage and skin of the surrounding area (▶ Fig. 6.10).[5]

6.5 Congenital Disorders of the External Ear

> The development of the external ear is a complex process and abnormalities, mostly minor, are common.

Approximately half of the malformations in the head and neck are in the region of the ear. Brent[7] reports one auricular malformation in approximately 6,000 neonates.

Abnormalities may be isolated or may be part of an inherited syndrome such as Franceschetti's or Goldenhar's syndrome. Exogenous factors are presumed to be the cause of the malformation in approximately 10% cases. These include maternal toxins such as thalidomide, alcohol, maternal rubella, and other viral infections.[8]

6.5.1 Auricular Appendages

These are thought to be due to excess of the mandibular arch (first branchial or pharyngeal arch) formations along the edge of the first branchial (pharyngeal) cleft (▶ Fig. 6.12).[9,10] They include minor skin tags and accessory auricles. In the presence of normally developed ears, appendages are best excised in the relaxed skin tension lines.

6.5.2 Fistulas and Sinuses

Congenital auricular fistulas, preauricular fistulas, and sinuses are formed by entrapped remnants of epithelium found in similar locations to those described for auricular appendages (▶ Fig. 6.12, ▶ Fig. 6.13, ▶ Fig. 6.14). If they have no tendency to recurrent inflammation, they may not require treatment. They may, especially if the orifice is below the tragus, be intimately associated with the facial nerve and surgery can be very challenging (see Chapter 12).[11]

For a fistulogram, aqueous contrast agent should be used. Before surgery, we employ staining of the outline of the fistula with methylene blue.

6.5.3 Auricular Dysplasias

Classification of auricular dysplasias is shown in ▶ Table 6.2 and ▶ Fig. 6.15.

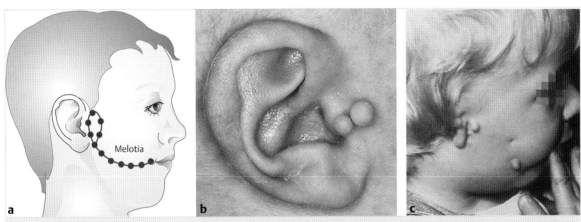

Fig. 6.12 Auricular appendages. **(a)** Location of preauricular appendages (as described by Otto in Weerda [1994])[9,10] along the edge of the first branchial cleft. **(b)** Preauricular appendages associated with a normally developed ear. **(c)** Preauricular appendages associated with anotia. (Reproduced from Weerda H. Surgery of the Auricle: Tumors, Trauma, Defects, Abnormalities. Stuttgart/New York, NY: Thieme Publishing Group; 2007, with permission.)

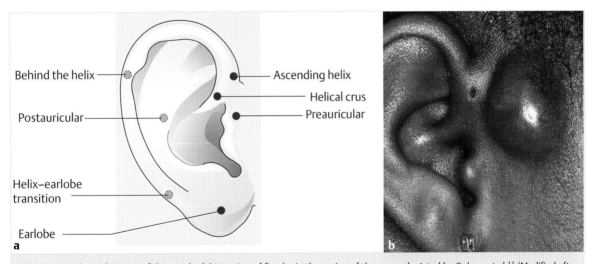

Fig. 6.13 Fistulas and sinuses of the auricle. **(a)** Location of fistulas in the region of the ear as depicted by Gohary et al.[11] (Modified after Gohary A, Rangecroft L, Cook R. Congenital Auricular and Preauricular Sinuses in Childhood. Z Kinderchir 1983;38:81–82, with permission.) **(b)** Infected congenital preauricular sinus, with opening. (Reproduced from Weerda H. Surgery of the Auricle: Tumors, Trauma, Defects, Abnormalities. Stuttgart/New York, NY: Thieme Publishing Group; 2007, with permission.)

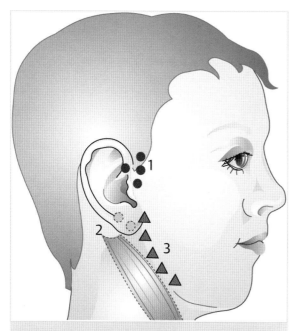

Arrested development or failures of differentiation of parts of the auricular primordium or the pharyngeal cleft can result in various types of malformation of the external ear (▶ Fig. 6.2 and ▶ Fig. 6.15). The most severe manifestation is anotia or complete absence of the external ear (grade III microtia). Lower grade microtia represents a less severe deformity where some of the components of the ear are present, but they are rudimentary and often greatly malformed. The different types of auricular malformations are related to embryological maldevelopment in the region of the mesenchymal hillocks 1 to 6 (▶ Fig. 6.2).[12] Malformations represent an aesthetic impairment that can produce "a significant psychosocial burden during the development of the personality."[13]

Prominent Ears

The normal auricle varies with body height and gender. Its length in adults is approximately 62 to 64 mm and its width is approximately 32 to 34 mm. The ear of children in the fifth or sixth year (preschool age) reaches nearly 90% of the size of an adult ear (▶ Fig. 6.16).

Fig. 6.14 Location of fistula openings in the region of the ear and neck as described by Otto.[10]1: anterior auricular surface: group comprising congenital, preauricular fistulae. 2: postauricular surface: group comprising fistulae of the neck and ear region, also referred to as a "duplication of the external auditory canal." 3: proximal group of lateral cervical fistulae. (Reproduced from Weerda H. Surgery of the Auricle: Tumors, Trauma, Defects, Abnormalities. Stuttgart/New York, NY: Thieme Publishing Group; 2007, with permission.)

> The maximum normal helix-to-mastoid distance is 20 mm.
> The normal maximum ear-to-mastoid plane angle is 30 degrees (▶ Fig. 6.16).

Table 6.2 Weerda's classification of auricular malformations arranged in increasing severity of the malformation (▶ Fig. 6.15)[9]

Degree of dysplasia	Definition	Subgroup
I: low-grade malformations (▶ Fig. 6.15)	General: most of the structures of a normal auricle are present Surgical: additional skin and cartilage are only occasionally required for reconstruction	Prominent auricle Macrotia Cryptotia (pocket ear) Cleft ear (transverse cleft) Stahl's ear Scaphoid ear (Satyr ear) Small deformities • Very pronounced Darwin's tubercle • Absent helical crus • Hyperplasia of the helical crus • Tragus deformities Lobule deformities: • Adherent earlobe • Macrolobule • Cleft earlobe • Microlobule • Aplasia of the lobule Tanzer's type I, IIA, and IIB cup-ear deformities
II: grade II microtia—moderate malformations (▶ Fig. 6.15; II)	General: the auricle still displays some structures of a normal auricle Surgical: additional skin and cartilage required for partial reconstruction	Tanzer's type III cup-ear deformity[24] Mini ear (Nagata's concha-type microtia)[25]: • Hypoplasia of the upper auricle • Hypoplasia of the middle third of the auricle • Hypoplasia (aplasia) of the lower auricle
III: grade III microtia with anotia; severe malformations (▶ Fig. 6.15; III)	General: structure of a normal auricle no longer present Surgical: additional skin and cartilage required for total reconstruction	Unilateral grade III microtia (Nagata's lobule-type microtia) Bilateral grade III microtia Anotia Normally congenital aural atresia will be found

Source note: Reproduced from Weerda H. Anomalien des äusseren Ohres. In: Naumann et al, Hrsg. Otorhinolaryngologie in Klinik und Praxis. Stuttgart/New York. Thieme; 1994: 488–499. Vol. I, with permission.

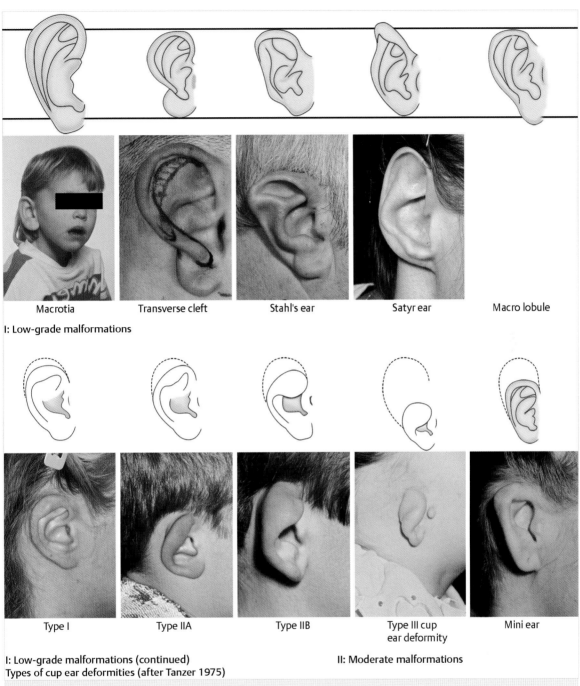

Macrotia   Transverse cleft   Stahl's ear   Satyr ear   Macro lobule

I: Low-grade malformations

Type I   Type IIA   Type IIB   Type III cup ear deformity   Mini ear

I: Low-grade malformations (continued)
Types of cup ear deformities (after Tanzer 1975)

II: Moderate malformations

Fig. 6.15 Different types of malformations (see also ▶ Table 6.2).

6

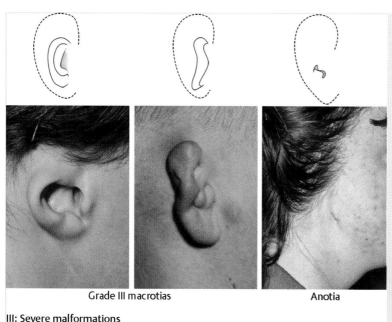

Fig. 6.15 (*Continued*) Different types of malformations (see also ▶ Table 6.2).

Grade III macrotias   Anotia

III: Severe malformations

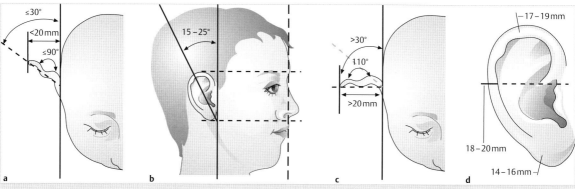

Fig. 6.16 Measurements of the normal and the prominent auricle. **(a)** In the normal ear, the angle between ear and mastoid is approximately 30 degrees, and the distance between the anterior helical rim and the mastoid is less than 20 mm. The scaphoconchal angle is less than 90 degrees. **(b)** The axis of the ear is angled 15 to 25 degrees posteriorly relative to the profile axis. **(c, d)** Prominent auricle with an angle between the ear and the mastoid plane of approximately 90 degrees; distance between the anterior helical rim and the mastoid is significantly larger than 20 mm; the scaphoconchal angle is 110 degrees (or > 90 degrees). Average distances of the anterior helical rim to the mastoid at the upper, middle, and lower auricle (always measured before and after setback operations). (Reproduced from Weerda H. Surgery of the Auricle: Tumors, Trauma, Defects, Abnormalities. Stuttgart/New York, NY: Thieme Publishing Group; 2007, with permission.)

It is the author's practice to offer surgery for prominent ears (setback otoplasty) before the child starts school. Elly[14] described the first operation in 1881 and we know approximately more than 100 different techniques to date.[15]

> In this book, I only want to give a short overview of the standard operations for prominent ears.

Setback Otoplasty Techniques

Suture Technique (Mustarde Technique)

The Mustarde technique was described in 1963. It can be used if there is a soft cartilage (▶ Fig. 6.17)[16]:

- The cartilage is exposed through a postauricular incision (▶ Fig. 6.17 a).
- The antihelix and superior crus are raised into a fold with 4–0 braided nonabsorbable sutures (▶ Fig. 6.17 a, b) and the skin incision is closed.

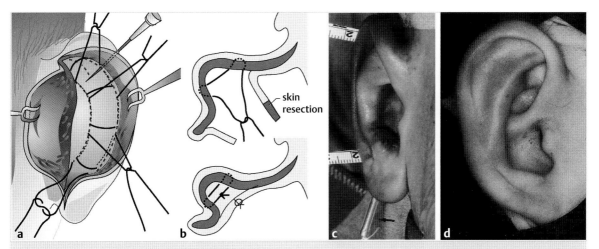

Fig. 6.17 Suture technique (Mustarde technique, 1963).[16] **(a,b)** After elevating the posterior skin and marking the antihelical fold, sutures are placed and tied. The skin will be closed by resorbable sutures (Vicryl rapide, Ethicon). **(c,d)** Postoperative outcome; measurement of distances between the mastoid and the superior helical rim **(c)**. (Reproduced from Weerda H. Surgery of the Auricle: Tumors, Trauma, Defects, Abnormalities. Stuttgart/New York, NY: Thieme Publishing Group; 2007, with permission.)

- An antihelical fold can be created with internal mattress sutures placed through small incisions when exposing the posterior auricular cartilage (▶ Fig. 6.17 b).
- Ointment-impregnated gauze is molded into the recesses of the corrected auricle, which is protected with a windowed foam pad.

The disadvantage, especially in ears with thick cartilage, is that the sutures may pull the helix back too far behind the antihelix, causing an unsightly appearance. They may also create a wavy scaphal line instead of a smooth contour.

Folding techniques without long incisions are described by Kaye (1967), Fritsch (1995), and Merck (1999).[5]

Incision Technique of Stenström

Stenström[17,18] showed, also in 1963, that scoring the anterior side of the antihelix could impart a natural contour to the auricle, generally without the need for retention sutures (▶ Fig. 6.18 a–e).

- Posterior incision (▶ Fig. 6.17 a).
- The anterior side of the antihelix is scored longitudinally (to no more than one-third the cartilage thickness; ▶ Fig. 6.18 c, d) or abraded with a rasp.
- The skin incision is closed with fine suture material.

The distances from the mastoid surfaces (maximum 20 mm) are measured before and after the setback procedure (▶ Fig. 6.17 c, ▶ Fig. 6.19 c).

---

i

Blind rasping of the cartilage or scoring the cartilage too deeply can easily lead to sharp edges or deformities of the auricle that require tedious reconstruction.[5]

Chongchet,[19] and Crikelair and Cosman[20] recommend incising the scaphoid cartilage and elevating the skin and anterior perichondrium after making the posterior skin incision so that the cartilage can be scored under vision (▶ Fig. 6.18 c, d). The cartilage can also be exposed through an anterior skin incision in the scapha. An additional conchal setback can now be done without great difficulties (▶ Fig. 6.18 e).

Incision Technique of Converse

- In this most widely used and modified technique (▶ Fig. 6.19),[21] the posterior skin is incised approximately 1 cm below the helical rim (or in the postauricular sulcus) and dissected from the posterior side of the auricle.
- The incision lines along the scaphoid and conchal rim (▶ Fig. 6.19 a) are marked with needles passed from the anterior to the posterior side of the auricle, and incisions are made through the cartilage to the anterior perichondrium with a no. 15 blade (▶ Fig. 6.18 d, ▶ Fig. 6.19 a).

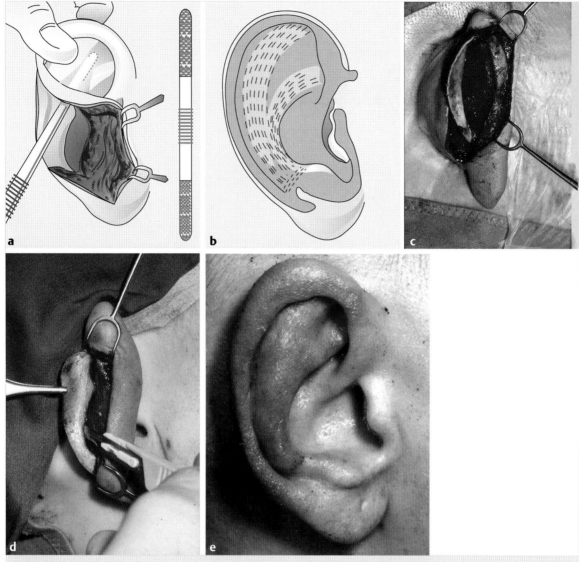

Fig. 6.18 Modification of Stenström's technique.[18] **(a)** Extended posterior approach through the scapha. Elevation of the anterior perichondrium–skin flap. **(b)** The marked region is rasped with an otoabrader, which has surfaces of varying degrees of coarseness. **(c, d)** Alternatively, the anterior aspect of the cartilage is scored with a no. 11 or no. 15 blade. The cartilage is bending without sutures. **(e)** Result. (Parts a and b reproduced from Weerda H. Surgery of the Auricle: Tumors, Trauma, Defects, Abnormalities. Stuttgart/New York, NY: Thieme Publishing Group; 2007, with permission. Parts c–e reproduced from Weerda H, Siegert R. Surgery of the Auricle. Part I: Surgery of Auricular Malformations. An Introduction with Clinical Examples. Tuttlingen, Germany: Endo-Press; 2012, with permission.)

- A series of 4–0 braided nonabsorbable mattress sutures (e.g., Ethibond, Ethicon; Gore-Tex, W. L. Gore & Associates, Inc.) are then placed to create the desired antihelical fold (▶ Fig. 6.19 b, c, e).
- The skin is closed with fine suture material.
- In ears with thick cartilage, the antihelix can be carefully thinned somewhat with a diamond wheel, burr, or brush.
- The skin is closed, and the critical distances are measured on both sides (▶ Fig. 6.19 c).
- Finally, a dressing is applied.

We find that this procedure, while somewhat complex, provides a smooth transition between the scaphoid and conchal lines (▶ Fig. 6.19 c, e).[22]

The incisions must be accurately planned to avoid unsightly sharp contours. Suture dehiscence leads to reprotrusion.

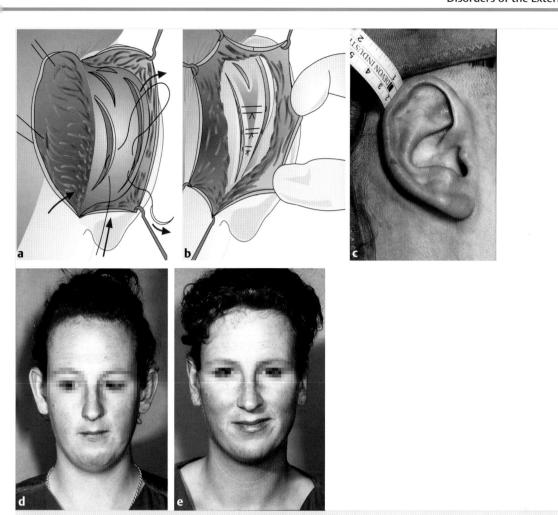

Fig. 6.19 Incision-suture technique of Converse et al.[21] **(a)** Posterior approach, incisions through the cartilage. **(b)** The antihelical fold is formed with 4–0 braided white polyester sutures (Mersilene, Ethicon) or Gore-Tex (Gore) sutures. **(c)** The distance (< 20 mm) between the helical rim and the mastoid is measured after the setback. Postoperative auricular contours are good. **(d)** Preoperative appearance. **(e)** Appearance after otoplasty. (Parts a and b reproduced from Weerda H. Surgery of the Auricle: Tumors, Trauma, Defects, Abnormalities. Stuttgart/New York, NY: Thieme Publishing Group; 2007, with permission. Parts c–e reproduced from Weerda H, Siegert R. Surgery of the Auricle. Part I: Surgery of Auricular Malformations. An Introduction with Clinical Examples. Tuttlingen, Germany: Endo-Press; 2012, with permission.)

Complications of Surgery to the Pinna

The incidence, cause, and treatment of early and late complications of setback otoplasty are given in ▶ Table 6.3 and ▶ Table 6.4, respectively.

- *Poor aesthetic results*: careful preoperative measurement of distances is important so that postoperative results can be quantified (▶ Fig. 6.16, ▶ Fig. 6.19 c). Revision surgery may be needed.
- *Suture fistula and granuloma*: suture fistulas (▶ Fig. 6.20) have been reported in approximately 10% of cases to be caused by hypersensitivity to suture material or knots placed too close to the surface of the ear. They are treated by removal of suture material.

- *Hypertrophic scars and keloid*: unlike keloids, *hypertrophic scar* formations (▶ Fig. 6.21) are limited to the original scar region and should regress over the course of several years. The consensus is that although the hypertrophic scar is indeed raised and bulging, it remains confined to the scar area (▶ Fig. 6.21) and may spontaneously regress within 1 to 2 years. Watchful waiting is recommended. If needed, they can be treated by corticosteroid infiltration. For this purpose, 10-mg triamcinolone acetonide diluted in 2-mL Ringer's solution is used. Steroids may also be introduced into the scar by needleless injection (Dermojet [Akra Dermojet]).
- *Keloids*, on the other hand, encroach on healthy skin (▶ Fig. 6.22). They are referred to as intradermal

Table 6.3 Early complications: up to 14 days after surgery (meta-analysis)[5] and therapy

Complications	Literature synopsis	Cause	Treatment
Hypersensitivity: pain, pressure, cold			
Bleeding Hematoma	11/712 = 1.5%		Hemostasis, drainage
Allergic reactions		Disinfectant, ointment, suture material	Elimination of the irritant
Infection: local defects (perichondritis); pressure sores (pressure necrosis)	22/593 = 3.6%	Type of dressing	Antibiotics, fenestrated gauze dressings
Auditory canal stenosis		Rotation of the concha	Cartilage excision
Narrow, high-riding auriculocephalic sulcus Ear setback too far		Excessive removal of postauricular skin	Skin graft
Defects Residuals Recurrence Partial or total asymmetry		Infection, iatrogenic cause, surgical error	Reoperation and reconstruction

Source note: Reproduced from Weerda H. Surgery of the Auricle: Tumors, Trauma, Defects, Abnormalities. Stuttgart/New York, NY: Thieme Publishing Group; 2007, with permission.

Table 6.4 Late complications: more than 14 days after surgery (meta-analysis)[5] and therapy

Complications	Literature synopsis	Cause	Treatment
Hypersensitivity: pain, pressure, cold	7/213 = 3.3%	Disappears after 6–12 mo	None needed
Suture fistulae, granulomas (▶ Fig. 6.20)	53/533 = 9.9%		Remove suture material
Obstructed sebaceous cyst (rare)		Everted suture	
Hypertrophic scar formation (▶ Fig. 6.21) Keloids (▶ Fig. 6.22)	14/775 = 1.8%		Steroid, excision, skin graft (full thickness), silicone gel sheet, pressure dressing, radiotherapy (up to 20 Gy)
Deformation of the ear: • Asymmetry • Overcorrection (pinned back, flat ears) • Telephone ear deformity (upper and lower auricle projecting too far); reverse telephone ear deformity (inadequate medialization of the central portion of the auricle) • Formation of sharp ridges ("catastrophic ear": destroyed cartilage, deformation in every plane; ▶ Fig. 6.23)	255/3,100 = 8.2%	Wrong technique, excessive scoring, excessive skin excision, infection	Reoperation, skin graft, revision, reconstruction with skin flaps, with fascia, with cartilage Limitation of damage by corrective surgery

Source note: Reproduced from Weerda H. Surgery of the Auricle: Tumors, Trauma, Defects, Abnormalities. Stuttgart/New York, NY: Thieme Publishing Group; 2007, with permission.

neoplasms, but fibroblasts in keloids demonstrate no histological difference from normal fibroblasts or those in hyperplastic scars. The collagen filaments form a network of atypical nodules and whirls. Many authors consider increased wound tension to be the cause of increased collagen synthesis. Furthermore, an abnormal rise in melanocyte-stimulating hormone is presumed, which could explain the increased frequency of keloids in dark-skinned patients. The keloid develops after approximately 1 to 2 months and practically never regresses spontaneously. A number of causes have been cited, including immune deficiency, medications, smoking, hormone abnormalities, connective-tissue diseases, age, skin color, and inheritance. Patient-independent factors are the location of the wound and operative technique.

• *Perichondritis*: perichondritis of the pinna may lead to a suppurative destruction of ear cartilage, which can sometimes lead to total destruction of the auricle, most frequently by *P. aeruginosa*. The lobule is typically free from infection as it contains no cartilage. Treatment is with antibiotic therapy after wound swabbing and culture, incision and drainage with careful changing of dressing daily, and excision of necrotic material and cartilage. Reconstruction after healing (▶ Fig. 6.23 b, d) may sometimes be needed.

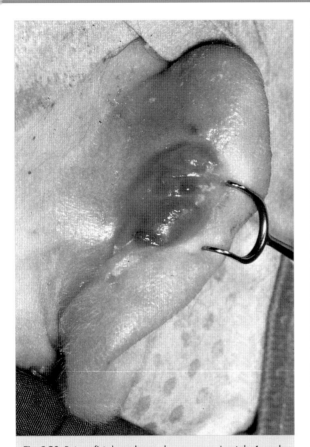

Fig. 6.20 Suture fistula and granuloma, approximately 4 weeks after surgery using the so-called incisionless technique. (Reproduced from Weerda H. Surgery of the Auricle: Tumors, Trauma, Defects, Abnormalities. Stuttgart/New York, NY: Thieme Publishing Group; 2007, with permission.)

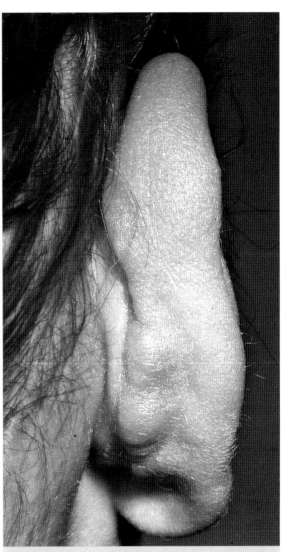

Fig. 6.21 Scar hypertrophy. (Reproduced from Weerda H. Surgery of the Auricle: Tumors, Trauma, Defects, Abnormalities. Stuttgart/New York, NY: Thieme Publishing Group; 2007, with permission.)

- *Deformation of the auricle* (▶ Fig. 6.23): if there is severe destruction after perichondritis or extensive scarring after otoplasty, the ears have to be reconstructed using different techniques.[5]

Management of Other Low-Grade, Moderate, and Severe Malformations (Microtia)

The child should have a thorough and early audiological evaluation to determine the level of hearing in the affected ear(s). Detailed imaging, including CT scanning and if appropriate MRI scanning, may help to determine the status of the middle ear including the ossicles and assists in planning treatment (see Chapter 1).

> The surgical management of microtia is highly specialized, and expertise tends to be concentrated in a few centers. A multidisciplinary approach may involve liaison with plastic surgeons, maxillofacial surgeons, prosthetists, audiologists, and pediatricians.

Many children will have complex medical histories, including learning disabilities, syndromic disorders, and craniofacial abnormalities. Hemifacial microsomia may need a specific management plan. A serial plan for the maxillofacial treatment of hemifacial microsomia is outlined in ▶ Table 6.5.[26] Early parental

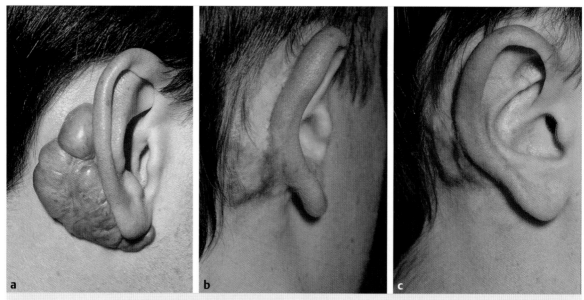

Fig. 6.22 Keloid. (a) Large keloid of the postauricular region. (b, c) Appearance 1 year after excision, coverage with full-thickness skin and radiotherapy.

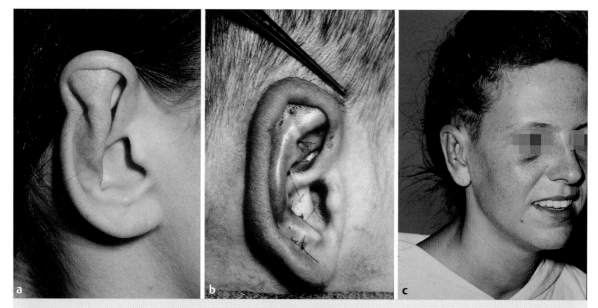

Fig. 6.23 Cartilage destruction. (a) Appearance after otoplasty demonstrating destruction of the cartilaginous structure, with the right ear worse than the left (c). (b) Reconstruction of the auricle with costal cartilage, which was fashioned and inserted through posterior incision. Skin and perichondrium are dissected off the cartilage in the region of the antihelix. Appearance after insertion of the cartilage, and temporal fascia molding of the form achieved with the aid of a few structures. (c) Appearance after reconstruction. (Reproduced from Weerda H. Surgery of the Auricle: Tumors, Trauma, Defects, Abnormalities. Stuttgart/New York, NY: Thieme Publishing Group; 2007, with permission.)

involvement and taking cognizance of the views of the child make for the best outcomes. Prosthetic ears are now of extremely high quality and when anchored to the skull using osseointegrated implant technology, they can offer excellent aesthetic result

but *fitting them involves destroying the surrounding skin and no subsequent reconstructive surgery can be carried out.*

The reconstruction of one or both auricles in severe microtia is carried out in one to five stages to improve

Table 6.5 Serial plan for the maxillofacial treatment of hemifacial microsomia[26]

Type of treatment	Treatment age (y)	Anatomical region	Duration	Indication
Distraction (extraoral)	1	Mandible	1 mm/day + consolidation time (~ 3 wk)	Mandibular malformation obstructing airways
	3–4	Mandible	1 mm/day + consolidation time (~4 wk)	Severe mandibular hypoplasia
Distraction (intraoral) + orthodontic treatment	7–9	Mandible	1 mm/day + consolidation time (~6 wk)	Moderate to mild mandibular hypoplasia
Sagittal split osteotomy	17	Mandible	~ 2 wk	Ramus shortening < 10% Correction for reduced growth after distraction Dysgnathias
		Maxilla	~ 2 wk	1. Inadequate spontaneous correction during growth after distraction 2. After maxillary distraction treatment of adults
Transplantation	5–8	Mandible	~ 2 wk	Extreme hypoplasia and aplasia of the head of the temporomandibular joint or the mandibular ramus
	17	Maxilla	~ 2 wk	For stabilization after sagittal split osteotomy with > 4 mm of osteotomy gap
		Malar bone	~ 2 wk	Partial or complete agenesis of the malar bone or malar arch
Augmentation	17	Malar bone, orbital ring	~ 2 wk	Hypoplastic malar bone/orbital ring
Genioplasty	16	Chin	1 wk	1. Malformation with dorsal or oblique chin position 2. Isolated progenia 3. As auxiliary measure for dysgnathias

Source note: Reproduced from Hasse A. Maxillofacial management of hemifacial microsomia. In: Weerda H. Surgery of the Auricle: Tumors, Trauma, Defects, Abnormalities. Stuttgart/New York: Thieme; 2007:271–275, with permission.

6

aesthetic appearance (▸ Fig. 6.24). The earliest operations are carried out at an age of 5 or 6 years, especially in moderate malformations. Brent[7] prefers an age of 10 years because we can harvest a stable costal cartilage to get a "three-dimensional" high framework (▸ Fig. 6.24 a). At this age the children are able to express their own desires.[5,23,24,25] Several techniques for autologous reconstruction are described. The creation of their "own" auricle, that is, not a pro sthesis, may improve self-confidence and self-esteem (▸ Fig. 6.24).[13]

Management of Hearing

> In children with unilateral/bilateral microtia and atresia, the inner ear usually is intact and hearing loss is purely conductive.

Typically there will be a 45- to 60-dB conductive hearing loss (▸ Fig. 6.27, WHA, without hearing aid) in each of the affected ears. If possible in case of unilateral or bilateral aural atresia, one or two conventional air-conduction hearing aids can be fitted during the first weeks of life (▸ Fig. 6.25).[27] If it is not possible to use an air-conduction hearing device, then the provision of a bone-conduction (BC) hearing aid is necessary. Since conventional BC hearing aids have their disadvantages, the aim should be to provide a bone-anchored hearing aid (BAHA) as soon as possible (▸ Fig. 6.26, ▸ Fig. 6.27). Surgical reconstruction of the sound apparatus can also be undertaken in stages together with auricular reconstruction (▸ Fig. 6.28). This is highly demanding surgery, and given the improvements in modern BAHA technology, it is now rarely done other than by a small number of experts.[5,13,26,28,29] The implantation of different sound transducers is also possible. (see Chapter 13, Chapter 14, Chapter 15 for more information on management of deafness in children.)

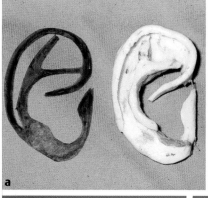
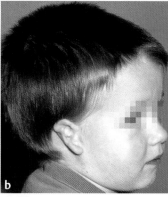
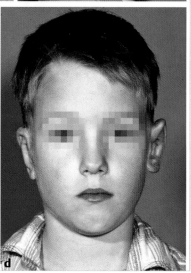
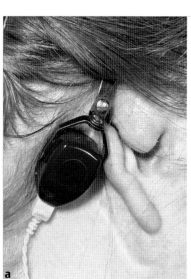

Fig. 6.24 Surgical result in a child with grade III microtia (right ear). **(a)** Three-dimensional Nagata-type framework[25] with tragus and framework template. **(b)** Third-degree malformation. **(c,d)** Some weeks after reconstruction with a cartilaginous framework from the sixth to ninth rib. (Reproduced from Weerda H, Siegert R. Surgery of the Auricle. Part I: Surgery of Auricular Malformations. An Introduction with Clinical Examples. Tuttlingen, Germany: Endo-Press 2012, with permission.)

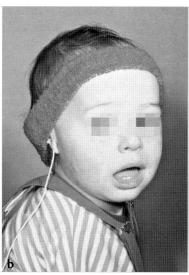

Fig. 6.25 Bilateral provision with a bone-conduction hearing aid (▶ Fig. 6.27). **(a)** Bone-conduction receiver with clip. **(b)** Bone-conduction receiver integrated in a headband. (Reproduced from Weerda H. Surgery of the Auricle: Tumors, Trauma, Defects, Abnormalities. Stuttgart/New York, NY: Thieme Publishing Group; 2007, with permission.)

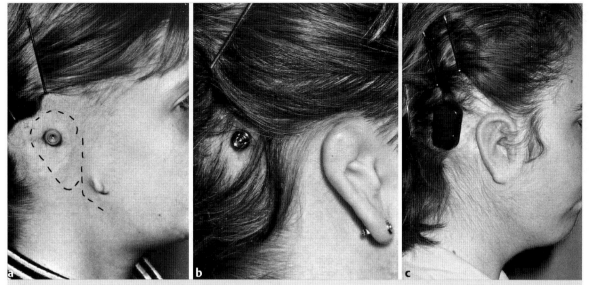

Fig. 6.26 Child with grade III microtia. **(a)** The remnant was removed and split skin transplanted. The bone screw was implanted in an incorrect anterior position. An auricular reconstruction was nearly impossible. **(b)** Bone screw in correct position in the hair. **(c)** The bone-anchored hearing aid was adapted; here we have been able to reconstruct the auricle. (Reproduced from Weerda H. Surgery of the Auricle: Tumors, Trauma, Defects, Abnormalities. Stuttgart/New York, NY: Thieme Publishing Group; 2007, with permission.)

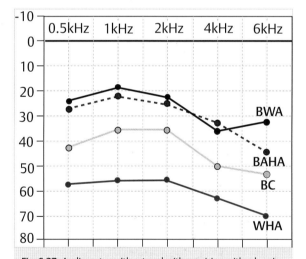

Fig. 6.27 Audiometry without and with provision with a hearing aid. Hearing threshold in the unilateral free-field sound audiogram without and with hearing-aid provision; comparison of the various types of hearing aids. BAHA, Bone-anchored hearing aid; BC, bone-conduction spectacles; BWA, body-worn aid; WHA, without hearing aid. (Modified after Weerda H. Surgery of the Auricle: Tumors, Trauma, Defects, Abnormalities. Stuttgart/New York, NY: Thieme Publishing Group; 2007, with permission.)

Audiometry with Hearing Aids

There is excellent improvement of hearing thresholds with bone-conduction hearing aids and BAHAs (▶ Fig. 6.27; see Chapter 15).

6.6 Key Points

- Different *inflammatory diseases* of the auricle need treating, often with antibiotic therapy based on culture results.
- The exposed position and bradytrophic structure of the auricle predisposes it to a large number of *traumata*, including penetrating and blunt traumata, chemical and thermal burns, and avulsions.
- Auricular *appendages, fistulae, and sinuses*, as well as small congenital disorders can occur.
- The *auricular dysplasias* can be classified in relation to increasing embryonal development and severity. The classification into three groups (first-degree or low-grade malformations, second-degree or moderate malformations, and third-degree or severe malformations and anotia) allows a useful overview for management and surgical repair.

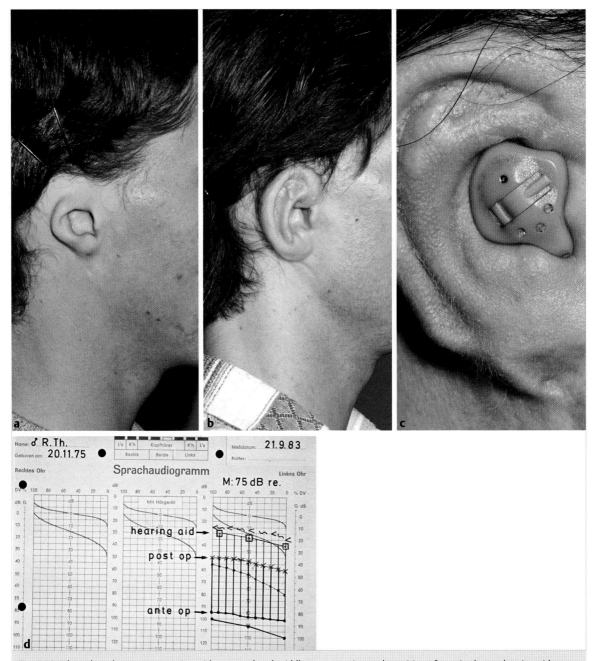

Fig. 6.28 Bilateral total ear reconstruction with ear canal and middle ear operation and provision of two in-the-ear hearing aids (a) before and (b, c) after surgery. (d) Audiogram before and after operation and with hearing aid. (Reproduced from Weerda H. Surgery of the Auricle: Tumors, Trauma, Defects, Abnormalities. Stuttgart/New York, NY: Thieme Publishing Group; 2007, with permission.)

References

[1] Leiber B. Ohrmuscheldystopie, Ohrmuscheldysplasie und Ohrmuschelmissbildung – klinische Wertung und Bedeutung als Symptom. Arch Otorhinolaryngol. 1972; 202:51–84

[2] Probst R, Grevers G, Iro H. Hals-Nasen-Ohrenheilkunde. 3rd ed. Stuttgart: Thieme; 2008

[3] Wall GM, Stroman DW, Roland PS, Dohar J. Ciprofloxacin 0.3%/dexamethasone 0.1% sterile otic suspension for the topical treatment of ear infections: a review of the literature. Pediatr Infect Dis J. 2009; 28 (2):141–144

[4] Bergstrom LV. Diseases of the external ear. In: Bluestone Ch, Stool S, Arjona P, eds. Pediatric Otolaryngology. Philadelphia, PA: Saunders; 1983

[5] Weerda H. Surgery of the Auricle: Tumors, Trauma, Defects, Abnormalities. Stuttgart: Thieme; 2007

[6] Weerda H. Reconstructive Facial Plastic Surgery: A Problem- Solving Manual. 2nd ed. Stuttgart: Thieme; 2015

[7] Brent B. The pediatrician's role in caring for patients with congenital microtia and atresia. Pediatr Ann. 1999; 28(6):374–383

[8] Eavery RD. Microtia and significant auricular malformation. Ninety-two pediatric patients. Arch Otolaryngol. 1995; 121:57–62

[9] Weerda H. Anomalien des äusseren Ohres. In: Naumann et al, ed. Otorhinolaryngologie in Klinik und Praxis. Vol. I. Stuttgart: Thieme; 1994: 488–499

[10] Otto HD. Pathogenese der Aurikularanhänge, Melotie und Polyotie. Arch Otorhinolaryngol. 1979; 225(1):45–56

[11] Gohary A, Rangecroft L, Cook RC. Congenital auricular and preauricular sinuses in childhood. Z Kinderchir. 1983; 38(2):81–82

[12] Davis J, ed. Aesthetic and Reconstructive Otoplasty. Berlin: Springer-Verlag; 1987

[13] Siegert R. Psychological aspects of severe microtia. In: Weerda H, ed. Surgery of the Auricle: Tumors, Trauma, Defects, Abnormalities. Stuttgart: Thieme; 2007:278–282

[14] Elly ET. An operation for prominence of the auricle. Arch Otolaryngol. 1881; 10:97

[15] Schmidt H. Die Ohrmuschel in der Medizin des 19 und des 20. Jahrhunderts und die Entwicklung der Anlegeplastik [dissertation]. Lübeck, Germany: Medizinischen Universität Lübeck; 2000

[16] Mustarde JC. The correction of prominent ears using simple mattress sutures. Br J Plast Surg. 1963; 16:170–178

[17] Stenstroem SJ. "Natural" technique for correction of congenitally prominent ears. Plast Reconstr Surg. 1963; 32:509–518

[18] Stenström SJ. Cosmetic deformities of the ear. In: Graff WC, Smith JW, eds. Plastic Surgery. 2nd ed. Boston, MA: Little, Brown Co; 1973: 603–604

[19] Chongchet V. Method of anthelix reconstruction. Br J Plast Surg. 1963; 16:268–272

[20] Crikelair GF, Cosman B. Another solution for the problem of prominent ear. Ann Surg. 1964; 160:314–324

[21] Converse JM, Nigro A, Wilson FA, Johnson N. A technique for surgical correction of lop ears. Plast Reconstr Surg (1946). 1955; 15(5):411–418

[22] Weerda H, Siegert R. Surgery of the Auricle. Part I: Surgery of Auricular Malformations. An Introduction with Clinical Examples. Tuttlingen: Endo-Press; 2012

[23] Weerda H, Walter C. Surgery of the pinna and surrounding area. In: Ward PH, ed. Plastic and Reconstructive Surgery of the Head and Neck. St. Louis, MO: CV Mosly; 1984:827–846

[24] Tanzer RC. Congenital deformities. In: Converse JM, ed. Reconstructive Plastic Surgery. Philadelphia, PA: Saunders; 1977: 1671–1719

[25] Nagata P. Modification of the stages in total reconstruction of the auricle: Part II. Grafting the three-dimensional costal cartilage framework for concha-type microtia. Plast Reconstr Surg. 1994; 93(2):231–242; discussion 267–268

[26] Hasse A. Maxillofacial management of hemifacial microsomia. In: Weerda H, ed. Surgery of the Auricle: Tumors, Trauma, Defects, Abnormalities. Stuttgart: Thieme; 2007:271–275

[27] Sommer H, Schoenweiler R. Provision of hearing aids for congenital aural atresia. In: Weerda H, ed. Surgery of the Auricle: Tumors, Trauma, Defects, Abnormalities. Stuttgart: Thieme; 2007:260–262

[28] Jarsdoerfer A, Kim JHN. Treatment of the malformed middle ear – techniques and results. In: Weerda H, ed. Surgery of the Auricle: Tumors, Trauma, Defects, Abnormalities. Stuttgart: Thieme; 2007: 245–254

[29] Siegert R. Surgery of the middle ear for grade III microtia in the presence of congenital aural atresia. In: Weerda H, ed. Surgery of the Auricle: Tumors, Trauma, Defects, Abnormalities. Stuttgart: Thieme; 2007:255–259

6

7 Acute Otitis Media

William P. L. Hellier

7.1 Introduction

> ℹ
>
> Acute otitis media (AOM) is one of the most common diseases diagnosed in the pediatric population.

In the United States, it is the most common indication for antibiotic therapy, generating more than 30 million prescriptions annually.[1] In the United Kingdom, 30% of children under the age of 3 years see their general practitioner with AOM each year,[2] and in a recent study in Europe, the incidence of AOM in children under the age of 6 years was found to be 256/1,000 child-years. The natural history of AOM can vary from that of a self-limiting disorder which resolves completely with analgesia alone, giving rise to no long-term adverse consequences, to a life-threatening condition with intracranial sepsis, often leading to serious and prolonged neurologic morbidity. In the preantibiotic era, the complications of AOM were greatly feared; in modern times, serious sequelae of AOM are uncommon, but the need for active management of AOM and the possibility of extensive spread beyond the middle ear (ME) must be borne in mind by the doctors of today.

7.2 Definitions and Classification of Otitis Media

Otitis media (OM) is defined as an inflammation of the ME cleft.

> ℹ
>
> OM does not refer to a specific etiology or pathogenesis.

It is useful to further subclassify OM, and the most common classifications used are based on the study by Bluestone et al.[3] Acute otitis media (AOM) differs from recurrent otitis media (ROM), otitis media with effusion (OME), and chronic suppurative otitis media (CSOM), each requiring a specifically tailored management approach.

7.2.1 Acute Otitis Media

AOM is defined as a condition with acute inflammation of the ME cleft and the presence of an effusion, and is associated with the onset of the signs and symptoms of acute infection. The pathological definition is straightforward,

but the clinical definition can be more difficult. Children can present with specific (otalgia or ear discharge) or more general (fever and irritability) symptoms. In the early stages there is inflammation of the tympanic membrane and the ME mucosa, but there is no ME effusion or fluid. The eardrum is thickened or erythematous, but moves well with pneumatic otoscopy or tympanometry. This early inflammatory stage may resolve or may progress to a full-blown empyema of the ME, which becomes filled with mucopus, often under tension and causing severe pain, sometimes relieved as the drum perforates and pus discharges from the ME (▶ Fig. 7.1).

Myringitis is characterized by inflammation of the tympanic membrane alone. This may be associated with either OM or possibly an external ear canal infection, but can occur in isolation due to viral infections with blistering or fluid-filled bullae on the drum—bullous myringitis (▶ Fig. 7.2).

7.2.2 Recurrent Acute Otitis Media

Many children will suffer multiple episodes of AOM. When does this become a separate pathological process and merits the term *recurrent acute otitis media* (ROM or RAOM), is moot point; but most authors would accept

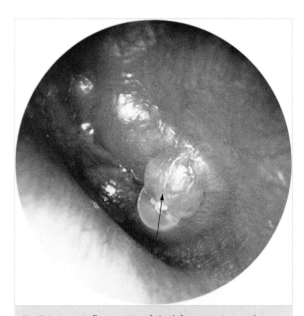

Fig. 7.1 Acute inflammation of the left tympanic membrane. The tympanic membrane is bulging and erythematous. Incipient perforation with discharge is evident in the posteroinferior quadrant (*arrow*). (Reproduced with permission of Probst R, Grevers G, Iro H. Basic Otorhinolaryngology: A Step-by-Step Learning Guide. Stuttgart: Thieme; 2006.)

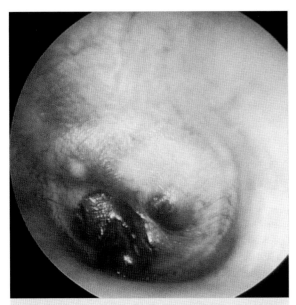

Fig. 7.2 Bullous myringitis with hemorrhagic blebs (left ear). (Reproduced with permission of Sanna M, Russo A, DeDonato G. Color Atlas of Otoscopy. Stuttgart: Thieme; 1999.)

that 3 or more episodes of AOM in a 6-month period, or 4 or more episodes in a 12-month period constitutes RAOM. The ME returns to normal in-between the episodes of AOM, otherwise the child has OME or CSOM, each of which has a different natural history and warrants a different therapeutic approach. There is increasing evidence that ROM in childhood may be associated with hearing loss in adult life.[4]

7.2.3 Otitis Media with Effusion

OME is characterized by inflammation of ME with an effusion that is usually serous or mucoid but not purulent, and is not associated with the signs and symptoms of acute infection. OME may follow an episode of AOM or may supervene in children with RAOM; it is discussed in detail in Chapter 8.

7.3 Epidemiology, Prevalence, and Risk Factors

7.3.1 Gender and Age

Teele et al reported that the incidence of AOM is higher in males but other studies have shown little difference between the sexes.[1]

> **i**
>
> AOM is primarily a disease of younger (preschool) children.

In the United States, approximately 30 to 60% of children will have an episode in their first year of life, up to 70 to 80% by the time they are 3 years old, and more than 90% by the age of 5 years. The highest prevalence is in the second 6 months of life.[1] A first episode of AOM before 6 months of age does independently make further episodes more likely. This could be due to the inflammatory episode leaving changes, scarring, or residual inflammation in the ME, making recurrent episodes more common, or could suggest that the child has an innate predisposition to AOM.

Younger children have short, wide, and immature Eustachian tubes (ETs) associated with aggregates of lymphoid and adenoidal tissue that can harbor bacteria close to the ascending ET, which can infect the ME space. They have immature immune systems and are more prone to upper respiratory tract infections (URTIs).

After the age of 7 years, the incidence seems to decrease (see Chapter 8).

7.3.2 Geographical and Ethnic Factors

It appears that there has been an increase in the prevalence of AOM over the last few decades. There is a greater incidence of AOM in native Americans, Canadian Inuits, and Australian Aboriginal children. This may be due to anatomical factors, but also could be related to other factors such as socioeconomic conditions or access to healthcare. In Europe, there seems to be some variation between countries, with Italy seemingly having a lower incidence than average.[5]

7.3.3 Environmental Factors

A number of environmental factors have been shown in population studies to influence the incidence of AOM, some of which are potentially reversible.

- AOM has a higher incidence in autumn and winter than in summer. This could be related to the increased prevalence of URTIs and/or the crowding of children inside over these periods.
- Many studies have shown an increase in AOM in children who attend nursery or day-care facilities especially from an early age. Again, the increased exposure to other children and viral infections is thought to be the cause.
- Children who are breast-fed compared to those who are artificially fed have a lower incidence of AOM. A number of factors have been suggested to explain this, but the transfer of protective maternal antibodies is probably the most accepted.
- There is a significant increase in children with AOM who are passively exposed to smoke by parental cigarette use in the home environment.

7

II

7.3.4 Anatomical Factors and Comorbidity

Anatomical changes of the head and neck, or host defense deficiencies have a significant influence on the incidence of AOM. Children with cleft palate, craniofacial abnormalities, and congenital or acquired immune or immunoglobulin deficiencies are all at higher risk for AOM.

> *Adenoidal hyperplasia* is also thought to predispose children to AOM, not as previously thought by a direct effect on the ET, but most probably by harboring the bacterial responsible for AOM possibly in the form of *biofilms*.

Some studies have suggested that there may be a genetic predisposition in children with RAOM.

7.4 Pathophysiology of Acute Otitis Media

The ME cleft is connected to the nasopharynx by the ET, which is responsible for the ventilation of the ME cleft. The ME is not sterile as it is directly associated with the nose and hence the outside world, and there seems to be a balance between the host defenses and the viral/bacterial agents that contaminate the system. When this balance is disturbed, an acute infection and the associated inflammatory response occurs. The balance can be altered by many factors, some of which have been discussed previously.

> The classic scenario for an episode of AOM is a child who catches a viral upper respiratory tract infection. This leads to mucosal inflammation and functional ET dysfunction, mucociliary stasis, and ME inflammation with effusion formation.

Pathologically the stages of AOM are well recognized.
- It begins with *inflammation* and *hyperemia* of the ME mucosa. There may be similar findings in the mucosa of the ET, and these may precede (ascending infection) or follow the changes in the ME.
- The swollen ME mucosa and dilated capillaries allow *exudation* of blood products including proteins, inflammatory cells, and mediators into the ME.
- There is an increase in ME goblet cells that produce more mucous.
- The bacterial and inflammatory cells produce toxic factors that together with the pressure of the

mucopurulent exudate can lead to a perforation of the pars tensa of the drum and discharge into the external ear.

AOM is usually benign and often can be self-limiting, with resolution and healing at any point in this process. In a small number of cases, progression of the pathological process occurs, as discussed later in this chapter.

> Major factors in the pathogenesis of AOM that influence progression in an individual case are the function of the ET, the child's immune response, and the bacterial or viral load. The biggest contributing factor involved in any one child is difficult to ascertain, and a combination of many factors may well be at work.

7.4.1 Eustachian Tube Function

The ET ventilates the ME. It helps to provide protection by remaining closed for much of the time to prevent microbial ingress and by helping to clear secretions from the ME by the action of its mucociliary lining. In a child, the ET is anatomically different to that in an adult, that is, being shorter and more horizontal, but it can also be functionally immature. It is difficult to know whether AOM may be caused initially by functional tubal obstruction, with a viral upper respiratory tract infection leading to tubal edema and mucociliary clearance breakdown, or by the failure of the tube to stop pathogens ascending into the ME. There have been some studies that have shown reflux from the nasopharynx into the ME in some children during swallowing, and this may predispose to AOM.

7.4.2 Immune Response

The nasopharynx naturally carries bacteria, and there is often colonization of the adenoids in children. There is, however, an innate immune defense system in the upper airway and ME that prevents invasion of the pathogens. The mucosa secretes numerous antimicrobial molecules, lysozymes, and antibodies including immunoglobulin M (IgM), and there is systemic production of bacteria-specific immunoglobulin G (IgG). In children, maternal IgG is transferred in the cord blood, but the levels decline after 6 months, before there has been a compensatory rise in the child's own IgG. This "window" of lower IgG levels probably explains, in part, the rise in the incidence of AOM at 6 months, with the peak age incidence of AOM being 6 to 12 months. Any failure or reduction in the systemic or epithelial immune defense system will make bacterial entry and AOM more likely.

7.4.3 Bacterial or Viral Load

> ⓘ
>
> It has recently been found that bacteria can exist in two states: active or planktonic. In the planktonic state, bacterial activity reduces and the cells congregate in groups surrounded by a matrix termed a *biofilm*. Biofilms are relatively inert, can lay dormant on the mucosa, and are not well penetrated by antibiotics.

Biofilms are found in the nasopharynx and ME and are thought to be reservoirs of infection that can become quickly active if stimulated. They are more resilient in areas of low-oxygen tension, which may exist in the ME when there is ET dysfunction as may often be seen with the immature tube in infants. The persistence of biofilms in the nasopharynx and ME, which are activated by viral inflammation of the area, may be the cause of some episodes of both AOM and RAOM.

7.5 Flora

> ⓘ
>
> Knowledge of the potential microbiology of AOM is vital to inform the clinician of the most appropriate antimicrobial treatment. This is discussed further in Chapter 7.7.3.

The role of bacteria in AOM is well recognized, but in many cases, viral infection plays a major part. In approximately 40% of cases of AOM, respiratory viruses are found in the nasopharyngeal secretions. The commonest viruses are respiratory syncytial virus and rhinovirus, but parainfluenza, influenza, and adenovirus are also involved. Viral infection alone is probably the cause of AOM in up to 20% of cases.

7.6 Clinical Features

7.6.1 Symptoms and Signs

The clinical features of AOM parallel the pathological process described.

- Symptoms often start with features of a viral URTI associated with nasal congestion, rhinorrhea, and a sore throat, but symptoms of AOM can occur quite rapidly with no obvious cause.
- Inflammation of the ME mucosa and tympanic membrane are either preceded by or follow ET dysfunction and ME effusion. Ear discomfort may be present from the start or slowly get worse with the increase in inflammation. The ear feels blocked or pressured, with a conductive hearing loss.
- There may be no ME fluid, but as the condition continues, the drum becomes dull and the ME mucosa thickens. The pressure of the mucopurulent effusion slowly builds, and at this point, the tympanic membrane is dull, thickened, and bulging. Otalgia at this stage of AOM is usual and is an indicative clinical symptom, but is not present in all children.
- The toxic effect of the infection and factors released by the bacteria and immune response often give rise to more systemic symptoms with a rising fever, and often, in smaller children, lethargy, malaise, vomiting, and possibly diarrhea.

7.6.2 Otoscopic Findings

> ⓘ
>
> On examination in this early stage, the tympanic membrane is hyperemic with injected vessels over the attic and malleus handle (▶ Fig. 7.3). If there is a continued buildup of pressure from the infected effusion in the ME, perforation of the pars tensa may occur (▶ Fig. 7.4).

Perforation of the Pars Tensa

This is noticed as a mucopurulent discharge from the ear, often with a reduction in the child's otalgia. Sometimes, this discharge is blood-stained, and a swab of this otorrhea can be taken for microbiological analysis. The

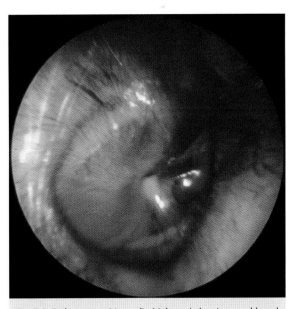

Fig. 7.3 Early acute otitis media (right ear) showing a reddened vascular strip along the manubrium. (Reproduced with permission of Wigand ME. Restitutional Surgery of the Ear and Temporal Bone. Stuttgart: Thieme; 2001.)

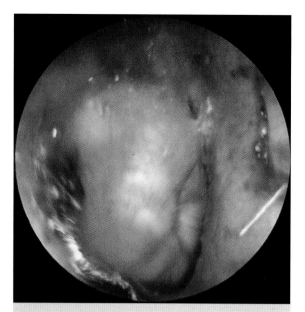

Fig. 7.4 Advanced acute otitis media (left ear) showing a thickened, bulging drumhead. Spontaneous perforation is imminent. (Reproduced with permission of Wigand ME. Restitutional Surgery of the Ear and Temporal Bone. Stuttgart: Thieme; 2001)

perforation of the drum is often seen as the natural "bursting of the abscess"; the child usually feels better, and the disease process starts to improve. In some cases, possibly more with virulent *S. pneumoniae* strains, there is not only a pinpoint perforation of the tympanic membrane, but also a degree of necrosis, leaving a much larger perforation.

Most small perforations heal spontaneously as the inflammatory process abates. Larger perforations may not heal and can become chronic defects (CSOM; see Chapter 9).

If the drum does not perforate, AOM can resolve spontaneously as the child's immune system regains the upper hand, but AOM can remain active with continuing symptoms or progress with further spread of infection and inflammation outside the confines of the ME and mastoid mucosa (▶ Fig. 7.5).

Mastoiditis and other complications are discussed later in this chapter.

7.6.3 Diagnostic Uncertainty

In older children, the diagnosis of AOM is usually relatively straightforward. They often present with classic symptoms of localized otalgia and are able to describe

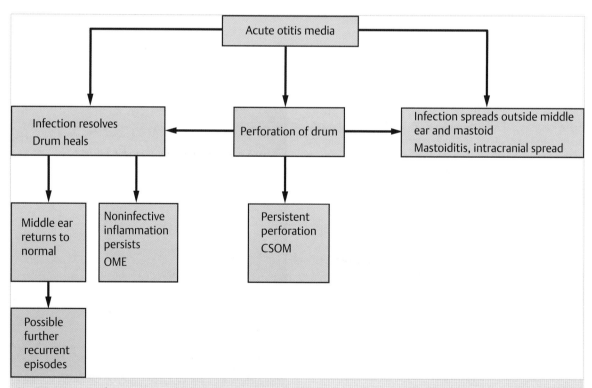

Fig. 7.5 Outcomes of acute otitis media. OME, Otitis media with effusion; CSOM, chronic suppurative otitis media.

their pain and hearing loss. Examination of the larger ear canal, with a better view of the drum, makes confirmation of the bulging, reddened tympanic membrane far easier (► Fig. 7.3, ► Fig. 7.4).

> Contrary to much traditional teaching, the diagnosis of AOM in young children is neither easy nor certain.

In 1990, a study in the British Medical Journal[6] found that the self-reported diagnostic certainty in a group of general practitioners of their diagnosis of AOM in the under 12-month age group was only 58%. In children under the age of 2 years, the symptoms can be vague, and they often cannot give a meaningful history. A child may pull at their ear, but pain is not always present, and nonspecific systemic symptoms such as fever, vomiting, loss of appetite, and even diarrhea may be the only signs of AOM.

> The most important sign is the state of the eardrum, and in a crying and upset 12-month-old child with a small ear canal and a little wax, getting an adequate view of the tympanic membrane may not be possible.

The peak age for the incidence of AOM is 6 to 18 months, so there can be diagnostic uncertainties in this largest group of children with AOM. Not all ear pain in these children is necessarily AOM, so a careful history and examination is essential in an unwell child, especially if he/she is "pulling an ear," with the potential for AOM as a diagnosis being borne in mind at all times.

> The presence of ear discharge with a history consistent with AOM certainly helps to confirm the diagnosis.

The ME, and not the external ear, contains mucous secreting glands, so the presence of mucopus in the external canal confirms that the drum has perforated. In the absence of mucopurulent otorrhea, the only true way of absolutely confirming the diagnosis of AOM is to perform a tympanocentesis, taking a small aspirate of ME fluid for microbiological diagnosis. This is generally not practical in the awake child and is rarely done in routine clinical practice.

Tympanometry can sometimes be used to assist with the diagnosis, but it can only give an indication as to the presence or absence of ME effusion and does not distinguish between the infected bulging effusion of AOM and the chronic noninfected effusion seen with OME. It should be used only as an aid to the clinical history and examination.

7.7 Treatment

7.7.1 Analgesia and Symptom Control

AOM is a painful and distressing condition for the parents and the child, and adequate symptom control, particularly analgesia, is essential. Pain may be controlled by simple analgesia such as paracetamol, with the addition of a nonsteroidal anti-inflammatory drug such as ibuprofen, if needed. In younger children, systemic symptoms such as fever and vomiting may occur, and it is important that hydration is maintained in this age group.

> There is no evidence base for the use of decongestants and antihistamines in the treatment of AOM.

Sometimes, topical decongestants when used in the short term can relieve the nasal symptoms caused by the viral nasal infection that preceded AOM, but they are not an effective treatment for AOM itself.

7.7.2 Antimicrobial Therapy

The natural history of AOM in many cases is that of a relatively benign self-limiting condition that resolves without major sequelae. It can progress to cause a chronic perforation, hearing loss, or the serious complications discussed later. A study from the preantibiotic era reported mastoiditis in 17% of cases of AOM,[7] and many older ear, nose, and throat (ENT) surgeons remember wards full of children needing surgery for AOM and its complications. In the postantibiotic era, the use of antimicrobial drugs has made the more serious sequelae of AOM fortunately very uncommon, but they are still seen, and some data suggest that possibly with the reduced use of antibiotics for AOM, these complications are being seen more often.

> The difficulty for the treating clinician is that currently there is no predictive test that can determine whether AOM affecting the child in front of them will resolve spontaneously or whether the infection if left untreated will progress. The use of antibiotics is therefore still the mainstay of treatment, but the clinical decision about how to treat a child with suspected or definite AOM may be finely balanced.

7

There have been a number of studies including a Cochrane review[8] that have shown that antibiotics have only a small effect on the resolution of AOM in many children. The role of early antimicrobial therapy is uncertain.[9] Most published guidelines emphasize that the great majority of children will recover from AOM without antimicrobial treatment, but compliance with guidelines is highly variable.[10]

With the growing concerns over the number of bacteria that are becoming antibiotic-resistant, a policy of a "watchful waiting" period is being increasingly used by many clinicians in a number of countries, notably in the Netherlands, in the treatment of AOM.

A child seen with early AOM who is otherwise systemically well is prescribed analgesia to control any otalgia, but not antibiotics at the initial consultation. If the ear pain subsides, then no further treatment at that stage is suggested as it would seem AOM has resolved. However, if the pain continues for more than 24 to 48 hours, the child becomes systemically unwell, or there are other worrying symptoms, then the child should be returned to the doctor for review and antibiotics. Topical antimicrobial therapy may be indicated, especially if the drum has perforated.[11]

> The decision to adopt a "watch and wait" policy for AOM should be carefully considered by the clinician and discussed with the child's parents. It is not suitable for children with other underlying medical conditions, for those that are systematically unwell, when follow-up care at 24 to 48 hours cannot be guaranteed, or when the child is under the age of 2 years. In these cases probably antibiotics should be the mainstay of treatment.

Children under the age of 2 years have the highest incidence of not only AOM, but also the complications of AOM, and as exact diagnosis is difficult, antibiotics should be used as the first line of treatment if there is any suspicion of complications.

7.7.3 Choice of Antibiotic

All antibiotics carry the risk of allergic reactions, gastrointestinal disturbance, and other reactions. Their use is not without unwanted side effects. The benefit of treatment need always be weighed against the risks.

The antibiotic used to treat AOM should take into account the three main bacteria involved: *S. pneumoniae*, *H. influenzae*, and *M. catarrhalis*. If there are microbiological data available, for example, from a swab of otorrhea post-AOM, then this information should be used to inform which antimicrobial is used.

> The three main organisms are generally sensitive to amoxicillin, which is a broad-spectrum penicillin, and so this is usually the antibiotic of choice. It is safe, well tolerated in children, available as a liquid, and inexpensive. In children who are allergic to penicillin, a good alternative is one of the macrolide group, for example, azithromycin, or a cephalosporin, which again are usually well tolerated.

There is a growing problem of bacterial resistance to antibiotics, especially with the emergence of β-lactamase-producing bacteria. Approximately 20 to 30% of *H. influenzae* and up to 100% of *M. catarrhalis* are now found to produce β-lactamase, and in certain parts of the developed world, 30 to 50% of *S. pneumoniae* are penicillin-resistant. A growing number of *S. pneumoniae* and *H. influenzae* species are showing growing resistance to macrolides.

> Where there are great concerns about such bacterial resistance, amoxicillin–clavulanate or a cephalosporin is probably the first-line antibiotic of choice.

Treatment with antibiotic therapy should continue for at least 5 days (5–7 days usually) in uncomplicated cases of AOM. There is usually an improvement in the child's symptoms over the first 1 to 2 days, with a slow resolution of the ME inflammation. Many children continue to have a noninfective effusion in the ME for up to 6 weeks after an episode of AOM, and the ear should be examined at 4- to 6-week intervals to make sure of full resolution. If the eardrum has perforated, the child will need to keep the ear dry until it has healed. Healing usually occurs rapidly once the infection has resolved, but the eardrum needs to be checked when the child is reviewed at the follow-up appointment.

7.8 Treatment Failure

7.8.1 Antimicrobial Therapy Modification

> The majority of children with AOM will have symptomatic improvement within 24 to 48 hours of antimicrobial therapy. If symptoms are ongoing or worsening after 48 to 72 hours, then this represents a failure of response to the antibiotics used.

This may be due to antibiotic resistance of one of the usual AOM bacteria, an unusual pathogenic agent, failure of penetration of the antibiotic into the ME, or progression of the infection. If the child's clinical state has not improved, then consider an alternative antibiotic. Amoxicillin–clavulonate should be used if amoxicillin has failed, and a fourth-generation cephalosporin such as ceftriaxone has support in the literature as a second-line antibiotic but needs parenteral administration.

7.8.2 Surgery

Those children who fail with the second antibiotic agent and are still symptomatic may need admission to hospital for myringotomy. This procedure involves incision of the tympanic membrane to aspirate and drain the infected ME effusion. It can be done under local anesthesia in older children, but younger ones will need a general anesthetic.
- The tympanic membrane is viewed using a speculum and an operating microscope.
- A myringotomy blade is used to cut a radial incision in the anteroinferior quadrant of the drum, as incising this area minimizes the risks to the ME structures and allows wide drainage of the ME (▶ Fig. 7.6).

Myringotomy allows decompression of the ME, which gives symptomatic relief, and importantly allows collection of fluid for microbiological analysis. In the preantibiotic era, it was the mainstay of treatment for AOM, but studies have found no major differences in outcomes in children with AOM treated with antibiotics alone or antibiotics with myringotomy. It still, however, retains its place in certain circumstances, especially when there has not been a response to antibiotics and

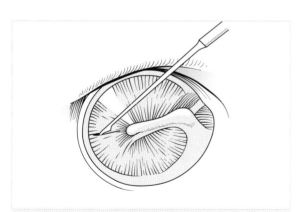

Fig. 7.6 Myringotomy. A radial incision is made in the anteroinferior quadrant of the tympanic membrane with a sickle knife. In acute otitis media, it can be difficult to identify landmarks in the inflamed drum. (Reproduced with permission of Theissing J, Werner JA, Rettinger G. ENT—Head and Neck Surgery: Essential Procedures. Stuttgart: Thieme; 2011.)

drainage of the effusion and microbiological testing is needed (Box 7.1).

> ### Box 7.1 Indications for Myringotomy in AOM
>
> - Failure to respond to adequate antimicrobial therapy.
> - Unwell toxic child with AOM.
> - Severe intractable otalgia despite adequate analgesia.
> - AOM occurring when child already on antibiotics.
> - Suspected suppurative complications.
> - Children with immunodeficiency.

If there is deterioration in the clinical state of a child with AOM with increasing fever and malaise, mastoid swelling, or any focal or general neurologic signs, for example, altered consciousness or fitting, spread of infection outside the temporal bone with a suppurative complication should be suspected. Urgent referral to a hospital unit is required for further investigations, imaging, and myringotomy or more extensive surgery, depending on the pathology.

7.9 Recurrent Acute Otitis Media

7.9.1 Definition

> ℹ️
>
> A group of children suffer from repeated AOM, with three or more episodes in 6 months, or four or more in 12 months.

The underlying cause of the RAOM is not fully known, but it may be due to host factors such as immaturity of the immune system, specific immunodeficiencies, nasal obstruction due to adenoidal hypertrophy, or immaturity of ET function. Consideration of these factors is important and investigation is sometimes needed if there is suspicion of an immune defect. In a child with infective episodes at other anatomical sites, investigation of the immune pathway, including specific pneumococcal antibodies and the complement system, is required under the supervision of a pediatrician. Recent studies have highlighted the presence of bacterial biofilms in the ME and nasopharynx, which may play a part in recurrent infections.

7.9.2 Management

Treatment of RAOM can be *expectant*, with observation to see if the child "grows out" of the infections with antibiotic and analgesic treatment of the individual events.

> The great majority of children with RAOM will "grow out" of the condition and parents can usually be reassured that symptoms improve greatly, typically at the age of 2 to 3 years when the child's immune system matures and susceptibility to URTIs becomes much less.

In recalcitrant children or where symptoms are especially severe, more active treatment is considered:
- Antimicrobial prophylaxis.
- Adenoidectomy.
- Tympanostomy tube insertion.

Antimicrobial Prophylaxis

Regular prophylactic antibiotics have been shown to be effective in reducing the number of episodes of AOM.[12] Previously sulphonamides have been used, but generally these have been discontinued due to the high risk of hypersensitivity reactions. A number of clinicians use a single dose of trimethoprim (2–3 mg/kg at night) or amoxicillin (20 mg/kg) at night for a 2- to 3-month period. However, studies have suggested that the average reduction in the overall number of episodes is only small (0.12 episodes per year).[13] Any reduction in the number of episodes needs to be weighed against the possibility of antibiotic-resistant bacteria in the child and also in the population as a whole. A trial of antimicrobial prophylaxis is reasonable in a child with severe RAOM, especially if the parents are not keen on surgical intervention straight away.

Adenoidectomy

This has been shown to reduce the number of episodes of AOM in children in a number of studies by as much as three episodes per year.[13] It is possible that removal of the hypertrophic lymphoid tissue improves ET function, but many believe that the adenoid acts a reservoir for bacterial infection, and adenoidectomy helps to reduce the bacterial load. These bacteria may exist in a free state or as a biofilm. Adenoidectomy does carry the small risk of hemorrhage and very rarely palatal insufficiency (see Chapter 18).

Tympanostomy Tube Insertion

> The mechanism of action of tympanostomy tubes in RAOM seems to be that of ventilating the ME space.

This may counteract the effects of ET dysfunction, but may also act directly on the bacterial biofilms in the ME cleft. There is evidence that these survive better in areas of lower oxygen concentration and therefore may be affected by the increased ventilation of the ME by the tympanostomy tube. A number of studies have found that tubes lead to a significant reduction in the number of episodes of AOM (one[14] showing a reduction of 1.5 episodes in 6 months and another[15] showing a relative decrease of AOM to be ~50%), and this has been confirmed by a recent Cochrane collaboration report. The risks of tube insertion are small, such as occasional otorrhea, and the surgery is quick and well tolerated (see Chapter 8).

7.10 Complications of Acute Otitis Media

> Serious complications of AOM are unusual, but the possibility of spread of infection beyond the ME cleft needs to be borne in mind by any doctor treating children. Children with complications need to be admitted to hospital for management under the care of an ENT surgeon.

Serious complications are classically divided into *extracranial* and *intracranial*, and are detailed in ▸ Table 7.1.
- Most cases of AOM will involve infection of both the ME cleft and mastoid air cells (tympanomastoiditis) with mucosal edema and a purulent exudate.
- In serious episodes due to mastoid obstruction, bacterial virulence, inadequate treatment, or reduced host defenses, infection may spread beyond the ME or mastoid mucosa.
- This leads to an infective osteitis followed by involvement of the periosteum, either by direct spread or through venous channels, to cause an acute mastoiditis.
- If the infiltrative and destructive infective process continues, progression to what is often termed *coalescent*

Table 7.1 Complications of acute otitis media

Intratemporal complications	Acute mastoiditis
	Facial paralysis
	Labyrinthitis
	Sensorineural hearing loss
	Petrositis/Gradenigo's syndrome
Extratemporal complications	Subperiosteal mastoid abscess Bezold's abscess
Intracranial complication	Extradural abscess
	Subdural abscess
	Cerebral/cerebellar abscess
	Sigmoid sinus thrombosis
	Otitic hydrocephalus
	Meningitis

mastoiditis may occur with breakdown of the normal mastoid architecture due to the lytic enzymes and toxic bacterial products.

- Infection can then spread beyond the mastoid either intracranially or extracranially, by direct spread through infected osteitic bone or through a septic thrombophlebitis of the blood vessels between the dural aspect of the temporal bone and the mastoid and ME.

7.10.1 Extracranial Complications

Mastoiditis

Epidemiology and Presentation

Acute mastoiditis is the most common of the serious complications of AOM. The classic presentation is that of a child with a history of AOM who develops a reddened, tender posterior auricular sulcus often with a degree of effacement and protrusion of the auricle (► Fig. 7.7, ► Fig. 7.8). This occurs due to the underlying osteitis and periostitis. If left untreated, this will progress, and pus will collect under the periosteum forming a *subperiosteal abscess* (► Fig. 7.9) or infection may spread further, potentially intracranially.

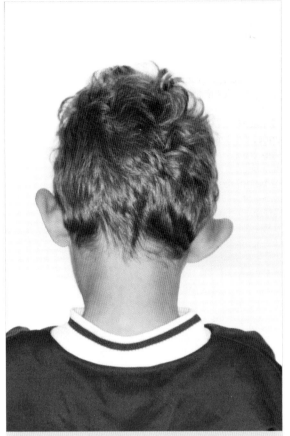

Fig. 7.7 Acute mastoiditis causing the pinna to project outward and downward.

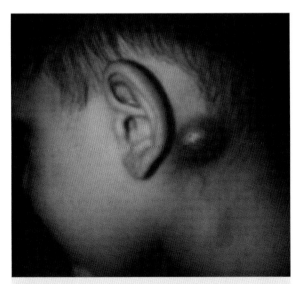

Fig. 7.8 Subcutaneous abscess secondary to acute mastoiditis.

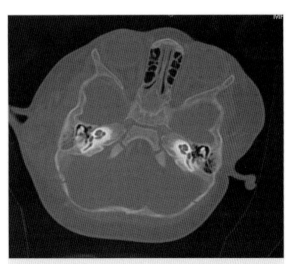

Fig. 7.9 Computed tomography showing subperiosteal abscess.

7

There have been a number of studies that have examined the incidence of mastoiditis in different populations. In Norway, the incidence of mastoiditis from 1999 to 2005 was found to be 4.3 to 7.1 per 100,000 in the 2- to 16-year-old age group, but 13.5 to 6.8 in the under 2-year-old age group.[16] In the United Kingdom, a recent study has estimated the incidence as 0.15/1,000 child-years.[17] Other studies have quoted incidences of 1.1 to 12 per 100,000. Most have found higher rates in children under the age of 2 years. AOM is, of course, commonest in this group. The incidence of mastoiditis after AOM has also been studied, and in the United Kingdom, it is found to be approximately 2.4 cases of mastoiditis per 10,000 cases of AOM (0.024%), but this was higher in children not treated with antibiotics (0.038%).[17]

Historically, Rudberg[7] in 1954 reported mastoiditis occurring in 17% of cases of AOM. Palva and Pulkkinen[18] in 1959 described the incidence of mastoiditis after AOM in Finland as 0.3%. Palva et al in 1985 reported[19] the incidence of mastoiditis to be 4/100,000, which they described as a marked reduction attributed to the increased use of antibiotics. There may have been other factors, such as a change in living standards over this time, which may have also influenced the rate of AOM.

There has been some debate over recent years whether there has been an increase in the incidence of mastoiditis as there has been a growing trend in primary care for withholding antibiotics for AOM. Van Buchem published a paper examining this subject,[20] finding only a small effect of antibiotic use on the rate of mastoiditis. However, children under the age of 2 years were excluded from the study, and this is the most common age group to suffer from complications of AOM. Other recent studies have shown a reduced incidence of mastoiditis in countries where antibiotic prescribing is higher (rates in Holland where antibiotic use is low are 3.8/100,000, in contrast with 1.2–2.0/100,000 in countries with high rates of prescribing).[21] There have been a number of papers that have suggested no change in mastoiditis rates (including a recent publication from the United Kingdom comparing 1991–1998 and 1990–2006 [Thompson et al[17]]), but a few suggest a rise in cases over the last few years. The picture is therefore a little mixed. This issue is further confused when one examines the literature, as in most series, approximately 40 to 60% of children admitted with a complication of AOM had already been started on antibiotics by their primary care physician for the preceding AOM. Although 50% of children have had no prior treatment, it would seem that a high proportion of cases of complications have occurred despite oral antibiotic therapy. This could be related to the virulence of the bacteria involved, an inappropriate antibiotic, or poor patient compliance.

Bacteriology and Management

Reviews of the bacteriology of mastoiditis show that in up to 50% of cases, no growth will be found on microbio-logical swab analysis.[22,23] This is possibly due to the previous administration of antibiotics. Of those cases with positive microbiology, *S. pneumoniae* is the most frequent bacteria isolated. *Streptococcus pyogenes*, *Staphylococcus aureus*, and *H. influenzae* are the next most common, with *Pseudomonas aeruginosa* and a mixture of anaerobes and other bacteria found infrequently. Antibiotic therapy for mastoiditis or a complication of AOM must therefore be targeted at these organisms.

> Children with suspected acute mastoiditis should be assessed by an experienced otolaryngologist and, if the diagnosis is confirmed clinically, admitted for intravenous antibiotic treatment. Some will need surgery.

In the preantibiotic era, surgery—mastoidectomy with myringotomy—was the mainstay of treatment. In the modern antibiotic era, there has been a marked change in management. A number of recent series have shown that the percentage of children with mastoiditis who need to undergo mastoidectomy has fallen from 16 to 34.5%.[24] The majority of cases of mastoiditis, especially if treated early in its course, will resolve with intravenous antibiotics, with or without myringotomy. Some studies[25,26] have shown that myringotomy does not always need to be performed but should be considered if the tympanic membrane is still intact to allow ME drainage and also to collect microbiological samples. If a subperiosteal mastoid abscess is present at admission or develops, this will need drainage. Imaging may help delineate the extent of an abscess and is particularly good at showing intracranial spread including involvement of the venous sinuses. Approximately 10% of children with a subperiosteal abscess have an intracranial complication, so preoperative imaging is important. Decompression is usually performed by formal surgical incision; some series have described management with simple needle aspiration in addition to myringotomy and antibiotics.

Careful observation of a child with mastoiditis is needed because if the condition does not improve or deteriorates, further intervention with cortical mastoidectomy may be needed. This will probably be required if the child has developed an intracranial or severe extracranial complication. However, there are a number of children where the decision to perform a mastoidectomy is more finely balanced. If there is a subperiosteal abscess, the child is systemically unwell, or there is failure of resolution after more than 24 to 48 hours, many otologists would argue that mastoidectomy, with drainage of the abscess, should be carried out. However, some series have managed such patients medically with high-dose intravenous antibiotics. In the modern era of subspecialization, not all otolaryngologists may be entirely comfortable exploring the mastoid of a 14-month-old child. A number of studies have looked at features of mastoiditis that predict the need for mastoidectomy. A high white cell blood count and C-reactive protein seem to be suggestive, but none have shown any absolute predictors and there remains a degree of clinical judgment. There is also no information that suggests whether a complete cortical mastoidectomy or a purely drainage procedure is more appropriate. The following surgical techniques are helpful:

- In a younger child, the postauricular incision is kept above the level of the mastoid tip to avoid inadvertent damage to a lateral facial nerve.
- A facial nerve monitor, if available, should be used.
- The mastoid air cell system in a child has variable development, so a burr is carefully used to remove the outer cortex of the mastoid.
- It is useful to carefully identify but not expose the dural plate and then to open the mastoid air cells down to the level of the lateral semicircular canal. It is unusual to find frank pus, more often one find very erythematous and inflamed mastoid mucosa.
- A swab should be taken for microbiological testing, and a drain left in the mastoid for 2 to 3 days.

Mastoiditis with Intracranial Sepsis

Some children with AOM and mastoiditis will have established intracranial sepsis when they present. Others will develop this during the course of their disease.

The classic symptom of intracranial complications is an unwell child with high fever, spiking pyrexias, the so-called picket fence chart. The child may be drowsy or lethargic, occasionally with focal neurologic signs.

Children presenting in this way or whose mastoiditis is not resolving need radiological investigation to assess the temporal bone and intracranial compartment. In the era of broad-spectrum antibiotics, it must be remembered that not all children with an intracranial complication will present with classic signs, and a high index of suspicion and a low threshold for radiological investigations are important.

Computed tomography (CT) scanning with contrast will give good bony information and can show intracranial sepsis. Magnetic resonance imaging (MRI) scanning gives far more brain and dural detail and will show peridural infection, cerebritis, or cerebral abscess (▶ Fig. 7.10, ▶ Fig. 7.11). Adding magnetic resonance angiography (MRA) gives more information about the sigmoid sinus, especially showing thrombus formation or cerebral sinus occlusion.

Treatment of the intracranial complication will depend upon its nature but may need involvement of the neurosurgeons or pediatric neurologists.

7

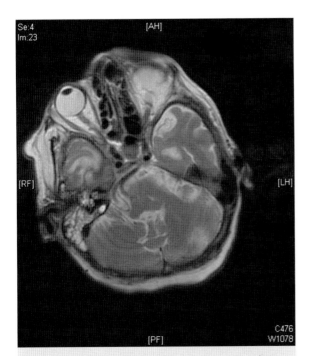

Fig. 7.10 Magnetic resonance imaging showing mastoiditis.

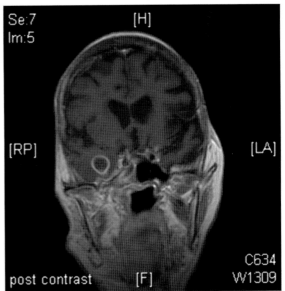

Fig. 7.11 Magnetic resonance imaging showing temporal lobe abscess.

- Extradural abscesses may be treated by complete cortical mastoidectomy with drilling down of the posterior or middle fossa plate to expose the extradural pus and allow drainage of this into the cranial cavity.
- Subdural abscesses may be drained in a similar way but with needle aspiration through the exposed dura in combination with the neurosurgeons.
- Intracerebral or cerebellar abscesses are often drained by the neurosurgery team through a separate burr hole.

A common finding in these cases is generalized dural inflammation with granulation tissue.

> All intracranial complication will need a prolonged course of intravenous antibiotics.

Facial Nerve Palsy

Facial palsy with AOM is uncommon. A Danish study found an incidence of 0.005%, mainly in children under the age of 3 years.[27] In the preantibiotic ear, this was far higher with rates of approximately 0.5%. A facial palsy may occur with a simple episode of AOM, but can also be associated with other complications notably mastoiditis. AOM is one of the more common causes of facial palsy in children, making up 30% of all pediatric facial paralyses.[28]

The facial nerve travels in the Fallopian canal through the ME cleft and is probably affected by the infective process occurring with AOM. Baxter[29] found that there were dehiscences in the bony canal in 55% of the 535 temporal bones studied, and this would certainly provide a route of infection spreading to the nerve from the ME. However, the rate of facial palsy in AOM is not nearly 55%, so other factors, such as host immunity, and not just direct spread of infection are probably involved.

> Treatment of a child with a facial palsy secondary to AOM is with admission for intravenous antibiotics and usually myringotomy.

There is little evidence that myringotomy confers a much greater benefit than antibiotics alone, but is probably justified in view of the significant effect of a facial palsy on a child and the need to decompress the pus in the ME if a perforation has not occurred. Antibiotics, myringotomy, and surgical exploration of the mastoid are needed in cases where AOM is complicated by a facial palsy and mastoiditis. The outcome however is usually good, with more than 95% of children having a full clinical remission and normal facial function.[27]

Petrous Apicitis and Gradenigo's Syndrome

Spread of infection and inflammation in AOM often occurs laterally presenting as mastoiditis, but far less frequently can occur medially to involve the pneumatized air cells of the petrous apex of the temporal bone. Petrous apicitis may occur subclinically with mastoiditis or may present as Gradenigo's syndrome with the triad of:
- Deep pain (often behind the eye) in the distribution of the trigeminal nerve.
- Diplopia due to an abducens nerve palsy.
- AOM (originally described as a discharging ear).

The trigeminal and abducens nerves lie in close proximity to the bone of the petrous apex, so a petrous osteitis can cause nerve irritation and dysfunction.

In the preantibiotic ear, petrous apicitis was frequently fatal but is now uncommon. It seems to occur in a slightly older age group, 6 to 7 years of age, than the peak age incidence for AOM.[30] Diagnosis is made on clinical symptoms and signs, followed by CT and MRI, which show increased enhancement at the petrous apex. There may be other complications of AOM associated with petrous apicitis, especially intracranial, so a careful clinical examination and review of the MRI is important.

> Petrous apicitis is treated by admission to hospital and high-dose intravenous antibiotics.

Before antibiotics, there were many operations described for petrous apex drainage around the osseous labyrinth, but surgery is extremely challenging, is associated with significant morbidity, including a high risk of facial paralysis and iatrogenic intracranial pathology, and is nowadays far less often needed. Most centers will perform a myringotomy if the ear is not discharging, and if there are concerns, a cortical mastoidectomy will be performed. However, there are reports of resolution with intravenous antibiotics alone, so treatment will depend upon the clinical state of the child and his/her response to therapy. Serial imaging and careful monitoring of the child's clinical condition determines the need for further intervention. If surgery is contemplated, seek the help of an experienced specialist otologist.

Bezold's Abscess

Freidrich Bezold in 1881 described a complication of mastoiditis with an abscess forming in the neck caused by suppuration in the mastoid eroding the mastoid cortex around the digastric ridge. The infection spreads between the digastric and sternocleidomastoid muscles, leading to an abscess below the sternocleidomastoid muscle or in the deep lateral neck space. Bezold described this as occurring in 20% of cases of mastoiditis after AOM, but today it is a rare occurrence, although there are still some cases reported.[31]

Bezold's abscess presents with neck pain associated with, or after, AOM. Neck swelling and erythema may not be marked initially as the abscess is in the deeper compartment of the neck. Clinical awareness of the possible diagnosis is important, and CT scanning or ultrasound is needed to image the deep neck. Treatment is with intravenous antibiotics and cortical mastoidectomy, and myringotomy if the tympanic membrane is intact, with neck exploration to drain the abscess.

Labyrinthitis

Infection and suppuration in the ME cleft can spread to the osseous labyrinth causing a serous or suppurative labyrinthitis. The usual pathway of spread is through the round window membrane, but invasion through the oval window niche may occur. Spread of infection is aided if there are abnormal communication routes between the ME and inner ear as can be seen in some congenital labyrinthine dysplasias such as the Mondini deformity. Labyrinthitis caused by AOM is not common, making up only 4% of the intratemporal complications in a recent report.[32]

A serous labyrinthitis occurs when there is inflammation in the labyrinth but no active bacterial invasion, and suppurative labyrinthitis occurs when there is active intralabyrinthine bacteria and pus formation.

The diagnosis is clinical and the main symptoms are vestibular with vertigo often followed by nausea and vomiting. Nystagmus is seen usually directed toward the opposite ear. The acute vertigo may continue for 1 to 2 days, with a slow improvement over 2 to 3 weeks, as the brain compensates for the loss of vestibular function. Hearing is commonly affected with a sensorineural hearing loss, but this is masked at first by the presence of the ME effusion, which has already caused a conductive hearing change. Some hearing can remain after a serous labyrinthitis, but total sensorineural hearing loss is the normal outcome after suppurative labyrinthitis.

> ℹ
>
> Treatment is with intravenous antibiotics, but once a labyrinthitis has started, even with immediate antibiotics, total hearing loss on the affected side is the usual result.

7.10.2 Intracranial Complications

The most serious adverse effects of AOM are undoubtedly intracranial septic complications, where there may be high morbidity and potential mortality. The significance of mastoiditis is that this is the "staging post" to intracranial complications.

> ℹ
>
> In all series, intracranial sepsis occurs in nearly all cases as a combination with or after mastoiditis (the only exception is meningitis that may occur without signs of mastoiditis). This is the reason mastoiditis must be treated seriously and urgently.

- Intracranial complications occur due to direct spread of infection from the mastoid osteitis, but also through a septic thrombophlebitis of the local venous system or mastoid emissary veins.
- Inflammation of the neighboring middle or posterior fossa dura may occur with localized abscess formation.
- Thrombophlebitis from the inflamed dura may lead to intracerebral or intracerebellar abscess collections.
- The walls of the sigmoid sinus are formed by dural folds, infection or inflammation of which leads to localized mural thrombus formation that may progressively reduce or totally obstruct venous flow.
- Propagation of this sigmoid sinus thrombosis (SST) may extend into the internal jugular vein, the transverse sinus, or other venous sinuses.
- This thrombus may become infected leading to frank pus or cause obstruction of the cerebral venous drainage system leading to hydrocephalus (otitic hydrocephalus).

In the preantibiotic era, the mortality of SST and intracranial abscess was almost 100%. In modern times, this mortality has fallen sharply, but death still occurs.

The incidence of intracranial complications after mastoiditis varies between modern series but is in the order of 4 to 20%.[22,23] There seems to be reasonably even distribution between extra-/intradural abscesses and infective SST. However, there may well be a combination of these complications.

Sigmoid Sinus Thrombosis

> ℹ
>
> The diagnosis of an SST can be difficult by clinical means alone. The most common feature is of a child who is more unwell that one would expect from a simple AOM, with high and often spiking pyrexia. Drowsiness, headache, and general malaise are often associated with SST, and in any child where there is a suspicion of this or any other intracranial infection, proceed to urgent imaging. CT scanning with contrast may show absence of flow in the sigmoid (the so-called Delta sign; ▶ Fig. 7.12), and MRI/MRA is also an excellent modality for imaging blood flow through the sinus (▶ Fig. 7.13).

7

II

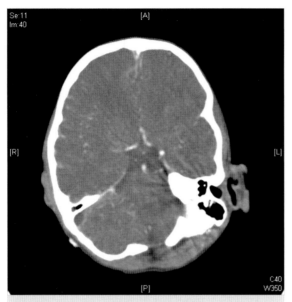

Fig. 7.12 Contrast computed tomography scan showing absence of flow in the sigmoid sinus (the Delta sign).

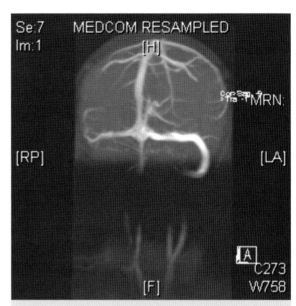

Fig. 7.13 Magnetic resonance angiography showing absence of flow in suspected right sigmoid sinus thrombosis.

SST is not usually managed by the neurosurgeons as it is usually seen in children with coagulopathies and presents to the pediatric medical neurologists where it is managed medically, typically with anticoagulation. The treatment of SST secondary to AOM is different, however, and has slowly changed over the years.

In the pre- and early antibiotic era, thrombus extension and septic emboli were not uncommon, and internal jugular vein ligation (IJVL) with sigmoid venotomy, thrombus removal, and packing were performed regularly. More modern series have shown that IJVL is now rarely needed, and surgical treatment has become more conservative, although there is still discussion over the optimum management.[33,34,35,36]

- Cortical mastoidectomy can be indicated, and it is important to fully expose the sigmoid sinus walls and some of the posterior fossa dura. This allows drainage of any perisinus collections or granulation tissue.
- Many papers have suggested that placing a needle into the sinus gives information about whether there is any blood flow, but this may be unnecessary as MRA now gives excellent preoperative information regarding flow and sinus patency.
- A number of series have indicated that in the presence of thrombus, the sinus should be opened and a thrombectomy be performed.[36,37,38] Recent studies, however, have shown that this may not be needed, and if the thrombus is not infected, the sinus can be left intact and recanalization may occur in a number of cases.[33,34,35]
- If there is infection of the intrasinus thrombus, then the sinus must be opened and the pus drained. It is usually

the case that with thrombus alone, the dural walls of the sigmoid sinus are thickened with granulations and can be left in situ, but where the thrombus has become infected, the dural walls have already thinned and the area of the sinus may be filled with purulent material and gas.

- If an SST has occurred, there is debate in the literature whether anticoagulation is needed.[34,35,38] A number of earlier case series recommended anticoagulation but there have been reports of hemorrhagic complications. A number of recent series where anticoagulation has not been instituted have reported good outcomes with no progression of the thrombus and no septic emboli.[34,35] The need for anticoagulation needs consideration and discussion with the pediatric neurology team, but the indication is certainly not absolute.

7.11 Acute Otitis Media and Chronic Suppurative Otitis Media

CSOM is the presence of a persistent nonintact tympanic membrane. The most common etiology for CSOM is a perforation following an acute ME infection and therefore represents the most common pathological complication of AOM. (see Chapter 9 for more detail.)

The prevalence of CSOM in children is high in some populations, such as the Maori or Aboriginal, where it may be as high as 5%. Browning and Gatehouse[39] in the United Kingdom found a tympanic membrane perforation rate of more than 4% in the adult population. CSOM may be inactive, but may also be persistently active with regular ear discharge, and with this the risk of possible spread of infection outside the temporal bone. Hearing loss due to the perforation and also postinfective ossicular damage can occur. Surgery is often needed to graft the tympanic membrane and close the ME, so this complication of AOM is not entirely benign. CSOM with cholesteatoma probably has a more complex etiology, but AOM may well play a part.

7.12 Key Points

- AOM is one of the most common diseases diagnosed in childhood usually occurring in the preschool age group.
- AOM is defined as a condition with acute inflammation of the ME cleft and the presence of an effusion and is associated with the rapid onset of the signs and symptoms of acute infection.
- The most common bacterial causes of AOM are *S. pneumoniae*, *H. influenzae*, and *M. catarrhalis*. Many cases of AOM have a viral etiology.
- AOM usually presents with otalgia, often following a viral URTI, but in younger children, it can present with more systemic symptoms such as fever, lethargy, malaise, and vomiting.
- AOM is usually a benign and self-limiting condition but can uncommonly lead to spread of infection outside the ME and serious complications.
- Many children with AOM can be managed with pain control alone, with natural disease resolution.
- Children with AOM who have persistent pain for more than 48 hours, more systemic symptoms, or are unwell should be considered for antibiotic therapy.
- Children with AOM who fail to respond to two courses of antibiotics may need admission to hospital for myringotomy.
- AOM may resolve by the eardrum perforating, leading to discharge of mucopus. In some cases, this can result in a persistent perforation of the tympanic membrane.
- RAOM is generally defined as three or more episodes of AOM in a 6-month period, or four or more episodes in a 12-month period.
- Most children with RAOM will "grow out" of it, but prophylactic antibiotics, adenoidectomy, or insertion of tympanostomy tubes have been shown to reduce the number of episodes of AOM.
- Complications of AOM are unusual but potentially life-threatening. They can be classified as intra- or extracranial complications.
- Mastoiditis occurs when there is spread of infection outside the ME cleft causing an osteitis. It is the most common serious complication of AOM.
- Mastoiditis is characterized by a reddened, swollen, tender posterior auricular sulcus often with protrusion of the pinna.
- Intracranial infective complications of AOM usually follow mastoiditis. It is important that if mastoiditis occurs, it is treated urgently with intravenous antibiotics and possibly surgery.
- Intracranial sepsis is usually characterized by an unwell, drowsy, or lethargic child with spiking pyrexias and, occasionally, focal neurologic signs.
- SST can follow mastoiditis and may require surgery and possibly anticoagulation, although this is an area of debate.
- A child with a complication of AOM should have radiological imaging to assess the ear and the intracranial structures.
- Other complications of AOM include facial nerve palsy, petrous apicitis, labyrinthitis, and Bezold's abscess.

References

[1] Teele DW, Klein JO, Rosner B. Epidemiology of otitis media during the first seven years of life in children in greater Boston: a prospective, cohort study. J Infect Dis. 1989; 160(1):83–94

[2] O'Neill P. Acute otitis media. BMJ. 1999; 319(7213):833–835

[3] Bluestone CD, Gates GA, Klein JO, et al. Committee report: terminology and classification of otitis media and its complications and sequelae. In: Lim DJ, Bluestone CD, Casselbrandt ML, et al, eds. Seventh International Symposium on Recent Advances in Otitis Media: report of the research conference. Ann Otol Rhinol Laryngol 2002;111(3 Suppl 188 Pt 2):8–18

[4] Aarhus L, Tambs K, Kvestad E, Engdahl B. Childhood otitis media: a cohort sutyd with 30-year follow-up of hearing (the HUNT study). Ear Hear. 2015; 36(3):302–308

[5] Liese JG, Silfverdal SA, Giaquinto C, et al. Incidence and clinical presentation of acute otitis media in children aged < 6 years in European medical practices. Epidemiol Infect. 2014; 142(8):1778–1788

[6] Froom J, Culpepper L, Grob P, et al. Diagnosis and antibiotic treatment of acute otitis media: report from International Primary Care Network. BMJ. 1990; 300(6724):582–586

[7] Rudberg RD. Acute otitis media; comparative therapeutic results of sulphonamide and penicillin administered in various forms. Acta Otolaryngol Suppl. 1954; 113 Suppl 113:1–79

[8] Venekamp RP, Sanders SL, Glasziou PP, Del Mar CB, Rovers MM. Antibiotics for acute otitis media in children. Cochrane Database Syst Rev. 2015; 1(6):CD000219

[9] Siddiq S, Grainger J. The diagnosis and management of acute otitis media: American Academy of Pediatrics Guidelines 2013. Arch Dis Child Educ Pract Ed. 2015; 100(4):193–197

[10] Wright H, Skinner AC, Jhaveri R. Evaluating guideline-recommended antibiotic practices for childhood respiratory infections: is it time to consider case-based formats? Clin Pediatr (Phila). 2016; 55(2):118–121

[11] Venekamp RP, Prasad V, Hay AD. Are topical antibiotics an alternative to oral antibiotics for children with acute otitis media and ear discharge? BMJ. 2016; 352:i308

[12] Leach AJ, Morris PS. Antibiotics for the prevention of acute and chronic suppurative otitis media in children. Cochrane Database Syst Rev. 2006; 18(4):CD004401

[13] Williams RL, Chalmers TC, Stange KC, Chalmers FT, Bowlin SJ. Use of antibiotics in preventing recurrent acute otitis media and in treating otitis media with effusion. A meta-analytic attempt to resolve the brouhaha. JAMA. 1993; 270(11):1344–1351

[14] McDonald S, Langton Hewer CD, Nunez DA. Grommets (ventilation tubes) for recurrent acute otitis media in children. Cochrane Database Syst Rev 2008;4:CD004741

7

[15] Le CT, Freeman DW, Fireman BH. Evaluation of ventilating tubes and myringotomy in the treatment of recurrent or persistent otitis media. Pediatr Infect Dis J. 1991; 10(1):2–11

[16] Kvaerner KJ, Bentdal Y, Karevold G. Acute mastoiditis in Norway: no evidence for an increase. Int J Pediatr Otorhinolaryngol. 2007; 71 (10):1579–1583

[17] Thompson PL, Gilbert RE, Long PF, Saxena S, Sharland M, Wong ICK. Effect of antibiotics for otitis media on mastoiditis in children: a retrospective cohort study using the United Kingdom general practice research database. Pediatrics. 2009; 123(2):424–430

[18] Palva T, Pulkkinen K. Mastoiditis. J Laryngol Otol. 1959; 73:573–588

[19] Palva T, Virtanen H, Mäkinen J. Acute and latent mastoiditis in children. J Laryngol Otol. 1985; 99(2):127–136

[20] van Buchem FL, Peeters MF, van 't Hof MA. Acute otitis media: a new treatment strategy. Br Med J (Clin Res Ed). 1985; 290(6474):1033–1037

[21] Van Zuijlen DA, Schilder AGM, Van Balen FAM, Hoes AW. National differences in incidence of acute mastoiditis: relationship to prescribing patterns of antibiotics for acute otitis media? Pediatr Infect Dis J. 2001; 20(2):140–144

[22] Dhooge IJM, Albers FWJ, Van Cauwenberge PB. Intratemporal and intracranial complications of acute suppurative otitis media in children: renewed interest. Int J Pediatr Otorhinolaryngol. 1999; 49 Suppl 1:S109–S114

[23] Luntz M, Brodsky A, Nusem S, et al. Acute mastoiditis—the antibiotic era: a multicenter study. Int J Pediatr Otorhinolaryngol. 2001; 57(1):1–9

[24] Tamir S, Shwartz Y, Peleg U, Shaul C, Perez R, Sichel JY. Shifting trends: mastoiditis from a surgical to a medical disease. Am J Otolaryngol. 2010; 31(6):467–471

[25] Geva A, Oestreicher-Kedem Y, Fishman G, Landsberg R, DeRowe A. Conservative management of acute mastoiditis in children. Int J Pediatr Otorhinolaryngol. 2008; 72(5):629–634

[26] Taylor MF, Berkowitz RG. Indications for mastoidectomy in acute mastoiditis in children. Ann Otol Rhinol Laryngol. 2004; 113(1):69–72

[27] Ellefsen B, Bonding P. Facial palsy in acute otitis media. Clin Otolaryngol Allied Sci. 1996; 21(5):393–395

[28] Evans AK, Licameli G, Brietzke S, Whittemore K, Kenna M. Pediatric facial nerve paralysis: patients, management and outcomes. Int J Pediatr Otorhinolaryngol. 2005; 69(11):1521–1528

[29] Baxter A. Dehiscence of the Fallopian canal. An anatomical study. J Laryngol Otol. 1971; 85(6):587–594

[30] Goldstein NA, Casselbrant ML, Bluestone CD, Kurs-Lasky M. Intratemporal complications of acute otitis media in infants and children. Otolaryngol Head Neck Surg. 1998; 119(5):444–454

[31] Marioni G, de Filippis C, Tregnaghi A, Marchese-Ragona R, Staffieri A. Bezold's abscess in children: case report and review of the literature. Int J Pediatr Otorhinolaryngol. 2001; 61(2):173–177

[32] Bluestone CD. Clinical course, complications and sequelae of acute otitis media. Pediatr Infect Dis J. 2000; 19(5) Suppl:S37–S46

[33] Bales CB, Sobol S, Wetmore R, Elden LM. Lateral sinus thrombosis as a complication of otitis media: 10-year experience at the children's hospital of Philadelphia. Pediatrics. 2009; 123(2):709–713

[34] Christensen N, Wayman J, Spencer J. Lateral sinus thrombosis: a review of seven cases and proposal of a management algorithm. Int J Pediatr Otorhinolaryngol. 2009; 73(4):581–584

[35] Wong I, Kozak FK, Poskitt K, Ludemann JP, Harriman M. Pediatric lateral sinus thrombosis: retrospective case series and literature review. J Otolaryngol. 2005; 34(2):79–85

[36] Lee JH, Choi SJ, Park K, Choung YH. Managements for lateral sinus thrombosis: does it need the ligation of internal jugular vein or anticoagulants? Eur Arch Otorhinolaryngol. 2009; 266(1):51–58

[37] Manolidis S, Kutz JW, Jr. Diagnosis and management of lateral sinus thrombosis. Otol Neurotol. 2005; 26(5):1045–1051

[38] Bradley DT, Hashisaki GT, Mason JC. Otogenic sigmoid sinus thrombosis: what is the role of anticoagulation? Laryngoscope. 2002; 112 (10):1726–1729

[39] Browning GG, Gatehouse S. The prevalence of middle ear disease in the adult British population. Clin Otolaryngol Allied Sci. 1992; 17(4):317–321

II

8 Otitis Media with Effusion

Marie Gisselsson Solén

8.1 Introduction

> ℹ Otitis media with effusion (OME), also called secretory otitis media, is an effusion behind the tympanic membrane without signs of acute inflammation.

Short-lived middle ear effusions are common, for example, following an acute otitis media (AOM), and need no treatment. Therefore, OME is usually taken to mean an effusion that has persisted for at least 3 months.

8.2 Epidemiology and Prevalence

> ℹ Middle ear effusion is the most common ear disease that occurs in children and practically all are affected at some point.[1,2] This is also the most common cause for transitory hearing loss in children.

The highest prevalence is found in children aged 1 to 5 years, but after the age of 8 years, OME is much less frequent.[1,2,3] It has been estimated that 50 to 80% of 4-year-olds in Europe and the United States have been affected by OME at least once,[2,4] and one study in the United Kingdom showed 5% of 5-year-olds to have persistent (at least 3 months) bilateral hearing impairment due to OME.[5]

There are two age peaks for OME, the first by 2 years of age and the second by 4 to 5 years of age, with a prevalence of approximately 16 to 20%.[4] During the former peak, the OME can usually be related to an episode of AOM, whereas during the latter, it more often cannot.[6,7,8] There is a strong seasonal variation with the disease being more common during the winter months, when the incidences of viral infections and AOM are higher.[9] Though no causal connection has been proven, numerous studies have shown an association between OME and allergic rhinitis.[10]

8.3 Etiology and Risk Factors

8.3.1 Etiology

OME can develop after an episode of AOM, after a viral infection, or without a previous infection. It is a multifactorial disease depending on endogenous factors (e.g., age, genetics, immunology, anatomy) as well as exogenous factors (e.g., siblings, day care, season).[11]

There are different theories as to how and why the middle ear fluid develops:

- The *ex vacuo theory* suggests that a dysfunctional Eustachian tube causes a low pressure in the middle ear, which in turn causes the middle ear mucosa to produce fluid.[12,13]
- The *inflammation theory* suggests that the inflammatory changes that occur in the middle ear mucosa during a viral or bacterial infection lead to upregulation of mucin-producing genes and thus to a production of fluid.[14,15]
- The *biofilm theory* suggests that it is bacterial biofilms in the middle ear that cause an inflammatory response, leading to the production of fluid. A biofilm is a bacterial community enclosed in a polymeric matrix. Bacteria within a biofilm differ from their planktonic counterparts in many ways. For example, they are less susceptible to antibiotics and do not grow in conventional cultures, which would explain why OME fluids are often culture negative.[16] Biofilms found in the middle ears of children receiving tympanostomy tubes for OME have been shown to contain ordinary AOM pathogens, such as *Streptococcus pneumoniae* and *Haemophilus influenzae*.[17] The adenoid often harbors biofilms, which could possibly, as discussed later, explain the beneficial effect of adenoidectomy in persistent cases of OME.

8.3.2 Risk Factors

Several risk factors for OME have been identified (▶ Table 8.1).

In twin studies, heredity has clearly been shown to play a role in the development of OME.[18,19] The same is true for having siblings and attending day care.[20] Both these factors lead to an increased mixing with other children, resulting in an increased probability of contracting upper airway infections. AOM is also a risk/etiological factor for developing OME.[21] Other factors that have been discussed but have not been proved to have a causal connection with OME are artificial feeding or a short duration of breast-feeding, parental smoking,[22,23] allergy,[24] and gastroesophageal reflux.[25]

Children with Down's syndrome almost universally suffer from OME from an early age. This OME is of a chronic nature and often persists to an older age than in healthy children. Another group of children who almost always suffer from OME are those with a cleft palate. This malformation affects the muscles that are engaged in opening the Eustachian tube, leaving the children particularly prone to OME.

Table 8.1 Risk factors for otitis media with effusion

Risk factor		Possible mechanism
Proven risk factors	Heredity	Anatomy, genetic susceptibility, immunological factors
	Siblings	Increased exposure to viral infections
	Day-care attendance	Increased exposure to viral infections
	AOM	Residual effusion, biofilm formation
	Down's syndrome	Impaired opening of Eustachian tube, increased susceptibility to infections
	Cleft palate	Impaired opening of Eustachian tube
	Ciliary dysfunction	Increased risk for infections due to reduced clearing of debris
Unclear risk factors	Short period of breast-feeding	Increased susceptibility to infections, earlier onset of AOM
	Passive smoking	Increased risk for AOM
	Allergy	Inflammatory changes in mucous membranes
	Gastroesophageal reflux	Inflammatory changes in mucous membranes

Abbreviation: AOM, acute otitis media.

8.4 Clinical Presentation

> The symptoms associated with OME are often mild. The main complaint is of hearing loss, but young children often present with vague symptoms such as irritability, bad sleep, and a loud voice.

An impairment of receptive and expressive language might occur during preschool years. However, older children with previous chronic OME do not differ in linguistic skills from age-matched children without a history of OME.[26] Older children may complain of a sense of fullness in their ears. Ear pain can be present, but is usually much milder than in AOM. Balance problems were long considered not to be associated with OME, but it now seems clear that some children with OME do have a vestibular dysfunction, as measured by electronystagmography and posturography. This dysfunction has been shown to improve after treatment of the OME with ventilation tubes.[27]

The mechanism behind the vestibular dysfunction is so far unknown, but the following three different explanations have been suggested:
- Ionic transfer through the round window alters the composition of inner ear fluids.
- The fluid in the middle ear causes serous/toxic labyrinthitis.
- The negative pressure in the middle ear is transferred to the inner ear, causing redisposition of inner ear fluids.

8.5 Clinical Findings

> The diagnosis of OME requires inspection of the tympanic membrane and evaluation of its mobility. Otomicroscopy combined with evaluation of the tympanic membrane mobility gives the most accurate diagnosis, whereas otoscopy alone is associated with overdiagnosis as well as underdiagnosis.[28]

The tympanic membrane is typically retracted, slightly thicker than normal, opaque, and with clearly visible blood vessels. The fluid behind the tympanic membrane can be either serous (yellow and clear) or mucoid (opaque; "glue ear"). Sometimes, a gas-fluid level or air bubbles can be seen through the tympanic membrane (▶ Fig. 8.1). Due to the fluid in the middle ear, the mobility of the tympanic membrane is reduced, which can be demonstrated by pneumatic investigation or by tympanometry.

Tympanometry is an objective way of measuring the mobility of the tympanic membrane by sending a sound wave into the external ear canal and then assessing the amount of movement this sound wave causes to the tympanic membrane and middle ear structures. The typical tympanometry result for a child with OME is a type B or C tympanogram. Whereas, a normal type A tympanogram shows a curve with a narrow peak of approximately 0 mm Hg, a type B curve is flat, indicating no or very little movement of the tympanic membrane, and a type C curve has a peak below 0 mm Hg, indicating a negative middle ear pressure (▶ Fig. 8.2, ▶ Fig. 8.3).

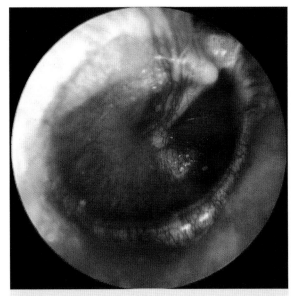

Fig. 8.1 Otitis media with effusion.

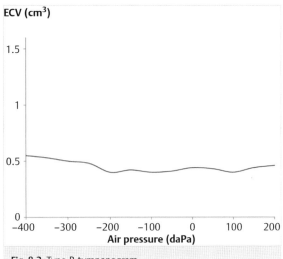

Fig. 8.2 Type B tympanogram.

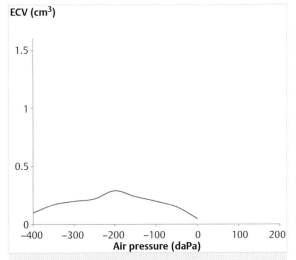

Fig. 8.3 Type C1 tympanogram.

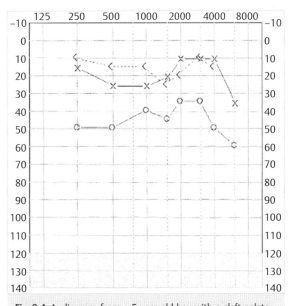

Fig. 8.4 Audiogram from a 5-year-old boy with a cleft palate and otitis media with effusion. He has a functioning ventilation tube in the left ear.

Tympanometry alone cannot be relied upon to select children for surgery,[29] and the hearing level should be assessed whenever there is a suspicion of hearing loss or when the OME condition has persisted for more than 3 months. After the age of 4 years, most children are able to perform regular audiometry, but age-adapted audiometry can be done by specially trained audiologists even in very young children. Screening audiometry at 20 dB is commonly used in children to assess that they hear at sound levels sufficient for speech development. Otoacoustic emissions are typically absent in OME due to the reduced transmission of sound waves in the middle ear. The typical audiometry result in a child with OME is a conductive hearing loss of 10 to 40 dB, often most prominent in low frequencies (▶ Fig. 8.4). The reason for the hearing loss is that energy is lost when sound waves pass from air to fluid, and the mobility of the ossicular chain is reduced. A summary of diagnostic methods and associated clinical findings can be found in ▶ Table 8.2.

Table 8.2 Summary of diagnostic methods and associated clinical findings

Diagnostic method	Typical finding
Otomicroscopy	Retracted tympanic membrane, fluid in the middle ear
Pneumatic otomicroscopy	Reduced/absent mobility
Tympanometry	Type B or C tympanogram
Audiometry	Conductive hearing loss of 10–40 dB, especially low frequencies
Otoacoustic emissions	Absent

8.6 Natural History

> The spontaneous resolution rate for middle ear effusions is very high, with 40% of cases resolving within 7 days, and 75 to 90% within 4 weeks.[30]

The longer the fluid has persisted, the less likely it is to resolve spontaneously.[31] The fluid per se is not harmful to the middle ear, and there is no evidence that OME in itself increases the risk for cholesteatoma; however, a dysfunctional Eustachian tube is common to both conditions. In the case of cholesteatoma, the dysfunction causes low middle ear pressure that results in a retraction pocket and subsequent accumulation of squamous epithelium. There is no evidence that temporary hearing loss due to OME should cause persistent damage to a child's linguistic skills,[26] although there is some evidence of an association between recurrent otitis media with tympanostomy tubes, and behavioral and learning difficulties in later childhood.[32]

8.7 Management

Treatment strategies for OME could be conservative, pharmacological, or surgical.[33] Two things decide what action should be taken in an otherwise healthy child with OME:

- The duration of the disease.
- The degree of symptoms (i.e., hearing loss).

> Thus, it is the hearing loss rather than the OME per se that calls for action.

Children with comorbidity factors such as Down's syndrome, cleft palate, or learning or speech disorders are more sensitive to the consequences of OME and, in some cases, less likely to recover spontaneously; therefore, they should be treated and monitored more actively. These children may benefit from early amplification and need regular audiological surveillance.

8.7.1 Expectant Treatment

> Since the spontaneous resolution rate is high, the first step to take in an otherwise healthy child with newly diagnosed OME is to apply "watchful waiting."

The concept of watchful waiting is often used in the context of mild conditions with a high spontaneous resolution rate, such as OME and AOM. It is not simply "no treatment"; it implies an active follow-up after diagnosis and subsequent action if the condition does not resolve by itself.

- It is important to evaluate the duration of symptoms before the child has visited the doctor. There is often a considerable delay between the first appearance of symptoms and the first doctor's visit.
- Every 3 or 6 months, the child's condition should be reevaluated through otomicroscopy, tympanometry, and, whenever hearing impairment is suspected, audiometry. Older children could be instructed to perform auto-inflation, either by Valsalva's maneuver or by using special medical equipment such as the Otovent balloon (Invotec). Repeated autoinflation has been proven to have a beneficial effect in OME.[34]
- Concerning children who have started school, teachers and school leaders should be informed of any hearing impairment and be given strategies for coping with this. There are simple facilitating measures that can be taken, such as ensuring the speaker gets the child's attention before speaking, allowing the child to sit close to the teacher with a view of the teacher as well as of the other children, and reducing background noise.

8.7.2 Medical Treatment

- An updated Cochrane review from 2016[35] showed that children treated with antibiotics for 23 months are more likely to have resolution of the middle ear fluid, however, they are also more likely to suffer side effects, and there is no evidence of improved hearing. In addition, the risk of increased bacterial resistance has to be considered, wherefore antibiotics are generally not a recommended treatment in OME.
- The effects of *antihistamines*, *decongestants*, and combinations of the two have been evaluated in a Cochrane analysis from 2011. None of the studied substances had an effect on the resolution of OME; however, treated subjects suffered from more side effects, wherefore the conclusion was to advise against the use of these treatments in OME.[36]

- *Steroids* could be used intranasally or systemically. There is no evidence that intranasal steroids have an effect on middle ear fluid, hearing loss, or subjective symptoms, but children with OME may, of course, have allergic rhinitis that warrants treatment. Systemic steroids, particularly in combination with antibiotics, reduce middle ear fluid in OME for a short period. However, the effect on hearing loss has not been studied and there is no evidence for long-term effects; besides, continuous treatment with systemic steroids is not an attractive solution in children. The conclusion of a Cochrane analysis from 2011 was thus that there is no evidence for a beneficial effect of steroids in OME beyond 1 month.[37]

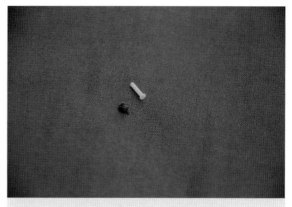

Fig. 8.5 Two examples of ventilation tubes.

8.7.3 Mechanical Treatment

Measures aiming to improve opening of the Eustachian tube have long thought to be one way of treating OME. Since it is difficult to explain Valsalva's maneuver to a child, devices for *autoinflation*, such as the Otovent balloon, have been developed to encourage successful opening of the Eustachian tube. Autoinflation in the treatment of OME has been evaluated in a Cochrane review that was updated in 2013.[34] Though the positive effects were relatively small (RR: 1.7) and the follow-up in most studies short, the low cost and absence of adverse events caused the authors to recommend autoinflation during the watchful waiting period.

Balloon dilatation of the Eustachian tube is used increasingly to treat various types of middle ear problems and has also been tried for OME. As yet, the literature consists of small noncontrolled case series of adult patients, and though results here are promising and without serious complications, according to a systematic review,[38] this procedure is not yet something to use in children.

8.7.4 Hearing Aids

Since the hearing impairment in OME is conductive, hearing aids have a good possibility of restoring hearing. A recent small study from the United Kingdom on OME children treated with either hearing aids or grommets concluded that the former group did not suffer from bullying or low self-esteem.[39]

8.7.5 Surgery

- *Myringotomy* (see ▶ Fig. 7.6) as a sole measure is not a recommended treatment in OME. The fluid can be suctioned from the middle ear, but the perforation usually heals after only a few days and the fluid reappears. Thus, myringotomy does not give a lasting improvement of hearing.[40]
- *Laser myringotomies* persist longer than conventional myringotomies but for a significantly shorter time than

ventilation tubes.[41,42] This procedure is therefore not recommended as a firsthand treatment for OME.

- *Ventilation (tympanostomy) tubes or grommets* exist in many different shapes (▶ Fig. 8.5). The tubes are usually spontaneously extruded from the tympanic membrane after a few months or occasionally years,[43,44,45] the time depending largely on the type of tube. After extrusion, spontaneous resolution of the OME condition has often occurred, and it is only a minority of children who need to have a second set of ventilation tubes. The current state of evidence for ventilation tubes in OME was evaluated in a 2010 Cochrane review. Using the high-quality trials for meta-analysis, a hearing benefit with ventilation tubes was seen at 6 to 9 months; however, no audiological differences were seen at 12 to 18 months.[46] A systematic review from 2011 showed strong evidence for a beneficial effect of ventilation tubes on hearing levels for at least 9 months, and likewise there was moderately strong evidence for an improved quality of life for up to 9 months.[45]

The most common tube-associated problem is tube otorrhea. Myringosclerosis is also common in patients who have had tubes (in approximately one-third of ears) but it seldom affects hearing. Persistent tympanic membrane perforations after tube extrusion occur in 2 to 16% of patients, largely depending on the type of tube used, but on average 5%.[47] For myringosclerosis as well as perforations, it is difficult to say if it is the tubes or the OME itself that is causative since most studies have been observational clinical studies without control groups.

- *Adenoidectomy*[48] has a significant effect on fluid resolution regardless of the size of the adenoid, but the effect on hearing levels is limited.[49] A possible explanation for the beneficial effect of surgery even when the adenoid is small could be that the adenoid supplies the middle ear with bacterial biofilms rather than that it causes mechanical obstruction of the Eustachian tube.[50] A recent systematic review and meta-analysis of children undergoing adenoidectomy with or without ventilation tubes and trying to identify groups who would benefit more from adenoidectomy than others found that children aged 4 years and older with persistent OME were likely to benefit from adenoidectomy more than others.[51]

8.7.6 Surgical Technique

As mentioned previously, there are several different types of ventilation tubes, and the insertion technique may differ somewhat between them, but the main principle for where and how to make the tympanocentesis basically remains the same.

- In children, ventilation tubes are usually inserted under general anesthesia. In an older, cooperative child, one might consider local anesthesia in the same way as in adults. The external ear canal can be filled with a local anesthetic cream, such as EMLA (AstraZeneca), for 30 to 60 minutes, after which the cream is removed by suction, leaving the external ear canal as well as the tympanic membrane anesthetized. Alternatively, one drop of phenol solution could be applied to the tympanic membrane using a thin cotton swab.
- The general rule is not to make the tympanocentesis in the upper posterior quadrant due to the assembly of middle ear structures behind this part of the tympanic membrane (hearing bones, chorda tympani, facial nerve), but otherwise it can be made where it seems most suitable. Different ears reveal different angles, giving more ready access to different parts of the tympanic membrane. In ears that show a severe tympanic membrane retraction, the easiest thing might be to try and make the tympanocentesis wherever there is some small collection of air.
- The tympanocentesis should preferably be made radially, that is, parallel to the fibers in the tympanic membrane (▶ Fig. 8.6), big enough to fit the chosen ventilation tube, but small enough to ensure that the tube is likely to stay in place even before the tympanic membrane has healed around it. If bleeding from the tympanic membrane vessels occur, which is common in severe and prolonged OME, the application of ear drops containing a mild corticosteroid and antibiotic is thought to prevent clotted blood from blocking the newly inserted ventilation tube. Ear drops could also be used for a few days after surgery in order to prevent a local infection and should be prescribed to all children with ventilation tubes to use in case of tube otorrhea.
- The choice of ventilation tube often depends on local traditions. One factor to consider is that **T**-shaped tubes tend to stay in place for longer periods than tubes with more shallow "collars," but they also tend to result more frequently in persistent perforations. Therefore, one might argue that this kind of tube should be reserved for children with long-standing OME who have previously tried other tubes that have been extruded prematurely.

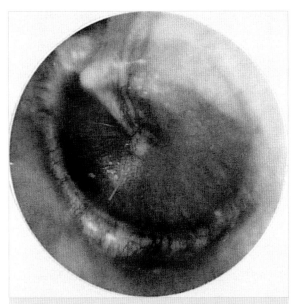

Fig. 8.6 Direction of a radial incision in the tympanic membrane.

8.7.7 Treatment Recommendations

The United Kingdom and the United States have both issued national guidelines on the treatment of OME in 2008 and 2004, respectively.[52,53] The guidelines agree on first applying a period of watchful waiting for approximately 3 months in children without any comorbidity. If the OME persists after this time point, audiometry should be performed, and if the hearing thresholds on the better ear are 25 to 30 dB, the child should be evaluated for surgery in the form of ventilation tubes (▶ Fig. 8.7). Primary ventilation tube insertion should be combined with adenoidectomy only in cases of nasal obstruction. However, children receiving ventilation tubes for the second time could be considered for adenoidectomy in order to prolong the effect of the tubes.

Hearing aids should be presented as an alternative in cases when surgery is less suitable. Some centers use Softband (Cochlear Ltd.) hearing aids, which make use of bone transmission and are worn with the amplifier behind the ear rather than in the external ear canal. Thus, these hearing aids do not require personal fitting, and can be borrowed for a period and then used by somebody else. The UK guidelines suggest hearing aids as the first-hand choice for children with Down's syndrome, based on the fact that the OME condition is likely to be long-lasting and that these children are more likely to have complications from ventilation tubes and to suffer from a simultaneous sensorineural hearing loss. Children with cleft palate may also be best treated with hearing aids as the OME tends to persist and tympanostomy tubes may need to be used for a prolonged period with an increased risk of infection and perforation.[52]

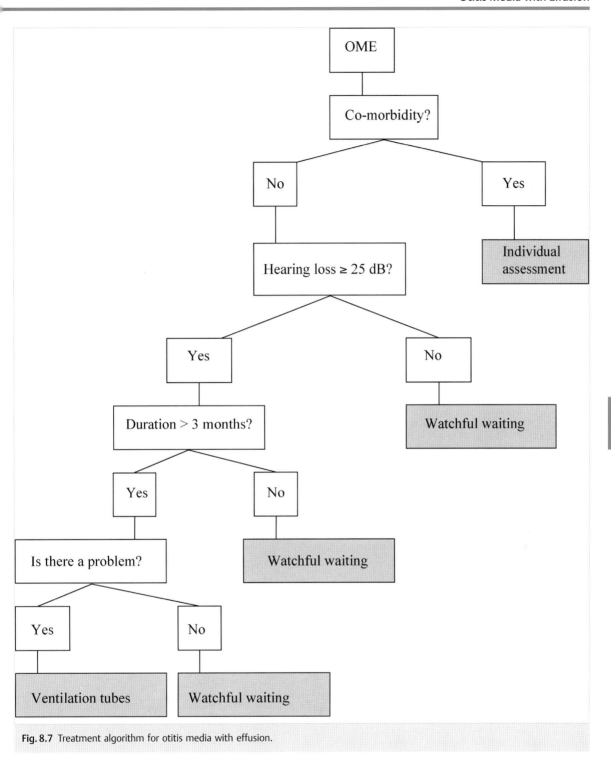

Fig. 8.7 Treatment algorithm for otitis media with effusion.

8

8.8 Key Points

- The duration and degree of hearing loss determine the treatment of OME.
- At present, there is no evidence for medical treatment of OME.
- Autoinflation can be considered during the watchful waiting period.
- There is evidence that ventilation tubes, sometimes accompanied by adenoidectomy, are efficient in improving hearing in OME for at least 9 months after surgery. Hearing aids could be an alternative, particularly in certain at-risk groups.

References

[1] Zielhuis GA, Rach GH, van den Broek P. Screening for otitis media with effusion in preschool children. Lancet. 1989; 1(8633):311–314

[2] Casselbrant ML, Brostoff LM, Cantekin EI, et al. Otitis media with effusion in preschool children. Laryngoscope. 1985; 95(4):428–436

[3] Cohen D, Tamir D. The prevalence of middle ear pathologies in Jerusalem school children. Am J Otol. 1989; 10(6):456–459

[4] Zielhuis GA, Rach GH, Van den Broek P. The occurrence of otitis media with effusion in Dutch pre-school children. Clin Otolaryngol Allied Sci. 1990; 15(2):147–153

[5] Williamson IG, Dunleavey J, Bain J, Robinson D. The natural history of otitis media with effusion—a three-year study of the incidence and prevalence of abnormal tympanograms in four South West Hampshire infant and first schools. J Laryngol Otol. 1994; 108(11):930–934

[6] Sadé J, Russo E, Fuchs C, Cohen D. Is secretory otitis media a single disease entity? Ann Otol Rhinol Laryngol. 2003; 112(4):342–347

[7] Ryding M, White P, Kalm O. Course and long-term outcome of 'refractory' secretory otitis media. J Laryngol Otol. 2005; 119(2):113–118

[8] Tos M. Epidemiology and natural history of secretory otitis. Am J Otol. 1984; 5(6):459–462

[9] Zielhuis GA, Heuvelmans-Heinen EW, Rach GH, van den Broek P. Environmental risk factors for otitis media with effusion in preschool children. Scand J Prim Health Care. 1989; 7(1):33–38

[10] Lack G, Caulfield H, Penagos M. The link between otitis media with effusion and allergy: a potential role for intranasal corticosteroids. Pediatr Allergy Immunol. 2011; 22(3):258–266

[11] Rosenfeld RM, Bluestone C, eds. Evidence-Based Otitis Media. 2nd ed. Ontario: Decker Inc.; 2003

[12] Alper CM, Tabari R, Seroky JT, Doyle WJ. Magnetic resonance imaging of the development of otitis media with effusion caused by functional obstruction of the eustachian tube. Ann Otol Rhinol Laryngol. 1997; 106(5):422–431

[13] Doyle WJ, McBride TP, Skoner DP, Maddern BR, Gwaltney JM, Jr, Uhrin M. A double-blind, placebo-controlled clinical trial of the effect of chlorpheniramine on the response of the nasal airway, middle ear and eustachian tube to provocative rhinovirus challenge. Pediatr Infect Dis J. 1988; 7(3):229–238

[14] Doyle WJ, Skoner DP, Hayden F, Buchman CA, Seroky JT, Fireman P. Nasal and otologic effects of experimental influenza A virus infection. Ann Otol Rhinol Laryngol. 1994; 103(1):59–69

[15] Buchman CA, Doyle WJ, Skoner DP, et al. Influenza A virus–induced acute otitis media. J Infect Dis. 1995; 172(5):1348–1351

[16] Post JC, Hiller NL, Nistico L, Stoodley P, Ehrlich GD. The role of biofilms in otolaryngologic infections: update 2007. Curr Opin Otolaryngol Head Neck Surg. 2007; 15(5):347–351

[17] Hall-Stoodley L, Hu FZ, Gieseke A, et al. Direct detection of bacterial biofilms on the middle-ear mucosa of children with chronic otitis media. JAMA. 2006; 296(2):202–211

[18] Casselbrant ML, Mandel EM, Fall PA, et al. The heritability of otitis media: a twin and triplet study. JAMA. 1999; 282(22):2125–2130

[19] Rovers M, Haggard M, Gannon M, Koeppen-Schomerus G, Plomin R. Heritability of symptom domains in otitis media: a longitudinal study of 1,373 twin pairs. Am J Epidemiol. 2002; 155(10):958–964

[20] Rovers MM, Zielhuis GA, Straatman H, Ingels K, van der Wilt GJ, van den Broek P. Prognostic factors for persistent otitis media with effusion in infants. Arch Otolaryngol Head Neck Surg. 1999; 125(11):1203–1207

[21] Alho OP, Oja H, Koivu M, Sorri M. Chronic otitis media with effusion in infancy. How frequent is it? How does it develop? Arch Otolaryngol Head Neck Surg. 1995; 121(4):432–436

[22] Blakley BW, Blakley JE. Smoking and middle ear disease: are they related? A review article. Otolaryngol Head Neck Surg. 1995; 112(3):441–446

[23] Williamson I.. Otitis media with effusion in children. BMJ Clin Evid 2007; 2007. pii: 0502.

[24] Hurst DS. The role of allergy in otitis media with effusion. Otolaryngol Clin North Am. 2011; 44(3):637–654, viii–ix

[25] Miura MS, Mascaro M, Rosenfeld RM. Association between otitis media and gastroesophageal reflux: a systematic review. Otolaryngol Head Neck Surg. 2012; 146(3):345–352

[26] Roberts JE, Rosenfeld RM, Zeisel SA. Otitis media and speech and language: a meta-analysis of prospective studies. Pediatrics. 2004; 113(3 Pt 1):e238–e248

[27] Casselbrant ML, Villardo RJ, Mandel EM. Balance and otitis media with effusion. Int J Audiol. 2008; 47(9):584–589

[28] Jones WS, Kaleida PH. How helpful is pneumatic otoscopy in improving diagnostic accuracy? Pediatrics. 2003; 112(3 Pt 1):510–513

[29] Knopke S, Irune E, Olze H, Bast F. The relationship between preoperative tympanograms and intraoperative ear examination results in children. Eur Arch Otorhinolaryngol. 2015; 272(12):3651–3654

[30] Mandel EM, Doyle WJ, Winther B, Alper CM. The incidence, prevalence and burden of OM in unselected children aged 1–8 years followed by weekly otoscopy through the "common cold" season. Int J Pediatr Otorhinolaryngol. 2008; 72(4):491–499

[31] Maw R, Bawden R. Spontaneous resolution of severe chronic glue ear in children and the effect of adenoidectomy, tonsillectomy, and insertion of ventilation tubes (grommets). BMJ. 1993; 306(6880):756–760

[32] Niclasen J, Obel C, Homøe P, Kørvel-Hanquist A, Dammeyer J. Associations between otitis media and child behavioural and learning difficulties: results from a Danish cohort. Int J Pediatr Otorhinolaryngol. 2016; 84:12–20

[33] Rosenfeld RM, Shin JJ, Schwartz SR, et al. Clinical Practice Guideline: Otitis Media with Effusion (Update). Otolaryngol Head Neck Surg. 2016; 154(1) Suppl:S1–S41

[34] Perera R, Glasziou PP, Heneghan CJ, McLellan J, Williamson I. Autoinflation for hearing loss associated with otitis media with effusion. Cochrane Database Syst Rev. 2013; 5(5):CD006285

[35] Venekamp RP1, Burton MJ, van Dongen TM, van der Heijden GJ, van Zon A, Schilder AG. Antibiotics for otitis media with effusion in children. Cochrane Database Syst Rev 2016;(6):CD009163. doi: 10.1002/14651858.CD009163.pub3

[36] Griffin G, Flynn CA. Antihistamines and/or decongestants for otitis media with effusion (OME) in children. Cochrane Database Syst Rev. 2011(9):CD003423

[37] Simpson SA, Lewis R, van der Voort J, Butler CC. Oral or topical nasal steroids for hearing loss associated with otitis media with effusion in children. Cochrane Database Syst Rev. 2011(5):CD001935

[38] Miller BJ, Elhassan HA. Balloon dilatation of the Eustachian tube: an evidence-based review of case series for those considering its use. Clin Otolaryngol. 2013; 38(6):525–532

[39] Qureishi A, Garas G, Mallick A, Parker D. The psychosocial impact of hearing aids in children with otitis media with effusion. J Laryngol Otol. 2014; 128(11):972–975

[40] Gates GA, Avery CA, Cooper JC, Jr, Prihoda TJ. Chronic secretory otitis media: effects of surgical management. Ann Otol Rhinol Laryngol Suppl. 1989; 138:2–32

[41] D'Eredità R, Shah UK. Contact diode laser myringotomy for medium-duration middle ear ventilation in children. Int J Pediatr Otorhinolaryngol. 2006; 70(6):1077–1080

[42] Youssef TF, Ahmed MR. Laser-assisted myringotomy versus conventional myringotomy with ventilation tube insertion in treatment of otitis media with effusion: long-term follow-up. Interv Med Appl Sci. 2013; 5(1):16–20

[43] Moon IS, Kwon MO, Park CY, et al. When should retained Paparella type I tympanostomy tubes be removed in asymptomatic children? Auris Nasus Larynx. 2013; 40(2):150–153

[44] Ichihara T, , Mori A, Kanazawa A, Nishikado A, Kawata R. Ventilation tube treatment in children with otitis media with effusion. Otolaryngol Head Neck Surg. 2012; 147 Suppl 2:225

[45] Hellström S, Groth A, Jörgensen F, et al. Ventilation tube treatment: a systematic review of the literature. Otolaryngol Head Neck Surg. 2011; 145(3):383–395

[46] Browning GG, Rovers MM, Williamson I, Lous J, Burton MJ. Grommets (ventilation tubes) for hearing loss associated with otitis media with effusion in children. Cochrane Database Syst Rev. 2010(10): CD001801

[47] Kay DJ, Nelson M, Rosenfeld RM. Meta-analysis of tympanostomy tube sequelae. Otolaryngol Head Neck Surg. 2001; 124(4):374–380

[48] Eliçora SS, Öztürk M, Sevinç R, Derin S, Dinç AE, Erdem D. Risk factors for otitis media effusion in children who have adenoid hypertrophia. Int J Pediatr Otorhinolaryngol. 2015; 79(3):374–377

[49] van den Aardweg MT, Schilder AG, Herkert E, Boonacker CW, Rovers MM. Adenoidectomy for otitis media in children. Cochrane Database Syst Rev. 2010(1):CD007810

[50] Park K. Otitis media and tonsils—role of adenoidectomy in the treatment of chronic otitis media with effusion. Adv Otorhinolaryngol. 2011; 72:160–163

[51] Boonacker CW, Rovers MM, Browning GG, Hoes AW, Schilder AG, Burton MJ. Adenoidectomy with or without grommets for children with otitis media: an individual patient data meta-analysis. Health Technol Assess. 2014; 18(5):1–118

[52] National Institute for Health and Care Excellency. Surgical Management of Otitis Media with Effusion in Children. 2008. Available at http://www.nice.org.uk/guidance/cg60/resources/guidance-surgical-management-of-otitis-media-with-effusion-in-children-pdf

[53] Rosenfeld RM, Schwartz SR, Pynnonen MA, et al. Clinical practice guideline: tympanostomy tubes in children. Otolaryngol Head Neck Surg. 2013; 149(1) Suppl:S1–S35

8

9 Disorders of the Middle Ear

Gavin A. J. Morrison

9.1 Introduction

This chapter will review the presentation, evolution, and management of disorders of the middle ear in children. Perforations and retractions of the tympanic membrane (TM) make up the great majority of these conditions, but rare pathologies such as atresia, otosclerosis, trauma, and neoplasms also occur. Cholesteatoma, involving both the middle ear and the mastoid air cells, is considered in Chapter 10.

9.2 Perforation

9.2.1 Prevalence and Classification

Perforation of the eardrum is a common childhood event (see Chapter 7). Box 9.1 shows the causes of TM perforations in children. The most common is perforation with an acute otitis media (AOM), which will usually heal quickly and spontaneously. Repeated infections can lead to a nonhealing perforation—one form of chronic suppurative otitis media (CSOM). In the developed world, the next most common cause of central persistent TM perforation is following extrusion of short-term ventilation tubes (grommets) and occurs in approximately 2.2% of ears or 4.4% of patients treated with grommets, and in 16.6% of those treated with long-term tympanostomy tubes (see Chapter 8).[1]

> **Box 9.1 Causes of Tympanic Membrane Perforations**
>
> - AOM and recurrent AOM.
> - Postventilation tubes (more than 2% per ear: Shah grommets).
> - Direct trauma to TM.
> - CSOM and specific CSOM such as tuberculosis, actinomycosis, and syphilis.
> - Barotrauma.
> - Otitis externa such as myringitis.
> - Blast injury (beware implantation cholesteatoma).

Factors that predispose to perforation are poverty, deprivation and low socioeconomic status, recurrent otitis media, Eustachian tube (ET) dysfunction, atrophic segments with poor drum vascularity, and the presence of retractions. Ethnicity also plays a role; the highest prevalence of recurrent otitis media is in Australian Aborigines, Native Americans, Indians, and Inuits.[2] Low rates are found in South Koreans. This ethnic variation is independent of socioeconomic factors.

CSOM has traditionally been classified as:
- *Tubotympanic*, where there is a central perforation (i.e., of the pars tensa), usually without cholesteatoma, that is, "mucosal" disease.
- *Atticoantral*, in which there may be a marginal retraction, marginal perforation, or attic (pars flaccida) disease with a greater likelihood of cholesteatoma.

The central perforation, tubotympanic, type is traditionally considered "safe", whereas atticoantral disease with cholesteatoma is considered "unsafe." If by safe we mean "unlikely to cause deeper erosion of the ossicular chain or temporal bone over the otic capsule," then this terminology is correct, but if by unsafe we mean a greater likelihood of complicated ear disease leading to meningitis or brain abscess, then the distinction is less clear. Browning[3] showed that both forms of CSOM can lead to brain abscess, although the risk is less after a modified radical mastoidectomy or in mucosal disease and greater in the presence of cholesteatoma.

> i
>
> The important factor is probably the presence or absence of cholesteatoma. For this reason, many now classify COSM as either of the following:
> 1. CSOM with cholesteatoma,
> 2. CSOM without cholesteatoma.

The risk of intracranial infection in the presence of an untreated active CSOM with or without cholesteatoma has been estimated in a 30-year-old adult to be 1 in 10,000 per annum or a lifetime cumulative risk of 1 in 200.[4] The risk for young children is probably higher as intracranial sepsis occurs mainly in children under the age of 3 years.

9.2.2 Pathophysiology and Flora

In association with a persistent perforation, mucosal changes in the middle ear include hyperplasia, metaplasia, increase in goblet cells, tympanosclerosis, bone destruction, and arrest of pneumatization of the mastoid air cells.

A perforation is often quiescent with no active infection but the most common pathogenic organisms cultured in a long-standing perforated ear are *Staphylococcus* species followed by *Proteus* species and then by *Pseudomonas* infections. *Escherichia coli* and *Klebsiella* species are also common. In contrast, otorrhea through a grommet is more likely to be caused by *Streptococcus pneumoniae*, *Pseudomonas*, *Haemophilus*, or *Moxarella* species.

9.2.3 Clinical Features of Tympanic Membrane Perforation

> Children with perforations frequently suffer recurrent infections with otorrhea. The perforation will also cause a chiefly conductive hearing loss.

The severity of the hearing loss is highly variable. The child with a small central perforation or anterior perforation may have normal hearing, whereas a large or subtotal perforation may cause a 50-dB conductive loss. In general, the larger the perforation, the larger the air-bone gap. The low frequencies are most affected. In one study,[5] the site of the perforation, anterior or posterior, was not a significant factor. Experience, however, suggests a definite trend toward greater conductive loss from posterior perforations. This is usually attributed to loss of the "baffle" effect when the round window membrane becomes exposed to direct in-phase sound waves. However, in the aforementioned study,[5] the severity of the conductive hearing loss depended upon the sound pressure differential across the TM, which is inversely proportional to the middle ear and the mastoid air volume. This can be measured from the tympanogram if a good seal is obtained. The smaller the middle ear volume, the greater the air-bone gap seen on the audiogram. ▶ Fig. 9.1 shows a large dry central perforation.

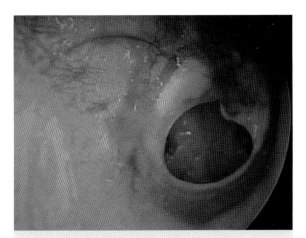

Fig. 9.1 Dry central perforation of pars tensa with myringosclerosis; right ear.

9.2.4 Management of Tympanic Membrane Perforations

Nonsurgical Management

> The small- or moderate-sized perforation, where the child has adequate hearing in at least one ear, and infrequent infections can be treated conservatively.

- Otorrhea is managed as needed if the discharge warrants it, with microsuction in a cooperative child, or by mopping the ear and prescribing topical nonototoxic eardrops with or without steroids.
- Use of aminoglycoside-containing ear drops three times daily is generally considered safe in an infected ear for 1 to 2 weeks, but should not be continued for fear of ototoxicity. Topical quinolone drops such as ciprofloxacin or ofloxacin (which in the United Kingdom are available as an eye drop formulation), either given alone or with a topical steroid drops such as *betnesol* is an effective alternative choice and carries no risks of ototoxicity.
- Persistent or repeated discharge despite treatment requires an ear swab for microbiology culture and sensitivity.
- If topical antimicrobials alone are insufficient, oral broad-spectrum antibiotics can be added. Co-amoxiclav will usually be effective unless the infection is caused by *Pseudomonas*, in which case oral ciprofloxacin for a week is advised and is generally safe.
- If the child has anything other than a very small perforation, parents should be advised to protect the ear with earplugs when the child is swimming. The author recommends the use of ear protection in the form of over-the-counter earplugs or custom-fitted water protective plugs from an audiologist for swimming in all children under the age of 2 years with a perforation, and in older children if the perforation is estimated to be 3 mm across or larger. Diving should be avoided without fitted plugs. In the bathroom, the head should not be immersed under the water or directly showered. Cotton wool with petroleum jelly (e.g., Vaseline, Unilever) as an earplug may be used in the younger children in the bathroom.
- In a child with bilateral perforations and a significant hearing impairment who is not yet suitable for surgical repair, amplification must be offered. If infections are infrequent, conventional acoustic air-conduction

hearing aids may be effective with an open or vented mould. Where infections are more frequent or become so, after a trial of an air-conduction hearing aid, a bone-conduction hearing aid, Softband (Cochlear Ltd.) (see Chapter 15) or very occasionally bone-anchored hearing aid (BAHA) can be considered.

- A child with unilateral perforation and significant hearing loss but a normal or nearly normal-hearing contralateral ear most commonly prefers to avoid the use of a hearing aid and manages well. The school should be informed about the side of the unilateral loss (see Chapter 14).

Surgery

Terminology

Surgical repair of a persistent TM perforation (myringoplasty) either on its own or in combination with middle ear surgery (tympanoplasty) at the appropriate age is usually a highly successful operation. The common indications for myringoplasty or tympanoplasty are shown in Box 9.2.

Box 9.2 Indications for Tympanoplasty

- Any ear with cholesteatoma.
- Recurrent otorrhea and nonhealing TM after 6 months.
- Disabling conductive hearing loss.
- To allow watersports.

In 1956, Wullstein described his classification of tympanoplasties[6]:

- Type I (myringoplasty) involves a repair of the TM only; the three ossicles are intact.
- Type II tympanoplasty is a reconstruction preserving the middle ear depth, but where there has been erosion of the malleus or incus, some form of ossiculoplasty is undertaken.
- Type III tympanoplasty involves a graft laid onto the stapes suprastructure with a shallower middle ear cleft.
- In type IV tympanoplasty, all three ossicles are lost, and the graft is on the footplate and covers the round window niche.
- Type V operation is for a fixed footplate, now being of historic interest; this was the '"fenestration" of the lateral semicircular canal used for otosclerosis before the popularization of stapedotomy and stapes prostheses.

Timing of Surgery

The medical literature does not give a clear answer as to the ideal age for reconstructive middle ear surgery. Randomized controlled trials have not been undertaken and expert opinion is derived from large case series and personal experience. Smyth and Hassard[7] reported successful surgery at a young age (5 years). Strong suggested that tubal cartilage and tensor palati muscles grow sufficiently after 7 years and so recommended surgery after this age.[8] However, Nagai et al felt that myringoplasty is warranted for younger children aged 7 to 12 years only if they have large mastoid pneumatization,[9] otherwise it is best to wait until children are 13 years and older. Most of the pediatric published series report a mean age of 10 or 11 years for myringoplasty.

A well-conducted study by Denoyelle et al showed that the success rate was not actually influenced by age at all.[10] Tympanoplasty surgery is certainly likely to be very successful in the child over 9 years of age. The decision to operate in younger children will depend upon the frequency of ear infections, whether there are bilateral or unilateral perforations, the child's desire to swim frequently, and the predicted ET dysfunction.

When an eardrum is repaired in a very young child, the risks of sequelae of hearing loss from recurrent persistent otitis media with effusion (OME) behind the repair and of continued AOM perhaps with reperforation become higher.

When the patient has a unilateral perforation, the decision is fairly straightforward. Repair is indicated if the child wishes to undertake frequent swimming, has a significant unilateral hearing loss, or is still getting infections, assuming that the contralateral ear is healthy with a normal or near-normal tympanogram and good ET function. A perforation that has resulted from a ventilation tube will typically show this clinical picture and can be repaired from the age of approximately 7 years. Factors such as a previously repaired cleft palate, a child with Down's syndrome, or a craniofacial anomaly need to be considered as they will adversely influence ET function, thus reducing the success rate.

The author will occasionally recommend tympanoplasty surgery at a much younger age, at the youngest 18 months, more typically at 3 or 4 years. The reason for operating early in these cases is substantial bilateral hearing loss from subtotal perforations, or unmanageably frequent and troublesome otorrhea. In the latter situation and with an intact eardrum albeit with the likely middle ear effusion, a dry ear will be much more acceptable to the family than chronic or very frequent discharge. Beware the child with a *persistent* purulent unilateral discharge. Not infrequently this will be caused by an attic cholesteatoma, which can be difficult to identify in a small and fractious child, and the management is very different, as covered in Chapter 10.

The medical literature has been equally contradictory with regard to whether the success rate is influenced by the presence of a discharging ear. The author's view concurs with that of Lau and Tos[11] that tympanoplasty results are poorer when the ear is actively infected at the time of surgery. A slightly moist but not purulent ear, however, can be operated upon without concern. Sometimes it proves almost impossible to achieve a dry ear preoperatively. Ear swabs, topical agents, and oral antibiotics are all helpful for a planned operation, which can then go ahead despite the discharging ear and with the use of postoperative antibiotics as well.

Adenoidectomy before or with Tympanoplasty

There is a nonsignificant trend in some published series suggesting that tympanoplasty surgery may have better outcomes if adenoidectomy has been undertaken.[12] The TARGET (Trial of Alternative Regimes in Glue Ear Treatment) trial data[13] clearly indicates that ET function is improved in the younger child by adenoidectomy. Therefore, if the clinical suspicion is of persistent adenoids or if tympanoplasty surgery is being undertaken at a young age, concurrent adenoidectomy may be advantageous.

Surgical Outcomes of Tympanoplasty

Most published series of pediatric myringoplasty show a high success rate in terms of closure of the perforation and graft take with figures from 71% to well over 90%.[14] Over a longer follow-up period, however, the success rates can fall off to approximately 65%. Hearing gain in the author's experience is usually exceptionally good in pediatric myringoplasty unless there is an ossicular problem or poor middle ear aeration, and normal or near-normal hearing can be expected. Published series, however show closure of the air-bone gap to within 10 dB in only two-thirds of cases.[10]

The risk of the OME persisting after the drum is repaired in the pediatric population will depend upon the patient's age, but one report gives a figure of 7.8%.[10] While early drum repair is usually highly successful, there is also a longer-term graft breakdown rate with reperforation, which has been estimated at 12.5% after 2 years.[15]

Smaller permeatal procedures such as "Gelfoam" and fat plug myringoplasty will carry lower success rates but may be suitable for small perforations, and have the advantages of taking little time and avoiding morbidity such as surgical scars.

Having a normal contralateral ear with good ET function is certainly a good prognostic factor for the outcome of myringoplasty. Denoyelle et al[10] found the following three prognostic factors for an abnormal postoperative TM (OME, retraction, or lateralization):

- Inflammatory changes to the middle ear mucosa.
- Contralateral perforation.
- Contralateral cholesteatoma.

Surgical Technique

The surgical approach for a tympanoplasty can be permeatal, endaural, or postaural. There is increasing interest in and experience with endoscopic techniques.[16]

Because of the relatively small meatus in childhood and for better access to the anterior mesotympanum, the author recommends a postaural approach. The graft material can be temporalis fascia or perichondrium, but periosteum taken from the immediate postaural mastoid bone also provides an ideal material. (The place for cartilage tympanoplasty is discussed later in relation to retractions.)

The edges of the perforation should be freshened, and an underlay technique with resorbable sponge support in the middle ear is fairly standard. If there is a small-to-moderate posterior perforation, then a "reverse through-lay" repair is very successful (▶ Fig. 9.2).

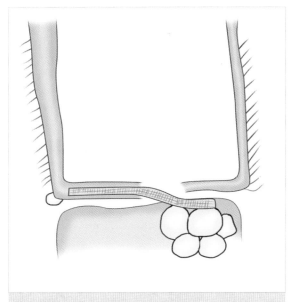

Fig. 9.2 Reverse through-lay myringoplasty: the graft sits on the fibrous layer posteriorly and under it anterior to perforation.

- In this technique, as the meatal flap is elevated to the annulus, a Plester D-knife is used to continue lifting the epithelial layer off the fibrous surface of the TM, without dislodging the annulus or entering the middle ear.
- This flap is continued toward the front of the perforation.
- Resorbable sponge is placed through the perforation only under the anterior margin, and the graft is then placed as an *onlay* on the fibrous layer of the drum posteriorly but under the lip of the perforation anteriorly with the sponge supporting it.

For a larger or anterior perforations and where the ossicular chain requires repair, an *underlay* technique is required.

> **i**
>
> It is important to trim the graft to the correct size. It should be larger than the perforation but not so wide that it folds and buckles. The TM is approximately 1 cm in diameter; therefore, the graft should be about this wide or less for a small perforation, but can usefully be longer to allow the posterior limb to extend a little way back up the ear canal. As a rough guide, the size of the surgeon's little fingernail will approximate to the TM dimensions. Placing the graft will be much easier if it has been thoroughly dried by leaving it on a glass slide.

Anterior perforations are technically more difficult to repair. There are two danger areas:
- First, a lot of sponge support is required anterosuperiorly in front of the lateral process of the malleus so that the graft can be tucked tightly under the drum remnant.
- The second area requiring attention is the anterior annulus where after freshening the perforation margin, there is only a tiny lip under which the graft can be placed. The option here is either to use a lot of sponge support and feed the anterior edge of the graft into a submucosal pocket down the ET or, as is the author's preference, to create an anterior canal wall tunnel and draw a small tongue of graft tissue up through this tunnel, thereby ensuring that the graft is secure and cannot fall away.

Finally, antibiotic or antiseptic ear packs are applied to the canal, and it may be helpful to carefully place a small dressing or silastic disc over the grafted drum before using multiple or longer dressings for the ear canal. If the child pulls out the accessible dressing, then the deeper ones will remain in situ. The author's preference is to use 1-cm-wide ribbon gauze soaked in bismuth iodoform paraffin paste (BIPP) for the ear dressings. Some surgeons do not employ any fiber-based dressings or packs (that need to be removed), instead preferring to fill the ear canal after surgery with antibiotic/antiseptic cream or ointment or even to insert absorbable gelatin sponges soaked in antimicrobial ointment. The wound is closed with resorbable subcuticular sutures so that they do not have to be removed at the first postoperative clinic visit.

9.3 Tubercular Otitis Media

This is now rare in western communities but still presents particularly in the developing world. Infection may occur through the blood-borne route or through the ET. Multiple perforations are described, and pale granulations in middle ear with visible sequestrated bone are typical. Facial palsy may result. Secondary infection and mastoid involvement with pyogenic organisms occurs. Diagnosis is through microbiology and culture and/or typical features on biopsy. Treatment is by limited surgery as dictated by the findings (e.g., removal of granulations and suction clearance) but primarily with antituberculous antimicrobial therapy under the supervision of a pediatric infectious diseases specialist.

9.4 Retraction Pockets

9.4.1 Classification and Natural History

It is helpful to grade the severity of both attic (pars flaccida) and pars tensa retractions in order to document progression or improvement and to allow comparison of treatment regimes in the medical literature. The most commonly accepted classifications are those of Tos and Poulsen for attic retractions (Box 9.3; ► Fig. 9.3)[17] and the Sadé classification (1979) for pars tensa retractions (Box 9.4; ► Fig. 9.4, ► Fig. 9.5).[18]

> **Box 9.3 Tos and Poulsen Classification of Pars Flaccida Retractions**
>
> - Type 1: retraction toward neck of malleus but airspace visible.
> - Type 2: retraction onto neck of malleus; no airspace visible behind membrane.
> - Type 3: retraction extends beyond osseous malleus full extent seen, limited attic wall erosion.
> - Type 4: more severe erosion of the outer attic wall.

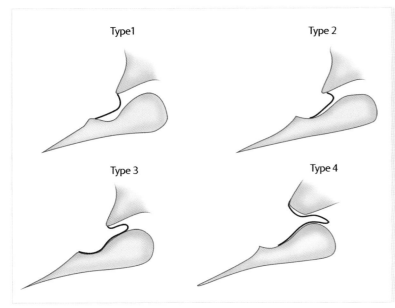

Fig. 9.3 Tos and Poulsen's classification of attic retraction pockets.

Type 1

Type 2

Type 3

Type 4

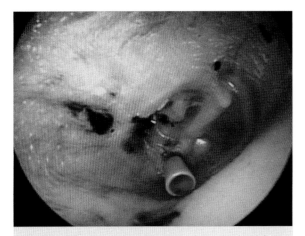

Fig. 9.4 Grade II pars tensa retraction pocket treated with long-term ventilation tube; right ear.

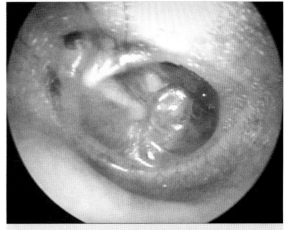

Fig. 9.5 Grade III retraction of pars tensa with effusion, left ear.

Box 9.4 Sadé Classification of Pars Tensa Retractions

- Grade I: mild retraction.
- Grade II: retraction onto the incus/incudostapedial joint.
- Grade III: retraction onto promontory.
- Grade IV: retraction and adhesion of the pars tensa to medial wall.

There are numerous other proposed classifications each with their merits. Charachon[19] employed the useful concept of whether a pocket is stable or collecting keratin.

The Erasmus atelectasis classification[20] proposes a system such that the stages fit the natural progressive evolution of the pathology.

It is said that retraction pockets fluctuate and can resolve. While this is certainly true for pars tensa retractions in the young child, it is not the case in the author's experience for attic retractions that either remain stable or progress. Likewise, deep and significant retractions in the pars tensa are highly unlikely to reverse spontaneously if they are still present by the teenage years. They can at this stage become and remain stable since the ET function has normalized. Understanding these natural histories allows for a logical treatment strategy.

9

9.4.2 Management of Attic Retraction

Conservative Management

In general, the management choice will depend upon the severity of the retraction. A careful microscope examination and the use of the otoendoscope in the office setting will greatly assist in the assessment.

> **i**
>
> Attic disease without infections can remain stable in the long term and may be managed conservatively (▶ Fig. 9.6).

If the limit of the retraction pocket can be seen, the hearing is good, and there is no build-up of keratin or infections, then a conservative approach is recommended. Active surveillance and recording of the findings ideally with otoendoscopy over numerous years is ideal.

Surgery

Attic Disease

If the limits of an attic retraction cannot be seen and if there is hearing impairment, keratin buildup, or infection, then a more interventional approach should be taken.

A fine-slice multiplanar computed tomography (CT) scan of the ears has a place as it may show more significant attic and mastoid soft-tissue disease. The assessment of bone destruction in the attic region can be misleading, for there is a normal notch or defect at the 12 o'clock position in the bone of the annulus. This becomes apparent only when the soft tissues of the pars flaccida retract or adhere to bone.

> **i**
>
> The indications for surgery in attic disease are periodic discharge, buildup of keratinous debris in the pocket, or conductive deafness with a type 3 or 4 Tos and Poulsen attic retraction.

The surgical options are as follows:
- Limited open atticotomy procedure.
- Closed surgery through a combined-approach tympanomastoidectomy (see Chapter 10).

In the latter procedure, the attic retraction and disease must be excised and the scutum attic bone defect should be reconstructed to avoid the otherwise, almost inevitable, re-retraction. If an atticotomy procedure is chosen, the attic shelf can be grafted (▶ Fig. 9.7) (e.g., with temporalis fascia). Alternatively, the bony attic defect can be reconstructed or even obliterated with a graft material such as cartilage or bone.

Undertaking attic surgery will involve the ossicular chain. It can be possible (with microinstruments, suction, and or laser) to remove all epithelium from the ossicular heads and leave the chain intact and mobile, but this is often not possible. The surgeon must therefore be prepared to remove the head of the malleus and the incus and undertake an ossicular reconstruction if necessary.

Pars Tensa Disease

The management of pars tensa retractions is less clearcut. A Cochrane review[21] concluded that no high-level

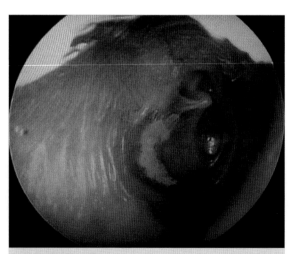

Fig. 9.6 Attic retraction type 3 without keratin or infections and good hearing; right ear.

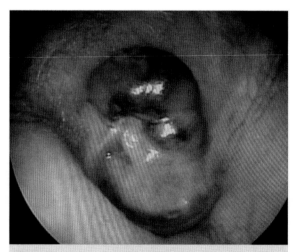

Fig. 9.7 Self-cleaning atticotomy; left ear.

evidence exists to support surgery (ventilation tubes or cartilage tympanoplasty) for TM retractions. This conclusion should not be read as support for nonintervention, as the review unfortunately both ignores attic retraction pockets entirely and only analyzes two randomized controlled trials. This misses the great wealth of important lower level evidence that remains essential to guiding good medical practice in surgery.

ET catheterization and balloon dilatation in an attempt to correct tubal blockage or dysfunction in the longer term have seen renewed interest. In the United Kingdom, the National Institute for Health and Clinical Excellence[22] suggested that this should currently be used only in a research setting in adults. It is not yet clear if it will have a long-term beneficial effect on ET dysfunction and hence a useful place in the management of retraction pockets. Once again, serial observation with otoendoscope and photo-endoscopy recordings, and use of the microscope will allow an accurate assessment of the natural history in the individual patient.

The management options will be as follows:
- Continued conservative observation.
- Insertion of a ventilation tube (grommet) for middle ear ventilation, which might elevate the retraction and improve hearing.
- A more invasive surgical approach of a reinforcement tympanoplasty with or without a ventilation tube or an ossiculoplasty.

> **i**
>
> The important factors in reaching a management decision are the hearing levels, and the severity and persistence of the retraction.

In association with more severe retractions, keratin buildup, infections, or bony erosions may be seen and are all indications for excision and tympanoplasty surgery. The patient's age and the assumed maturity of Eustachian tubal function can also be important.
- Mild, grade I retractions (Sadé classification) tend to be fully reversible if ET function normalizes with time. Unless they are associated with significant conductive hearing loss from a middle ear effusion (OME), they will normally be managed conservatively.
- If the retraction is grade II onto the incudostapedial joint and as is usually the case the hearing remains normal or nearly normal, then once again conservative management is usually recommended. This will involve serial observation (active surveillance).
- If over time the retraction appears to be leading to any erosion of the lentiform process of the incus or incudostapedial joint, then consideration should be given to ventilating the ear surgically with a grommet (ventilation tube). Again, the coexistence of persistent OME

with hearing loss is also an indication for a ventilation tube. Standard Shah or Shepard ventilation tubes tend to extrude early from atelectatic drums. Alternative longer-term ventilation tubes placed through the smallest myringotomy can be more successful, but, of course, carry a higher postextrusion perforation rate.
- Grade III or IV retraction pockets of the pars tensa require the surgeon to give careful consideration to the pros and the cons of surgery. The collapsed atelectatic TM lying on the promontory is likely to be associated with modest but significant hearing loss. If this is the finding in the child below the teenage years, then the first line of treatment is usually the insertion of a ventilation tube. Later, when it is felt that ET function should have improved at say 14 years of age, then excision of the atelectatic retraction pocket with a reinforcement tympanoplasty (commonly cartilage tympanoplasty of some sort) is the suggested management. Serial tympanograms can show that despite a fixed retracted drum, the ET is functioning adequately with a normal or modest negative middle ear pressure (type A or C1 tympanogram). At this time, in the author's experience, the reinforcement repair has every expectation of long-term success, and the reinforced TM should have little tendency to re-retract over many years.
- If a pars tensa retraction is deep and its limits cannot be seen even with an endoscope, in the region of the facial recess or sinus tympani, then unless hearing remains very good, the patient should be offered excision and repair, once again ideally waiting until the teenage years when it is hoped that ET function may be more normalized (▶ Fig. 9.8). If such an ear is left alone, then there is a greater risk in future years of progression to a frank pars tensa acquired cholesteatoma. The author therefore does consider reinforcement tympanoplasty a

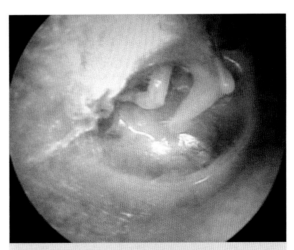

Fig. 9.8 Early grade III retraction, but into sinus tympani and facial recess with low-grade infection, represents good ear for excision and repair in teenage years.

9

preventative operation. The difficulty of recommending such an approach, however, is that there is no sound medical evidence that allows us to predict which patients will progress to cholesteatoma and which might remain simply a little hearing-impaired without infections for many years following conservative management.

There is good medical evidence that posterosuperior retractions do lead to primary acquired cholesteatomas.[23] Ideally, close surveillance should allow the otologist to pick up progression to an unstable status in the retraction with buildup of keratin and mild infections, permitting intervene before a full cholesteatoma forms. The decision should therefore be made following a reasonable period of time with good continuity of care and not on the basis of a single assessment in clinic unless a true cholesteatoma is already present. With this approach, it should be possible to undertake preventative surgery in the patients who need it.

When hearing is substantially impaired after erosion of the ossicular chain from long-term retraction or when the ear has an "out-of-sight" pocket with evidence of slight discharge or keratin buildup, then excision and reinforcement tympanoplasty with ossiculoplasty is more certainly indicated. Box 9.5 summarizes proposed indications for excision and reinforcement tympanoplasty surgery with or without ossiculoplasty.

Box 9.5 Indications for Pars Tensa Retraction Pocket Excision and Reinforcement Tympanoplasty

- Grade II: if erosion of long process of the incus (LPI) with significant conductive hearing loss.
- Grade III: if failed to stabilize after ventilation tubes, conductive loss, and once teenager.
- Grade IV: if retraction limit not seen, hearing loss, and teenager.
- Grade IV: if recurrent, even minor, infections.
- Grade IV: if debris accumulation in pocket.

Some children—especially those who have had severe recurrent middle ear infections and repaired cleft palates, those with Down's syndrome, and those with other craniofacial anomalies—may have lifelong severe ET dysfunction. These patients still represent the greatest challenge to the pediatric otologist. If their retraction pockets are deep and unstable with keratin buildup or recurrent infections or are progressive, then use of long-term ventilation tubes or excision and reinforcement tympanoplasty together with a new ventilation tube can be considered. Achieving a long-term nonretracted functioning TM without infections even with the aforementioned surgery may prove impossible. The primary aim in these children should be to achieve a safe ear, free of infections. Hearing reconstruction is a secondary consideration as the results are poorer. The atelectatic retracted drum with ossicular erosion but with no cholesteatoma keratin buildup or infections might in this situation be managed conservatively, and the hearing loss can be addressed through acoustic amplification or a bone-conduction hearing aid (Softband) or BAHA.

Techniques for Cartilage Reinforcement Tympanoplasty

Many different surgical techniques have been described in both children and adults.[24] Common techniques are the "butterfly" inlay method usually from a transcanal approach, "cartilage palisade" tympanoplasty, a full-thickness composite island cartilage tympanoplasty with attached perichondrium graft or a thinned cartilage with perichondrium, and "shield" cartilage grafts for total drum replacement. The butterfly inlay is suitable for small 2- to 3-mm central perforations, a disc of tragal cartilage can be punched out, its circular edge incised circumferentially and the resultant groove is "clipped" in to the freshened perforation. The other techniques are all underlay tympanoplasties, with the graft being palisades of thin parallel strips of cartilage alternating with strips of denuded exposed perichondrium. Cartilage islands and shields should ideally remain attached to a larger perichondrium tissue graft so that the whole composite graft can be stabilized and accurately positioned in relation to the annulus and meatal skin flaps.

Outcomes of Tympanoplasty

Yung[25] reviewed long-term results of fascia tympanoplasty, confirming that for the totally collapsed drum, the re-retraction rate was 50%. Cartilage (palisade) tympanoplasty especially for posterior retractions has since been shown to give a more favorable anatomical outcome without re-retraction compared with fascia grafting.[26] The Parisian group from l'Hopital Robert Debre[27] subsequently showed that when cartilage tympanoplasty was used for severe retraction, the re-retraction rate at 2 years was only 12% overall and yet significantly lower if the surgery was undertaken over the age of 10 years.

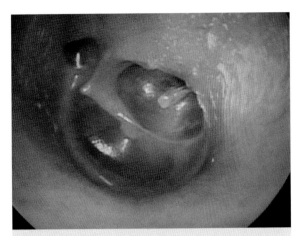

Fig. 9.9 Early grade III retraction, but into sinus tympani and facial recess with low-grade infection, represents good ear for excision and repair in teenage years.

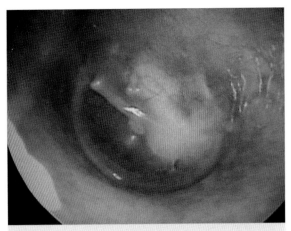

Fig. 9.10 Postoperative image, island cartilage tympanoplasty, and incus transposition; left ear.

The thickness of the cartilage could be one factor influencing hearing results. Results from various authors show quite variable hearing outcomes and rather poorer results than would be ideal. Theoretical considerations of sound transmission have shown that the optimal thickness of cartilage is 0.3 mm rather than full thickness from the pinna. Cartilage slicers (e.g., KURZ Precise Cartilage Knife Set, Heinz Kurz GmbH) can achieve precise cartilage sheets but not easily with an attached perichondrium, and the author's preference is to use a composite island technique, thinning the cartilage by hand with a blade and leaving a larger perichondrium sheet attached to the other side. It is then positioned with the reinforced cartilage under the posterosuperior or posterior drum, and the attached perichondrium can be positioned as a tongue extending over the posterior canal wall or attic wall for support. If the anterior half of the drum is normal, it does not require reinforcement (▶ Fig. 9.9, ▶ Fig. 9.10).

▶ Fig. 9.11 shows a flowchart for a proposed management strategy for pars tensa retraction pockets.

Excision of Retraction Pockets

Numerous authors have recommended excising a retraction pocket and leaving it unrepaired, or even excising a pocket and inserting a grommet in a different part of the TM.[28,29] This strategy gives up to 74% success rate in terms of spontaneous healing of the drum. The rationale is that the drum will show its high natural tendency to heal, and during the healing process, the middle ear pressure will be normal because of the perforation allowing time for ET function to improve as the middle ear mucosa is likely to be healthier. The author opines that this approach can be very successful in a patient with a relatively small isolated central retraction pocket. Typically, this will have developed at a site of previous perforations or more likely at the site of previous ventilation tubes. The totally collapsed atelectatic drum is not suitable for this approach.

Ossiculoplasty

Ossicular reconstruction can be undertaken in conjunction with myringoplasty and/or closed or open mastoidectomy if the air-bone gap is more than 15 dB and if other anatomical and audiometric factors are favorable. The ossicular chain tends to become eroded at the lentiform process of the incus as a result of previous acute infections behind a healthy drum or following chronic retraction onto the ossicles with or without infections. More detailed discussions can be found in manuals of operative otological surgery.

- When the stapes suprastructure is intact and mobile, the options are to use the drilled and sculpted incus, either horizontally in a mastoid cavity with a shallow middle ear depth or vertically in a normal depth middle ear, or to employ an "off-the-shelf" partial prosthesis such as the TTP-VARIAC System or a clip prosthesis. If titanium is used, then a cartilage interposition under the drum and on the titanium head is advised. The author usually quotes a 75% chance of a useful hearing improvement but a very small chance of a worse hearing ear.
- Small erosions of the long process of the incus can be repaired with bone cement or an interposition without removing the incus. The author prefers to avoid

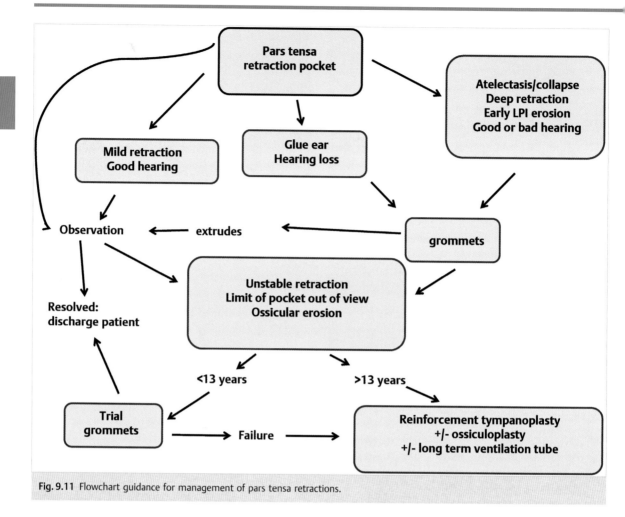

Fig. 9.11 Flowchart guidance for management of pars tensa retractions.

these methods as cement can show late fractures, and other assemblies can be unstable with "too many joints."

- When the stapes suprastructure is eroded and the footplate is mobile, the reconstruction requires a total replacement form the footplate to the underside of the drum or handle of malleus. Autologous bone is not recommended in this situation as it so readily fixes to the ponticulus bone. A total ossicular replacement prosthesis (TORP) is suggested. Numerous types are available. The surgery requires skill and patience since the TORP can easily dislodge. A shoe around the footplate made from titanium or cartilage, or even fascia wrapped around the shaft can help anchor it during the important healing period. Judgment of the exact length for the TORP and perfect positioning is critical to achieving a good hearing result. Success may be expected in 50% of cases, but there is a small risk of sensorineural deafness.

9.5 Congenital Disorders of the Middle Ear

9.5.1 Atresia and Congenital Ossicular Fixation

Atresia of the ear present from birth may be unilateral or bilateral. Commonly, the otic capsule is well formed, giving normal cochlear function and a maximal conductive deafness.

The infant with bilateral atresia requires immediate management, typically with assessment of hearing thresholds to confirm normal cochlear function, and a bone-conduction hearing aid or Softband.

Table 9.1 Syndromes with congenitally abnormal ears

Syndrome	Pinna	External meatus	Malleus/incus	Stapes	Facial nerve
Mandibulofacial dysostosis	Deformed	Atretic	Fused and fixed	deformed	Anomalous
Crouzon	Low-set	Atretic	Fixed	Deformed	Normal
Marfan	Collapsed	Narrow	Normal	Normal	Normal
Klippel–Feil	Deformed	Atretic	Deformed	Deformed	Normal
Osteogenesis imperfecta	Normal	Normal	Normal	Fixed	Normal
Rubella	Normal	Normal	Normal	Fixed	Normal

Unilateral atresia, with a normal-hearing contralateral ear, may also be managed with a hearing aid but the child can acquire speech and language without this.

The ear with microtia and atresia of the external meatus and middle ear is not suitable for surgical auditory reconstruction. The unilateral case should be managed in a multidisciplinary clinic where pinna surgical reconstruction or bone-anchored prostheses are offered. Staged rib graft reconstruction of the auricle or pinna would usually be offered from the age of approximately 9 to 10 years. Auditory aiding is offered from a very young age however (see Chapter 14).

If the child has a well-formed external meatus, TM, and good middle ear aeration, and the CT scan demonstrates a normal or near-normal facial nerve course, then ossicular anomalies or fixation can be corrected surgically with ossiculoplasty or stapedectomy procedures. In the bilateral case, surgery could be undertaken at a young age, but for the unilateral ear, the child should be old enough to understand the prospects for success and the risks before choosing such a reconstructive approach. ▶ Table 9.1 shows some of the common syndromic conditions that are frequently associated with congenital conductive hearing loss and the likely anatomical anomalies.

> This is extremely demanding surgery, and by far the greatest majority of patients with bilateral ear atresia will be best served initially with a Softband or bone-conduction hearing aid and subsequently with a BAHA or perhaps an implantable hearing device. Bilateral BAHAs provide some advantages.

Middle ear congenital anomalies can also occur with a normal or reasonably well-formed external ear, TM, and good middle ear aeration. The malleus and incus may be malformed, fused to each other, or fixed in bone at the annulus and in the attic. Isolated stapes fixation may also be encountered. The congenitally deformed stapes foot-plate may have a central defect with a perilymph or cerebrospinal fluid (CSF) fistula, from a preexisting congenital translabyrinthine fistula. These children may present with recurrent meningitis, and when unilateral, the preexisting hearing loss can have been missed.

- The principal management of the child with a congenitally abnormal middle ear or ears is amplification with acoustic hearing aid(s), a Softband, BAHA, or a middle ear implantable hearing device, if the canal is too narrow for normal aiding. Ideally, a specialist multidisciplinary clinic setting with an experienced otologist should be available if reconstructive surgery of the middle ear cleft is to be considered.

- If a child presents with recurrent meningitis, a source of acquired, developmental, or congenital CSF leak should be sought by examination and imaging of the anterior and lateral skull base, probably with fine-slice multiplanar CT imaging at first. Defects from the middle fossa at the tegmen or through the posterior fossa through the internal auditory meatus or the cochlear aqueduct, and from a labyrinthine fistula to the middle ear cleft will require surgical exploration and repair. An anterior skull base fistula with CSF rhinorrhea, likewise, would need surgical closure to minimize the risk of future meningitis.

9.5.2 The Facial Nerve

Congenital dehiscence of the facial nerve just superior to the oval window is a common finding and a normal variant. It is abnormal, however, for the unprotected nerve to herniate against the stapes and obscure the oval window. The facial nerve may also pursue an entirely abnormal course. Most commonly in the congenitally anomalous ear, it is far forward in the horizontal segment, and the nerve trunk tends to be shorter and therefore at a more acute angle. The nerve may encroach upon the stapes and oval window, or may be displaced inferiorly with a deformed stapes arch around the exposed nerve, which can cross the oval window, or may be displaced inferiorly with an absent oval window and lie across the promontory as a soft-tissue band.

9.5.3 Vascular Anomalies in the Middle Ear

A common vascular anomaly within the tympanic cavity is a high-riding herniation of the jugular bulb, seen as a smooth blue bulging structure. Rarely a stapedial artery (artery of the second pharyngeal or branchial arch) persists as a large vessel crossing the anterior stapes footplate.

9.6 Other Conditions Affecting the Middle Ear

9.6.1 Otosclerosis

Otosclerosis is a rare but well-recognized entity in the pediatric population. Presentation is often from the age of approximately 10 years, and the condition is more frequently bilateral. The first line of treatment will be hearing aids, but stapedotomy surgery can be highly successful and the author will offer it in teenage children. The literature reports surgery from the early teenage years but suggests it is best to wait until 15 or 16 years when the child has full understanding of the implications. A CT scan is recommended for diagnostic purposes and, in some cases, for bilateral congenital stapes fixation. The long-term outcome in expert hands is reasonably good,[30] but there is a slow progression over time with deterioration in bone thresholds. Denoyelle et al[31] reported that in a series of 35 pediatric stapedotomies, less than 20% had otosclerosis and the majority were undertaken for congenital stapes fixation.

9.6.2 Temporal Bone Fracture

- Most temporal bone fractures (80%) are longitudinal (▶ Fig. 9.12), with the fracture line running into the middle ear, and causing a hemotympanum or possibly tearing the drum and/or disrupting the ossicular chain. Facial palsy is rare. Early management is to keep the ear dry and free of infection. Audiometry and, if necessary, a CT scan of the temporal bone can be undertaken. Recovery can be complete but ossiculoplasty might be necessary at a later time.
- A transverse fracture of the temporal bone is less common and much more likely to run through the labyrinth producing a profound sensorineural hearing loss, vertigo, and a 50% probability of a facial palsy. A fine-slice multiplanar CT scan should define the fracture. Early management is focused on avoiding ascending infection and meningitis. Prophylactic antibiotics, especially if there is CSF otorrhea, are commonly prescribed for 1 to 2 weeks and the ear is kept dry. CSF otorrhea usually stops spontaneously, but if it continues after 3 weeks, then surgical repair is considered. If there is doubt about the nature of the fluid, a blood free sample

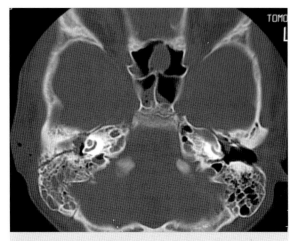

Fig. 9.12 Longitudinal fracture of the temporal bone is the most common injury.

should be collected and sent for analysis. CSF can be diagnosed by detection of β2-transferrin using protein electrophoresis. Another less commonly available test is β-trace protein quantitation using immunoassay. Both the new immune-fixation tests for β2-transferrin and the β-trace protein are effective at detecting CSF leaks.

> **i**
>
> Facial nerve management is usually undertaken based on clinical grounds. In all cases, systemic steroids to reduce edema around the nerve are prescribed.

If the facial palsy was complete and immediate, then early facial nerve decompression or repair surgically is indicated. A partial weakness (facial paresis) is much more likely to recover with conservative treatment. The CT scan, however, is very important as it may show an area of contusion or a fracture in the course of the facial nerve in which case decompression surgically is worthwhile. The entire course of the facial nerve can be decompressed if the fracture has caused a profound deafness, but where the hearing loss is conductive, only the horizontal and descending tympanomastoid segments of the nerve are readily accessed.

If the facial nerve palsy was definitely delayed in its onset, then conservative treatment is usually advisable as the nerve must be in complete continuity (neuropraxia).

9.6.3 Histiocytosis X

Histiocytosis comprises a number of disorders in which there is infiltration and accumulation of monocytes, macrophages, and dendritic cells in the affected tissues. It rarely involves the middle ear. Nomenclature to describe the various disorders has changed over time. Langerhans' cell histiocytosis (LCH) was initially subdivided into eosinophilic granuloma, Hand–Schüller–Christian's disease, and Letterer–Siwe's disease, but these are now unified under the term *histiocytosis X*.

The World Health Organization classifies histiocytosis X as:

- Class I: LCH.
- Class II: mononuclear phagocytes other than Langerhans' cells.
- Class III: malignant histiocytic disorders.

The condition is slightly more common in males and can occur at any age from neonates to adults, but it peaks in children from 1 to 3 years. It can be localized in an isolated bone such as the temporal bone or involve multiple organs and systems. The clinical presentation includes the skull bones in 49% of cases. When the ear is involved, the presentation may mimic purulent otitis media or mastoiditis. Lymph node enlargement may be found in the neck and elsewhere. A skull radiograph will show lytic skull lesion(s), and CT and magnetic resonance imaging (MRI) can show the extent of the lesion. Biopsy is required to establish the diagnosis. Langerhans' cells are seen in aggregates, and multinucleated giant cells are common.

Optimal management has not been established. Up to 20% of patients achieve spontaneous regression. Multidisciplinary care is required with hematologists and oncologists. Solitary bone lesions can be treated with curettage or excision but not at the expense of damaging hearing or facial nerve function. Intralesional steroid injection (triamcinolone) may be helpful.

The prognosis for unifocal disease is usually excellent but follow-up should be continued for 3 years after remission. Multisystem disease is treated with a combination of systemic steroids and cytotoxic drugs. Analgesics are helpful for pain, and biphosphonates have been used to inhibit bone resorption. Approximately 60% of patients with multifocal disease have a chronic course with a 10% mortality.

9.6.4 Malignant Disease of the Ear

Rhabdomyosarcoma is the most common soft-tissue sarcoma in children. Embryonal rhabdomyosarcoma makes up 55% of these cases. The presentation is with an expanding mass, hearing loss, and otorrhea. Facial nerve paralysis may be present. Any unusual ear condition requires biopsy for diagnosis. CT and MRI scanning will be required. Treatment should be in a specialist tertiary pediatric oncology center and comprises surgery, radiotherapy, and chemotherapy. The prognosis depends upon the histology and stage of the disease.

9.7 Key Points

- Persistent perforations in children most commonly result from recurrent AOM or following ventilation tube insertion.
- CSOM without cholesteatoma can be managed conservatively or surgically.
- Indications for pediatric tympanoplasty are to stop recurrent infections, to improve hearing, and to allow watersports.
- Pediatric tympanoplasty is usually undertaken from age of 10 to 11 years.
- Surgery for retraction pockets is debated, and indications are the presence of cholesteatoma, an unstable or progressive retraction, and poor hearing.
- Cartilage tympanoplasty is helpful for retraction pocket surgery and in ET dysfunction especially.

References

[1] Kay DJ, Nelson M, Rosenfeld RM. Meta-analysis of tympanostomy tube sequelae. Otolaryngol Head Neck Surg. 2001; 124(4):374–380

[2] Gunasekera H, Haysom L, Morris P. Craig. J Pediatr. 2008; 121 Suppl 1:S107–S107

[3] Browning GG. The unsafeness of 'safe' ears. J Laryngol Otol. 1984; 98 (1):23–26

[4] Nunez DA, Browning GG. Risks of developing an otogenic intracranial abscess. J Laryngol Otol. 1990; 104(6):468–472

[5] Mehta RP, Rosowski JJ, Voss SE, O'Neil E, Merchant SN. Determinants of hearing loss in perforations of the tympanic membrane. Otol Neurotol. 2006; 27(2):136–143

[6] Wullstein H. Theory and practice of tympanoplasty. Laryngoscope. 1956; 66(8):1076–1093

[7] Smyth GD, Hassard TH. Tympanoplasty in children. Am J Otol. 1980; 1(4):199–205

[8] Strong MS. The eustachian tube: basic considerations. Otolaryngol Clin North Am. 1972; 5(1):19–27

[9] Nagai M, Nagai T, Morimitsu T. Myringoplasty in children. Auris Nasus Larynx. 1991; 18(3):215–220

[10] Denoyelle F, Roger G, Chauvin P, Garabedian EN. Myringoplasty in children: predictive factors of outcome. Laryngoscope. 1999; 109(1): 47–51

[11] Lau T, Tos M. Tympanoplasty in children. An analysis of late results. Am J Otol. 1986; 7(1):55–59

[12] Charlett SD, Knight LC. Pediatric myringoplasty: does previous adenoidectomy improve the likelihood of perforation closure? Otol Neurotol 2009; 30(7):939–942

[13] MRC Multicentre Otitis Media Study Group. Adjuvant adenoidectomy in persistent bilateral otitis media with effusion: hearing and revision surgery outcomes through 2 years in the TARGET randomised trial. Clin Otolaryngol. 2012; 37(2):107–116

[14] Phillips JS, Yung MW, Nunney I. Myringoplasty outcomes in the UK. J Laryngol Otol. 2015; 129(9):860–864

[15] Westerberg J, Harder H, Magnuson B, Westerberg L, Hydén D. Ten-year myringoplasty series: does the cause of perforation affect the success rate? J Laryngol Otol. 2011; 125(2):126–132

[16] Cohen MS, Landegger LD, Kozin ED, Lee DJ. Pediatric endoscopic ear surgery in clinical practice: Lessons learned and early outcomes. Laryngoscope. 2016; 126(3):732–738

[17] Tos M, Poulsen G. Attic retractions following secretory otitis. Acta Otolaryngol. 1980; 89(5–6):479–486

9

[18] Sadé J, Berco E. Atelectasis and secretory otitis media. Ann Otol Rhinol Laryngol. 1976; 85(2) Suppl 25 Pt 2:66–72

[19] Charachon R. Classification of retraction pockets [in French]. Rev Laryngol Otol Rhinol (Bord). 1988; 109(3):205–207

[20] Borgstein J, Gerritsma TV, Wieringa MH, Bruce IA. The Erasmus atelectasis classification: proposal of a new classification for atelectasis of the middle ear in children. Laryngoscope. 2007; 117(7):1255–1259

[21] Nankivell PC, Pothier DD. Surgery for tympanic membrane retraction pockets. Cochrane Database Syst Rev. 2010(7):CD007943

[22] NICE Interventional procedure guidance [IPG409]: Balloon dilatation of the eustachian tube. National Institute for Health and Care Excellence. 2011 http://www.nice.org.uk/guidance/IPG409

[23] Sudhoff H, Tos M. Pathogenesis of sinus cholesteatoma. Eur Arch Otorhinolaryngol. 2007; 264(10):1137–1143

[24] Tos M. Cartilage tympanoplasty methods: proposal of a classification. Otolaryngol Head Neck Surg. 2008; 139(6):747–758

[25] Yung MW. Retraction of the pars tensa—long-term results of surgical treatment. Clin Otolaryngol Allied Sci. 1997; 22(4):323–326

[26] Cabra J, Moñux A. Efficacy of cartilage palisade tympanoplasty: randomized controlled trial. Otol Neurotol. 2010; 31(4):589–595

[27] Couloigner V, Molony N, Viala P, Contencin P, Narcy P, Van Den Abbeele T. Cartilage tympanoplasty for posterosuperior retraction pockets of the pars tensa in children. Otol Neurotol. 2003; 24(2):264–269

[28] Srinivasan V, Banhegyi G, O'Sullivan G, Sherman IW. Pars tensa retraction pockets in children: treatment by excision and ventilation tube insertion. Clin Otolaryngol Allied Sci. 2000; 25(4):253–256

[29] Blaney SP, Tierney P, Bowdler DA. The surgical management of the pars tensa retraction pocket in the child—results following simple excision and ventilation tube insertion. Int J Pediatr Otorhinolaryngol. 1999; 50(2):133–137

[30] Asik B, Binar M, Serdar M, Satar B. A meta-analysis of surgical success rates in congenital stapes fixation and juvenile otosclerosis. Laryngoscope. 2016; 126(1):191–198

[31] Denoyelle F, Daval M, Leboulanger N, et al. Stapedectomy in children: causes and surgical results in 35 cases. Arch Otolaryngol Head Neck Surg. 2010; 136(10):1005–1008

10 Cholesteatoma

Gavin A. J. Morrison

10.1 Introduction

Stratified squamous keratinizing epithelium in the middle ear cleft or mastoid represents cholesteatoma. This layer of skin is known as the matrix. Desquamated dead keratin forms the bulk of the central mass seen clinically. The active basal germ layer of skin lies on the outside of the cholesteatoma in contact with the middle ear or mastoid or ossicles. Unless this is removed surgically, and not just the keratin mass, the disease cannot be eradicated. Cholesteatoma frequently becomes infected and liquefied by opportunistic gram-negative organisms. The external surface of the cholesteatoma, in contact with perichondrium and bone leads to bony erosion, probably by expansion and from an enzymatic process.

10.2 Classification

10.2.1 Congenital Cholesteatoma

Cholesteatoma is categorized as congenital, primary acquired, and secondary acquired. Congenital cholesteatoma is a true inclusion epidermoid incorporated into the temporal bone during embryonic development. The original cell rests do not always originate in the middle ear and can be located anywhere in the temporal bone. Often these lesions are located in the anterosuperior mesotympanum, presenting initially as a white mass behind an intact drum and subsequently with conductive hearing loss. Progression can be rapid and extensive throughout the ear, the temporal bone, and the mastoid.

10.2.2 Primary Acquired Cholesteatoma

This refers to a lesion arising in the attic or posterosuperior part of the middle ear where there has been no previous history of otitis media. In the early stage, the disease is silent (▶ Fig. 10.1), but when the keratin becomes moist and infected, the erosive properties of the cholesteatoma become active.

10.2.3 Secondary Acquired Cholesteatoma

Secondary acquired cholesteatoma follows active middle ear infection usually with large posterior marginal defects and may present earlier because of an offensive smelling discharge.

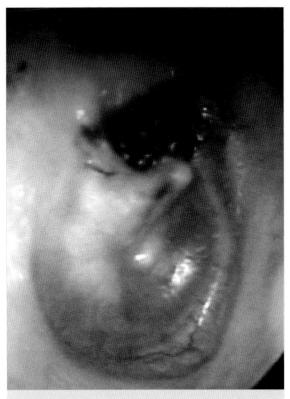

Fig. 10.1 Primary acquired attic cholesteatoma of right ear, presents with dry crust in attic.

10.2.4 Presentation, Early Management, and Imaging

The clinical presentations of cholesteatoma are otorrhea and conductive deafness.[1] The diagnosis is confirmed by otoscopy, supplemented by microscopy, as needed, when the presence of keratin or matrix ingress is seen (▶ Fig. 10.2). A pure-tone audiogram (PTA) with masking as appropriate to the findings is an essential baseline investigation in a child with a cholesteatoma. In children too young for a PTA or in children with comorbidity that makes PTA unsuitable, an accurate audiological assessment of hearing thresholds under the supervision of an experienced audiologist is mandatory before embarking on surgery. Definitive treatment is surgical but initial management includes medical treatment often with antibiotic–steroid eardrops and microsuction (Box 10.1). This aural toilet will allow better assessment of the disease and in the short term helps control the secondary infections.

10

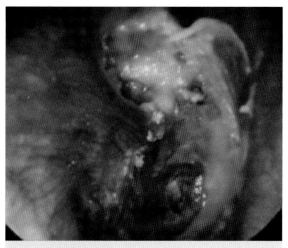

Fig. 10.2 Infected erosive attic cholesteatoma; right ear.

Box 10.1 Management of Pediatric Cholesteatomas

- Microscope and otoendoscope assessment.
- Preoperative air and bone PTA.
- Preoperative computed tomography (CT) scan of ears.
- Definitive surgery (closed or open).

A CT scan is recommended to identify the extent of the soft-tissue disease, the amount of pneumatization of the mastoid, and whether there is any bone erosion over the labyrinth. A fistula of the lateral semicircular canal is the most common such finding. The scan will allow planning of the best surgical approach for the disease. It will also assist in diagnosis when this is unclear as erosion of the scutum and the distribution of the soft tissue in the attic and antrum may all help to indicate likely cholesteatoma disease. The advantage CT scanning has in children is that images are acquired quickly, so a general anesthetic (GA) is often not required. Magnetic resonance imaging (MRI) scanning more often needs a GA and gives no fine anatomical detail of the mastoid and middle ear, so while diffusion-weighted (DW) scans can confirm keratin, they have a very limited place in preoperative assessment.

10.3 Treatment of Cholesteatoma

10.3.1 Aim of Treatment

The definitive treatment for all childhood cholesteatomas is surgical.

If left untreated, an ear with cholesteatoma will lead to progressive adjacent bone destruction risking sensorineural deafness, dizziness, facial nerve palsy, and intracranial spread with meningitis, lateral sinus thrombosis, extradural collections, and cerebral or cerebellar abscesses. The hearing will inevitably deteriorate. The untreated ear will continue to discharge offensively from time to time even if these more serious complications do not occur. The risk of serious intracranial complication from untreated cholesteatoma is very significant. In one adult retrospective study,[2] nearly 7.5% of patients suffering from chronic middle ear disease with cholesteatoma developed intracranial complications. The most frequent complication was meningitis, and the average duration of the disease was 11.9 years. If the risks were divided equally over time (which is unlikely), this equates to a 0.6% risk per annum.

The goal of surgery is to remove all the cholesteatoma matrix from the middle ear and mastoid air cells while retaining or improving hearing, preserving facial nerve function, and, if possible, the chorda tympani nerve.

The aim is to provide a safe dry ear, free of infections and with useful hearing. If possible, good natural ventilation of the middle ear cleft and prevention of future progression of disease should be sought as well.

10.3.2 Choice of Approach

There are two principal approaches to surgery for cholesteatoma:

- *Canal wall up* (CWU) or closed cavity surgery in which the posterior canal wall is left intact.
- *Canal wall down* (CWD) or open cavity surgery in which the canal wall is sacrificed to improve access and to permit a better view during follow-up.

There are advantages and disadvantages of both the closed and open cavity techniques[3]; these are summarized in ▶ Table 10.1. The big advantage of CWU or closed surgery is that a dry and self-cleaning ear is readily achieved. However, it is technically more difficult to remove the matrix completely and both residual disease and a recurrence of a new cholesteatoma from re-retraction means that further surgeries are likely to be needed. Typically, the author would plan a second-look revision tympanomastoidectomy at approximately 18 months after the first-stage combined-approach tympanoplasty (CAT) operation for an extensive cholesteatoma. The disadvantage of the open technique remains the greater likelihood of infections and the difficulty of repeated clinic visits and microsuction treatment of a child's ear in the clinic setting.

Table 10.1 Advantages and disadvantages of open and closed surgery for cholesteatoma

	CAT closed surgery	Open cavity surgery
Advantages	• Quicker postoperative healing • Increased likelihood of dry ear • Achieves a self-cleaning ear • Preserves normal middle ear depth for ossiculoplasty	• Shorter surgery time • Easier to remove whole matrix • Lower rates of recurrent cholesteatoma • Less likelihood of multiple operations
Disadvantages	• Longer surgery time • More demanding to eradicate matrix • Increased likelihood of residual or recurrent disease • Need for more surgical procedures over time • Requires 7-y surveillance	• Takes longer to heal postoperative • More outpatient visits for aural toilet required over long term • Increased frequency of ear infections • Hearing reconstruction might be less effective in shallow middle ear

Abbreviation: CAT, combined-approach tympanoplasty.

Ideally, the surgeon should be comfortable performing all available techniques and tailor the operation to the individual's needs.

> **i**
>
> A preoperative CT scan can provide invaluable information in planning surgery.

The author's preference in all cases with a well or moderately pneumatized mastoid bone is to employ a postaural approach and attempt a CWU (CAT) tympanomastoidectomy. If, however, the CT scan demonstrates a very small poorly pneumatized sclerotic mastoid bone, or an unusually low middle fossa dura or anterior sigmoid sinus, then an "inside-out" CWD atticoantrostomy operation is selected. As a rule of thumb, the distance from the posterior canal wall to the sigmoid sinus should be at least a little wider than the ear canal diameter to allow adequate access for combined-approach surgery. The surgical access from the mastoid to the attic will also require evaluation as the height of the middle fossa dura is very variable and may dip so low that the CAT is not the optimal choice.

10.3.3 Surgical Technique

A CAT allows access to the middle ear through the ear canal and also from a posterior tympanotomy (facial recess approach) through mastoidectomy. The posterior ear canal wall is left in situ, so the reconstructed ear retains a normally sized, self-cleaning ear canal and normal middle ear depth. When CAT surgery is undertaken and the ossicular chain is eroded, some surgeons like to attempt ossicular reconstruction at the first-stage operation. Others feel the results are better by waiting until the second-look surgery. The author prefers the former approach since, if successful, the child hears well immediately, and with modern scanning for surveillance (vide infra), a second surgery might be avoidable.

> **i**
>
> • In the CWD operation, the posterior bony canal wall is drilled away creating an open mastoid cavity. This is also termed *atticoantrostomy* or a modified radical mastoidectomy.
> • With this operation, while the cholesteatoma matrix is also fully removed, the open cavity will become lined with similar squamous epithelium.
> • The cartilaginous external meatus also needs to be enlarged with a meatoplasty, with the object of achieving a self-cleaning ear in which wax and desquamated epithelium may migrate outward. This is not always achievable, and the CWD mastoidectomy patient might typically require a couple of outpatient attendances per annum for aural toilet.

The surgical access for an open mastoid cavity can be from an end-aural or a postaural incision. If the mastoid is drilled first and then the canal wall is taken down, a modified radical mastoidectomy will result. The modified cavity involves grafting the tympanic segment as a tympanoplasty. Radical mastoidectomy with removal of all the ossicles and grafting onto the footplate of the stapes is now very rarely needed. When the open cavity is created from an "inside-out" drilling and dissection technique, the surgery progresses by widening and drilling away much of the bony canal wall to just expose the cholesteatoma limits, in the direction from which it has developed—middle ear to attic to aditus to mastoid antrum to other mastoid air cells. This operation is therefore known as an atticoantrostomy. If the disease is limited to the attic region, an *atticotomy* alone is performed and can readily achieve a self-cleaning ear with a small attic "shelf." The "inside-out" atticoantrostomy operation should therefore achieve the smallest possible mastoid cavity while fully removing the disease. With an adequate meatoplasty, these ears are frequently dry and healthy.

If a modified radical mastoidectomy technique is used, and especially if there is a well-pneumatized mastoid bone, then the mastoid cavity will tend to be much larger

10

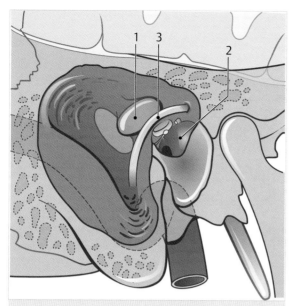

Fig. 10.3 Canal wall down mastoid cavity. 1, antrum; 2, middle ear/drum remnant; 3, facial nerve. (Modified with permission from Behrbohm H, Kaschke O, Nawka T, Swift A. Ear, Nose, and Throat Diseases: With Head and Neck Surgery, 3rd ed. Stuttgart/New York: Thieme; 2009.)

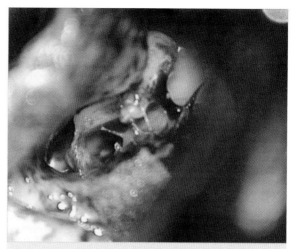

Fig. 10.4 Otoendoscopic view of left middle ear at second-stage CAT surgery.

and more kidney-shaped. These open cavities will have a greater likelihood of requiring multiple outpatient visits to remove wax and keratin and, in general, seem more likely to suffer repeated infections (▶ Fig. 10.3).

Endoscopic middle ear and mastoid surgery is gaining popularity, both for first-stage or primary operations and for second-look surveillance. Except for very limited cholesteatomas, the microscope and drill will normally be needed in addition; however, the range of new small and angled endoscopic ear instruments with microsuction allow disease clearance from inaccessible areas. Endoscopes as an adjunct to microsurgery are standard practice for most otologists.

10.3.4 Cavity Reconstruction

A further extension of open cavity surgery is to very radically exenterate all the mastoid air cells and remove the bony margins of the mastoid, especially at the mastoid tip. This is said to allow the soft tissues around the ear to collapse in leaving a smaller cavity in the long term. If a large mastoid cavity has been necessitated by very extensive cholesteatoma invading all areas of a well-pneumatized mastoid bone, then reconstruction with techniques to obliterate or partly obliterate the mastoid cavity or even to reconstruct the posterior canal wall with implanted materials can be employed. Thus, a smaller cavity is recreated and should generally be more trouble-free. This can be done at the time of the original mastoid surgery (primary reconstruction) or may be delayed.

Immediate or primary obliteration of a cavity does, like closed surgery, carry a risk of burying residual cholesteatoma inadvertently, so DW MRI scanning as well as serial otoendoscopic examination is recommended for a few years after this type of surgery.

10.4 Long-Term Management: Follow-Up

10.4.1 "Second-Look" Surgery

Because of the problem of recidivism, follow-up is important in all patients with both open and closed mastoidectomies. The author's preference for CAT surgery is to plan a second-look operation 18 months after the first one, unless the disease was very limited and the level of confidence of complete excision high. The timing of the second-stage surgery can be brought forward or extended according to the clinical assessment, appearance of the ear, and hearing. Some authors have advocated routine use of otoendoscopes for minimally invasive staged check-ups.[4,5] These techniques can avoid a large unnecessary exposure where the first surgery has been highly successful but require careful case selection and possibly a preoperative CT scan. The surgeon should consent the parent for a full exploration if necessary since the views can be difficult with limited access due to intramastoid adhesions, and if residual disease is encountered, endoscopic removal can be challenging. Endoscopy is very useful, however, as an adjunct during open second-stage surgery to allow fuller examination (▶ Fig. 10.4).

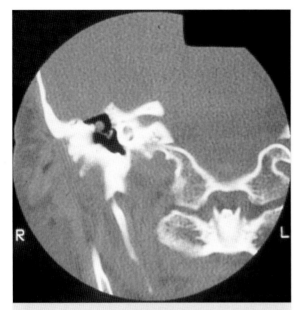

Fig. 10.5 Coronal CT showing enlarging attic residual keratin pearl after previous combined-approach tympanoplasty surgery.

Fig. 10.6 diffusion-weighted magnetic resonance imaging coronal plane image showing two high signal regions representing cholesteatoma.

10.4.2 Imaging

Scanning techniques now have an important and useful place in cholesteatoma surveillance.[6,7] A CT scan cannot differentiate the nature of the soft tissue, but sometimes a characteristic rounded mass will strongly suggest a keratin ball (▶ Fig. 10.5). Unnecessary radiation should be avoided and non-echo planar diffusion-weighted magnetic resonance imaging (non-EPI DW MRI) now has a positive predictive value of 93% for detection of cholesteatoma.[8] In another study, overall sensitivity and specificity for detection of cholesteatoma were 82 and 90%, respectively.[9] Cholesteatoma shows as a bright signal on DW images (▶ Fig. 10.6).

The author currently recommends planned interval non-EPI DW MRI scanning instead of a second-look operation if there was a limited cholesteatoma and a high degree of confidence that the excision was complete, no re-retraction on otoscopy, and good postoperative hearing. When these criteria are not met, however, especially when further hearing reconstruction can be attempted, second-stage surgery is advised instead. MRI scanning can then have an important role in avoiding unnecessary third-stage procedures.

> **i**
>
> Due to the late occurrence of recidivism and because the recidivism rate increases as time goes on, children should be periodically followed up for as long as possible.[10] As a minimum, the author recommends a 7-year disease-free period before considering stopping otological follow-up.

10.5 Surgical Outcomes

The debate about open versus closed ear surgery for cholesteatoma has continued for decades. Smyth reported long-term follow-up showing a 14% incidence of recurrent cholesteatoma with CWU surgery compared with a 1% figure for CWD,[11] but other studies challenge this and Roger et al[12] reported a multivariate analysis of risk factors for future disease in which the type of operation selected was not significant but the presence of ossicular chain interruption, disease in the posterior mesotympanum, and the experience of the surgeon were important.

In a recent study[13] with a mean follow-up period of 6 years, rates of cholesteatoma recurrence for CWU and CWD mastoidectomy groups were similar at 8 versus 6%.

There have been many publications reporting long-term follow-up in cholesteatoma for adults and children. Some usefully divide the incidence of recidivism into *recurrent* disease (that is a new cholesteatoma forming from re-retraction) and *residual* disease (that is, some keratin matrix inadvertently left and buried anywhere behind the drum or within the mastoid system). The author's own series showed no difference in recidivism rates for CWU versus CWD surgery. However, recurrent disease occurred in 9.1% of patients and residual disease in 5.5% overall from a series of 92 pediatric cholesteatoma mastoidectomies, followed over a 6-year period. The majority of cases were managed with closed techniques. The large posterior tympanotomy can give an excellent view of the middle ear and allow complete removal of facial recess cholesteatoma (▶ Fig. 10.7).

10

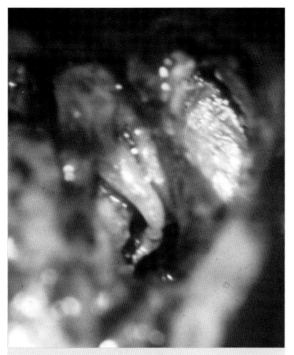

Fig. 10.7 Operative view after cholesteatoma removal through posterior tympanotomy; right ear.

Many other reports on children from well-known otological groups have demonstrated a high incidence of cholesteatoma recidivism in the long term, in the region of 30 to 47% over 5 to 7 years.

The use of a handheld laser (such as a potassium titanyl phosphate laser [KTP]) in the ear and mastoid has been recommended in recent years and can be helpful in removing or rendering nonviable, small areas of surgically inaccessible cholesteatoma matrix. This can help improve surgical success rates either by allowing the ossicular chain to be left intact or by reducing the rates of residual disease.[14]

10.6 Tips for Cholesteatoma Surgery

There are many excellent manuals of operative otological surgery, and this chapter cannot cover in detail all the surgical strategies employed. Outcomes in tympanomastoid surgery are highly dependent on good surgical technique, and the following tips may help to avoid residual and recurrent disease particularly where combined-approach closed surgery is undertaken:

- Ensure wide surgical exposure.
- Give meticulous attention to detail.
- Sacrifice the chorda tympani nerve, if necessary.
- Drill the bone of the posterior annulus to remove cholesteatoma from the sinus tympani or some of the facial recess, through the ear canal, if needed.

- If the ossicular chain is intact but enveloped in disease, disassemble it by removing the incus and head of malleus and then reconstruct the chain.
- Consider primary ossiculoplasty to avoid unnecessarily prolonged hearing loss and revise this, if necessary, at the second stage.
- Use otoendoscopes in assessing for residual disease and use the defocused laser to render small areas of adherent keratin nonviable in the most dangerous or inaccessible areas.
- Irrigate the whole surgical field with saline at the end of the procedure to wash out any loose keratin flakes and clean the field, making microscopic assessment of the mucosal status much easier.
- The attic bone (scutum) needs to be carefully and accurately reconstructed with bone or cartilage to avoid recurrent attic retraction.
- If there is Eustachian tube dysfunction with pars tensa retraction, then undertake cartilage reinforcement tympanoplasty to avoid re-retraction into the facial recess.

10.7 Key Points

- Cholesteatoma in children should be managed surgically.
- Preoperative CT scanning assists in planning the surgical approach.
- The goal of surgery is complete eradication of cholesteatoma matrix with a dry ear and preservation of useful hearing and facial nerve and chorda tympani nerve functions.
- Open and closed techniques are available, and microscope, otoendoscopes, and lasers all have a place.
- Residual and recurrent cholesteatoma rates remain significant in pediatric cholesteatoma and long-term follow-up should be maintained.
- Good middle ear and mastoid ventilation, and attic and posterior drum reinforcement are the mainstays for avoiding recurrence.
- Non-EPI DW MRI scanning is indicated at 1 to 2 years after primary surgery when the surgeon has a high confidence that the disease was fully removed, the ear is dry, and hearing is good.
- Second-look surgery is indicated when the ear is not dry or stable, hearing is poor, or the surgeon considers there is a risk of disease recidivism.

References

[1] Rosito LP, Netto LS, Teixeira AR, da Costa SS. Hearing impairment in children and adults with acquired middle ear cholesteatoma: audiometric comparison of 385 ears. Otol Neurotol. 2015; 36(8):1297–1300

[2] Maksimović Z, Rukovanjski M. Intracranial complications of cholesteatoma. Acta Otorhinolaryngol Belg. 1993; 47(1):33–36

[3] Harris AT, Mettias B, Lesser TH. Pooled analysis of the evidence for open cavity, combined approach and reconstruction of the mastoid

cavity in primary cholesteatoma surgery. J Laryngol Otol. 2016; 130 (3):235–241

[4] Barakate M, Bottrill I. Combined approach tympanoplasty for cholesteatoma: impact of middle-ear endoscopy. J Laryngol Otol. 2008; 122 (2):120–124

[5] Tierney PA, Pracy P, Blaney SP, Bowdler DA. An assessment of the value of the preoperative computed tomography scans prior to otoendoscopic 'second look' in intact canal wall mastoid surgery. Clin Otolaryngol Allied Sci. 1999; 24(4):274–276

[6] Yamashita K, Hiwatashi A, Togao O, et al. High-resolution three-dimensional diffusion-weighted MRI/CT image data fusion for cholesteatoma surgical planning: a feasibility study. Eur Arch Otorhinolaryngol. 2015; 272(12):3821–3824

[7] von Kalle T, Amrhein P, Koitschev A. Non-echoplanar diffusion-weighted MRI in children and adolescents with cholesteatoma: reliability and pitfalls in comparison to middle ear surgery. Pediatr Radiol. 2015; 45(7):1031–1038

[8] Dremmen MH, Hofman PA, Hof JR, Stokroos RJ, Postma AA. The diagnostic accuracy of non-echo-planar diffusion-weighted imaging in the detection of residual and/or recurrent cholesteatoma of the temporal bone. AJNR Am J Neuroradiol. 2012; 33(3):439–444

[9] Khemani S, Lingam RK, Kalan A, Singh A. The value of non-echo planar HASTE diffusion-weighted MR imaging in the detection, localisation and prediction of extent of postoperative cholesteatoma. Clin Otolaryngol. 2011; 36(4):306–312

[10] Kuo CL, Shiao AS, Liao WH, Ho CY, Lien CF. How long is long enough to follow up children after cholesteatoma surgery? A 29-year study. Laryngoscope. 2012; 122(11):2568–2573

[11] Smyth GD. Canal wall for cholesteatoma: up or down? Long-term results. Am J Otol. 1985; 6(1):1–2

[12] Roger G, Denoyelle F, Chauvin P, Schlegel-Stuhl N, Garabedian EN. Predictive risk factors of residual cholesteatoma in children: a study of 256 cases. Am J Otol. 1997; 18(5):550–558

[13] Shirazi MA, Muzaffar K, Leonetti JP, Marzo S. Surgical treatment of pediatric cholesteatomas. Laryngoscope. 2006; 116(9):1603–1607

[14] Hamilton JW. Systematic preservation of the ossicular chain in cholesteatoma surgery using a fiber-guided laser. Otol Neurotol. 2010; 31(7):1104–1108

10

11 Disorders of Balance

Gundula Thiel

11.1 Introduction

Children fall. Children are clumsy. That is part of normal development. The question for the medical professional is: "When do I have to worry?"

> Clearly the most worrying differential diagnosis of dizziness and imbalance at any age is a central nervous system (CNS) tumor. This is reassuringly rare; it almost never presents with imbalance as the sole symptom,[1] and it accounts for less than 1% of cases[2] even in a specialist pediatric balance clinic.

Most children and young adults (more than 55% of cases) who present with disorders of balance will be diagnosed with migraine or a disorder on the "migraine precursor spectrum."[1,3,4,5] Others will have benign and self-limiting conditions such as orthostatic reactions or otitis media with effusion (OME).

It can be difficult to tell if a child really has a pathological balance problem or is just on a different level of motor maturity to his/her age-matched peers. Although causes of imbalance are manifold, true vestibular pathology is uncommon in children.

> Even if there is peripheral vestibular dysfunction, the plasticity of the neuronal system is such that children compensate surprisingly quickly and completely for vestibular losses. Peripheral vestibular disorders that would cause significant and prolonged morbidity in adults resolve very quickly in children, and medical help is often neither sought nor necessary.

The etiology of balance problems is nonvestibular in the great majority of cases.

Diagnosis and management mainly rely on thorough history taking and examination, most of which can be achieved in the outpatient setting without the need for specialist equipment.

11.2 Physiology of Balance in Children

11.2.1 Maturation and Development

In children, as in adults, the maintenance of equilibrium depends on sensory input from three major systems:
- Proprioceptive.
- Visual.
- Vestibular.

In addition, cognitive function plays an important role.

Motor control of movement rests in the cerebral cortex, and the responses to afferent input are modified and processed in the brainstem and the cerebellum (▶ Fig. 11.1). Pathology in any of these systems can and does cause dysequilibrium.

In order to achieve postural control, these visual, vestibular, and proprioceptive inputs need to develop and be successfully integrated.

The balance system constantly improves and matures from birth to adulthood. Although all systems are anatomically present from birth, they need time to mature during childhood and adolescence.

A successful balance strategy includes inputs from each of the three systems, and the relative importance of visual, proprioceptive, and vestibular system changes during development. Growth and postural maturity proceeds cephalocaudally, with the baby achieving head control first and standing stability later.

The relative predominance of each of the three systems that control the physiology of balance at any one time during childhood is uncertain, but it seems that very young children in the process of acquiring balance rely much on visual input. Adults in contrast rely much more on somatosensory inputs.[1,6]

The mature vestibular system can suppress incongruent information, but this maturity is probably not reached until the age of 12 years, so children are less well able to select and control misleading visual information.[7] Among the three sensory inputs, the vestibular system is the least efficient and the last to develop in children, not reaching maturity before the age of 10 to 15 years.[6,8,9]

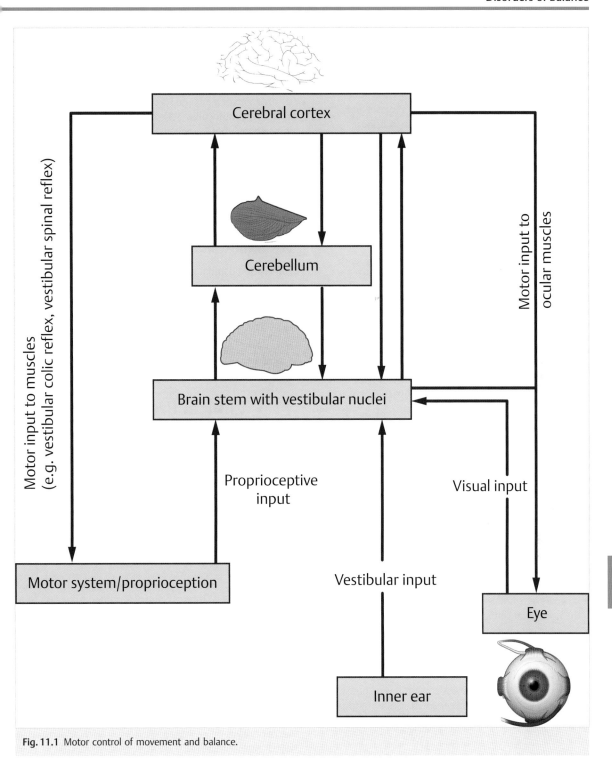

Fig. 11.1 Motor control of movement and balance.

Cerebral cortex

Cerebellum

Brain stem with vestibular nuclei

Motor input to muscles
(e.g. vestibular colic reflex, vestibular spinal reflex)

Motor input to ocular muscles

Proprioceptive input

Visual input

Motor system/proprioception

Vestibular input

Inner ear

Eye

11

Adultlike postural stability and maturation of all three systems cannot be assumed in young adolescents. It is estimated that the balance system does not reach full maturity before the age of 15 years and there may be considerable variation in individual children.[1,8]

The relative dominance of different components of the system varies not only during development but also from child to child. This variable maturation helps to explain the changing patterns of differential diagnosis of imbalance in children.

11.2.2 Vestibular Reflexes

Afferent impulses from the visual, vestibular, and somatosensory/proprioceptive systems are processed in the vestibular nuclei and the cerebellum and are converted into efferent impulses to the muscles controlling the eyes, neck, and spinal cord (▶ Fig. 11.1).

These vestibular reflexes (*vestibulo-ocular, vestibulocollic*, and *vestibulospinal*) allow us to maintain balance.

The responses differ between various age groups, and their examination can provide diagnostic help in evaluating the complaint of dizziness and disequilibrium. Their assessment can guide us in the diagnosis of vestibular pathology.

Vestibulo-Ocular Reflex

The vestibulo-ocular reflex (VOR) stabilizes the image on the retina during head movement through a reflexive eye movement opposite to the direction of head movement.

Both semicircular canals and the otolith organs are involved in this reflex arc.
- It can be assessed by caloric testing, which mainly tests the horizontal semicircular canal.
- A simple but effective way to measure vestibular function in the older child in the office is the "head impulse test," which involves the examiner moving the patient's head to the left to stimulate the semicircular canal in the left ear, observing the eye movement response while the patient tries to keep looking at a stationary target straight ahead, and repeating the maneuver for the right ear.

The VOR is present at birth but develops throughout childhood. Full maturity might only happen in preadolescence,[1] but an absent VOR by the age of 10 months is considered abnormal.

Vestibulocollic Reflex

This helps to stabilize vision while the body is in motion by minimizing head movement and head bobbing through engagement of neck muscles. The main vestibular organ involved is the saccule.

The vestibulocollic reflex can be specifically tested through vestibular evoked myogenic potentials (VEMPs). This gives information about saccular and inferior vestibular nerve function but these are specialized and rarely needed in everyday clinical practice.

The reflex is present at birth but continues to mature into adolescence.

Vestibulospinal Reflex

The vestibulospinal reflex helps stabilize the body in relationship to gravity. The afferents combine proprioceptive input from the periphery, as well as visual and labyrinthine afferents. It is tested with basic balance tests like Romberg's test.

It is also present at birth and continues to mature into adolescence.

11.3 Clinical Presentation

Children and their parents seldom complain directly of "dizziness," as particularly young children are unable to articulate this.

True "vertigo," defined as an illusion of movement, is especially rare in children.

The incidence from large epidemiological studies and even from special interest clinics is quoted to be less than 1%.[10,11]

The consultation will typically be initiated by parents who might have noticed the child being "clumsy" or not meeting the milestones his/her peers or siblings have.

The presentation can be varied and includes unsteadiness, clinginess and fretfulness, crying, and torticollis. The older child and teenager can be more precise in their description of the symptoms, but even here difficulties in verbalization arise.

Through a combination of history and examination in most cases, a diagnosis can be reached in the outpatient department and treatment or appropriate referral instigated.

11.3.1 History

A systematic approach to questioning can lead to important clinical information (► Table 11.1).

> **i**
>
> A differentiation between a vestibular and a nonvestibular cause of symptoms can often be inferred by eliciting "what does it feel like?"

Table 11.1 Targeted history

Question	Finding	Clinical information
What does it feel like?	Vertigo	Vestibular
	Lightheaded Pain Loss of consciousness	Nonvestibular (migraine, orthostatic, seizure, syncope)
Are there other associated symptoms?	Tinnitus Hearing loss Aural fullness	Endolymphatic hydrops Congenital
	Declining hearing after head trauma	Enlarged vestibular aqueduct
	Cranial nerve weakness	Intracranial lesion
	Headaches Torticollis	Migraine BPVC Paroxysmal torticollis
	Sweating Palpitations Dyspnea	Orthostasis Anxiety Panic attack
	CHL	OME CSOM
	Nausea Vomiting	Vestibular Migraine
Duration of symptoms	Seconds to minutes	BPPV
	Hours	Hydrops
	Days	Vestibular neuritis Labyrinthitis
Aggravating factors	Movement	Vestibular
	Turning over	BPPV
	Valsalva	"Third window"
Background history	Head trauma	
	Tumor	
	Surgery to the brain/ear	
	Ototoxic medications	
	Cardiac disease	
	Otological disease	
	Vascular disease	
	Ophthalmological disease	
	Family history	NF2 Acoustic neuroma Migraine
	Anxiety/depression Stress at school/work	
	Headaches	Migraine
	SNHL	Syndromic Nonsyndromic Congenital Acquired

Abbreviations: BPPV, benign paroxysmal positional vertigo; BPVC, benign paroxysmal vertigo of childhood; CHL, conductive hearing loss; CSOM, chronic suppurative otitis media; NF2, neurofibromatosis type 2; OME, otitis media with effusion; SNHL, sensorineural hearing loss.

11

True vertigo points toward a vestibular origin, but this level of clarity and accuracy in the description and characterization of symptoms is rare, even in adults. If the imbalance is aggravated by movement, this points further to a vestibular origin of the problem. Turning over in bed or other quick head movements worsen or set off benign paroxysmal postural vertigo (BPPV), and straining worsens the vertigo caused by the very rare "third window" phenomena such as perilymph fistula.

The duration of symptoms can be divided into:
- Seconds to minutes.
- Hours.
- Days to weeks.

Very short-lived episodes (typically seconds) indicate BPPV. Endolymphatic hydrops symptoms last for hours or occasionally days but the pattern can be similar for the more common migrainous disorders, and the symptoms of vestibular neuritis or labyrinthitis can last for days to weeks.

It is important to note that children will compensate much more quickly than adults and will often recover in days rather than in weeks and months.

Associated symptoms are of particular importance and will help delineate between otological, neurologic, and other origins of symptoms.
- *Nausea* and/or *vomiting* are indicative of vestibular involvement but can also be associated with migraines.
- *Syncope*, *loss of consciousness*, *headaches*, and *seizures* or "fitting" point to a central (i.e., neurologic) origin of symptoms.
- *Tinnitus*, *aural fullness*, and *hearing loss*, particularly when these symptoms are fluctuant, can be an indication of endolymphatic hydrops.
- *Sweating, palpitations, lightheadedness*, or *dyspnea* in association with balance dysfunction can point toward orthostatic reactions. Adolescent girls are particularly susceptible to this, probably because of the rapid physiological changes associated with puberty and the commencement of menstruation, but endocrine and metabolic changes in boys can also precipitate balance dysfunction.
- A history of *sensorineural hearing loss* (SNHL) may be related to a syndromic, nonsyndromic, congenital, or acquired cause of deafness, and such presentations warrant further investigations.

"Dizzy spells," sometimes with hyperventilation, are a common component of anxiety or panic attacks in both sexes.

The most common diagnoses in children with balance disorders involve the migrainous spectrum including migraine precursors such as:
- Migrainous vertigo.
- Benign paroxysmal vertigo of childhood (BPVC).
- Paroxysmal torticollis.

Headaches can be very variable or even absent and do not necessarily have to be in a specific location or to have a typical temporal relation to the dizziness.[12]

The background medical and family history may provide obvious pointers to the differential diagnosis.

Neurologic deficit and declining hearing after head trauma should prompt neuroimaging to exclude a CNS lesion or malformation such as enlarged vestibular aqueduct.

Medications and known otological vascular or ophthalmological disease may be implicated. Head trauma (temporal bone fracture) and intracranial/otological surgery can cause balance disturbances, but children often compensate quickly and completely for unilateral vestibular losses. In contrast with adults, even children with a known temporal bone fracture and SNHL will not usually have vestibular complaints.[13]

Take a careful and detailed social history, focusing on the child's interaction with teachers and peers at school. Anxiety, depression, stress, and bullying at school can all manifest with symptoms of dizziness. Adolescent girls are particularly susceptible to eating disorders and may present with features such as syncope, dizzy spells, or unexplained episodes of loss of balance. The eating pattern can be surreptitious and the family may not be aware that the girl is undernourished. If such conditions are suspected, prompt and sensitive referral to the child mental health service can greatly improve outcome.

A positive family history might support a diagnosis of migraine or very rarely point to conditions such as neurofibromatosis type 2 (NF2) or acoustic neuroma.

11.3.2 Examination

A thorough examination of the child is paramount (▶ Table 11.2). This should include a basic neurologic as well as a full ear, nose, and throat (ENT) assessment.

Clinical examination can prove challenging particularly in the younger child, but with time and patience, most of the important physical findings can be elicited.

Otoscopy and Audiology

Examination of the ears is particularly important and must include an age-appropriate hearing assessment.

OME, chronic suppurative otitis media (CSOM), acute otitis media, and mastoiditis can cause balance disturbances.

Table 11.2 Targeted examination

Examination	Technique	Finding	Diagnostic relevance
Nystagmus	Fixing gaze on object in neutral position	Spontaneous Directional fixed, horizontal (Worse in direction of fast phase of nystagmus)	Vestibular pathology Irritation: fast phase toward affected labyrinth Damage: fast phase away from affected labyrinth
	Fixing gaze on object 20–30 degrees to the left and right and up and down of neutral	Vertical, torsional, pendular, direction changing	Cerebellum; brainstem; drugs
Smooth pursuit	Follow object with eyes	Not smooth; catch up saccades	Central pathology
Saccades	Rapid refixation from one object to another (examiner fingers at various positions)	Over- or undershooting	Central pathology
Romberg	Stand with feet together, eyes closed	Swaying or toppling over	Vestibular or proprioceptive weakness
Sharpened Romberg	Stand with feet in heel to toe position, eyes closed	Swaying or toppling over	Vestibular or proprioceptive weakness
Fukuda (Unterberger)	Step on the spot with eyes closed for ~20 s	Rotation to of > 45 degrees to one side	Rotation toward the side of vestibular lesion
Head shake	Shake head with closed eyes for 30 s, then open eyes, and look straight ahead	Nystagmus	Peripheral vestibular lesion; nystagmus beating away from affected ear
Head thrust (impulse)	Quick head-shake lateral while looking at examiner's nose	Corrective saccades	Peripheral vestibular lesion; corrective saccades when thrust toward side of vestibular lesion
Dix–Hallpike (Frenzel glasses)	Quick lay down from sitting position to supine with head hanging over the edge of the bed, turned 45 degrees down	Geotropic nystagmus, latency, fatigable	BPPV

Abbreviation: BPPV, benign paroxysmal positional vertigo.

Balance Assessment

A thorough yet speedy balance examination can be carried out in the outpatient setting and does not require specialist equipment. As the child enters the consulting room, observe his/her gait, stance, balance, and overall age-appropriate motor function.[14] This can be expanded by performing Romberg's test. The "sharpened" (tandem) Romberg test and the Fukuda stepping test are also useful.

Romberg and "Sharpened Romberg" Test

Romberg's test is carried out with the patient standing eyes open and then closed, arms in neutral position and feet together. In the sharpened Romberg test, the feet are placed in a heel to toe position.

Swaying or toppling when visual control is removed is considered a positive test and indicates a vestibular disorder or proprioceptive deficit.

Fukuda (Unterberger) Stepping Test

The patient is asked to march on the spot with her eyes closed for 20 seconds. Deviation/rotation to one side of more than 45 degrees is considered pathological. The deviation is toward the side of vestibular dysfunction, but the reliability of this test has been disputed.

Testing Eye Movements

A full neuro-ophthalmological examination is complex and beyond the scope of this chapter, but a basic examination should be carried out and may give important diagnostic aid in the ENT clinic. Examine the child's eye movements and record if there is nystagmus, smooth pursuit, and/or saccades.

> Nystagmus most commonly consists of a slow drift and a quick corrective phase (jerk nystagmus). Its direction is described by the quick phase, a corrective saccade bringing the eye back on target.

- Look for spontaneous nystagmus, and in the older child, look for gaze-evoked nystagmus by asking him/her to look in a particular direction, for example, by following the examiner's finger.

- Testing for nystagmus can be made even more sensitive by removing visual fixation. This can be done in the clinic by getting the child to wear Frenzel glasses while testing. Nystagmus due to a unilateral peripheral vestibular lesion (e.g., labyrinthitis or a vestibular neuronitis) can be suppressed by visual fixation and only becomes apparent when this is removed.

Pathological nystagmus can be caused by vestibular or central disorders, drug toxicity, or metabolic disorders.

Nystagmus can be formally recorded using electro- or videonystagmography but these tests are rarely needed.

Vestibular Nystagmus

Nystagmus due to a peripheral vestibular lesion (i.e., pathology in the inner ear rather than in the vestibular nuclei in the brainstem or any other brain lesion) is typically horizontal or mixed (horizontal–torsional) and suppressed by visual fixation.

Vestibular nystagmus increases when the gaze is directed toward the fast phase of the nystagmus (Alexander's law). It can be described as follows:

- First degree (only when looking in the direction of the fast phase).
- Second degree (present in neutral/straight ahead gaze as well).
- Third degree (also evident when looking in the direction of the slow phase).

The degree of nystagmus is a measure of the severity of a vestibular lesion and will reduce as compensation progresses.

In presence of a destructive vestibular lesion, the fast phase will be directed *away* from the affected ear and in the presence of an irritative lesion *toward* the affected ear.

Post Head-Shake Nystagmus

With the child's eyes closed, the examiner quickly rotates (shakes) the child's head laterally from left to right for approximately 30 seconds (▶ Fig. 11.2). If this induces nystagmus, then the direction of the fast component of the nystagmus is *away* from a paretic lesion.

Head Thrust (Impulse) Testing

Ask the child to look at the examiner's nose and quickly rotate (thrust) his/her head laterally. Eyes drifting away from the target and corrective saccades point to a periph-

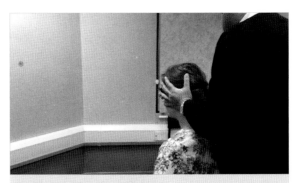

Fig. 11.2 Testing for post head-shake nystagmus.

eral lesion located on the side the head was moved toward.

Vertical (up or down beating) or purely torsional nystagmus is usually due to CNS lesions. This should prompt rapid investigations, for example, computed tomography or magnetic resonance imaging and appropriate referral.

Pursuit Testing

Ask the patient to track a target, for example, the examiner's finger, as it is moved in front of him/her while he/she keeps his/her head still. Halting movements or catch-up saccades are abnormal and point to a central lesion.

Saccades

Ask the patient to fix on alternating stationary targets, for example, the examiner's left and right index fingers presented in sequence at the periphery of vision, without moving his/her head.

Inability to find the target, overshooting and undershooting, indicates a central lesion.

The Dix–Hallpike Test

Seat the patient on an examining couch with enough room to lie backward so that he/she is in a position of the head hanging over the edge of the couch, turned 45 degrees downward (▶ Fig. 11.3). Bring him/her quickly from sitting to this position with the head tilted first to the right and then to the left.

The test is positive if this maneuver induces a geotropic, rotational nystagmus when the affected ear is turned downward. This is classical for BPPV. As in adults, an Epley's particle-repositioning maneuver can be carried out and is curative in approximately 80% of cases at the first attempt.

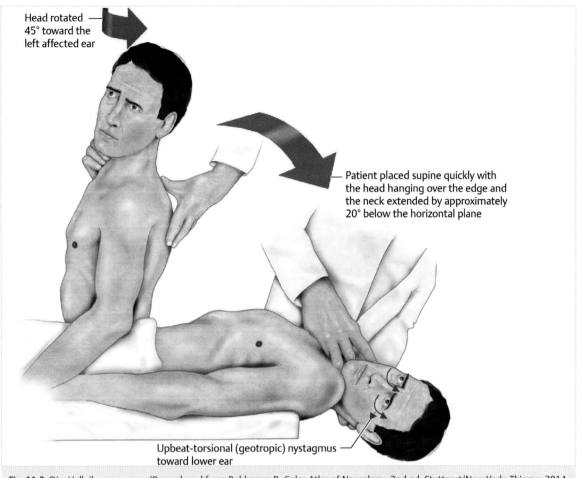

Head rotated 45° toward the left affected ear

Patient placed supine quickly with the head hanging over the edge and the neck extended by approximately 20° below the horizontal plane

Upbeat-torsional (geotropic) nystagmus toward lower ear

Fig. 11.3 Dix–Hallpike maneuver. (Reproduced from Rohkamm R. Color Atlas of Neurology, 2nd ed. Stuttgart/New York: Thieme; 2014, with permission.)

11.3.3 Investigations

Audiology

> ℹ
>
> Assessment of the child's hearing is an integral part of clinical examination. Balance disorders can be broadly categorized into those with and those without hearing impairment, with important etiological implications.

Imaging

Intracranial lesions are rare. It is even rarer for them to present with balance problems as the only symptom, but they are the most worrying of possible underlying causes of balance dysfunction. Cranial nerve palsy, evidence of nystagmus of central origin, or a focal neurologic deficit requires neuroimaging (▶ Fig. 11.4).

Vestibular Function Testing

A good assessment of vestibular function can be made in the outpatient setting using the aforementioned tests. More specialist balance testing is not widely available. A further problem is that there are very few normative data on children and so interpretation of results is difficult.

Tertiary pediatric center investigations might include caloric testing, videonystagmography (▶ Fig. 11.5), cervical and ocular VEMPs, electrocochleography, and blood tests or serology, as dictated by individual circumstances. If so, referral to pediatric neurology or specialist vestibular services should be considered.

11.4 Differential Diagnosis and Management

While the differential diagnosis of balance impairment in children includes the range of conditions know in adult practice, some differences are important (▶ Fig. 11.6, ▶ Fig. 11.7; ▶ Table 11.3).

11

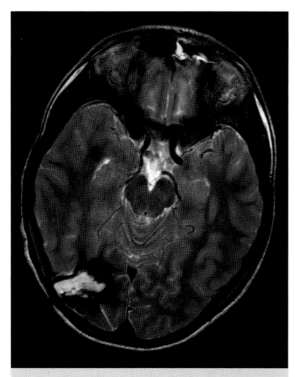

Fig. 11.4 Magnetic resonance imaging scan of a 13-year-old boy who presented with dizzy spells and brief episodes of visual disturbance. He was initially treated for migraine. Note the large right occipital mass, a cavernous hemangioma. A rare case of multiple intracranial "cavernomas."

The majority of children, in some series more than 55%, are diagnosed with disorders of the migrainous or migraine precursor spectrum. Orthostatic reactions are also particularly common, especially in adolescent females.

> **i**
>
> Depression and anxiety disorders are prevalent in the teenage population and may present with disorders of equilibrium.

- The majority of young children suffer from OME at some stage in their lives and this can lead to balance impairment.
- Head trauma is also more common in the pediatric setting.
- The differential diagnosis of balance impairment in children can be divided into etiologies with and without hearing impairment.

11.4.1 Balance Disorders with Normal Hearing

Migraine and Migraine Precursor Disorders

Migrainous Vertigo

Migrainous vertigo is increasingly recognized in adults and children alike.[12,15]

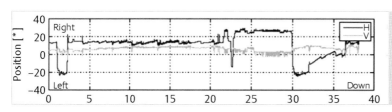

Fig. 11.5 Electronystagmogram. Electrodes at the inner and outer canthus record ocular movements. Fast (saccades) and slow movements are shown on the trace.

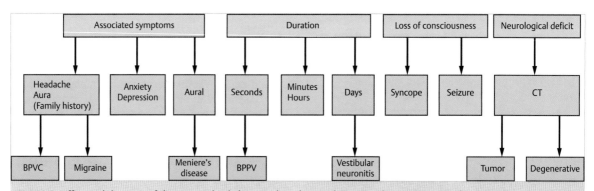

Fig. 11.6 Differential diagnosis of dizziness and imbalance without hearing loss. BPPV, benign paroxysmal positional vertigo; BPVC, benign paroxysmal vertigo of childhood.

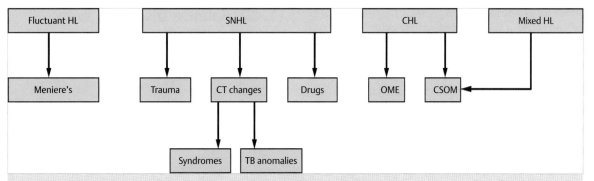

Fig. 11.7 Differential diagnosis of dizziness and imbalance with hearing loss. CHL, conductive hearing loss; CSOM, chronic suppurative otitis media; HL, hearing loss; OME, otitis media with effusion; SNHL, sensorineural hearing loss.

Table 11.3 Treatment of balance impairment in children

Diagnosis		Treatment[a]
ENT	OME	Grommets
	CSOM	Mastoid exploration
	Meniere's disease	Stepwise as for adults
	BPPV	Otolith repositioning (Epley's maneuver)
	Vestibular neuritis	Symptomatic, vestibular rehabilitation
	Cochlear implant	Symptomatic, vestibular rehabilitation
	Labyrinthitis (viral)	Steroid (oral or intratympanic) Symptomatic, vestibular rehabilitation
	Labyrinthitis (bacterial)	Antibiotics, surgical Vestibular rehabilitation
Non-ENT	Migraine	Underlying condition
	BPVC	Underlying condition
	Paroxysmal torticollis	Underlying condition
	Basilar migraine	Underlying condition
	Central tumors	Neurosurgical/oncological
	Trauma	Supportive, vestibular rehabilitation
	Ototoxic medication	Supportive, vestibular rehabilitation
	Seizure disorder	Underlying condition
	Vascular/cardiac disease	Underlying condition
	Autoimmune disease	Underlying condition

Abbreviations: BPPV, benign paroxysmal positional vertigo; BPVC, benign paroxysmal vertigo of childhood; CSOM, chronic suppurative otitis media; ENT, ear, nose, and throat; OME, otitis media with effusion.
[a]For non-ENT diagnoses, treatment should be by the relevant specialty.

The temporal relationship between headaches and vertigo can be variable. Vertigo might precede, be concomitant with, or follow the dizziness/vertigo. Associated symptoms might include photo/phonophobia, nausea, and sensory aura (visual, olfactory, vestibular). Headaches are not always typical[16] and are often frontal, occipital, and of shorter duration than in adults (less than 2 hours).[12] There may be no clear history of headache and presentation can vary considerably from that of adults.[12]

Management is largely supportive but treatment strategies for migraine may be appropriate.[17]

Benign Paroxysmal Vertigo of Childhood

This usually occurs in children between the ages of 3 and 8 years and is characterized by very brief (seconds to minutes) attacks of vertigo associated with spontaneous nystagmus, pallor, anxiety, nausea, and vomiting. Pain is not a feature and children usually revert to normal activity once the attack has run its course.[12]

These attacks usually stop after a few years. However, children can go on to develop classical migraines in later life. A significant number (reported up to 43%) have a family history positive for migraine.[12] Treatment is medical and aimed at the underlying condition.

Paroxysmal Torticollis

This condition is characterized by brief and self-limiting episodes of head tilt, associated with nausea and vomiting. It is considered to be in the same spectrum as BPVC and affects children under the age of 3 years. Symptoms usually resolve after this age.[12] Management is supportive and the condition resolves as the child gets older.

Anxiety/Psychogenic Balance Disorders

Evidence of possible secondary gain as well as a mismatch between patient complaints/symptoms and objective clinical findings including vestibular testing should prompt a particularly careful examination of the social and psychological background.

Vestibular complaints may be associated with a variety of disorders including anxiety, depression, attention disorders, autism, and psychosis. Referral to psychological support services may be helpful.

In some cases, children may be feigning illness (malingering) or may develop symptoms related to bullying, social exclusion, or exam pressures.

Vestibular Neuritis

Sometimes referred to as acute vestibulopathy, this is thought to result from a viral infection or similar insult of the labyrinth or vestibular nerves and is common in adults and children alike.

It causes sudden onset of severe vertigo without loss of hearing. Severe symptoms usually last for days but milder symptoms usually persist for weeks to months. In children, however, much quicker recovery is reported, probably owing to increased neuronal plasticity and central compensation. The management is expectant.

Benign Paroxysmal Positional Vertigo

BPPV is one of the most common conditions causing balance disorder in adulthood. It is characterized by short spells of vertigo associated with movement, particularly head turning. It is thought to be caused by displaced otoconia in the semicircular canals.

It usually recovers spontaneously, but canalith-repositioning maneuvers (e.g., Epley's maneuver) can be curative in more than 80% of cases.[18]

In children, this is very rare and often preceded by trauma or vestibular neuritis.

11.4.2 Balance Disorders with Hearing Impairment

Otitis Media With Effusion

One of the most common problems in the pediatric population is OME. This can lead to hearing loss and recurrent acute otitis media and is also implicated in balance impairment.

The mechanisms are unclear and explanations range from pressure effects to effects of bacterial toxins on the vestibular system (see also Chapter 8).

Chronic Suppurative Otitis Media

CSOM with or without cholesteatoma can cause balance impairment. The semicircular canals might be affected by pressure or infection or directly damaged by disease.

Management is that of the primary condition (see Chapter 9 and Chapter 10).

Surgery

Surgery to the brain or the middle/inner ear can lead to imbalance by damaging either the peripheral vestibular system or the central pathways.

These conditions will most likely be permanent and treatment should focus on vestibular rehabilitation.

Trauma

Trauma, in particular temporal bone fractures, can lead to vestibular loss.

Skull fractures can involve the otic capsule and SNHL, and balance impairment can ensue.

Children usually compensate very quickly for unilateral vestibular losses and might never complain about imbalance. If recovery is slow, vestibular rehabilitation should be considered.

Intracranial Lesion

Tumors, particularly of the posterior fossa, can cause balance disturbance. Hearing loss is not always present but can be.

Prompt imaging and immediate referral to the pediatric neurosurgeon is indicated.

A positive family history for NF2 should alert the physician to the possibility of hereditary acoustic neuroma and other brain tumors and again prompt imaging and referral is indicated.

Meniere's Disease

Endolymphatic hydrops and related conditions are characterized by vertigo lasting hours to days associated with otological signs including aural fullness and pressure, tinnitus, and fluctuant hearing loss. The latter is typically predominant in the low frequencies. The condition is much rarer in children than in adults.

Treatment is similar in both but hearing conservation is clearly of great importance in children.

Ototoxic Drugs

Administration of ototoxic medication, for example, aminoglycosides (e.g., gentamycin), can lead to SNHL and loss of balance function. This is usually irreversible.

Labyrinthitis

This is thought to be caused by an acute inflammation of the vestibular labyrinth, which is assumed to be due to viral infection. Symptoms can be auditory (sudden deafness, sometimes tinnitus) and vestibular with varying severity.

The outcome is usually good, but hearing may not recover and occasionally vestibular rehabilitation is indicated.

Bacterial labyrinthitis is more severe and can be the result of middle ear or meningeal infection. Treatment is with broad-spectrum antibiotics, steroids, and possible surgical intervention to treat the infective source.

11.5 Key Points

- Control of balance relies on successful integration of visual, vestibular, and proprioceptive inputs. These systems may not reach maturity until the age of 10 to 15 years and are characterized by neuronal plasticity and central compensation.
- The most common diagnoses in children with balance disorders are migraine or a disorder on the "migraine precursor spectrum."
- Intracranial lesions are rare in childhood and almost never present with imbalance as the *sole symptom*. The presence of other neurologic symptoms should prompt imaging.
- Diagnosis and management mainly rely on thorough history taking and examination.
- A differentiation between vestibular and nonvestibular symptoms can often be inferred by asking "What does it feel like?"

- It is important to ask about the duration of symptoms, any associated symptoms or conditions, and medical and family history.
- Examination and investigation should include otoscopy, audiology, balance assessment, and tests of eye movements.
- Cranial nerve palsy, evidence of nystagmus of central origin, and a focal neurologic deficit require neuroimaging.
- Tertiary pediatric center investigations might include caloric testing, videonystagmography, cervical and ocular VEMPs, electrocochleography, blood tests, and serology.
- Balance disorders with normal hearing may be caused by migraine (particularly BPVC or paroxysmal torticollis); anxiety/psychogenic balance disorders, vestibular neuritis, and BPPC.
- Balance disorders with hearing impairment may be caused by OME, CSOM, surgery to the brain or middle/inner ear, trauma, intracranial lesion, Meniere's disease, ototoxic drugs, or labyrinthitis.

References

[1] O'Reilly R, Grindle C, Zwicky EF, Morlet T. Development of the vestibular system and balance function: differential diagnosis in the pediatric population. Otolaryngol Clin North Am. 2011; 44(2):251–271, vii

[2] Wiener-Vacher SR. Vestibular disorders in children. Int J Audiol. 2008; 47(9):578–583

[3] Choung YH, Park K, Moon SK, Kim CH, Ryu SJ. Various causes and clinical characteristics in vertigo in children with normal eardrums. Int J Pediatr Otorhinolaryngol. 2003; 67(8):889–894

[4] Ravid S, Bienkowski R, Eviatar L. A simplified diagnostic approach to dizziness in children. Pediatr Neurol. 2003; 29(4):317–320

[5] Langhagen T, Albers L, Heinen F, et al. Period prevalence of dizziness and vertigo in adolescents. PLoS ONE. 2015; 10(9):e0136512

[6] Hirabayashi S, Iwasaki Y. Developmental perspective of sensory organization on postural control. Brain Dev. 1995; 17(2):111–113

[7] Ionescu E, Morlet T, Froehlich P, Ferber-Viart C. Vestibular assessment with Balance Quest Normative data for children and young adults. Int J Pediatr Otorhinolaryngol. 2006; 70(8):1457–1465

[8] Cherng RJ, Chen JJ, Su FC. Vestibular system in performance of standing balance of children and young adults under altered sensory conditions. Percept Mot Skills. 2001; 92(3 Pt 2):1167–1179

[9] Steindl R, Kunz K, Schrott-Fischer A, Scholtz AW. Effect of age and sex on maturation of sensory systems and balance control. Dev Med Child Neurol. 2006; 48(6):477–482

[10] O'Reilly RC, Morlet T, Nicholas BD, et al. Prevalence of vestibular and balance disorders in children. Otol Neurol. 2010; 31(9):1441–1444

[11] Riina N, Ilmari P, Kentala E. Vertigo and imbalance in children: a retrospective study in a Helsinki University otorhinolaryngology clinic. Arch Otolaryngol Head Neck Surg. 2005; 131(11):996–1000

[12] Langhagen T, Schroeder AS, Rettinger N, Borggraefe I, Jahn K. Migraine-related vertigo and somatoform vertigo frequently occur in children and are often associated. Neuropediatrics. 2013; 44(1):55–58

[13] Vartiainen E, Karjalainen S, Kärjä J. Vestibular disorders following head injury in children. Int J Pediatr Otorhinolaryngol. 1985; 9(2):135–141

[14] Wiart L, Darrah J. Review of four tests of gross motor development. Dev Med Child Neurol. 2001; 43(4):279–285

11

[15] Lagman-Bartolome AM, Lay C. Pediatric migraine variants: a review of epidemiology, diagnosis, treatment, and outcome. Curr Neurol Neurosci Rep. 2015; 15(6):34

[16] McCaslin DL, Jacobson GP, Gruenwald JM. The predominant forms of vertigo in children and their associated findings on balance function testing. Otolaryngol Clin North Am. 2011; 44(2):291–307, vii

[17] National Institute for Health and Care Excellence. Headaches in over 12s: diagnosis and management. NICE guidelines [CG150]. London: NICE; September 2012. Available at https://www.nice.org.uk/guidance/cg150?unlid=8704789772016714201857

[18] Richard W, Bruintjes TD, Oostenbrink P, van Leeuwen RB. Efficacy of the Epley maneuver for posterior canal BPPV: a long-term, controlled study of 81 patients. Ear Nose Throat J. 2005; 84(1):22–25

12 Facial Palsy Reconstruction in Children

Amir Sadri and Adel Y. Fattah

12.1 Introduction

Facial paralysis is a complex clinical problem with functional, psychological, and aesthetic components. The facial nerve is responsible for the tone and dynamic activity that is vital to ocular protection, nasal airflow, articulation of speech, and oral continence. Although functional impairment may be a significant issue in children, the effect on facial expression has a greater impact on social interaction with those perceived as "different" potentially suffering at the hands of their peers. Psychological stress rather than functional deficit is the critical factor in predicting social handicap and the main reason for seeking corrective surgery.[1,2] Nonverbal communication conveyed by facial expression is essential in normal social engagement, and spontaneous dynamic smile is critical for such communal interaction. As a result, restoration of facial nerve function is able to achieve great psychosocial benefits in addition to solving specific functional issues. Following permanent injury to the facial nerve, the aim of reconstruction is therefore not only to restore function, but also to recreate the smile. Our experience has led us to believe that it is an altered smile that is the primary cause of morbidity in children, and that in contrast to adults, the eye is often spared from the functional sequelae of facial nerve dysfunction. In this chapter, we provide a synopsis of how to systematically assess, investigate, and manage facial palsy in children and we outline options for reconstruction and rehabilitation.

12.2 Anatomy of the Facial Nerve

The facial nerve is a second pharyngeal (hyoid) arch derivative and therefore supplies structures derived from the same arch.[3] These include the muscles of facial expression, and taste sensation to the anterior two-thirds of the tongue (▶ Table 12.1). An understanding of the anatomy of the facial nerve (▶ Fig. 12.1) allows prediction of deficits and directs clinical diagnosis. The facial nerve comprises two nerves: the *facial motor nerve*, which is a purely motor nerve, and the *nervus intermedius*, which carries afferent taste and parasympathetic secretomotor fibers. These unite at the genu to form the common facial nerve in the temporal bone. To highlight this, the preceding terminology will be used throughout this chapter.

Table 12.1 Second pharyngeal arch derivatives

Arch	2
Cranial nerve	Facial
Muscle	Facial muscles Stapedius Stylohyoid Posterior belly of digastric
Skeletal	Stapes Styloid process Stylohyoid ligament Lesser cornu and body of hyoid
Aortic arch	Stapedial artery
Pharyngeal groove	Cervical sinus
Pharyngeal pouch	Faucial tonsil

12.3 Central Course

12.3.1 The Facial Motor Nerve

Corticobulbar (upper motor neuron) fibers descend from the precentral motor cortex toward the facial nerve nucleus in the caudal pons. These fibers cross over in the caudal pons, but those innervating the upper facial muscles also synapse in the ipsilateral facial motor nucleus. Sparing of the upper facial muscles in a facial palsy suggests a cortical or corticobulbar lesion. Lower

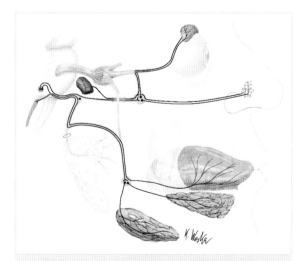

Fig. 12.1 The facial nerve and the nervus intermedius. (Reproduced from Gilroy and MacPherson, Atlas of Anatomy, 3rd edition, © 2016, Thieme Publishers, New York. Illustration by Karl Wesker.)

12

motor neuron nerve fibers wind around the abducens nucleus to emerge from the brainstem at the pontomedullary junction in concert with the nervus intermedius.

The Nervus Intermedius

The nervus intermedius is a smaller mixed nerve carrying afferent taste and parasympathetic secretomotor fibers. It is best considered as comprising two nerves (the greater superficial petrosal nerve and the chorda tympani; ▶ Fig. 12.1) that hitchhike alongside the facial motor nerve in the temporal bone. The nerve fibers arise in the superior salivary nucleus medial to the facial motor nucleus where the cell bodies of the preganglionic parasympathetic fibers lie. Afferent taste fibers run alongside these and synapse in the nucleus tractus solitarius in the medulla.

At their exit from the brainstem, the nerves lack epineurium and bridge an interval to enter the internal auditory meatus. Here they lie at the cerebellopontine angle closely related to the vestibulocochlear nerve. At this point, cranial nerves V to VIII are at risk from space-occupying lesions. Combined palsies strongly suggest this diagnosis and urgent imaging is mandatory.

12.3.2 Intratemporal Course

Upon entering the internal auditory meatus, the facial nerve courses through the petrous temporal bone within the Fallopian canal (▶ Fig. 12.2). Here the nerve is readily

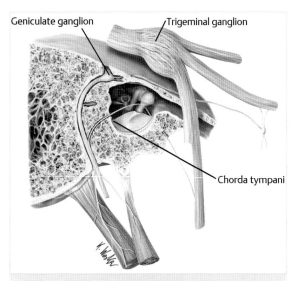

Geniculate ganglion   Trigeminal ganglion

Chorda tympani

Fig. 12.2 Intratemporal course of the facial nerve. (Reproduced from Gilroy and MacPherson, Atlas of Anatomy, 3rd edition, © 2016, Thieme Publishers, New York. Illustration by Karl Wesker.)

susceptible to compression from neoplastic, inflammatory, and traumatic events. In children, the nerve occupies proportionally less of the lumen of the canal than in adults; therefore, there is theoretically less likelihood of facial nerve compression. The intratemporal components of the facial nerve can be divided into the following three segments:
- Labyrinthine.
- Tympanic.
- Mastoid.

Labyrinthine Segment

The labyrinthine segment courses from the internal acoustic meatus to the geniculate ganglion where the nervus intermedius and facial motor nerve unite. The labyrinthine segment is the shortest and narrowest segment and lies posterior to the cochlea; any compression occurs initially at this point. After traversing the labyrinthine segment, the common facial nerve suddenly changes direction, forming a knee-shaped bend (genu) and thereafter running posteroinferiorly. The main branch of this portion is the *greater petrosal nerve.*

Tympanic Segment

The tympanic segment extends from geniculate ganglion to the bend at the lateral semicircular canal; here the thin lateral wall of the Fallopian canal separates the nerve from the tympanic cavity.

Mastoid Segment

The mastoid segment is the longest part and runs from the second bend to the stylomastoid foramen; the branches from this portion are the *nerve to stapedius* and the *chorda tympani.* The facial nerve runs vertically down the anterior wall of the mastoid process to exit at the stylomastoid foramen.

i

In younger children, the mastoid segment lies very superficial, virtually subcutaneously. This is because the tympanic part of the temporal bone has not ossified and the mastoid portion has yet to pneumatize (over the first year). It is due to the postnatal growth of these structures that the facial nerve eventually has a deeper location in the adult.

12.3.3 Branches of the Nervus Intermedius

Greater Petrosal Nerve

Also known as the *greater superficial petrosal nerve*, it leaves the common facial nerve and passes through the petrosal bone to enter the middle cranial fossa by running forward in a groove on the petrous temporal bone beneath the dura mater. It exits the cranial cavity through the foramen lacerum until it reaches the opening of the pterygoid canal. Here it is joined by the deep petrosal nerve, which is derived from the sympathetic plexus about the internal carotid artery. They unite to form the nerve of the pterygoid canal (vidian nerve) that will course toward the pterygopalatine fossa where parasympathetic fibers synapse in the pterygopalatine (sphenopalatine) ganglion. Postganglionic fibers join the maxillary nerve and are distributed to the lacrimal gland, nose, and palate through its branches.

Chorda Tympani

The chorda tympani traverses the middle ear along the superior inner surface adjacent to the tympanum. At the anterior border of the tympanum, it enters the petrotympanic fissure and turns downward and forward to reach the infratemporal fossa to join the lingual nerve, which distributes taste fibers to the anterior two-thirds of the tongue, and the parasympathetic secretomotor fibers, which synapse in the submandibular ganglion, to the submandibular and sublingual glands. It is these branches that are responsible for the intraoral eruption of herpes zoster in Ramsay Hunt syndrome. The chorda tympani is at risk in the middle ear and mastoid surgery. Trauma to the nerve, which can be caused by transection or by excessive manipulation and stretching, leads to alteration in taste sensation (dysgeusia) typically manifest as a metallic taste; this is much more severe when bilateral and is a significant but underreported cause of morbidity following tympanomastoid surgery.

12.3.4 The Facial Motor Nerve in the Face

Upon exiting the stylomastoid foramen, the facial nerve gives a posterior auricular branch and lies between the posterior belly of digastric and the stylohyoid muscles giving a branch to each before entering the substance of the parotid gland. In infants and young children, the intraparotid portion lies very superficial, where it can easily be damaged (see ▶ Fig. 26.4).

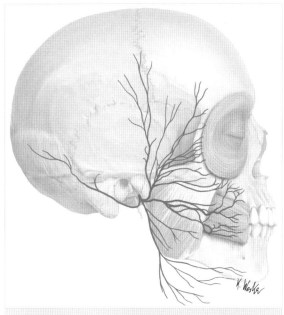

Fig. 12.3 Divisions of the facial nerve. (Reproduced from Gilroy and MacPherson, Atlas of Anatomy, 3rd edition, © 2016, Thieme Publishers, New York. Illustration by Karl Wesker.)

Within the parotid gland, the facial nerve divides into the five main divisions of the facial nerve: *temporal (frontal)*, *zygomatic*, *buccal*, *mandibular*, and *cervical* (▶ Fig. 12.3). These provide motor control to the 18 paired muscles of facial expression and to orbicularis oris.

All the facial muscles are supplied from their deep surface with the exception of buccinator, mentalis, and depressor anguli oris.[4] There are several common branching patterns, but each patient has a unique arrangement of branches, making knowledge of such patterns of limited value. There are surface anatomy landmarks that are helpful in identifying specific divisions.[5] A caveat is that such landmarks are determined in adults and the relative proportions in children are different, nonetheless they are a useful guide. The temporal branch that innervates the frontalis and orbicularis oculi muscles can be located using a line drawn from 1 cm below the inferior border of the tragus to a finger's breadth behind the eyebrow. This is termed *Pitanguy's line* and represents the vector along which the temporal division runs immediately under the temporoparietal fascia. In reality, it comprises numerous smaller branches over a defined area[6] and clinically its function is manifest by raising the eyebrows and by eyelid closure.

12

The midpoint of a line that runs from the root of the helix to the oral commissure is termed *Zuker's point*, which is the point at which a buccal or zygomatic branch innervates the oral (smile) musculature. The buccal and zygomatic divisions have overlapping innervation of the midfacial musculature. Evaluation of the zygomatic division is by assessing lower eyelid tone, eye closure, and the smile. The buccal division is examined by puckering the lips and blowing out the cheeks to establish lip seal.

The mandibular division (*marginal mandibular nerve*) may be at risk during surgery in the submandibular region, for example, in removal of lymph nodes, excision of the submandibular gland, or drainage of septic neck swellings. The nerve runs deep to platysma and is best avoided by ensuring that incisions are kept at least 2 cm below the inferior mandibular border.[5] In this way, the nerve is kept out of harm's way as it is lifted upward in the superior flap as dissection progresses in the subplatysmal plane. This nerve innervates the depressor anguli oris and damage is manifest as an asymmetric smile, where the lower lip rides higher than the contralateral normal side. The cervical branch can be located 1 cm below the angle of the mandible on a line perpendicular to that drawn from the mentum to the mastoid process. Dysfunction of the cervical branch is of far less clinical or aesthetic importance.

12.4 Classification of Facial Palsy

Facial palsy is a sign with many causes, and comprehensive classification systems have been proposed.[7] The most efficient method to classify causes for diagnostic purposes is to consider the anatomical location of the nerve (central, temporal, and facial) and then apply the "surgical sieve" (▶ Table 12.2). Rare systemic causes, such as fetal acetylcholine receptor inactivation syndrome,[8] may be considered further down the diagnostic pathway.

Facial palsy at birth occurs in approximately 0.2 to 2% of live births, 80 to 90% of which are due to birth trauma. Overall, a cause for pediatric facial palsy is determined in 70% of cases.[9] Acquired idiopathic facial palsy is a diagnosis of exclusion and termed *Bell's palsy*. In children, additional weight should be given to considering a congenital cause, but the commonest etiology

overall is obstetric birth injury and most recover within a month.[10,11] Congenital idiopathic isolated palsy of the mandibular division is a typical presentation, but the true incidence is hard to define. Syndromic facial palsy is infrequent but is most commonly part of hemifacial microsomia where there is hypoplasia affecting one side of the face, often in association with other congenital anomalies of the head and neck. The most common causes of facial palsy in children are outlined as follows.

12.4.1 Congenital

This term refers to facial palsy present at birth that does not rapidly improve; supportive management is indicated with consideration of reconstruction when the child is older.

Idiopathic Facial Palsy

In children, the most common congenital cause is idiopathic facial nerve palsy. There are a number of presentations typically affecting the mandibular division (discussed next) or multiple divisions; the lower face is most obviously affected during animation.

Neonatal Asymmetric Crying Facies

The term *neonatal* indicates that the condition is present at birth rather than acquired. It classically presents as normal appearance at rest but an asymmetric lower lip position with crying or smiling.

> **i**
>
> Parents and clinicians will typically complain of the lip being "pulled down" but this is the unaffected side where the normal depressor anguli oris muscle is functioning. The defect is due to a failure of the contralateral muscle to counteract the normal upward pull of the midfacial musculature during smiling.

It affects 0.6% live births, and in approximately 10% of cases, there are significant associated malformations. Whether the defect is due to muscle hypoplasia or nerve dysfunction is the subject of debate; electrodiagnostic studies have suggested muscle hypoplasia, whereas an

Table 12.2 Constructing a differential diagnosis for acquired facial palsy (in adults and children)			
Sieve	**Anatomical location**		
	Central	**Temporal**	**Facial**
Trauma	Penetrating trauma	Skull-base fracture	Laceration
Neoplasia	Medulloblastoma	Cholesteatoma	Adenocarcinoma
Inflammatory	Lyme disease	Bell's palsy	Bell's palsy
Vascular	Stroke	Vascular malformation	Vascular malformation

ultrasonographic study (USS) found that six of seven patients had normal muscles.[12] Cayler's (cardiofacial) syndrome is asymmetric crying facies in association with cardiac malformations; fluorescence in situ hybridization (FISH) analysis has demonstrated the 22q.11 microdeletion in these instances. Positive FISH testing is an indication for echocardiogram and referral to pediatric cardiologist. Electrodiagnostic testing and USS of muscle is of little practical value and difficult to perform in infants.

Hemifacial Microsomia

This is a spectrum of morphogenetic anomalies of the tissues derived from the first and second pharyngeal arches. Facial palsy has been reported to be present in 22 to 45% of patients[13] and forms part of the OMENS (orbit, mandible, ear, nerve, soft tissue) classification,[14] whereby the palsy is classified as upper face, lower face, or complete involvement. It is managed in the same way as other cases of established facial palsy. One consideration is that these patients typically require orthognathic surgery at skeletal maturity, and planning of a cross-facial nerve graft should be undertaken with care.

Möbius' Syndrome

Möbius' syndrome is a rare sporadic congenital form of cranial nerve palsy that affects the abducens and facial nerves bilaterally, together with numerous other cranial and extracranial anomalies in a variable fashion (▶ Fig. 12.4). It is estimated that it affects 1 per 300,000 live births and approximately 200 cases of all ages are present in the United Kingdom. At birth, severe strabismus is noted together with a "masklike" facies; ophthalmology is often the first surgical specialty to have contact with these babies either due to the strabismus or lagophthalmos necessitating corneal protection. Other cranial nerve palsies lead to swallowing and feeding difficulties necessitating nasogastric feeding, percutaneous gastroenterostomy, or even tracheostomy for airway protection in severe cases. Other signs include the Poland's syndrome of chest and hand malformations and lower limb malformations such as talipes.

In addition to the lack of facial expression, a delay in speech development and hearing loss can add to the impression of learning disabilities, which is present in 10 to 75%,[15] the wide range in percentage indicating that the very low numbers in the study groups make it difficult to ascertain a true incidence.

> **i**
>
> These patients require coordinated care by a specialist team with supportive and surgical management individualized to the patient and family.

The facial palsy in these patients is bilateral but typically has a mixed picture with partial activity in some divisions of the facial nerve in an asymmetric pattern. Like most cases of congenital pediatric facial palsy, the lower face has a greater impact to the overall appearance upon animation. Therapy may be of some benefit in these patients, but if the child desires a smile, surgical reconstruction can be considered around the age of 7 years or above.

CHARGE Syndrome

CHARGE syndrome (coloboma, heart defects, atresia of the choanae, retardation of growth/development, genitourinary, and ear malformations) is a rare genetic syndrome affecting 1 to 3 per 10,000 live births and the acronym refers to the clinical features. There are specific clinical criteria for diagnosis, and a mutation in the CHD7 gene occurs in approximately two-thirds of patients. Facial palsy occurs in some cases, typically as part of multiple cranial nerve anomalies with consequent hearing loss and swallowing problems. As a consequence of the choanal atresia, the otolaryngologist will often be the first surgical specialty to assess these children; airway and feeding considerations take precedence (see Chapter 16).

12.4.2 Acquired

An acquired facial palsy may present at birth after traumatic delivery and rapidly improves, or presents later following a period of normal function.

Obstetric Facial Palsy (Trauma/Facial)

> **i**
>
> The most common form of facial palsy in children is obstetric facial palsy.[10,11]

This is caused by the posterior blade of the forceps or maternal sacral promontory exerting pressure on the facial nerve as it exits the stylomastoid foramen, resulting in a neurapraxia manifest as a facial palsy affecting multiple divisions. It resolves completely in 90% of cases. By the time the child is seen by the surgical specialist, the palsy is already rapidly improving. Low birth weight (> 3,500 g) is a risk factor and there is an association with other birth injuries such as brachial plexus palsy and clavicular fractures. Initially, it is difficult to differentiate from a congenital palsy and is sometimes classified as such; the delivery history and rapid improvement allow diagnosis after monitoring for a couple of months.

Otitis Media (Infectious/Temporal)

This is a common cause, and children with otitis media present with signs of middle ear infection such as

12

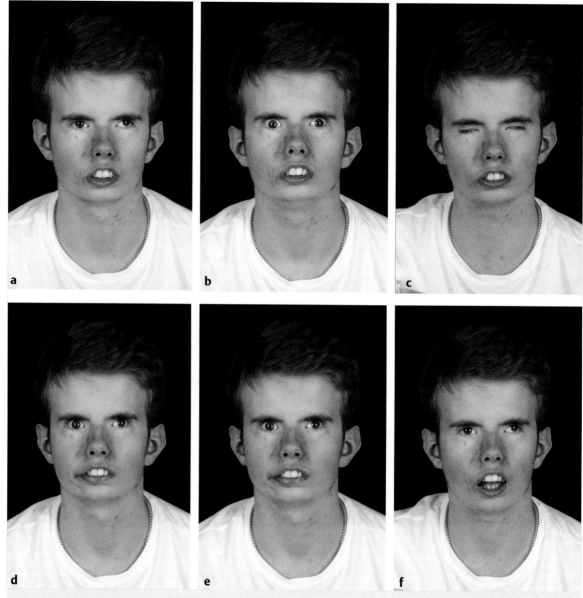

Fig. 12.4 Möbius' syndrome: bilateral facial and abducens nerve palsy. Standardized views. **(a)** Repose. **(b)** Raised eyebrows. **(c)** Gentle eye closure. **(d)** Small smile. **(e)** Full smile. **(f)** Pucker lips.

earache, deafness, injection of the tympanum, effusion, discharge, or even acute mastoiditis. Ear signs typically present a week prior to manifestation of facial nerve weakness. If the tympanum remains intact, myringotomy and antibiotic therapy may be indicated to relieve pressure on the nerve.

> **i**
>
> Neurapraxia typically resolves and the prognosis is excellent in promptly managed cases.

Ramsay Hunt syndrome is varicella zoster infection of the geniculate ganglion manifest as a more severe facial palsy with a vesicular eruption of the external auditory meatus and the ipsilateral palate and tongue. It was Hunt's clinical descriptions that lead to the recognition of the somatosensory function of the facial nerve. In contrast to acute otitis media, these patients suffer a more dense facial palsy and are less likely to recover. Additionally, a large retrospective study determined that the palsy preceded the rash, making differentiation from Bell's palsy challenging. The incidence in children above the age of 6 years is comparable to that in adults, and prompt

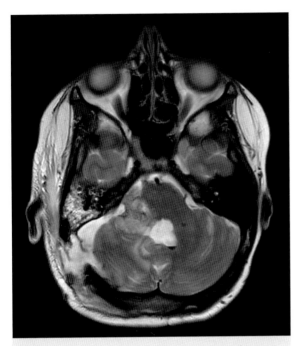

Fig. 12.5 Magnetic resonance imaging scan showing large mass (ependymoma) in the right cerebellopontine angle in a 14-year-old girl. Clinical features included complete facial palsy and vocal cord palsy.

initiation of combined antiviral and corticosteroid therapy are key to treatment.[16]

Brain Tumors (Central/Neoplasia)

Space-occupying lesions of the posterior fossa and their surgical treatment can present with facial palsy and often multiple cranial nerve palsies. The most common tumors resulting in facial palsy are medulloblastomas (20% of pediatric brain tumors), cerebellar astrocytomas, and ependymomas (▶ Fig. 12.5); all are generally treated surgically to achieve curative resection. A period of monitoring postsurgery is worthwhile to determine if there is any improvement in facial nerve functioning; thereafter, surgical reconstruction can be planned following oncological multidisciplinary team (MDT) discussion. If planned resection is likely to cause facial nerve palsy, the specialist team can provide preoperative counseling and potentially perform immediate reconstruction as part of the primary procedure.

Iatrogenic Facial Palsy

The facial nerve trunk and its branches are at risk during tympanomastoid surgery, parotid surgery, and surgery in the upper part of the neck where trauma to the marginal mandibular nerve is an ever-present risk. It is important to remember that the nerve and its branches are extremely superficial in young children, and the site of exit from the stylomastoid foramen is much higher than in adults as the mastoid process has not yet developed. The nerve and its branches can be easily damaged if, for example, a postauricular incision to approach the mastoid is made too low, if the surgeon in parotidectomy is unfamiliar with the anatomy, or if an incision to approach a lesion in the submandibular region is not made well below the inferior border of the mandible (see Chapter 26). Management of iatrogenic facial palsy is outlined in Box 12.1.

Box 12.1 Management of Iatrogenic Facial Palsy (Immediately Postoperatively)

- Review operation note (was the nerve seen/protected? If so, it is likely neurapraxia).
- If the nerve is likely to have been cut consider reexploring with a colleague/specialist.
- Is there pressure on the nerve? If so, remove pack/drain hematoma.
- If neurapraxia, wait 6 weeks with regular review to look for improvement.
- If no improvement, consider referral to a specialist for reexploration.
- Maintain ocular competence throughout the surveillance period and involve ophthalmology.

Bell's Palsy

Acquired idiopathic facial palsy in children is a diagnosis of exclusion; it is much less common in children below the age of 16 years but is treated in the same manner as for adults. It is thought to be viral. The American Academy of Otolaryngology – Head and Neck Surgery Foundation have published guidelines for management (see Chapter 12.7.2).[17]

12.5 History and Examination

History and examination is important to determine the cause of facial palsy and to assess the degree of deficit and the need for supportive and reconstructive management. A systematic approach is key to accurate documentation of the degree of deficit, subsequent monitoring of facial nerve function, and planning for reconstruction (see Box 12.2).

Box 12.2 Examination in Children

Inspect the following:

- Scars from previous surgery, for example, bicoronal, lateral skull base, parotidectomy.
- Eyebrow: ptosis, asymmetry of eyebrow position.
- Upper lid: lagophthalmos, lid retraction.
- Globe: corneal abrasions, Bell's phenomenon (► Fig. 12.6).
- Lower lid: ectropion, tear pooling, snap test.
- Cheek ptosis, compare nasolabial folds.
- Nose: nasal valve inspection, assess nasal patency.
- Mouth: commissure symmetry at rest, tooth show, assess bilabial speech, blisters of Ramsay Hunt's syndrome, bimanual palpation of parotid gland.
- Ear: hyperacusis and examine external auditory meatus for blisters and middle ear pathology.

Examine the facial nerve:

- Temporal branch: raise eyebrows (frontalis); close eyes tight (orbicularis oculi).
- Zygomatic branch: smile and compare tooth show (zygomaticus).
- Buccal: blow out cheeks (buccinator/orbicularis oris).
- Mandibular: Lip ride with smile and/or tooth show (depressor anguli oris).

Look for multiple cranial nerve palsies: "I would now like to examine the remaining cranial nerves…"

- V (a potential motor for reconstruction): Bite teeth together (feel masseter and temporalis contraction).
- VIII: cerebellopontine angle tumor, consider audiometry.
- IX, X, XI: multiple palsies may preclude cranial nerve transfer for reconstruction.
- XII: a potential motor for reconstruction.

Investigations:

- Ophthalmic assessment if any corneal pathology.
- Consider formal speech assessment.
- Consider formal psychological assessment.
- Consider electromyography (EMG) if you suspect viable facial musculature remains.

Discussion:

- The principal aim of early treatment is ocular protection; thereafter, discuss the patient's primary concerns and his/her goals for treatment, all the time asking "is this an achievable muscle-specific goal?"

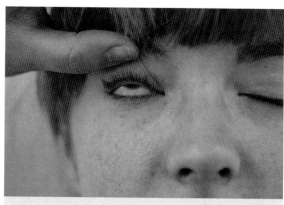

Fig. 12.6 Bell's phenomenon. Eyelids are closed tightly and the upper lid is lifted: the globe is rotated upward indicating an intact protective phenomenon. Up to 10% of the population do not have this and the reflex is "not intact."

The clinical features in children differ from adults: age-related ptosis of the facial tissues in adults makes any asymmetry more obvious, especially around the eyes. In children, the eyes are often much less obviously affected, becoming an issue in later life. Facial ptosis is not so evident such that a child with idiopathic facial palsy may look almost symmetrical at rest, but asymmetric upon facial animation.

Absence of frontalis activity results in brow ptosis and (in adults) there may be "excess" of upper lid skin (dermatochalasis). This is not true excess, and in many cases, lifting the eyebrow will correct this. Upper lid blepharoplasty should not be performed in isolation, as subsequent eyebrow lift will leave the eye unable to close. Weak innervation of the orbicularis oculi muscle leads to lagophthalmos, an inability to close the eye. The oculomotor-innervated levator palpebrae superioris may overcome the orbicularis tone and create a wider palpebral aperture: *lid retraction*. There may be a paralytic ectropion of the lower eyelid. The combination of these deficits leaves the globe at risk of exposure, and patients may complain of ocular surface symptoms and exhibit scleral injection, chemosis, corneal abrasions, and ulceration. Some patients may have dry eyes due to loss of parasympathetic secretomotor input to the lacrimal gland. By contrast, reduced effective blink reflex leads to a dry eye that drives paradoxical epiphora.

In contrast to adults who show premature age-related changes in the face, such as deepening of the nasolabial folds, children will often have a reduced nasolabial crease. Paralysis of the perioral musculature can produce asymmetry of the oral commissures, drooling, and oral incontinence. Inability to hold the lips sealed will affect bilabial sounds such as /b/, /p/, and /m/. These features are not universal, especially if the child has no other neurodevelopmental pathology, and the asymmetric smile is nearly always the main issue. Psychological morbidity is significant, often underestimated by the surgeon, and may lead to underperformance and bullying at school. Holistic care and an MDT (otolaryngologist, ophthalmologist, plastic surgeon, neurosurgeon, psychologist, speech and

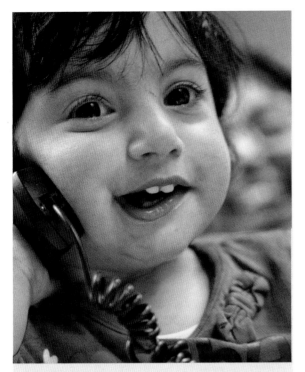

Fig. 12.7 Asymmetric crying facies. Reduced activity in the mandibular division of the facial nerve on the affected side allows the lower lip to ride up creating asymmetry (patient's left).

language therapists, and physical therapists)[18] are the key to optimum outcomes.

Facial palsy can affect one or more divisions of the facial nerve and be either complete (total loss of function) or partial (some function remains); thus, *asymmetric crying facies* (▶ Fig. 12.7) may be described as a unilateral complete mandibular division facial palsy. Such terminology rapidly communicates the deficit between clinicians.

12.5.1 Secondary Features: Synkinesis, Spasm, and Contracture

Synkinesis (Greek translation: joined movement) refers to uncontrolled facial contractions away from the site of voluntary motion. It is thought to occur due to aberrant regeneration of facial nerve axons along incorrect pathways, or it may be due to facial nerve nucleus hyperexcitability. Typical patterns include oral-ocular synkinesis (eye closure with mouth movement) and the reverse (oculo-oral synkinesis). "Crocodile tears" (Bogorad's syndrome) is an uncommon result of the faulty regeneration of facial nerve fibers whereby motor fibers are directed erroneously to the lacrimal gland resulting in epiphora during mastication. It is a specific example of synkinesis and analogous to Frey's syndrome. Occasionally, painful facial spasm and contractures can result from a partially recovered facial palsy.

> **i**
> A range of nonsurgical therapies is directed to controlling these symptoms.

12.5.2 Documenting the Severity of Facial Palsy: Grading Systems, Standardized Photography and Patient-Reported Outcome Measures

Accurate documentation of facial nerve function is important to monitor progress and appraise the results of medical and surgical interventions. Facial nerve grading scales were introduced to provide a more uniform and accurate method for assessing facial nerve function. Numerous scales have been introduced, the most commonly used being the House–Brackmann system,[19,20] but it is generally agreed that it is not effective for determining changes in facial nerve function following therapeutic intervention. A recent systematic review found that the Sunnybrook scale[21] fulfilled the desired criteria for a facial grading scale (▶ Fig. 12.8).

In addition to objective assessment of facial nerve function, standardized photography should be performed documenting the movements animated by each of the facial nerve divisions (▶ Fig. 12.9).

Finally, as facial nerve dysfunction has a significant psychological morbidity associated with it, a patient-reported outcome measure allows documentation of the subjective effects of the palsy on the patient. There are now validated measures, for example, the Facial Clinimetric Evaluation Scale[22] and the Facial Disability Index, to assess the quality of life in patients with facial assymetery.[23]

12.6 Investigations

12.6.1 Diagnostic

Congenital Palsy

A child born with facial palsy is most likely to have an acquired obstetric or idiopathic palsy. In such cases, monitor and observe carefully for recovery: rapid recovery and a history of difficult vaginal, particularly forceps, delivery would suggest injury. If the child appears syndromic, investigate as indicated by the clinical features. Magnetic resonance imaging (MRI) requires a general anesthetic for young children to remain motionless long

12

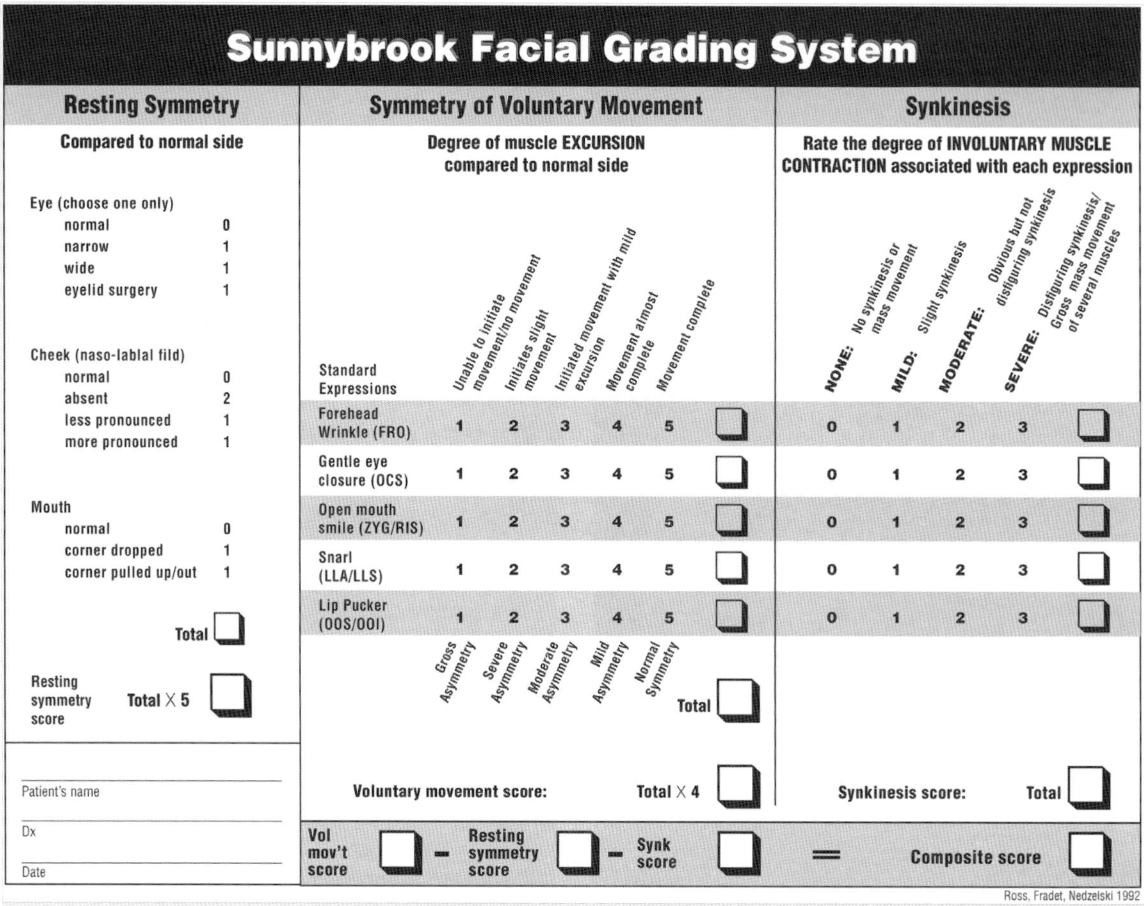

Sunnybrook Facial Grading System

Resting Symmetry

Compared to normal side

Eye (choose one only)	
normal	0
narrow	1
wide	1
eyelid surgery	1

Cheek (naso-labial fild)	
normal	0
absent	2
less pronounced	1
more pronounced	1

Mouth	
normal	0
corner dropped	1
corner pulled up/out	1

Total ☐

Resting symmetry score — Total X 5 ☐

Symmetry of Voluntary Movement

Degree of muscle EXCURSION compared to normal side

Standard Expressions	Unable to initiate movement/no movement	Initiates slight movement	Initiated movement with mild excursion	Movement almost complete	Movement complete	
Forehead Wrinkle (FRO)	1	2	3	4	5	☐
Gentle eye closure (OCS)	1	2	3	4	5	☐
Open mouth smile (ZYG/RIS)	1	2	3	4	5	☐
Snarl (LLA/LLS)	1	2	3	4	5	☐
Lip Pucker (OOS/OOI)	1	2	3	4	5	☐
	Gross Asymmetry	Severe Asymmetry	Moderate Asymmetry	Mild Asymmetry	Normal Symmetry	Total ☐

Voluntary movement score: Total X 4 ☐

Synkinesis

Rate the degree of INVOLUNTARY MUSCLE CONTRACTION associated with each expression

	NONE: No synkinesis or mass movement	MILD: Slight synkinesis	MODERATE: Obvious but not disfiguring synkinesis	SEVERE: Disfiguring synkinesis/ Gross mass movement of several muscles	
Forehead Wrinkle (FRO)	0	1	2	3	☐
Gentle eye closure (OCS)	0	1	2	3	☐
Open mouth smile (ZYG/RIS)	0	1	2	3	☐
Snarl (LLA/LLS)	0	1	2	3	☐
Lip Pucker (OOS/OOI)	0	1	2	3	☐

Synkinesis score: Total ☐

Patient's name

Dx

Date

Vol mov't score ☐ – Resting symmetry score ☐ – Synk score ☐ = Composite score ☐

Ross, Fradet, Nedzelski 1992

Fig. 12.8 Sunnybrook facial grading scale. This is a regional-weighted system based on the evaluation of facial symmetry at rest, voluntary facial movements, and synkinesis; each is evaluated on point scales, and a composite score (0–100) is generated as a continuous scale. This is in contrast to a ranked scale (e.g., House-Brackmann Scale [HBS]), which attempts to categorize into specific groups. Changes in score can be used to chart recovery or response to therapy. (Reproduced from Ross BG, Fradet G, Nedzelski JM. Development of a sensitive clinical facial grading system. Otolaryngol Head Neck Surg 1996;114(3):380–386, with permission.)

enough to capture images; there is no indication for a scan for diagnostic purposes unless there is a history of worsening paralysis or there is some other focal neurologic deficit.

Acquired Palsy

Imaging is indicated in almost all cases of acquired palsy in children or if there are any *red flag* signs (see Box 12.3). MRI with contrast is the modality of choice and will detect not only neoplastic lesions but also enhancement of the nerve in Bell's palsy. Imaging need not be performed within the first week of a sudden onset palsy without other neurologic signs, as diagnostic specificity is reduced. If otoscopic examination suggests a mass or if there is a history of chronic otitis media, mastoiditis, or a suspected skull base fracture, CT scan with bone windows of the temporal bone is recommended (▶ Fig. 12.10). Serological testing for Lyme disease is indicated if there has been a history of foreign travel to endemic areas. In the vast majority of acquired cases, either imaging will determine a discrete lesion or a normal scan will suggest Bell's palsy as a diagnosis of exclusion, or Ramsay Hunt's syndrome in cases of vesiculation.

Box 12.3 Red Flag Signs

- Bilateral palsy.
- Slow onset (over 3 weeks) with progressive deterioration.
- Multiple cranial nerve palsies.
- Strabismus.
- Hearing loss/tinnitus.

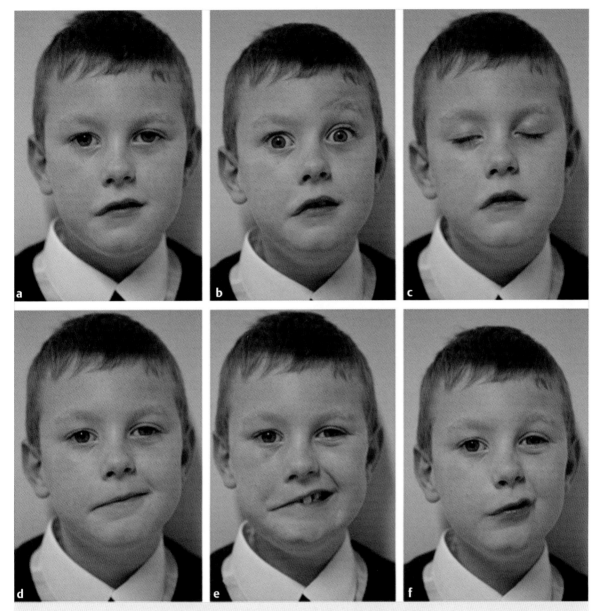

Fig. 12.9 Standardized facial palsy views. **(a)** Repose. **(b)** Raised eyebrows (note the asymmetry). **(c)** Gentle eye closure (there is 3-mm lagophthalmos on the right). **(d)** Small smile. **(e)** Full smile. **(f)** Pucker lips.

12.6.2 Prognostic

Evoked EMG (EEMG) or electroneurography (ENoG) can be used to investigate cases of facial nerve paralysis that fail to improve.[24] However, these tests are only valuable during the early stages of disease (< 3 weeks), which presents logistical problems in terms of time from referral.

EEMG records postsynaptic potentials with electrodes in the nasolabial fold. Poor prognosis is associated with a decreased EEMG response to < 10% of normal. If this response is elicited early, surgical decompression may be of value, although the evidence is limited. ENoG works by stimulating the facial nerve as it exits the temporal bone and measuring the muscular response (evoked compound muscle action potential). The higher the ENoG value, the better the prognosis. However, the key question is, "what will the investigation tell you and what will you do about it?" If it is Bell's palsy, there is no indication for surgical decompression and medical or expectant management is needed. If a discrete pathology has been found, then surgical therapy is directed toward alleviating this.

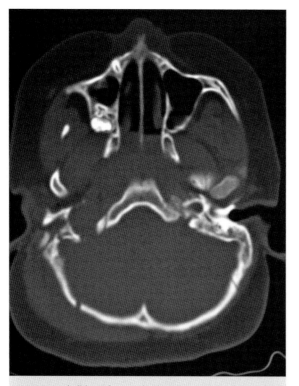

Fig. 12.10 Skull-base fracture leading to right complete facial palsy of all divisions. Skull-base fracture that involves the right occipital and petrous temporal bones.

Electrophysiology is rarely used in our center.

12.7 Treatment

12.7.1 Supportive Management

Corneal protection is the clinician's primary concern.

Ocular surface symptoms, such as redness, itching, and dryness, are indication for immediate lubrication and referral to an ophthalmologist for assessment. Generally, *preservative-free* hypromellose eye drops are used during the day and simple eye ointment at night. Patients and parents can be taught to tape the lid shut at night to pro-

tect the eye. The importance of the Bell's phenomenon (upward rolling of the globe with eye closure; ▶ Fig. 12.6) is evident in these cases as it protects the cornea when the eye cannot be completely closed.

Specialized (facial rehabilitation) physical therapists can provide support and education, such as teaching patients massage and stretching exercises to counteract muscle tightness and spasm. Neuromuscular retraining and biofeedback exercises to those patients with partial paralysis of the facial nerve have been shown to reduce and control synkinesis.[25] In specific cases, electrical stimulation therapy under specialist guidance is of value in maintaining muscle activity, but many children have difficulty maintaining compliance.

Psychological impact of facial palsy can be dramatic, and appropriate support or cognitive behavioral therapy from a psychologist can improve patient well-being, compliance with treatment, and expectation of outcomes.[26] Support groups such as Facial Palsy UK (www.facialpalsy.org.uk) are available, and there are some for the very rare syndromes such Möbius' syndrome (www.moebiusresearchtrust.org) and CHARGE syndrome (www.charge-syndrome.org.uk).

12.7.2 Medical Management

Traditionally, corticosteroids and antivirals (e.g., acyclovir) have formed the mainstay of medical therapy in patients with Bell's palsy.[27,28]

There is good evidence that oral steroids alone given within 72 hours of facial paralysis in patients with Bell's palsy promotes faster nerve recovery.[29,30,31,32] There is also some evidence that the addition of antiviral therapy provides additional benefits, although this merits further investigation.[33]

12.7.3 Reconstructive Management

Classification for Reconstruction

When considering reconstruction, dysfunction is classified in a manner that helps guide management, that is, by division and partial versus complete loss of function. Key factors to consider are outlined in Box 12.4. Simplistically, one has to determine whether to restore symmetry to the face at rest or restore movement.

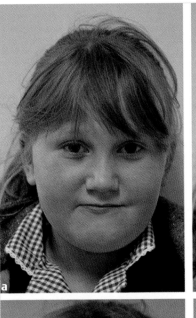
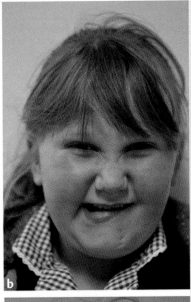
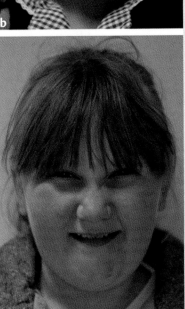

Fig. 12.11 Asymmetric crying facies treatment with botulinum toxin A. **(a,b)** Pretreatment. **(c,d)** Posttreatment. Depressor anguli oris on the left fails to counteract the upward motion of the face with smile. Treatment of the muscle on the right (unaffected side) restores symmetry to the smile.

Box 12.4 Key Factors to Consider in Facial Palsy Reconstruction

- Corneal protection is a priority.
- What are the patient's primary concerns?
- Are there muscle-specific goals?
- Is it a partial palsy? If so, is function adequate?
- Is there a proximal nerve stump?
- Is there viable facial muscle?

Reconstructive Management Options

If function is adequate, botulinum toxin type A can be used to weaken the contralateral side to restore symmetry (▶ Fig. 12.11). If not, facelifts and slings in the form of synthetic (Gore-Tex, Gore) and nonsynthetic (fascia lata or palmaris longus tendon) material can be used to improve nasal airflow, elevate the cheek, support the lower eyelid, and elevate the oral commissure to restore symmetry. Such procedures require reoperation at intervals as they slowly give way over time and are generally not required or recommended in children.

> Restoration of movement requiring a muscle and a nerve is often needed in children, and a variety of combinations of muscle and nerve can be used to restore motion.

12

Table 12.3 Reconstructive management of established facial palsy

Type of injury	Facial nerve viability	Management options
Partial	Adequate nerve function	Weaken normal side
	Inadequate nerve function	Augment affected side with cross-facial nerve graft or cranial transfer
Early (viable facial muscle)	Proximal stump	Direct repair; ipsilateral nerve grafting
	No proximal stump	Cross-facial nerve graft; cranial nerve transfer
Late (no viable facial muscle)	Proximal stump	Free muscle transfer to ipsilateral facial nerve; local muscle flap
	No proximal stump	Free muscle transfer with cross-facial nerve graft or cranial nerve transfer; local muscle flap

The key issue is whether viable facial nerve remains in the face; if so, the contralateral facial nerve or another cranial nerve can be used to reestablish innervation.[34] After 18 months, most authors would consider the degree of muscle atrophy too great to consider reinnervation and muscle will need to be imported into the face (► Table 12.3).

Local Muscle Transfers

Local or free muscle transfers can be used to reestablish movement in the face. Local transfers include the temporalis or masseter muscles powered by a functioning trigeminal nerve. The Labbé modification of temporalis transfer releases both attachments of the muscle, increasing its reach to the corner of the mouth.[35] The masseter muscle transfer is performed by repositioning the attachment of muscle from the mandible into the upper and lower lips, but is recognized as a poor option in most hands.[36]

Free Muscle Transfers

Free muscle transplantation can be employed. To achieve facial reanimation with free muscle transfer, a suitably sized muscle must be positioned on the face and neurotized either with the contralateral normal facial nerve (cross-facial nerve graft) or with other cranial nerve (trigeminal or hypoglossal nerve).

Several muscles have been used to reanimate the face, but the gracilis muscle due to its size, expendability, and ease of dissection is the most frequently used (► Fig. 12.12). Once harvested, the muscle is transposed and tensioned along the nasolabial crease into the oral commissure. The muscle is motored using either a cross-facial nerve graft or cranial nerve. The choice of neural input depends on patient and surgeon factors: using the contralateral facial nerve gives a spontaneous but weaker smile. By contrast, using the motor nerve to masseter gives a stronger smile upon biting, but cortical adaptation means that the conscious need to bite is often lost over time.[37] The results of free muscle transfer are currently considered superior to regional muscle or nerve transfers.[18]

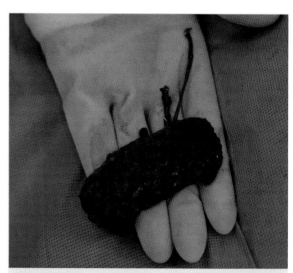

Fig. 12.12 Free gracilis muscle transfer for facial reanimation. This 20-g, 10-cm-long portion of the gracilis muscle is transplanted into the face to recreate a dynamic smile for the patient.

12.8 Key Points

- Facial palsy in children differs from that in adults in etiology, symptomatology, and reconstructive requirements.
- Children require an MDT approach, careful assessment, and treatment that take their psychosocial requirements into account.

References

[1] VanSwearingen JM, Cohn JF, Turnbull J, Mrzai T, Johnson P. Psychological distress: linking impairment with disability in facial neuromotor disorders. Otolaryngol Head Neck Surg. 1998; 118(6):790–796

[2] Bradbury ET, Simons W, Sanders R. Psychological and social factors in reconstructive surgery for hemi-facial palsy. J Plast Reconstr Aesthet Surg. 2006; 59(3):272–278

[3] Fattah AY, Meara JG, Britto JA. Craniofacial development and congenital anomaly: a contemporary review of processes and pathogenesis. In: Bluestone CD, Simons JP, Healy BG, eds. Bluestone and Stool's

Pediatric Otolaryngology. 5th ed. Shelton, CT: People's Medical Publishing House; 2014:1–18

[4] Freilinger G, Gruber H, Happak W, Pechmann U. Surgical anatomy of the mimic muscle system and the facial nerve: importance for reconstructive and aesthetic surgery. Plast Reconstr Surg. 1987; 80(5): 686–690

[5] Davies JC, Agur A, Fattah AY. Anatomic landmarks for localisation of the branches of the facial nerve. OA Anatomy. 2013; 1(4):1–9

[6] Davies JC, Fattah A, Ravichandiran M, Agur AM. Clinically relevant landmarks of the frontotemporal branch of the facial nerve: a three-dimensional study. Clin Anat. 2012; 25(7):858–865

[7] Westin LM, Zuker R. A new classification system for facial paralysis in the clinical setting. J Craniofac Surg. 2003; 14(5):672–679

[8] Oskoui M, Jacobson L, Chung WK, et al. Fetal acetylcholine receptor inactivation syndrome and maternal myasthenia gravis. Neurology. 2008; 71(24):2010–2012

[9] Shargorodsky J, Lin HW, Gopen Q. Facial nerve palsy in the pediatric population. Clin Pediatr (Phila). 2010; 49(5):411–417

[10] Hughes CA, Harley EH, Milmoe G, Bala R, Martorella A. Birth trauma in the head and neck. Arch Otolaryngol Head Neck Surg. 1999; 125 (2):193–199

[11] Duval M, Daniel SJ. Facial nerve palsy in neonates secondary to forceps use. Arch Otolaryngol Head Neck Surg. 2009; 135(7):634–636

[12] Sapin SO, Miller AA, Bass HN. Neonatal asymmetric crying facies: a new look at an old problem. Clin Pediatr (Phila). 2005; 44(2):109–119

[13] Gougoutas AJ, Singh DJ, Low DW, Bartlett SP. Hemifacial microsomia: clinical features and pictographic representations of the OMENS classification system. Plast Reconstr Surg. 2007; 120(7):112e–120e

[14] Vento AR, LaBrie RA, Mulliken JB. The O.M.E.N.S. classification of hemifacial microsomia. Cleft Palate Craniofac J. 1991; 28(1):68–76, discussion 77

[15] Singham J, Manktelow R, Zuker RM. Möbius syndrome. Semin Plast Surg. 2004; 18(1):39–46

[16] Sweeney CJ, Gilden DH. Ramsay Hunt syndrome. J Neurol Neurosurg Psychiatry. 2001; 71(2):149–154

[17] Baugh RF, Basura GJ, Ishii LE, et al. Clinical practice guideline: Bell's palsy. Otolaryngol Head Neck Surg. 2013; 149(3) Suppl:S1–S27

[18] Fattah A, Borschel GH, Manktelow RT, Bezuhly M, Zuker RM. Facial palsy and reconstruction. Plast Reconstr Surg. 2012; 129(2):340e–352e

[19] House JW, Brackmann DE. Facial nerve grading system. Otolaryngol Head Neck Surg. 1985; 93(2):146–147

[20] Fattah AY, Gavilan J, Hadlock TA, et al. Survey of methods of facial palsy documentation in use by members of the Sir Charles Bell Society. Laryngoscope. 2014; 124(10):2247–2251

[21] Ross BG, Fradet G, Nedzelski JM. Development of a sensitive clinical facial grading system. Otolaryngol Head Neck Surg. 1996; 114(3): 380–386

[22] Kahn JB, Gliklich RE, Boyev KP, Stewart MG, Metson RB, McKenna MJ. Validation of a patient-graded instrument for facial nerve paralysis: the FaCE scale. Laryngoscope. 2001; 111(3):387–398

[23] Ho AL, Scott AM, Klassen AF, Cano SJ, Pusic AL, Van Laeken N. Measuring quality of life and patient satisfaction in facial paralysis patients: a systematic review of patient-reported outcome measures. Plast Reconstr Surg. 2012; 130(1):91–99

[24] Byun H, Cho Y-S, Jang JY, et al. Value of electroneurography as a prognostic indicator for recovery in acute severe inflammatory facial paralysis: a prospective study of Bell's palsy and Ramsay Hunt syndrome. Laryngoscope. 2013; 123(10):2526–2532

[25] Pourmomeny AA, Zadmehre H, Mirshamsi M, Mahmodi Z. Prevention of synkinesis by biofeedback therapy: a randomized clinical trial. Otol Neurotol. 2014; 35(4):739–742

[26] Walker DT, Hallam M-J, Ni Mhurchadha S, McCabe P, Nduka C. The psychosocial impact of facial palsy: our experience in one hundred and twenty six patients. Clin Otolaryngol. 2012; 37(6):474–477

[27] Youshani AS, Mehta B, Davies K, Beer H, De S. Management of Bell's palsy in children: an audit of current practice, review of the literature and a proposed management algorithm. Emerg Med J. 2015; 32(4): 274–280

[28] Kang HM, Jung SY, Byun JY, Park MS, Yeo SG. Steroid plus antiviral treatment for Bell's palsy. J Intern Med. 2015; 277(5):532–539

[29] Sullivan FM, Swan IRC, Donnan PT, et al. Early treatment with prednisolone or acyclovir in Bell's palsy. N Engl J Med. 2007; 357(16):1598–1607

[30] Engström M, Berg T, Stjernquist-Desatnik A, et al. Prednisolone and valaciclovir in Bell's palsy: a randomised, double-blind, placebo-controlled, multicentre trial. Lancet Neurol. 2008; 7(11):993–1000

[31] de Almeida JR, Al Khabori M, Guyatt GH, et al. Combined corticosteroid and antiviral treatment for Bell palsy: a systematic review and meta-analysis. JAMA. 2009; 302(9):985–993

[32] Holland NJ, Weiner GM. Recent developments in Bell's palsy. BMJ. 2004; 329(7465):553–557

[33] Gagyor I, Madhok VB, Daly F, et al. Antiviral treatment for Bell's palsy (idiopathic facial paralysis). Cochrane Database Syst Rev. 2015; 11 (11):CD001869

[34] Fattah A, Borschel GH, Zuker RM. Reconstruction of facial nerve injuries in children. J Craniofac Surg. 2011; 22(3):782–788

[35] Labbé D, Huault M. Lengthening temporalis myoplasty and lip reanimation. Plast Reconstr Surg. 2000; 105(4):1289–1297, discussion 1298

[36] Baker DC, Conley J. Regional muscle transposition for rehabilitation of the paralyzed face. Clin Plast Surg. 1979; 6(3):317–331

[37] Manktelow RT, Tomat LR, Zuker RM, Chang M. Smile reconstruction in adults with free muscle transfer innervated by the masseter motor nerve: effectiveness and cerebral adaptation. Plast Reconstr Surg. 2006; 118(4):885–899

12

Part III

The Hearing Impaired Child

13 Introduction, Detection, and Early Management

An N. Boudewyns and Frank Declau

13.1 Introduction

This chapter deals with permanent childhood hearing impairment (PCHI). This is defined as a unilateral or bilateral permanent hearing impairment greater than or equal to 40 dB HL averaged over the frequencies 0.5, 1, 2, and 4 kHz. PCHI is considered a major individual and public health problem not only because of its prevalence but also because of the potential impact of unidentified and therefore untreated hearing loss on speech and language development, academic achievements, and the child's social and emotional development.

Speech development is impaired by delayed age at diagnosis of hearing loss. The greater the delay, the worse the effect.[1] Impairment is measurable as early as 3 years of age and has consequences throughout life, leading to lower reading abilities, poorer school performance, and under- or unemployment.

13.2 Epidemiology and Prevalence

> Hearing loss is the most common sensorineural deficit. Bilateral hearing loss ≥ 40 dB HL is present in 1.33 per 1,000 newborns. When unilateral hearing loss is included, the incidence figures raise to 1.86 per 1,000 at birth.[2]

In developing countries, the prevalence of congenital hearing loss may be as high as 6 neonates per 1,000 live births.[3,4] The risk for PCHI is 10 times higher in infants from the neonatal intensive care unit (NICU), with a prevalence of 2 to 4%. Bilateral severe hearing loss (> 70 dB HL) was documented in 1.9% of NICU graduates at 3 years of age.[5]

Nearly 20 to 30% of affected children have profound hearing loss (> 90 dB HL). Approximately 30% of children with bilateral hearing loss have additional disabilities, most frequently generalized learning difficulty or intellectual disability.[6]

Hearing loss may become manifest postnatally. The child passes the neonatal hearing-screening test and hearing loss becomes apparent later in childhood. It can be categorized as delayed onset, progressive, or acquired. Delayed-onset hearing loss results from adverse medical conditions that are present during the pre- or perinatal period (intrauterine infections, asphyxia). Their effects become manifest over time. Progressive hearing loss is usually caused by viral infections, hereditary factors, or neurodegenerative disorders. Acquired hearing loss results from external factors occurring in the postnatal period, such as meningitis, use of ototoxic drugs, trauma, and noise exposure.

Consequently, the prevalence of PCHI increases during childhood with values of 2.7 per 1,000 children around 5 years (prelingual hearing loss) and up to 3.5 per 1,000 during adolescence.[2] Postnatal impairment may account for 25% of all bilateral PCHI at the age of 9 years.[7]

13.3 Etiology

Hearing loss present at birth is termed *congenital hearing loss*.

> In approximately 50% of the cases with congenital hearing loss, a *genetic* or *inherited cause* can be identified; the remaining are related to *environmental factors* (► Fig. 13.1).[8]

The hearing loss may be an isolated defect, may occur in association with one or more congenital defects that do not constitute a defined syndrome, or may be one feature of a group of congenital anomalies that form a defined and recognized pattern (syndromic hearing loss). More than 450 genetic syndromes that include hearing loss have been described.[9] Nonsyndromic inherited hearing loss is often difficult to differentiate from environmental or multifactorial causes of hearing loss. Ototoxic medication, especially aminoglycosides, may cause hearing loss in newborns. Patients carrying an A1555G mutation in the mitochondrial 12S ribosomal gene are more sensitive to aminoglycoside ototoxicity.[10]

13.3.1 Genetic Causes of Permanent Childhood Hearing Impairment

> Inherited deafness is extremely heterogeneous genetically and shows considerable phenotypic variability.

More than 175 different loci/genes have been identified over the last decades. For a full summary of loci and genes associated with inherited hearing loss, the reader is advised to consult the Hereditary Hearing Loss homepage at http://hereditaryhearingloss.org/.

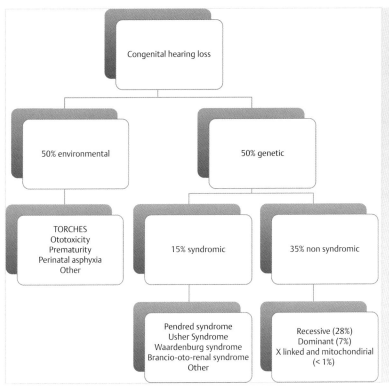

Fig. 13.1 Relative contribution of environmental and genetic causes to congenital hearing loss. (Modified after Smith RJ, Bale JF, Jr, White KR. Sensorineural hearing loss in children. Lancet 2005; 365(9462):879–890, with permission.)

The pattern of inheritance is *autosomal recessive* in approximately 75% of cases, *autosomal dominant* in approximately 20%, *X-linked* in approximately 5%, and *mitochondrial* in less than 1%.[11]

In general, prelingual, profound, nonprogressive deafness is inherited as an autosomal recessive trait.

The genetic causes may be subdivided into syndromic and nonsyndromic forms.

Syndromal Hearing Loss

Syndromal hearing loss accounts for 30% of all cases of genetic hearing impairment.[12] A list of the most common syndromic causes for PCHI is presented in ▶ Table 13.1.

In the following sections, we briefly describe three syndromic forms of PCHI. A basic knowledge of these syndromes is required to understand the rationale of the standard diagnostic protocol for infants/children with PCHI as described further in this chapter. For more detailed information and more rare syndromes, refer to the Hereditary Hearing Loss Homepage.

Pendred's Syndrome

The most common syndromic form is Pendred's syndrome (▶ Fig. 13.2). This syndrome combines inner ear malformations, in particular a bilateral enlargement of the endolymphatic duct and sac (LEDS) with or without coch-

lear hypoplasia with thyroid dysfunction as manifested by an abnormal perchlorate test or a goiter. Most frequently, Pendred's syndrome is linked to mutations in the *SLC26A4* gene (Pendrin) on chromosome 7. A finding of bilateral LEDS should prompt thorough investigations for Pendred's syndrome. Children with nonsyndromic LEDS carry a single SLC26A4 mutation in 61% of the cases.[2] Children with LEDS are at risk for sudden hearing loss following head injury or sudden changes in intracranial pressure. Parents of these children should be advised about minimizing the risk of head injury, for example, by avoiding contact sports and diving.

Usher's Syndrome

Usher's syndrome is a heterogeneous autosomal recessive inherited disorder with a prevalence of 3.5 per 100,000 children. It is characterized by sensorineural hearing loss (SNHL) of varying severity associated with progressive pigmentary retinal degeneration. Approximately 3 to 6% of all children who are deaf and another 3 to 6% of children who are hard of hearing have Usher's syndrome.

Usher's syndrome type I (USH1) is distinguished from the other infantile form (USH2) on the basis of severity of hearing loss and the extent of vestibular involvement: USH1 is characterized by profound congenital deafness, absent vestibular function, and progressive visual loss starting in the first decade of life.[13]

13

Table 13.1 Limitative list with the most prevalent syndromic causes for permanent childhood hearing impairment

Syndrome	Gene	Inheritance pattern	Phenotype
Waardenburg			
Type 1 (most common)	PAX3	AD	Unilateral (10%) or bilateral (90%) hearing loss, patches of hypopigmentation in skin, eye, hair, dystopia canthorum, synophrys, pinched nares
Type 2	MITF, SNAI2	AD	As type 1 but without dystopia canthorum
Klein-Waardenburg syndrome (Type 3)	PAX3	AD and AR	As type 1 but with limb abnormalities
Waardenburg-Shah syndrome (Type 4)	EDNRB, EDN3, and SOX10	AD and AR	As type 2 but with Hirschprung disease
Branchio-otorenal	EYA1, SIX1, and SIX5	AD	Hearing loss, preauricular pits, dysplastic ears, branchial fistulae, renal abnormalities
Treacher Collins	TCOF1, POLR1C, and POLR1D	AD	Conductive hearing loss, ossicular anomalies, microtia, cleft palate, micrognathia, downward slanting eyes, coloboma
Pendred	SLC26A4, FOXI1, and KCNJ10	AR	Sensorineural hearing loss, enlargement of the vestibular aqueduct, thyromegaly
Usher			
Type 1	MYO7A, USH1C, CDH23, PCDH15, CIB2, and SANS	AR	Profound HL, vestibular symptoms, RP from first decade
Type 2	USH2A, VLGR1, and WHRN	AR	Nonprogressive, moderate-to-severe HL, RP from first to second decade
Type 3	CLRN1 and PDZD7	AR	Progressive HL, variable vestibular symptoms, variable onset of RP
Jervell and Lange-Nielsen	KVLQ1 and KCNE1	AR	Profound bilateral hearing loss, QTc prolongation, syncope, sudden death

Abbreviations: AD, autosomal dominant; AR, autosomal recessive; HL, hearing loss; QTc, corrected QT; RP, retinitis pigmentosa.

Jervell and Lange-Nielsen's Syndrome

Jervell and Lange-Nielsen's syndrome, also known as long QT syndrome (LQTS), is a rare autosomal recessive disorder with an estimated incidence of 1.6 to 6 cases per million, thought to result from mutations in genes that encode proteins forming the delayed rectifier potassium channel. The responsible genes have been identified as *KVLQ1* and *KCNE1*, located on chromosomes 11 and 21, respectively.[14] Mutations in these genes encoding cardiac ion channels result in delayed myocellular repolarization. The syndrome consists of congenital bilateral profound deafness and prolongation of the QT interval as detected by electrocardiography (ECG; abnormal corrected QT [QTc] > 440 ms). Affected individuals have syncopal episodes and may have sudden death.

Nonsyndromal Inherited Hearing Loss

Nonsyndromal inherited hearing loss accounts for 70% of genetic causes.[12]

Despite the tremendous heterogeneity of deafness, mutations in one gene, encoding the gap junction β_2 protein, connexin 26 (*GJB2*), are responsible for more than half of hereditary prelingual SNHL in the white population.[8]

> Particularly when both parents have normal hearing, connexin-related deafness will be strongly suspected.

Connexin 26 is a gap junction protein expressed in supporting cells and connective tissue of the inner ear. These gap junctions are critical for recycling of potassium ions and maintenance of a normal endocochlear potential. More than 100 mutations involving *GJB2* have been identified. They often cause a profound and nonprogressive hearing loss, although phenotypic variations and milder variants are known. A single variant known as 35delG accounts for up to 70% of all pathogenic mutations. Homozygous* 35delG mutations result in profound hearing loss. Heterozygous mutations in connexin 26 may contribute to hearing loss when there is a simultaneous mutation in connexin 30 (*GJB6*) (compound heterozygosity).

---

* Homozygous: having two identical alleles at a given gene locus; heterozygous: having two different alleles at a given gene locus; compound heterozygous: having two different mutant alleles at the same gene locus.

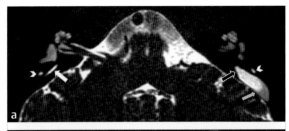

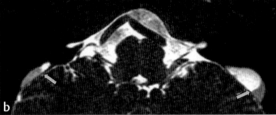

Fig. 13.2 A 12-year-old boy with severe high-frequency sensorineural hearing loss on the left side and moderate on the right side. Axial 0.3 mm thick heavily T2-weighted driven equilibrium (DRIVE) images at the level of the labyrinth (a) and lower in the posterior fossa (b). (a) A prominent endolymphatic duct can be seen on the right side (*white arrow*) with a width similar to the cross-section through the posterior semicircular canal (*white arrowhead*). On the left side the endolymphatic duct (*black arrow*) is clearly larger than the cross-section of the posterior semicircular canal (*white arrowhead*) and hence clearly widened. The widened endolymphatic duct continues posteriorly in an enlarged endolymphatic sac. (b) The extension of the enlarged endolymphatic sac in the posterior fossa on the left side can be seen and although the dimensions of the right endolymphatic duct were borderline, the endolymphatic sac is clearly enlarged and its extension in the posterior fossa can also be seen (*gray arrow*). The more extensive enlargement on the left side explains also the more dominant hearing loss on this side. Note that both high-signal clear fluid and low-signal proteinaceous fluid and/or fibrous areas can be seen in the enlarged endolymphatic sacs (*gray arrows*). Courtesy of Jan Casselman, AZ St. Jan Hospital, Department of Radiology, Bruges, Belgium.

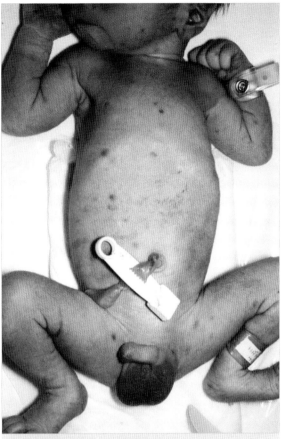

Fig. 13.3 Newborn baby with congenital rubella. The skin lesions are characteristic. Other features include profound sensorineural hearing loss, cataracts, microcephaly, and hepatosplenomegaly. Vaccination has virtually eliminated this condition in the developed world.

13.3.2 Environmental Causes of Permanent Childhood Hearing Impairment

> **i**
>
> Various infectious pathogens may result in SNHL when they infect the mother during pregnancy. These agents are quoted as TORCHES (toxoplasmosis, others, rubella [▶ Fig. 13.3], cytomegalovirus [CMV], and herpes simplex virus [HSV]).

Congenital Rubella Infection

In countries without universal rubella vaccination, congenital rubella infection is the most common environmental cause.

The earlier the infection is acquired during pregnancy, the more severe the effect on the fetus. Nearly 90% of the infants with the congenital rubella syndrome have SNHL. Hearing loss is usually bilateral, severe to profound, affecting all frequencies, and may be progressive and/or asymmetric. Other findings include pigmentary retinitis (most common and consistent finding), cataract, microcephaly, intellectual disability, cardiovascular abnormalities, intrauterine growth retardation, and hyperbilirubinemia.[15]

13

Congenital Cytomegalovirus Infection

This infection represents the most important cause of SNHL in the developed countries where universal rubella vaccination is available, having an incidence of approximately 1 in 100 births. At birth, 3.9% of infants with congenital CMV infection have hearing loss.[2] Intrauterine transmission of primary CMV infection, especially during 4th to 22nd week of gestation, has the most potential to cause significant fetal damage. The rate of transmission to infants born to mothers who had a primary infection or a recurrent infection during pregnancy is 30 to 40% and 1.4%, respectively (▶ Fig. 13.4). The risk of congenital CMV with recurrent infection (i.e., in a mother who had a previous CMV infection) is lower.

Transmission of CMV

People who are infected with CMV shed the virus from infected body fluids such as saliva, urine, blood, and semen. For pregnant women, the most common exposures to CMV are through sexual contact and through contact with the urine or saliva of young children with CMV infection. A pregnant woman may pass the virus to her baby as the virus can cross the placenta and infect the fetus's blood. CMV can also be shed in breast milk but infections that occur from breast-feeding usually do not cause symptoms or disease in the infant. Pregnant women should be counseled to take preventive measures with the aim to avoid getting urine or saliva of children on the hands or in the nose, eyes, and mouth.

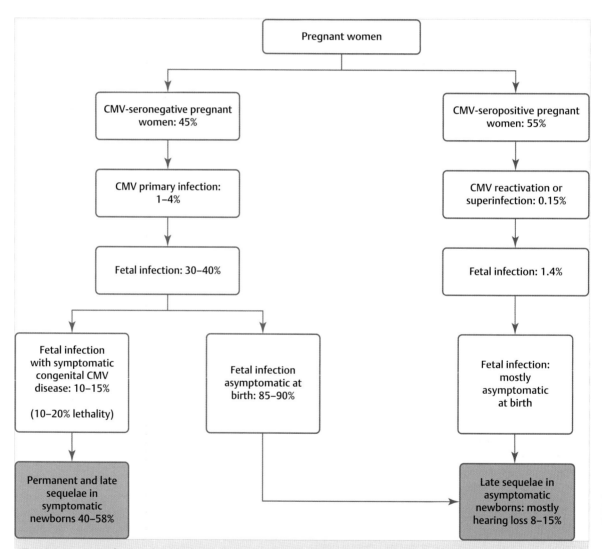

Fig. 13.4 Frequency of maternal and fetal cytomegalovirus infections and morbidity of infected children. (After Stagno S, Pass RF, Cloud G, Britt WJ, Henderson RE, Walton PD, et al. Primary cytomegalovirus infection in pregnancy. Incidence, transmission to fetus, and clinical outcome. JAMA 1986;256(14):1904–1908; and Ludwig A, Hengel H. Epidemiological impact and disease burden of congenital cytomegalovirus infection in Europe. Euro Surveillance European Communicable Disease Bulletin 2009;14(9):26–32.)

Primary intrauterine CMV infections are a leading cause of SNHL and second only to Down's syndrome as a known cause of intellectual disability. Approximately 10 to 15% of infants with congenital CMV infection are symptomatic at birth. These infants may present with jaundice (conjugated hyperbilirubinemia), hepatosplenomegaly, petechiae (thrombocytopenia), microcephaly, lethargy, hypotonia, and seizures.[16]

Symptomatic children are at particularly increased risk for SNHL with a cumulative prevalence of 36% at 6 years.[17] In a recently published systematic review, it was concluded that 1 out of 3 symptomatic children and 1 out of 10 asymptomatic children, will experience hearing loss (▶ Fig. 13.4).[18] There is no pathognomonic configuration for the hearing loss caused by congenital CMV infection. Unilateral and bilateral hearing losses at any frequency may occur in children with congenital CMV infection, with loss varying from mild to profound, the latter being more common in symptomatic infants. In addition, progressive and fluctuating hearing loss has been observed in 29.4% of symptomatic and 54.1% of asymptomatic babies with congenital CMV infection. In fact, approximately half of the cases of hearing loss due to congenital CMV infection are late onset and/or progressive and, therefore, will not be detected at birth through newborn hearing screening.[19]

Toxoplasma Gondii

Toxoplasma Gondii ⓘ

Infection of the mother may be detected by serological testing during pregnancy.

Rates of congenital infection range from less than 0.1 to 1 per 1,000 live births. At birth, 90% of toxoplasmosis babies will have no clinical features at birth, although many will develop visual or learning disabilities later in life.[20,21] The prevalence of toxoplasmosis associated hearing loss in affected babies ranges from 0 to 28% and seems to depend on prior treatment.[22] Early identification and treatment are the key to minimizing morbidity. In children who received 12 months of antiparasitic treatment initiated prior to 2.5 months of age and with serologically confirmed compliance, the prevalence of SNHL was 0%. This is in strong contrast with those children receiving no or limited treatment and in whom a prevalence figure for SNHL of 28% was documented. Other findings caused by congenital toxoplasmosis include chorioretinitis, hydrocephalus, intracranial calcifications, lymphadenopathy, and pulmonary lesions.[15]

Transmission of Toxoplasma ⓘ

Toxoplasma can be transmitted to a pregnant woman by ingestion of raw or inadequately cooked infected meat or by exposure to cat litter, dog feces, or soil containing oocysts. Toxoplasma infection can be prevented by cooking meat at temperatures high enough to kill the protozoan parasite, by avoiding contact with raw meat, poultry or seafood, unwashed vegetables or fruit, and pet excrement.

Syphilis

An annual incidence of 0.1 per 1,000 live births is reported. Congenital syphilis can be found in two entities: an infantile form (early), which is usually fatal in outcome, and a tardive form (late). The late form expresses itself with sudden SNHL in childhood that tends to be profound and symmetric and associated with vestibular symptoms.

A recently published literature search on the prevalence of SNHL following congenital syphilis infection concluded that there are no reports of confirmed congenital SNHL secondary to in utero syphilis infection.[23] This conclusion was largely based upon a prospective study in 75 neonates born with serological evidence of congenital syphilis who all had normal auditory brainstem responses (ABRs) in the newborn period.[24]

Herpes Simplex Virus

Neonatal HSV infection has an annual incidence of less than 0.01 to 0.33 cases per 1,000 live births.[15] Infections are very rarely caused by in utero exposure. They present as disseminated infection, encephalitis, or localized infection.[25] SNHL related to congenital HSV infection has, however, only been described in disseminated disease in which other obvious clinical sequelae of HSV infection and comorbid conditions were present.

Noninfectious Environmental Causes Of PCHI

- Ototoxic medication, especially aminoglycosides, may cause hearing loss in newborns. Patients carrying an A1555G mutation in the mitochondrial 12S ribosomal gene are more sensitive to aminoglycoside ototoxicity.[10]
- Perinatal factors associated with PCHI include peripartum hypoxia, hyperbilirubinemia with kernicterus, or

13

III

the need for exchange transfusion and extracorporeal membrane oxygenation (ECMO). These risk factors are typically found in infants staying in the special care baby unit or the NICU.

- Alcohol abuse during pregnancy may result in fetal alcohol syndrome and associated hearing loss. Use of chemotherapy during pregnancy may also cause hearing loss in the newborn.[26]

13.4 Risk Factors for Hearing Loss

The Joint Committee on Infant Hearing (JCIH) from the American Academy of Pediatrics identified several risk factors for congenital or late-onset childhood hearing loss (Box 13.1).[27] Three of these are considered as major risk factors for congenital hearing impairment:

1. NICU stay > 48 hours.
2. Family history of permanent hearing impairment.
3. Craniofacial anomalies.

One or more of these three risk factors were found in only 58.9% of children with bilateral congenital hearing impairment.[28] This means that a large number of babies with PCHI will not be identified if screening is confined to those at high risk.

Box 13.1 Risk Factors for Permanent Congenital, Delayed, or Progressive Hearing Loss in Childhood[27]

- Caregiver concern regarding hearing, speech, language, or developmental delay.
- Family history of hearing loss.
- Neonatal intensive care > 5 days or any of the following regardless of length of stay: ECMO, assisted ventilation, use of ototoxic drugs (gentamycin, tobramycin) or loop diuretics, or hyperbilirubinemia requiring exchange transfusion.
- In utero infections (TORCHES).
- Craniofacial anomalies including those that involve the outer ear, ear canal, ear tags, ear pits, and temporal bone anomalies.
- Physical findings associated with a syndrome known to include permanent hearing loss (e.g., white forelock).
- Syndromes associated with hearing loss or progressive or late-onset hearing loss.
- Neurodegenerative disorders or sensorimotor neuropathies.
- Confirmed bacterial or viral (especially herpes and varicella) meningitis.
- Head trauma, especially basal skull or temporal bone fractures that require hospitalization.
- Chemotherapy.

Robertson et al[5] found a 3.1% prevalence of permanent hearing loss in a cohort of 1,279 NICU survivors (≤ 28 weeks of gestation and < 1,250 g of birth weight) at the age of 3 years. In this study, all children with delayed-onset hearing loss and 82% of those with progressive hearing loss had required prolonged supplemental neonatal oxygen use. An association was suggested between prolonged need for oxygen/respiratory failure and permanent hearing loss through ototoxicity. Recent investigations of risk factors for SNHL in NICU infants found that dysmorphic features, low APGAR* scores at 1 minute, sepsis, meningitis, cerebral bleeding, and cerebral infarction should be considered as risk factors for SNHL, independent of postconceptional age, gender, and NICU admittance.[29]

In addition, recent data from a large epidemiological study in 103,835 screened non-NICU babies showed that sociodemographic factors such as gender (boys), increasing birth order, birth length, feeding type (higher risk with formula), low level of education, and Eastern European origin of the mother are independent risk factors for permanent hearing impairment.[30] Many of these risk factors are associated with poverty and deprivation.

13.5 Identification of Hearing Loss

More than 50% of cases of PCHI may be detected shortly after birth through a program of neonatal hearing screening. However, as mentioned earlier, a pass on the neonatal hearing test does not preclude late-onset hearing loss. Less severe congenital hearing loss (< 30–40 dB) is not detected in most screening programs. Progressive or late-onset hearing impairment, as seen with congenital CMV infection or in some inherited conditions, is also not detected by a newborn screening program. Up to now, postnatal identification will remain dependent upon the interaction between parents and professionals and on pathways that allow ready access to audiology services. Continued surveillance, screening, and referral of infants and toddlers are needed.

Health care providers, educators, and parents must remain attentive to the developmental progress of children, especially in expressive and receptive language domains.

A hearing (re)assessment is recommended for all children experiencing developmental or learning difficulties.

---

* APGAR: score used for evaluation of the newborn based upon five items: A (appearance), P (pulse), G (grimace), A (activity), and R (respiration).

13.5.1 Neonatal Hearing Screening

To be successful, a neonatal hearing-screening program should endeavor to be universal since selective screening based on high-risk criteria fails to detect at least half of all infants with congenital hearing loss. According to Declau et al, in a retrospective study of 170 referred neonates after universal neonatal hearing screening (UNHS), risk factors were also statistically not different between the normal-hearing and hearing loss groups. On the other hand, the presence of a high-risk factor predicts hearing loss in 68%.[31]

Screening Methods

In UNHS programs, two types of tests are commonly used: otoacoustic emissions (OAEs) and automated ABR (A-ABR). A detailed description of these tests may be found in Chapter 13.6.1. In the past, many centers used the Ewing test. This test is based upon an orientation reflex where the baby turns his/her head in the direction of a presented sound stimulus. This reflex is most evident at 9 to 12 months of age and disappears later on. In comparison with the Ewing test, both A-ABR and OAEs (transient OAE [TEOAE] or distortion product OAE) yield far better sensitivity and specificity, are easy to use, and are cost-effective.

- OAEs are highly sensitive but show less specificity. There is a higher rate of false-positive results due to middle ear pathology. Detection of OAEs implies a normal function of the auditory system up to the level of the outer hair cells. Hearing loss caused by auditory neuropathy/auditory dyssynchrony (Box 13.2) will be missed with this technology.
- A-ABR has a higher specificity. False-positives may result from an immature central nervous system.[32] Automated algorithms eliminate the need for individual test interpretation, reduce the effects of screener bias and errors on test outcome, and ensure test consistency across all infants, test conditions, and screening personnel.

The JCIH recommends ABR technology as the only appropriate screening technique for use in the NICU. For infants who do not pass A-ABR testing in the NICU, referral should be made directly to an audiologist for rescreening and, when indicated, comprehensive evaluation including standard ABR. For rescreening, a complete screening on both ears is recommended, even if only one ear failed the initial screening.

For readmissions in the first month of life for all infants (NICU or well infant), when there are conditions associated with potential hearing loss (e.g., hyperbilirubinemia that requires exchange transfusion or culture-positive sepsis), a repeat hearing screening is recommended before discharge.

Box 13.2 Auditory Neuropathy/ Dyssynchrony

Some children will have normal OAEs but absent or abnormal ABR readings. This condition is referred to as "auditory neuropathy/auditory dyssynchrony" (AN/AD). Rapin and Gravel suggested that the term AN/AD should be limited to cases in which the pathology is located at the spiral ganglion cells, their processes, or the eighth cranial nerve.[33] This condition may be related to structural abnormalities of the auditory nerve such as cochlear nerve aplasia/hypoplasia, and in bilateral cases, mutations in the *OTOF* gene should be excluded.

Some infants with an initial diagnosis of AN/AD may demonstrate improved auditory function and even "recovery" on ABR testing.[34] Particularly in high-risk neonates, a repeat ABR testing is recommended at the age of 6 months.

For those infants who "recover" from AN/AD, regular surveillance of developmental milestones, auditory skills, parental concerns, and middle ear status is recommended consistent with the JCIH 2007 Position Statement.[27] Because the residual effects of transient AN/AD are unknown, ongoing monitoring of the infant's auditory, speech, and language development, as well as global (e.g., motor, cognitive, and social) development is critical. Those infants and young children whose speech and language development is not commensurate with their general development should be referred for speech and language evaluation and audiological assessment.

13.5.2 Screening Strategies

In most European countries, UNHS is now well established and typically uses a two-phase screening paradigm. Either TEOAEs repeated twice, TEOAEs followed by A-ABR, or A-ABR repeated twice have similar identification rates for congenital hearing loss of 0.45%, 0.25%, and 0.42%, respectively. However, the referral rate is lowest (0.8%) for the A-ABR protocol, with increasing referral rates of 1.6% for a combined TEOAE/A-ABR protocol and the highest referral rate of 5.8% for the TEOAE twice protocol,[35] reflecting the higher rate of false-positives with TEOAE screening. In parallel, the overall economic cost is lowest for the A-ABR protocol.

False-positive rates vary among centers and depend on the strategy and timing of testing.

- In the Wessex study,[36] a false-positive rate of the overall screening procedure (TEOAE followed by A-ABR) of 1.5% (specificity: 98.5%) has been found (postnatal day 1, 1.9%, to postnatal day 4, 1.1%).
- If an infant has a positive result on the screening test (uni- or bilateral), the likelihood that the infant has indeed a bilateral moderate-to-profound hearing loss is

expressed by the positive predictive value (PPV: number of infants with bilateral hearing loss and a positive test divided by the total number testing positive).

- In the Wessex study,[36] the overall PPV of UNHS has been estimated 6.7%. In the well-baby nursery, the PPV was 2.2%, whereas for high-risk babies, the PPV was 20%. This means that for the well-baby nursery, 1 of every 45 infants referred for outpatient audiological evaluation eventually proved to have moderate-to-profound bilateral SNHL and 1 in 5 infants for the high-risk babies.

A patient-tracking system with central data management is crucial to effectively manage the screening and rehabilitation process. In many UNHS programs, the screening-to-therapy coordination is the weakest point of the pathway with the proportion of children lost to follow-up (and treatment) as high as 2 to 52% of those referred.[37]

A stringent cooperation protocol is needed to guarantee the most optimal follow-up. Seamless coordination between the screening program on the one hand and the health and rehabilitation services on the other is of the utmost importance for a successful treatment strategy.

Beyond the quality of life and psychosocial benefits of improved language, communication, and learning, there are increasing data on the cost-effectiveness of UNHS. The actual costs of screening vary according to region. In general, there is agreement that the lifetime costs of deafness, particularly prelingual, are very high. Costs of UNHS are comparable with other newborn screening programs[37] and, even with wide modeling parameters, the benefits of UNHS outweigh the costs.[38]

For more information, visit the NHS Web site at hearing.screening.nhs.uk.

13.6 Diagnostic and Etiological Work-Up Following Referral from Screening

The gold standard for validation of the screening results is a combination of ear, nose, throat (ENT) and audiological consultation performed with electrophysiologic testing such as diagnostic ABR, auditory steady-state responses (ASSRs), and/or behavioral testing. A test battery is required to cross-check results of both behavioral and physiological measures.[35]

An otolaryngologist in close collaboration with the medical geneticist and pediatrician performs the medical evaluation. The purpose of this multidisciplinary team is not only to determine the etiology of hearing loss, but also to identify related medical conditions and to provide recommendations for medical treatment as well as referral to other services.[12] This team may also advise on further investigations and molecular genetic testing and can provide counseling with expertise in genetic pre- and posttest discussions.

13.6.1 Audiological Assessment

When a child fails on a neonatal hearing screening test, a complete audiometric test battery is required to confirm the presence of a hearing loss and to assess its severity (mild/moderate/severe/profound) and laterality (uni- or bilateral). This has further implications for both the etiological work-up and treatment/rehabilitation.

By convention, the severity of hearing loss across the frequencies of 250 to 4,000 Hz is considered (▶ Table 13.2).[39]

The following hearing tests are routinely performed in the audiological work-up of neonatal/pediatric hearing loss.

Auditory Brainstem Responses

Auditory brainstem potentials reflect electrical events elicited by auditory stimuli and generated in the auditory pathway in its course through the brain. These potentials can be recorded from scalp electrodes using computer averaging techniques. In clinical practice, click-evoked ABR is most commonly used and is considered the gold standard for objective assessment of hearing.

Following the administration of a broadband click stimulus, typical deflections can be discerned and these are labeled as waves I to V with their specific amplitudes and latencies. Wave V is the most robust waveform. The auditory threshold is determined as the smallest sound intensity (dB nHL) for which wave V can be discerned in a reproducible way following the application of a click stimulus to the ear. ABR potentials are evoked mainly by signals containing acoustic energy above 2 kHz, and the obtained thresholds are within 10 dB of the average behavioral audiogram at the higher frequencies (2–4 kHz).

Table 13.2 Hearing loss classification according to severity[39]

Mean hearing threshold for 250–4,000 Hz (dB HL)	Hearing loss severity
26–40	Mild
41–55	Moderate
56–70	Moderately severe
71–90	Severe
>90	Profound

Bone-conduction ABR is a reliable method to assess cochlear function in cases with structural outer ear anomalies such as stenosis or atresia of the external auditory canal.

Auditory brainstem potentials can be recorded from preterm infants as young as 25 weeks of gestational age and reliable responses to a 65-dB SL click signal first appear at the 28th week of gestation. The wave latencies decrease as gestation proceeds and they continue to decrease throughout the first year of life. The maximal change in wave latencies is observed between the 28th and 34th week of gestation. There is also an increase in wave amplitude with maturation. The decrease in wave I latency to a constant click intensity and the decrease in central conduction time (difference between wave I and V) with gestational age represent maturation of the peripheral and central auditory pathways, respectively.[40] These maturational changes imply that care should be taken with the interpretation of ABR results in preterm babies. Particularly in high-risk babies, ABR testing should be repeated at a later age, at the age of 3 months and again between 6 and 8 months (postterm age) before making definitive conclusions about the hearing status.[41,42] An example of a normal ABR tracing in a newborn is presented in ▶ Fig. 13.5.

In cases with an abnormal ABR waveform morphology or when ABR waveforms are absent, the child should be tested for a cochlear microphonic. The constellation of abnormal or absent ABR in the presence of a cochlear microphonic (with or without the presence of OAEs) points toward a diagnosis of AN/AD.[42]

Auditory Steady-State Responses

ASSRs are elicited by AM/FM modulated tonal stimuli. The stimulus used for ASSR testing is a continuous signal, and higher average sound pressure levels can be delivered than with click stimuli. ASSR may be used to obtain hearing threshold information in children with profound hearing loss (> 90 dB HL). Therefore, ASSR is more suitable than ABR to determine residual hearing at high intensities.

The absence of ASSR thresholds at maximum intensities indicates no usable hearing and predicts poor results with hearing aids.[43] ASSR may assist in hearing-aid fitting and in the selection of young children for cochlear implantation.

The presence or absence of a response is determined by statistical (objective) methods. This eliminates the risk for interpretation bias by inexperienced clinicians.

Good correlations were found between ASSR-based threshold estimations and click-evoked ABR thresholds. For all types of hearing loss (conductive or sensorineural), a close correlation is found between click-evoked ABR and average ASSR thresholds at 2 and 4 kHz, respectively, and 76% of the thresholds correspond within 10 dB or less.[44]

- Interpretation of ASSR thresholds in normal-hearing individuals or those with mild-to-moderate hearing loss (up to 60 dB) should be done cautiously.
- Estimation of behavioral thresholds by ASSR in hearing loss less than 60 dB gives more variable results, especially at 0.5 kHz. In these cases, it may be more appropriate to consider the average ASSR threshold for 0.5 to 4 kHz to estimate behavioral thresholds.[45]
- If the average ASSR-based threshold estimations at 0.5, 1, 2, and 4 kHz exceed 40 dB HL, the ASSR thresholds estimation at individual frequencies is reliable and may be used to predict pure-tone thresholds.[46]
- The best correlations between ASSR and behavioral thresholds are found in more severe hearing impairments, a phenomenon that has been attributed to recruitment.[47]

ABR and ASSR are to the same degree affected by middle ear pathology[44] and by background electrical noise levels due to transient movements and electromyogenic potentials. The level of consciousness does not affect responses.

Since recordings are sensitive to muscle tension, in infants or children, these measurements are typically done in natural sleep after feeding (▶ Fig. 13.6), during sedated sleep (chloral hydrate), or during general anesthesia. The latter method also allows for performing a tympanocentesis to evacuate middle ear fluid when present.

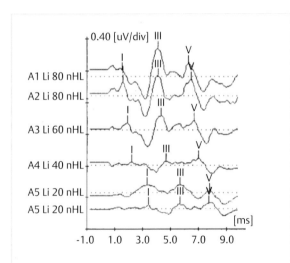

Fig. 13.5 Auditory brainstem response tracings in a newborn with normal hearing in the left ear, as indicated by a reproducible wave V at a stimulus intensity of 20 dB nHL.

13

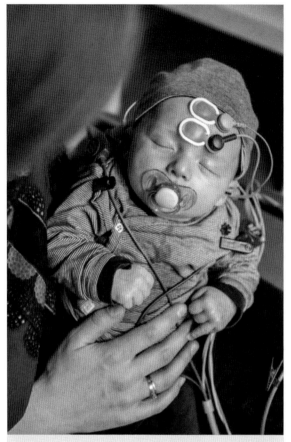

Fig. 13.6 Auditory brainstem response recordings using insert phones in an infant during natural sleep.

ABR and ASSR are complementary in the evaluation of pediatric hearing loss. If no ABR responses are obtained, ASSR is indicated to assess the presence of residual hearing at high stimulation intensities and to provide frequency-specific information in the severe versus profound hearing loss range.

A comparison between ABR and ASSR is presented in ▶ Table 13.3 and further illustrated in ▶ Fig. 13.7 and ▶ Fig. 13.8.

Tympanometry

Tympanometry measures tympanic membrane mobility. Reduced tympanic membrane mobility may be caused by cerumen impaction or the presence of middle ear fluid.

> **i**
>
> Assessment of middle ear function is important in the audiometric work-up of congenital hearing loss to distinguish SNHL from hearing loss caused by transient external ear or middle ear disorders.

In infants, the compliance of the middle ear is higher and the resonant frequency of the tympanic membrane is lower compared to adults. The use of conventional 226-Hz tympanometry in children below 7 months of age has a poor sensitivity (high proportion of false-negatives). In this age group, it was found that an abnormal tympanogram has the same significance as in older subjects. On the other hand, a "normal" type A tympanogram indicating a normal static compliance and normal middle ear pressure may be associated with a normally ventilated middle ear but has also been recorded in children with confirmed middle ear effusion.[48,49] Diagnostic accuracy for the detection of middle ear fluid can be improved by the use of a 1,000-Hz probe-tone frequency.

• In infants up to 3 months of age, 1,000-Hz tympanometry is the method of choice.

Table 13.3 Comparison of typical features for ABR and ASSR recordings

ABR	ASSR
Gold standard for objective hearing threshold detection	Not to be used for objective hearing assessment in patients who simulate hearing loss
Response detection is subjective	Responses are determined by statistical methods
No information at high stimulation intensities	Threshold information at intensity levels up to 120–130 dB
Information about hearing thresholds anywhere between 1 and 4 kHz	Frequency-specific thresholds but largest difference with behavioral thresholds at 0.5 kHz
Does not distinguish between severe and profound hearing loss	The absence of ASSR response at maximum stimulation intensity predicts poor results with hearing aid fitting
Absent click-evoked ABR does not rule out useful residual hearing	Most accurate in estimating behavioral thresholds for more profound hearing impairment
	Helpful in hearing aid fitting in young children
Accurate threshold detection in high-frequency range in normal-hearing individuals or those with mild-to-moderate hearing loss	Less reliable for behavioral threshold estimation in normal-hearing or mild-to-moderate hearing loss up to 60 dB
Abbreviations: ABR, auditory brainstem response; ASSR, auditory steady-state response.	

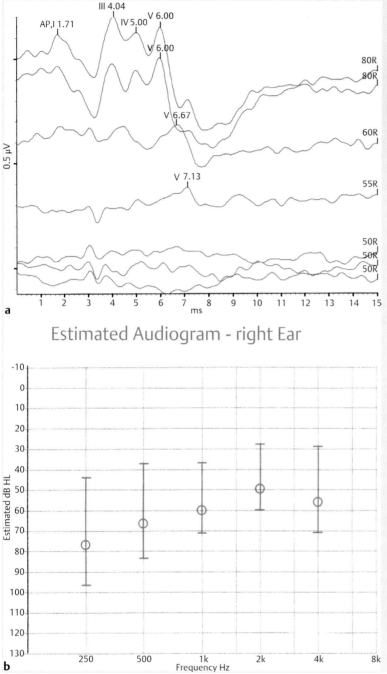

Fig. 13.7 (a) Auditory brainstem response (ABR) and **(b)** auditory steady-state response (ASSR) findings in a patient with unilateral moderately severe hearing loss in the right ear. ABR results indicate a hearing threshold at 55 dB nHL. ASSR show estimated hearing thresholds at a mean value of 57.5 dB HL for 0.5, 1, 2, and 4 kHz.

- In infants between 3 and 9 months of age, a two-stage evaluation is proposed with 1,000-Hz tympanometry followed by 226-Hz tympanometry in case of failure.
- In infants over 9 months of age and in children and adults, 226-Hz tympanometry is appropriate.

Normative data for the interpretation of 1,000-Hz tympanometry in different age groups including NICU graduates were published.[50,51] In selected populations, such as children with Down's syndrome, the use of 1,000-Hz tympanometry irrespective of age may improve the specificity of the test procedure (less chance for type B tympanogram in the absence of middle ear fluid).[52]

Tympanometry in neonates requires the use of specially designed neonatal probes since an inadequate probe seal may affect the success of tympanometry in this group. With the use of appropriate probes, success rates for getting an adequate seal between 87 and 99% have been reported (▶ Fig. 13.9).

13

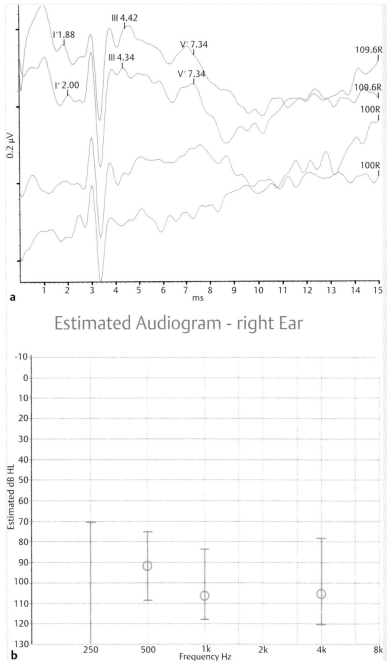

Fig. 13.8 (a) Auditory brainstem response indicates the absence of a reproducible response at stimulation intensities of 100 dB nHL for the right ear. **(b)** Auditory steady-state response recordings performed at the same day indicate hearing thresholds of 90 dB HL at 0.5 kHz, and 105 dB HL at 1 and 4 kHz.

Otoacoustic Emissions

Detection of OAEs requires adequate transmission of sound to and from the cochlea. However, click-evoked OAEs have been found in children with otitis media with effusion and a flat tympanogram. Therefore, the presence of click-evoked OAEs cannot be considered as the gold standard for normal middle ear function. Click-evoked OAEs represent outer hair cell function and are typically present in cases of AN/AD.

> Because of these considerations, detection of OAEs should not be used as a single test for assessment of normal-hearing status. The results of OAE testing should be interpreted together with data obtained from tympanoscopy, tympanometry, and ABR testing.

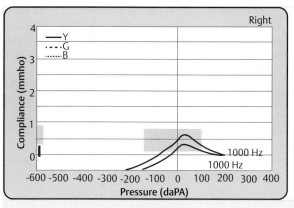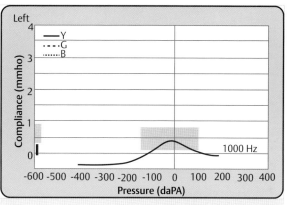

Fig. 13.9 Neonatal 1,000-Hz tympanogram.

Vestibular Examination

> Congenital hearing loss may be associated with various degrees of vestibular impairment. Signs of vestibular impairment are not usually present in newborns or infants but may become manifest between 1 and 2 years of age with delayed motor development.

In children with absent vestibular function, motor milestones are often delayed, and walking age is typically later than 18 months. Especially in the presence of congenital malformations of the vestibular system, such as enlarged vestibular aqueduct, vestibular dysplasia, anomalies of the semicircular canals, and some syndromic forms of congenital hearing loss such as Usher's syndrome, branchio-otorenal syndrome, and Pendred's syndrome, age-appropriate vestibular examinations should be planned as dictated by the clinical findings. For a detailed description of vestibular examination in infants/children, refer to Chapter 10.

13.6.2 Etiological Assessment

Upon confirmation of hearing loss, the child should be referred for an otological and medical evaluation with the aim of establishing an etiological basis for hearing loss.[27] A definite etiological diagnosis can be established in 55.2% of infants with congenital hearing loss identified through UNHS.[31]

This has important implications for prediction of the further evolution of the hearing loss and the follow-up of the infant as well as for counseling of the parents in the case of any wishes for another child.

A basic knowledge of the most common causes of PCHI and risk factors combined with information from family history, clinical findings, and auditory testing is essential for an evidence-based and patient-oriented evaluation strategy.

Genetic forms of hearing loss must be distinguished from acquired (nongenetic) causes of hearing loss. The genetic forms of hearing loss are diagnosed by otological, audiological, and physical examination, family history, ancillary testing, and molecular genetic testing. Molecular genetic testing, available in clinical laboratories for many types of syndromic and nonsyndromic deafness, plays a prominent role in diagnosis and genetic counseling.[12]

The following are investigations that are recommended, and of these, level 1 investigations must be carried out in all cases and level 2 investigations should be carried out in specific conditions. A summary is presented in Box 13.3 and Box 13.4.

> **Box 13.3 Standard Diagnostic Protocol for Infants/Children with Permanent Hearing Impairment (Level 1)**
>
> - Pediatric history.
> - Family history of deafness.
> - Clinical examination including tympanoscopy.
> - Developmental examination.
> - Referral to a medical geneticist and molecular genetic testing.
> - Laboratory testing for CMV infection.
> - Ophthalmological examination.
> - Magnetic resonance imaging (MRI).

13

Box 13.4 Complementary Investigations in Infants/Children with Permanent Hearing Impairment (Level 2)

- Urine dipstick.
- Hematology and biochemistry.
- Thyroid function tests.
- Immunology tests.
- Metabolic screen.
- Clinical photography.
- Chromosomal studies.
- Renal ultrasound.
- Vestibular examination.
- Family audiograms: first-degree relatives.
- ECG.
- Serological testing (rubella, herpes simplex, toxoplasmosis, syphilis).
- Computed tomography (CT).

Family History (Level 1)

The evaluation includes a detailed pedigree analysis for congenital hearing loss, medical history, and risk factors as identified by the JCIH 2007 Position Statement (see Box 13.1).[27]

The medical history should include details of pregnancy and maternal health, birth, and the postnatal period. These could be obtained from parents and from detailed examination of the mother's and child's medical notes and parent's health record.

Pedigree analysis of the family allows identifying the specific pattern of inheritance of the hearing loss. A three-generation family history with attention to other relatives with hearing loss and associated findings should be obtained.

Thorough familial history may reveal paternity issues as well as consanguinity and hearing impairment in other family members.

Clinical Examination (Level 1)

Clinical examination comprises not only a tympanoscopy and an examination of the head and face in search for outer ear anomalies (▶ Fig. 13.10), preauricular pits or tags (▶ Fig. 13.11), branchial/pharyngeal cleft pits, cysts, or fistulae, but also telecanthus, heterochromia iridis, white forelock, pigmentary anomalies, high myopia, pigmentary retinopathy, goiter, and craniofacial anomalies.

A systematic physical examination is performed to detect subtle dysmorphic features. It is also important to perform or arrange an age-appropriate developmental assessment.

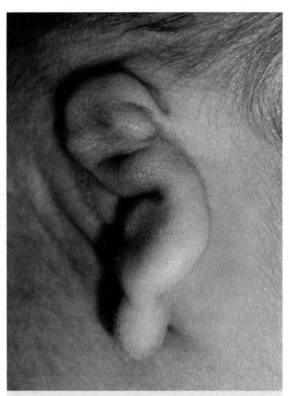

Fig. 13.10 Right ear microtia with typical peanut deformity (type 3 microtia according to Weerda's classification [1988]).

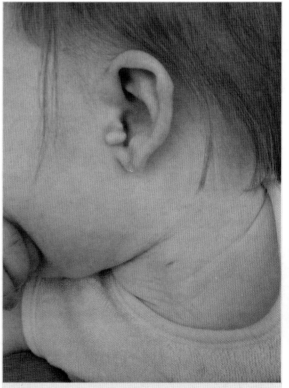

Fig. 13.11 A child with branchio-otorenal syndrome illustrating a branchial cyst and a preauricular pit (left side).

Molecular Genetic Testing

When single-gene testing is performed, prioritization of genes for testing can be based on epidemiological and/or phenotypic data.

- Mutation analysis of connexin 26 (*GJB2*) should be performed in every infant with bilateral hearing loss (level 1). If only one Cx26 mutation is identified, compound heterozygosity with a mutation in the neighboring gene *GJB6* that codes for connexin 30 has to be excluded. The incidence of children identified with Cx26/Cx30 mutations with other concurrent disease has been reported to be exceedingly low and supports the view that if the mutation is identified, additional testing can be avoided.[53]
- In case aminoglycoside therapy was administered or if there is a family history of hearing loss through maternal inheritance, screening for the presence of the mitochondrial 1555A > G mutation should be undertaken (level 2). Other mitochondrial mutations have to be considered depending on the family history (A7445G mutation).[54]
- Chromosomal anomalies and microdeletions may be responsible for up to 5.3% of SNHL in children.[61] If there is developmental delay, dysmorphic features or additional medical problems occur, and cytogenetic analysis and/or karyotyping are required (level 2).
- In cases of inner ear malformations such as an enlarged vestibular aqueduct and/or Mondini dysplasia (▶ Fig. 13.12), a test for the mutation in the *SLC26A4* gene (pendrin on chromosome 7) should be ordered. Mutations in this gene are the second-most frequent cause of autosomal recessive nonsyndromic hearing loss.
- An enlarged vestibular aqueduct may be seen in both nonsyndromic (DFNB4) and syndromic forms of

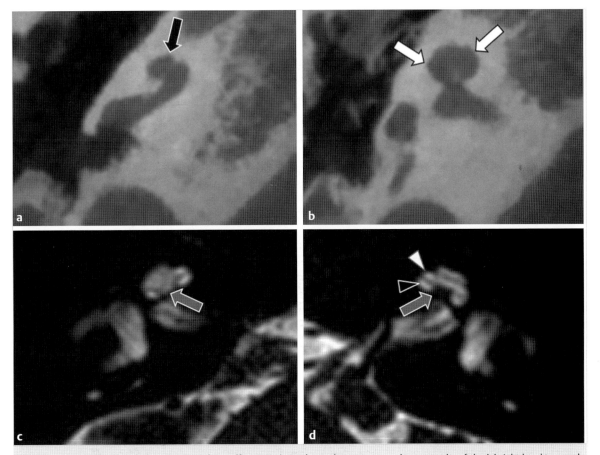

Fig. 13.12 Incomplete partition type II (Mondini malformation). Axial cone-beam computed tomography of the **(a)** right basal turn and **(b)** second/apical turn of the cochlea. Notice that the second/apical part of the cochlea is centered too far anterior on the basal turn (*black arrow*) and that the apical/second turn forms one cystic structure lacking a normal internal architecture or modiolus (*white arrows*). **(c, d)** Axial T2-weighted driven equilibrium (DRIVE) magnetic resonance images of both the inner ears. The normal modiolus (*gray arrow*) and separation between the cochlear turns and scalae are missing on the right side **(c)**. Compare with the normal modiolus (*gray arrow*) and separation between scala tympani (*black arrowhead*) and vestibuli (*white arrowhead*) on the normal left side. (Courtesy of Jan Casselman, AZ St Jan Hospital, Department of Radiology, Bruges, Belgium.)

13

deafness (such as Pendred's syndrome and branchio-otorenal syndrome [▶ Fig. 13.11]). Mutations in three known genes account for approximately half of Pendred's syndrome/DFNB4 cases: *SLC26A4* (~50% of affected individuals), *FOXI1* (< 1% of affected individuals), and *KCNJ10* (< 1% of affected individuals), suggesting further genetic heterogeneity. Sequence analysis of *SLC26A4* identifies disease-causing mutations in approximately 50% of affected individuals from either simplex or multiplex families. These persons are often compound heterozygotes for disease-causing variants in *SLC26A4* although, not infrequently, only a single variant is detected. Molecular genetic testing of *SLC26A4* is clinically available. Molecular genetic testing of *FOXI1* and *KCNJ10* is available on a research basis only.[55]

- Gene-specific mutation screening for other loci may be necessary, especially when there is suspicion of a syndromal deafness or a pedigree suggesting autosomal dominant inheritance. Alternatively, mutation screening may be negative, but does not exclude other types of genetic deafness. In patients with an unremarkable family history of deafness and a negative test result for connexin 26, the probability that the deafness is genetic can be given. The probability will vary based on the number of hearing siblings.

Counseling should focus on recurrence risk, the risk for medical comorbidity, and the evolution of the hearing loss.

Current genetic diagnostic tests consist of mutation screening by Sanger deoxyribonucleic acid (DNA) sequencing. This is a time-consuming laboratory technique relying on the use of DNA polymerase and limited because of low throughput. If Sanger sequencing were to be employed for sequencing all known NSHL disease-causing genes, the procedure would become prohibitively expensive. As only two genes (*GJB2* and *SLC26A4*) are now routinely tested in most laboratories, a diagnosis is obtained in only a subset of patients. Recent advances in the field of medical genetics are likely to change our approach to the etiological work-up of congenital hearing loss. The development of new techniques based on *next generation sequencing* (NGS), which make a complete screening of all the NSHL genes possible in a quick and cost-effective way with a high sensitivity and specificity, is likely to change the etiological work-up of hearing loss in the next few years. Recently, several strategies have been published to screen a large collection of hearing loss genes in one assay using a capture-based or polymerase chain reaction (PCR)-based target enrichment approach followed by NGS. Targeted NGS-based *gene panels* such as OtoSCOPE have been developed and allow for a comprehensive genetic testing for genes known to cause both nonsyndromic hearing and selected forms of syndromic hearing loss.[56] It is expected that within the next few years, similar molecular genetic tests will be available in several centers to screen all known disease-causing genes at a price comparable to the current diagnostic test in which only a few genes are analyzed using Sanger sequencing.

A recent guideline published by the American College of Medical Genetics and Genomics recommend the use of gene panels if initial genetic testing for DFNB1-related hearing loss (*GJB2* and *GJB6*) is negative.[57] However, it must be emphasized that the use of these technologies requires the results being discussed with a clinical geneticist to ensure correct interpretation of the data and appropriate genetic counseling.

If the hearing loss remains idiopathic, reevaluation at the age of 6 years is advised because certain stigmata may not be apparent until later in life and because of the emergence of new genetic tests.[58]

Viral Cultures and Serology

In asymptomatic children with hearing loss, congenital CMV infection should be excluded (level 1). The other infectious agents belonging to the TORCHES group should be suspected as a cause of the hearing loss when there is a suggestive history and clinical presentation since they are associated with severe and symptomatic disease.

Cytomegalovirus (Level 1)

> The gold standard to detect congenital CMV infection at birth is viral culture on fibroblasts or PCR within the first 3 weeks of life from urine or saliva. However, its use in the etiological work-up of SNHL is limited as a reliable test result can only be obtained in the first 3 weeks of life.

If the hearing impairment is diagnosed beyond 3 weeks of age, retrospective isolation of CMV-DNA in the dried blood spot of the neonatal screening is recommended.[59] Quality-control data indicate that sensitivity can vary widely depending on the gene being amplified and the technique being used for DNA extraction from cards. The marked difference in sensitivity and specificity reported between laboratories has led to a call for increased quality control of this diagnostic method.

As noted earlier, not all babies will be viremic in the newborn period, and as only approximately 50 to 100 µL of blood is spotted onto cards, detection is somewhat limited by sample volume; a negative result does not therefore exclude congenital CMV.

Serological testing for CMV-specific immunoglobulin M (IgM) antibody in sera from the mother and the child is more easily available but less sensitive (70% in newborns) and specific as viral isolation.

Rubella (Level 2)

From birth to 3 months of age, IgM will be present in clotted blood samples in all cases of congenital infection, and between 3 and 6 months in 90%.

Maternal immunization status may not be significant.

Toxoplasma Gondii (Level 2)

If IgM is present in a baby's blood up to 6 months of age, this indicates a congenital Toxoplasma infection.

Syphilis (Level 2)

FTA-Abs* serology can be carried out at any time.

Herpes Simplex Virus (Level 2)

Neonatal infection is diagnosed by virus cultures or PCR in skin lesions or other clinical specimens in case of a disseminated disease and by detection of IgM antibodies.

Laboratory Blood Testing

Standardized batteries of automated laboratory blood tests, such as urea and electrolytes, and liver function tests in infants failing UNHS are not helpful to identify the cause of hearing loss in newborns, except in the presence of a relevant history.[60]

Hematology (Blood Tests; Level 2)

Full blood count, hemoglobinopathy screening, and erythrocyte sedimentation rate rarely provide answers to the cause of a hearing loss, so these tests should be carried out with very low priority.[54]

Serum Biochemistry (Level 2)

Urea and electrolytes, and serum creatinine may be useful to assess renal function when the child is older or if conditions like Alport's syndrome are suspected.

The outcome of the neonatal blood spot should first be checked before requesting tests for congenital hypothyroidism.

Urine Examination (Level 2)

Dipstick for blood and protein can be done easily. Urinalysis may reveal renal involvement, but most syndromes involving hearing and renal impairment have significant clinical variability and manifest themselves later in life (e.g., Alport's syndrome).

Imaging

High-Resolution Computed Tomography (Level 2) and Magnetic Resonance Imaging (Level 1)

> ℹ️
>
> Either one or both examinations are requested in all children with confirmed unilateral or bilateral hearing loss of at least 60 dB HL or with craniofacial malformations. This audiological cutoff is set accordingly to the report of Bamiou et al.[61]

MRI of the inner ear and internal auditory meatus is the first-line radiological investigation in children. It will show most structural abnormalities except those of the ossicular chain. MRI will show soft tissues of the auditory pathways, for example, brain, seventh and eighth nerves and membranous labyrinth including the endolymphatic sac.

CT of the temporal bone will clearly show the bony structures including middle ear ossicles and should be considered when information on the bony structures is needed. However, CT scans do not show soft tissues such as the membranous labyrinth, the cochlear nerve and the brain itself and involves radiation.[61]

CT and MRI may be carried out from birth and the timing depends on when the parents are ready and what action is planned. Infants and children over 3 months will normally need sedation for radiological investigations and children over 2 years may require a general anesthetic.

McClay et al found that children with unilateral hearing loss had a greater percentage of inner ear anomalies than children with bilateral SNHL.[62] The overall incidence of inner ear abnormalities in ears of children with SNHL evaluated by MRI was 40%. The most common abnormalities seen are an abnormal cochlea and abnormal cochlear nerve, an enlarged vestibular aqueduct, and vestibular dysplasia. Children with severe and profound SNHL have a greater percentage of inner ear anomalies than children with mild or moderate SNHL. They also found that profound or progressive hearing loss and craniofacial abnormalities were significant predictors of abnormal CT findings.

Renal Ultrasound (Level 2)

This is indicated only if branchio-otorenal syndrome is suspected (i.e., conductive hearing loss with preauricular pits, branchial sinuses), if there are multiple or multisystem abnormalities, or if there is a family history of renal problems (level 2).[54]

---

* FTA-Abs: fluorescent treponemal antibody absorbed is a treponemal test specific for syphilis.

Ophthalmological Evaluation (Level 1)

Even if the overall quality of evidence in the literature concerning hearing-impaired children and their ophthalmic problems is very low, all children should be offered referral for detailed assessment by a pediatric ophthalmologist at the time of diagnosis to ensure correct visual acuity and to exclude associated pathology.

The prevalence of ophthalmic problems in hearing-impaired children seems to be very high (~40–60%). Although they may have a serious impact on children's acquisition of communication skills, speech development, and education, these problems may otherwise remain undetected for years. Eye problems may include nonspecific problems of squint and refractive errors. In some children, the eye examination may help to make or clarify a diagnosis such as CHARGE syndrome (*c*oloboma, *h*eart defects, *a*tresia of the choanae, *r*etardation of growth/development, *g*enitourinary, and *e*ar malformations), Usher's syndrome, Waardenburg's syndrome, or congenital CMV, toxoplasmosis, or rubella.[54]

A comprehensive ophthalmological assessment is required, which includes baseline assessment of visual acuity, indirect funduscopy, pupillary reflexes, and extraocular muscle assessment.[63]

Electrophysiologic testing to help identification of Usher's syndrome may also be required.

Electrocardiography (Level 2)

Although a screening ECG is not highly sensitive for detecting Jervell and Lange-Nielsen's syndrome, it may be suitable for screening hearing-impaired children.

High-risk children (i.e., those with a family history that is positive for sudden death, sudden infant death syndrome, syncopal episodes, or LQTS) should have a thorough cardiac evaluation. Mutations in two genes have been described in affected persons.[14]

13.7 Rehabilitation and Hearing Aids

Congenital deafness changes the functional properties of the auditory system and affects cortical development.[64] Interactions between brain areas involved in auditory, visual, and somatosensory processing may be altered and uncoupling of the auditory system from other systems may affect key cognitive functions.

Early detection of hearing loss will allow for early intervention and rehabilitation. The first 6 months of life have been found crucial for hearing acquisition. Introduction of hearing aids before the age of 6 months will improve subsequent hearing development and is now considered a standard goal in the management of hearing-impaired children.[27]

Adjustment of hearing aid settings in infants and young children requires special skills and dedicated audiologists. Especially during the first year of life, hearing thresholds may change due to maturation, or fluctuations may occur related to intercurrent otitis media. Close cooperation between the audiologist and ENT specialist is therefore needed, and hearing thresholds and middle ear status should be checked at regular intervals.

Once it becomes evident that hearing aids do not provide sufficient improvement in hearing status, cochlear implantation should be considered.

In children with profound hearing loss, cochlear implantation is more beneficial than conventional hearing aids for improving speech and language acquisition.[65]

Early implantation (before 12 months of age) seems to be more beneficial in terms of expressive/receptive language development and speech perception. However, cochlear implantation in very young children implies specific challenges to the cochlear implant team. Particular attention should be paid to the certainty of the diagnosis of hearing loss, an age-appropriate surgical and anesthetic technique, intraoperative testing, postoperative programming, and long-term safety.[66]

A detailed discussion of hearing rehabilitation is provided in Chapter 14.

13.8 Measures to Prevent Hearing Deterioration

13.8.1 Noise Trauma

Exposure to environmental noise should be avoided in infants and children with hearing loss. There is increasing evidence that noise-induced hearing loss also affects children with prevalence rates from 12 to 15% of school aged children in the United States. Noise-induced hearing loss may not only result from personal entertainment devices but may also be caused by noise generated by powered garden or domestic equipment, and the recreational use of firearms.[67]

13.8.2 Specific Preventive Measures

Identification of an etiological cause for the hearing loss may allow for specific preventive measures such as for the following circumstances:

- *Congenital CMV infection*: ganciclovir and valganciclovir should be considered in infants with symptomatic CMV infection and central nervous system manifestations. When started before the age of 1 month, this treatment prevents best-ear hearing deterioration during early childhood. Both drugs have equal therapeutic efficacy and toxicity (most frequently neutropenia), but oral administration of valganciclovir avoids the risks of indwelling catheters for drug infusion.[68] Treatment lasts for 6 weeks both with the oral or intravenous way of administration, and the effect on hearing is assessed by a control ABR/ASSR measurement.
- *m.15555A > G mitochondrial mutation*: children with these mutations are at increased risk for hearing loss following exposure to aminoglycosides. Consequently, administration of these drugs should be avoided in mutation carriers.
- *Congenital inner ear anomalies*: children with congenital inner ear malformations may suffer sudden hearing deterioration or leakage of cerebrospinal fluid after head trauma or rapid changes in barometric pressure. Contact sports and scuba diving should therefore be discouraged. When a sudden hearing loss occurs, a short course of oral steroids (e.g., prednisone) should be considered, although many may experience a spontaneous partial recovery even without treatment. Parents of these children should be counseled about the increased risk for meningitis and they should be instructed about early symptoms and signs of meningitis. The use of the pneumococcal vaccine following the schedule for high-risk patients is recommended.
- *Cochlear implants*: children with cochlear implants are at increased risk of bacterial meningitis. It is recommended that such children be vaccinated against pneumococcal disease.[69]

13.9 Key Points

- UNHS allows for early detection of congenital hearing loss.
- Upon referral from screening, these infants should undergo a comprehensive audiological and etiological work-up in order to determine the type, severity, and laterality of the hearing loss. The etiological work-up may provide information about the underlying cause of the hearing loss and would allow parental counseling,

guide treatment, and rehabilitation and allow for preventive measures to avoid further deterioration when applicable.
- Children in whom hearing loss is detected beyond the neonatal period should also undergo a similar audiological and etiological work-up.
- Based on current protocols, an etiological diagnosis may be established in approximately 50% of infants/children with congenital hearing loss—a figure that is likely to increase in the very near future due to recent advances in molecular genetics.

References

[1] Lustig LR, Leake PA, Snyder RL, Rebscher SJ. Changes in the cat cochlear nucleus following neonatal deafening and chronic intracochlear electrical stimulation. Hear Res. 1994; 74(1–2):29–37

[2] Morton CC, Nance WE. Newborn hearing screening—a silent revolution. N Engl J Med. 2006; 354(20):2151–2164

[3] Olusanya BO, Ruben RJ, Parving A. Reducing the burden of communication disorders in the developing world: an opportunity for the millennium development project. JAMA. 2006; 296(4):441–444

[4] Olusanya BO, Swanepoel de W, Chapchap MJ, et al. Progress towards early detection services for infants with hearing loss in developing countries. BMC Health Serv Res. 2007; 7:14

[5] Robertson CM, Howarth TM, Bork DL, Dinu IA. Permanent bilateral sensory and neural hearing loss of children after neonatal intensive care because of extreme prematurity: a thirty-year study. Pediatrics. 2009; 123(5):e797–e807

[6] Van Naarden K, Decouflé P, Caldwell K. Prevalence and characteristics of children with serious hearing impairment in metropolitan Atlanta, 1991–1993. Pediatrics. 1999; 103(3):570–575

[7] Weichbold V, Nekahm-Heis D, Welzl-Mueller K. Universal newborn hearing screening and postnatal hearing loss. Pediatrics. 2006; 117 (4):e631–e636

[8] Smith RJ, Bale JF, Jr, White KR. Sensorineural hearing loss in children. Lancet. 2005; 365(9462):879–890

[9] Alford RL, Friedman TB, Keats BJ, et al. Early childhood hearing loss: clinical and molecular genetics. An educational slide set of the American College of Medical Genetics. Genet Med. 2003; 5(4):338–341

[10] del Castillo FJ, Rodríguez-Ballesteros M, Martín Y, et al. Heteroplasmy for the 1555A > G mutation in the mitochondrial 12S rRNA gene in six Spanish families with non-syndromic hearing loss. J Med Genet. 2003; 40(8):632–636

[11] Smith RJH, Shearer AE, Hildebrand MS, Van Camp G. Deafness and hereditary hearing loss overview. In: Pagon RA, Bird TD, Dolan CR, Stephens K, Adam MP, eds. Seattle, WA: GeneReviews; 1993

[12] Sommen M, van Camp G, Boudewyns A. Genetic and clinical diagnosis in non-syndromic hearing loss. Hearing Balance Commun. 2013; 11(3):138–145

[13] Young NM, Mets MB, Hain TC. Early diagnosis of Usher syndrome in infants and children. Am J Otol 1996; 17: 30–34

[14] Tranebjaerg L, Samson RA, Green GE. Jervell and Lange-Nielsen syndrome. In: Pagon RA, Bird TD, Dolan CR, Stephens K, Adam MP, eds. Seattle, WA: GeneReviews; 1993

[15] Bale JF, Jr. Fetal infections and brain development. Clin Perinatol. 2009; 36(3):639–653

[16] Boppana SB, Pass RF, Britt WJ, Stagno S, Alford CA. Symptomatic congenital cytomegalovirus infection: neonatal morbidity and mortality. Pediatr Infect Dis J. 1992; 11(2):93–99

[17] Peckham CS, Stark O, Dudgeon JA, Martin JA, Hawkins G. Congenital cytomegalovirus infection: a cause of sensorineural hearing loss. Arch Dis Child. 1987; 62(12):1233–1237

[18] Goderis J, De Leenheer E, Smets K, Van Hoecke H, Keymeulen A, Dhooge I. Hearing loss and congenital CMV infection: a systematic review. Pediatrics. 2014; 134(5):972–982

13

[19] Fowler KB, Boppana SB. Congenital cytomegalovirus (CMV) infection and hearing deficit. J Clin Virol. 2006; 35(2):226–231

[20] Carter AO, Frank JW. Congenital toxoplasmosis: epidemiologic features and control. CMAJ. 1986; 135(6):618–623

[21] Wilson CB, Remington JS, Stagno S, Reynolds DW. Development of adverse sequelae in children born with subclinical congenital Toxoplasma infection. Pediatrics. 1980; 66(5):767–774

[22] Brown ED, Chau JK, Atashband S, Westerberg BD, Kozak FK. A systematic review of neonatal toxoplasmosis exposure and sensorineural hearing loss. Int J Pediatr Otorhinolaryngol. 2009; 73(5):707–711

[23] Chau J, Atashband S, Chang E, Westerberg BD, Kozak FK. A systematic review of pediatric sensorineural hearing loss in congenital syphilis. Int J Pediatr Otorhinolaryngol. 2009; 73(6):787–792

[24] Gleich LL, Urbina M, Pincus RL. Asymptomatic congenital syphilis and auditory brainstem response. Int J Pediatr Otorhinolaryngol. 1994; 30 (1):11–13

[25] Westerberg BD, Atashband S, Kozak FK. A systematic review of the incidence of sensorineural hearing loss in neonates exposed to Herpes simplex virus (HSV). Int J Pediatr Otorhinolaryngol. 2008; 72(7):931–937

[26] Cardonick E, Iacobucci A. Use of chemotherapy during human pregnancy. Lancet Oncol. 2004; 5(5):283–291

[27] American Academy of Pediatrics, Joint Committee on Infant Hearing. Year 2007 position statement: principles and guidelines for early hearing detection and intervention programs. Pediatrics. 2007; 120 (4):898–921

[28] Fortnum H, Davis A. Epidemiology of permanent childhood hearing impairment in Trent Region, 1985–1993. Br J Audiol. 1997; 31(6):409–446

[29] Coenraad S, Goedegebure A, van Goudoever JB, Hoeve LJ. Risk factors for sensorineural hearing loss in NICU infants compared to normal hearing NICU controls. Int J Pediatr Otorhinolaryngol. 2010; 74(9):999–1002

[30] Van Kerschaver E, Boudewyns AN, Declau F, Van de Heyning PH, Wuyts FL. Socio-demographic determinants of hearing impairment studied in 103,835 term babies. Eur J Public Health. 2013; 23(1):55–60

[31] Declau F, Boudewyns A, Van den Ende J, Peeters A, van den Heyning P. Etiologic and audiologic evaluations after universal neonatal hearing screening: analysis of 170 referred neonates. Pediatrics. 2008; 121(6):1119–1126

[32] Mc Cormick B, ed. Paediatric Audiology 0–5 Years. 3rd ed. London: Whurr Publishers; 2004

[33] Rapin I, Gravel J. "Auditory neuropathy": physiologic and pathologic evidence calls for more diagnostic specificity. Int J Pediatr Otorhinolaryngol. 2003; 67(7):707–728

[34] Psarommatis I, Riga M, Douros K, et al. Transient infantile auditory neuropathy and its clinical implications. Int J Pediatr Otorhinolaryngol. 2006; 70(9):1629–1637

[35] Lin HC, Shu MT, Lee KS, Lin HY, Lin G. reducing false positives in newborn hearing screening program: how and why. Otol Neurotol. 2007; 28(6):788–792

[36] Wessex Universal Neonatal Hearing Screening Trial Group. Controlled trial of universal neonatal screening for early identification of permanent childhood hearing impairment. Lancet. 1998; 352(9145):1957–1964

[37] Rohlfs AK, Wiesner T, Drews H, et al. Interdisciplinary approach to design, performance, and quality management in a multicenter newborn hearing screening project: introduction, methods, and results of the newborn hearing screening in Hamburg (Part I). Eur J Pediatr. 2010; 169(11):1353–1360

[38] Pimperton H, Blythe H, Kreppner J, et al. The impact of universal newborn hearing screening on long-term literacy outcomes: a prospective cohort study. Arch Dis Child. 2016; 101(1):9–15

[39] Clark JG. Uses and abuses of hearing loss classification. ASHA. 1981; 23(7):493–500

[40] Starr A, Amlie RN, Martin WH, Sanders S. Development of auditory function in newborn infants revealed by auditory brainstem potentials. Pediatrics. 1977; 60(6):831–839

[41] King AM. The national protocol for paediatric amplification in Australia. Int J Audiol. 2010; 49 Suppl 1:S64–S69

[42] King AM, Purdy SC, Dillon H, Sharma M, Pearce W. Australian hearing protocols for the audiological management of infants who have auditory neuropathy. Aust NZ J Audiol. 2005; 27(1):69–77

[43] Rance G, Briggs RJ. Assessment of hearing in infants with moderate to profound impairment: the Melbourne experience with auditory steady-state evoked potential testing. Ann Otol Rhinol Laryngol Suppl. 2002; 189 Suppl:22–28

[44] Swanepoel D, Ebrahim S. Auditory steady-state response and auditory brainstem response thresholds in children. Eur Arch Otorhinolaryngol. 2009; 266(2):213–219

[45] Swanepoel D, Erasmus H. Auditory steady-state responses for estimating moderate hearing loss. Eur Arch Otorhinolaryngol. 2007; 264 (7):755–759

[46] Scherf F, Brokx J, Wuyts FL, Van de Heyning PH. The ASSR: clinical application in normal-hearing and hearing-impaired infants and adults, comparison with the click-evoked ABR and pure-tone audiometry. Int J Audiol. 2006; 45(5):281–286

[47] Picton TW, Dimitrijevic A, Perez-Abalo MC, Van Roon P. Estimating audiometric thresholds using auditory steady-state responses. J Am Acad Audiol. 2005; 16(3):140–156

[48] Kei J, Allison-Levick J, Dockray J, et al. High-frequency (1000 Hz) tympanometry in normal neonates. J Am Acad Audiol. 2003; 14(1):20–28

[49] Paradise JL, Smith CG, Bluestone CD. Tympanometric detection of middle ear effusion in infants and young children. Pediatrics. 1976; 58(2):198–210

[50] Margolis RH, Bass-Ringdahl S, Hanks WD, Holte L, Zapala DA. Tympanometry in newborn infants—1 kHz norms. J Am Acad Audiol. 2003; 14(7):383–392

[51] Alaerts J, Luts H, Wouters J. Evaluation of middle ear function in young children: clinical guidelines for the use of 226- and 1,000-Hz tympanometry. Otol Neurotol. 2007; 28(6):727–732

[52] Lewis MP, Bradford Bell E, Evans AK. A comparison of tympanometry with 226 Hz and 1000 Hz probe tones in children with Down syndrome. Int J Pediatr Otorhinolaryngol. 2011; 75(12):1492–1495

[53] Morzaria S, Westerberg BD, Kozak FK. Evidence-based algorithm for the evaluation of a child with bilateral sensorineural hearing loss. J Otolaryngol. 2005; 34(5):297–303

[54] Working Group of BAAP/BAPA. Guidelines for aetiological investigation of infants with congenital hearing loss identified through newborn hearing screening. British Association of Audiovestibular Physicians and British Association of Paediatricians in Audiology; 2009

[55] Hilgert N, Smith RJ, Van Camp G. Forty-six genes causing nonsyndromic hearing impairment: which ones should be analyzed in DNA diagnostics? Mutat Res. 2009; 681(2–3):189–196

[56] University of Iowa Carver College of Medicine Molecular Otolaryngology and Renal Research Laboratories. Deafness/OtoSCOPE. Available at http://www.medicine.uiowa.edu/morl/deafnessclinical/. Accessed September 3, 2015

[57] Alford RL, Arnos KS, Fox M, et al. ACMG Working Group on Update of Genetics Evaluation Guidelines for the Etiologic Diagnosis of Congenital Hearing Loss, Professional Practice and Guidelines Committee. American College of Medical Genetics and Genomics guideline for the clinical evaluation and etiologic diagnosis of hearing loss. Genet Med. 2014; 16(4):347–355

[58] De Leenheer EM, Janssens S, Padalko E, Loose D, Leroy BP, Dhooge IJ. Etiological diagnosis in the hearing impaired newborn: proposal of a flow chart. Int J Pediatr Otorhinolaryngol. 2011; 75(1):27–32

[59] Boudewyns A, Declau F, Smets K, et al. Cytomegalovirus DNA detection in Guthrie cards: role in the diagnostic work-up of childhood hearing loss. Otol Neurotol. 2009; 30(7):943–949

[60] Mafong DD, Shin EJ, Lalwani AK. Use of laboratory evaluation and radiologic imaging in the diagnostic evaluation of children with sensorineural hearing loss. Laryngoscope. 2002; 112(1):1–7

[61] Bamiou DE, MacArdle B, Bitner-Glindzicz M, Sirimanna T. Aetiological investigations of hearing loss in childhood: a review. Clin Otolaryngol Allied Sci. 2000; 25(2):98–106

[62] McClay JE, Booth TN, Parry DA, Johnson R, Roland P. Evaluation of pediatric sensorineural hearing loss with magnetic resonance imaging. Arch Otolaryngol Head Neck Surg. 2008; 134(9):945–952

[63] Nikolopoulos TP, Lioumi D, Stamataki S, O'Donoghue GM. Evidence-based overview of ophthalmic disorders in deaf children: a literature update. Otol Neurotol. 2006; 27(2) Suppl 1:S1–S24, discussion S20

[64] Kral A, O'Donoghue GM. Profound deafness in childhood. N Engl J Med. 2010; 363(15):1438–1450

[65] Osberger MJ, Maso M, Sam LK. Speech intelligibility of children with cochlear implants, tactile aids, or hearing aids. J Speech Hear Res. 1993; 36(1):186–203

[66] Sampaio AL, Araújo MF, Oliveira CA. New criteria of indication and selection of patients to cochlear implant. Int J Otolaryngol. 2011; 2011:573968

[67] Harrison RV. Noise-induced hearing loss in children: a 'less than silent' environmental danger. Paediatr Child Health (Oxford). 2008; 13(5):377–382

[68] Nassetta L, Kimberlin D, Whitley R. Treatment of congenital cytomegalovirus infection: implications for future therapeutic strategies. J Antimicrob Chemother. 2009; 63(5):862–867

[69] Centers for Disease Control and Prevention. Fact Sheet: Use of vaccines to prevent meningitis in persons with cochlear implants. Available at http://www.cdc.gov/vaccines/vpd-vac/mening/cochlear/dis-cochlear-faq-hcp.htm

13

14 Nonsurgical Management of the Child with Hearing Loss

Priya Singh and Josephine Marriage

14.1 Introduction

Permanent childhood hearing impairment (PCHI) from early life occurs in approximately 1 per 1,000 live births in most populations. In approximately 50% of these cases, the hearing loss may be due to some factors around the birth, including prematurity, illness, or congenital infection. In the other half of the cases, the hearing loss is related to genetic factors, though not necessarily with experience of deafness in other family members, especially in autosomal recessive conditions.[1] Newborn hearing screening programs (NHSPs) have been implemented in many European countries to identify these cases early and to optimize auditory learning potential (see Chapter 13). The rationale for identifying babies with hearing loss and providing early intervention with hearing aids is to achieve optimum development of the auditory system during critical periods of early neural plasticity.[2] The aim is that speech, language, and academic outcomes for the majority of hearing-impaired (HI) children should be on a par with their peers with normal hearing by the time of school entry. This is not yet being fulfilled in most countries, but the academic and communication achievements have greatly improved for recent generations of HI children.[3]

In addition to the infants with hearing loss at or around birth, children may acquire debilitating hearing loss during childhood and adolescence. These include approximately 1 in 10 children who have intermittent or chronic hearing loss from middle ear effusion (otitis media with effusion [OME]; see Chapter 8), which may impact on talking and on learning development, and those with acute or recurrent ear infections (see Chapter 7). Another group of children acquire hearing loss over the years of childhood such that the prevalence of permanent loss of greater than 40 dB in at least one ear by teenage years is approximately 1.6 per 1,000. This compares with 1.1 per 1,000 at birth.[4] The commonest causes of late onset hearing loss include bacterial meningitis, congenital cytomegalovirus (CMV) infections, acquired infections (mumps, measles), ototoxic medication, and temporal bone fracture from head trauma.[5,6,7]

Congenital hearing losses with onset in childhood, rather than at birth, arise from genetic susceptibility to deterioration in cochlear hearing levels over time. This may be hearing loss in isolation or as part of a genetic syndrome. Example of genetic syndromes with progressive hearing loss include Alport's syndrome with renal abnormalities, Usher's syndrome with loss of vision, and Down's syndrome (trisomy 21) associated with early conductive hearing loss and abnormal aging.

> ℹ
>
> The onset of a hearing loss may be first indication of a wider genetic condition; therefore, careful and thorough investigation of each case is important.

14.2 What Is the Impact of Hearing Loss for Children?

> ℹ
>
> The period from birth to 3 years is the critical period for speech and language acquisition, and the aim of newborn hearing screening is for early identified children to have age-appropriate language by school entry.[8]

Speech is acquired through hearing and its more active counterpart of listening. There is no part of the child's day in which it is not important for the child to be able to hear sounds in the environment. The neural processes for binaural hearing, localization skills, listening in noise, and applying auditory attention are laid down in the early years of life. Even a fluctuating conductive hearing loss from middle ear effusion can delay or obstruct these processes for later auditory learning potential.[9] A typical vocabulary size at school entry is between 5,000 and 20,000 words, depending on the richness of language exposure at home, but, by adulthood, it may be 60,000.[10] Most of these words have not been taught but have been acquired through overhearing and tangential learning. Language level and hearing ability predict later acquired literacy skills as the school curriculum is mainly delivered through audition.[11] The scores by children in standardized attainment scores used in Britain for schools are influenced by the noise levels in the classroom, even when controlled for socioeconomic group.[12] This demonstrates the importance of being able to overhear speech by different talkers as a foundation skill for literacy, academic, and social achievement. One of the recent themes being reported in the research literature on hearing impairment is that children with hearing loss often have subtle difficulties in peer-group situations, even if their language skills are age-appropriate on assessment.[13] The evidence is clear: the impact of hearing loss in early life, even for short periods, is wide-ranging and has long-term effects on achievement and life choices.

> ### Tips and Tricks
>
> Avoid simplified phrases such as "speech is coming on well" unless there are specific measures from standardized evaluations such as language scores. Comments may be quoted out of context and be overinterpreted as meaning "no intervention is required." The medical doctor's statements carry very high credibility and may be hard to counterbalance by the relevant professional working with the family thereafter.

14.3 Diagnosis of Acquired Hearing Loss

As the focus of screening for hearing loss is now on identifying children with bilateral permanent hearing loss at birth (with concurrent improvements in outcomes for these infants), how is the much larger group of children, with later and possibly fluctuating hearing loss, picked up? Some may have had no period of illness, for example, those with later onset genetic deafness or chronic noninfective middle ear effusion. The screening of hearing at school entry is no longer standard practice in most countries. A wide-ranging yet methodical system of surveillance is necessary, usually through primary practitioners and family doctors leading on to ear, nose, and throat (ENT)/audiology and pediatric referrals.

> Hearing deficits may be noticed by parents and carers. When a parent expresses concern about their child's hearing, there is almost always a hearing or communication impairment.

The tendency is for families to assume that their child hears well unless they have clear indications to the contrary. Thus, if parents specifically express concerns about their child's hearing, this is a red flag for there being a problem. It may not be hearing—sometimes it is a more generalized communication difficulty—but it is *always* important to arrange hearing assessment if parents or carers are questioning hearing.

> ### Tips and Tricks
>
> If parents or teachers are concerned about hearing, this is a red flag. The child needs full and accurate assessment of hearing in each ear. A fuller communication assessment is needed if hearing is found to be normal. The converse is *not* true; parents, teachers, and carers may not always be aware that a child has poor hearing. If there is any doubt, refer for early assessment.

14.3.1 Objective Hearing Assessment in the Early Months of Life

Screening Tests

Otoacoustic emission (OAE) testing is a noninvasive and simple method for recording reflected sound generated by the normal activity of the outer hair cells in the cochlea (refer to Chapter 13 for more on screening tests). The OAE is typically absent for hearing loss of 25 to 30 dB HL or above or when there is middle ear effusion, which makes it highly suitable for screening for hearing loss in early life. OAEs are generated by the outer hair cells in the cochlea and therefore this test is not sensitive to cases with normal cochlear function but with an auditory neuropathy (refer to Chapter 13, Chapter 14.4.3, and ▶ Fig. 14.7) in which the transmission of neural information is compromised.

Objective Assessment of Hearing Loss

Auditory Brainstem Response or Brainstem Evoked Response Audiometry

> The techniques used for hearing assessment depend upon the age and developmental status of the child. In the first few months of life, up to approximately 4 months of age, auditory brainstem response (ABR) testing is used. This is typically needed for newborn babies who have failed the preliminary screening tests, typically OAE (see Chapter 13).

Electrodes are attached to the vertex, high forehead, and mastoid of the baby's head. These record the electroencephalogram (EEG) activity that is time-locked to the presentation of short acoustic signals, either clicks or tone bursts, to the ear. Use of averaging and filtering of the EEG allows the auditory neural potentials from the

14

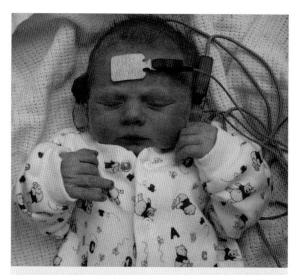

Fig. 14.1 Newborn undergoing auditory brainstem response.

Tips and Tricks

Cases in which a hearing impairment has been misdiagnosed tend to arise from overreliance on a single method of assessment without any functional observation, or when insufficient attention is paid to parents' report of poor hearing responses in the case history, regardless of whether the infant passed the NHSP screen at birth.

brainstem pathways to be extracted and analyzed in response to acoustic signals of different intensities and frequencies. ABR therefore reflects early hearing levels for detection and transduction of sound signals within the cochlea and onto the central neural pathways. This type of electrophysiologic testing is used to define the extent and type of hearing loss in each ear for infants referred from NHSPs. ABR testing is carried out in natural sleep (easier to arrange up to 12 weeks of age) or under sedation or general anesthetic in the older child (▶ Fig. 14.1).

Auditory Steady-State Responses and Cortical Evoked Response Audiometry

New methods of electrophysiologic testing are being developed including auditory steady-state responses (ASSRs) and cortical evoked response audiometry (CERA). CERA has the benefit of allowing speech sounds to be presented through hearing aids worn by the infant during the test to assess the effectiveness of the hearing aid fitting in the first months of life.[14]

Acoustic Reflex Thresholds and Auditory Neuropathy

Acoustic reflex thresholds give additional diagnostic information along with evoked potential measurement of the cochlear microphonic component of the ABR. Auditory neuropathy is present in approximately 1 in 10 children with permanent hearing loss from birth.[15] There are updated prevalence data from NHSPs and full information on all aspects relevant to a newborn hearing screening and follow-up assessment and habilitation services given on the UK Web site (hearing.screening.nhs.uk/publications).

14.3.2 Behavioral Hearing Tests

As the infant develops, from approximately 6 months of age, behavioral tests are used to measure hearing levels. The aim of all behavioral testing is to define the minimal sound levels detected across a range of frequencies, in each ear separately for air-conduction and bone-conduction signals, that is, to determine hearing thresholds for the child that correspond to pure-tone audiometric (PTA) readings in older children and adults.

Visual Reinforcement Audiometry

Visual reinforcement audiometry (VRA) is appropriate from approximately 6 months to approximately 30 months of developmental age.

In this test technique, the infant is conditioned to associate the presentation of a specific frequency of sound to a visual reward by turning his/her head toward the lighting up of a toy or activation of a video clip. Once the association of sound has been paired to the visual reward, the intensity level of the signal is reduced until the child no longer responds. The intensity is then increased in incremental steps until the infant makes a head turn on hearing the signal. There is a skill in providing the appropriate engagement of attention for the child for this type of testing and an established test protocol is followed to avoid for random head turns being interpreted as hearing responses by well-intentioned but invalid testing.[16] Sounds are presented to each ear separately through inserts for air conduction and for bone conduction to derive a full audiogram for each child. This type of testing has now replaced traditional techniques of unconditioned testing, for example, distraction testing or observation of responses in the sound field.[17]

Conditioned Play Audiometry

From approximately 2 years of age, conditioned play audiometry (CPA) responses in which the child learns to make play-based responses when a sound is presented are used. Testing with headphones or insert earphones and bone conduction is necessary to determine whether the hearing loss is conductive, mixed, or sensorineural in nature. Once a child reaches approximately 5 years of age, he/she will typically be able to perform the PTA similar to an adult, possibly pressing a button or making a response with a toy.

Tips and Tricks

It is important to be aware that children with sensorineural hearing loss (SNHL) will also have episodes of middle ear effusion and that flat tympanometry does not imply that a hearing loss is solely due to middle ear effusion. If a mixed hearing loss is misidentified as a conductive hearing loss, grommet insertion may be arranged with only limited improvements in hearing, and the opportunity to identify and treat more severe hearing loss may be delayed.

All test techniques require the first signal to be clearly audible to demonstrate the child's role in the game. Thus, the starting stimulus must be demonstrably audible to the child, and the toys need to be engaging and appropriately motivating for the developmental age of the child. A clear understanding of typical developmental milestones and profiles through infancy and early life is a great asset for people carrying out efficient pediatric audiology, as 40% of the cases with PCHI have additional cognitive, sensory, and developmental impairments.

Pure-Tone Audiogram

The audiogram is a chart showing the sensitivity of hearing in each ear, mainly across the frequency range important for understanding speech (Box 14.1). The reduced sensitivity is measured in decibels hearing level (dB HL), with the standard for normal hearing shown by a straight line at zero (0 dB) on the y-axis.

Box 14.1 Interpreting the Audiogram

The PTA defines the lowest (quietest) level at which a pure-tone signal is detected, in each ear, when other sounds are absent. Standards are applied for test rooms so that they are appropriately quiet (BS EN ISO 8253–1:1998) and there is a specified procedure that must be used for results to be comparable across different test sessions (e.g., BSA, 2011).[18] Most decisions on management for hearing loss are predicated on the hearing thresholds shown by the audiogram. It is therefore crucial that the audiogram is an accurate representation of hearing thresholds, regardless of the test technique used to derive it. It is much more important that there are two or three frequencies reliably derived than that more frequencies are represented but with poor

---

reliability. Common sources of error in testing are that visual cues are available to the child, (e.g., seeing hand movements for presenting the sound, or that the tester looks toward the child) or that a poor tester presents tones with regular timing patterns so the child is able to correctly guess when to make a response. It is crucial that in the initial conditioning of the child's response to the presented signal, the tone is clearly audible to the child and that no assumptions are made about the child's hearing status prior to completing the testing.

The full audiogram may be derived by VRA or by conditioned responses over several test sessions. The audiogram reflects the hearing detection levels for the child and therefore also the sounds that are inaudible. The constraints on the child's listening skill development arising from lack of experience in hearing speech and environmental sounds are important. Limited hearing inevitably also restricts the auditory feedback that a child has for his/her own vocalizations in his own babbling and early speech sounds.[21]

However, the audiogram does not measure an individual child's potential ability to differentiate and recognize complex signals of speech in daily life once hearing amplification or surgery is performed. The range of variables that are known to impact on speech understanding include use of visual cues, cognitive ability, speech and language level, personality type, parent engagement, and communication modes at home. Thus, a mild or moderate audiogram configuration may be debilitating for one child, but have relatively less impact on another child. In a study by Taylor,[22] no correlation was found between the three-frequency pure-tone average and performance on speech in noise scores for 100 adult listeners, thus highlighting the variable impact of hearing loss for different individuals.

The extent of hearing loss is traditionally described as normal, mild, moderate, severe, and profound, in line with categories shown in ▶ Fig. 14.2. However, hearing loss tends to vary across frequencies and so may be normal in the low frequencies, mild to moderate in the midfrequencies, and severe in the high frequencies (as shown in ▶ Fig. 14.2 for a typical age-related hearing loss configuration), making audiometric categorization meaningless.

Quantifying Extent of Hearing Loss

In the United Kingdom, the British Society Audiology (BSA) guidelines[18] quantify hearing loss according to the thresholds obtained in a PTA with similar categories given by the American Speech-Language-Hearing Association guidelines in the United States.[19] However, these have limited value in understanding the impact of hearing loss for a child on the basis of these simple

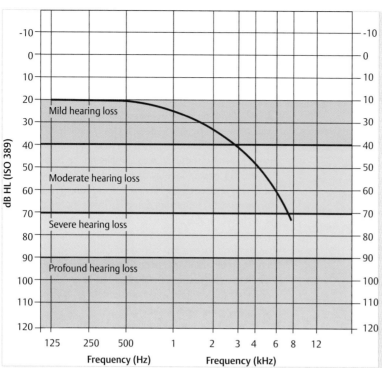

Fig. 14.2 Audiometric classifications for extent of hearing loss.

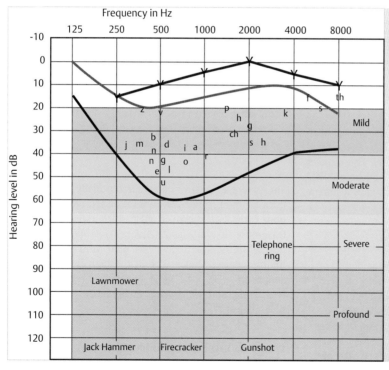

Fig. 14.3 An audiogram with the average speech spectrum for conversational-level speech shown between the two curved lines with different speech sounds of English and some environmental sound sources.

descriptors. ▶ Fig. 14.3 shows the typical speech spectrum for conversational-level speech on the audiogram format, with different speech sounds (or phonemes) included to represent their acoustic features across intensity and frequency.

In terms of the functional effect of hearing loss categories, it can be seen that a mild hearing loss may reduce half of the audible information in conversational-level speech, or more for quiet speech or when at a distance. A moderate loss may make distant speech inaudible and

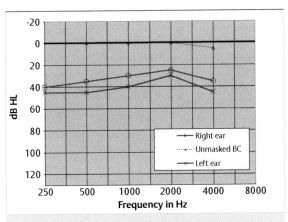

Fig. 14.4 Audiometric examples of bilateral conductive hearing loss, mild to moderate on the left and mild on the right.

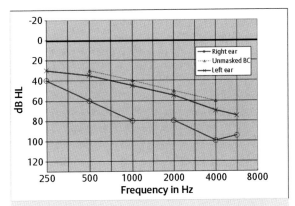

Fig. 14.5 Audiometric examples of bilateral sensorineural loss, moderate to severe on the left and severe to profound on the right.

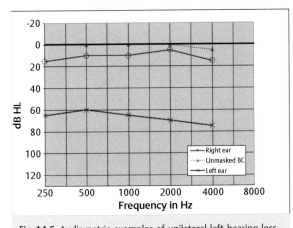

Fig. 14.6 Audiometric examples of unilateral left hearing loss, no masking done. Triangles relate to right hearing levels. Needs masking to define true left hearing, which is the dead ear.

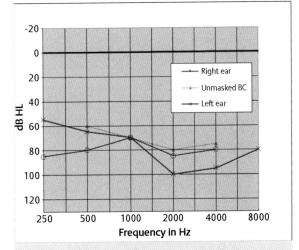

Fig. 14.7 Possible configuration of auditory neuropathy spectrum disorder audiogram, with otoacoustic emission present and absent auditory brainstem responses.

degrade the quieter parts of conversational speech even at close range. A severe hearing loss makes speech inaudible even at close range, though the child may be able to hear some of his/her own vocalizations. A profound hearing loss prevents the child from hearing his/her own speech or that of others at all without hearing aid or cochlear implant (CI) amplification.

The hearing loss may be:

- Conductive (▶ Fig. 14.4).
- Sensorineural (▶ Fig. 14.5, ▶ Fig. 14.6).
- Mixed conductive and sensorineural.
- Auditory neuropathy (▶ Fig. 14.7).

Knowing the type of hearing loss is crucial for considering appropriate options for management and also for predicting the levels of amplification required to reduce the sound deprivation from hearing loss. Children need to experience sound in both ears to derive localization skills and meaning as the basis of speech understanding and also to alert them to oncoming sounds. The development of the brain and neural networks for audition is highly influenced by exposure to the auditory environment and so preschool hearing loss impacts on the rate and progress of sound learning, with the size of a child's vocabulary in the first year of school predicting future reading comprehension.[20]

Tips and Tricks

Be careful with the use of the word *mild* based on audiogram thresholds. This can be misinterpreted by parents and carers as implying a condition with minimal impact on the child. Parents look to medical practitioners to give clear, evidence-based information for their options for interventions.

14

Speech Discrimination Testing

The use of speech recognition testing is important within the test battery as a more holistic measure of the functional impact of hearing loss on the child. Assessment of the child's speech discrimination can be included, using live voice testing, from approximately 3 years' development age to demonstrate the impact on speech understanding and to provide audiological certainty across different audiology test techniques. This is usually done by presenting a set of pictures or items that are familiar to the child. An item is asked for ("Where's the duck?") without giving lipreading cues or looking toward the target item. The lowest speech level at which the child can consistently identify all the items is measured on a sound-level meter. The choice of items is important: a choice between "coat, goat, note, and boat" gives much more specific information than a choice between "cup, shoe, biscuit, and butterfly," in which the target items have different vowels and syllable numbers. Speech testing is important in that it demonstrates to parents the impact of hearing loss on the child, which may be subtle in real-life situations, and gives a measure of disability for considering urgency of intervention.

Speech Intelligibility Index

A helpful way of predicting the impact of a level of hearing loss for a child is to consider the proportion of speech information that is inaudible to him/her with his/her hearing deficit on the audiogram. The speech spectrum can be represented on the audiogram as a shaded area covering the frequencies range 125 to 8,000 Hz and the intensity range from 20 to 60 dB (▶ Fig. 14.8).

All of the shaded speech area needs to be audible for a child to accurately follow conversational-level speech in quiet listening conditions. If a child has a flat hearing loss of 60 dB, it is more meaningful to say that only 10% of the information in speech (or SII) is audible than to say that he/she has 60% hearing loss, which might be interpreted as meaning he/she hears 40% of speech (see Boothroyd and Gatty[23] for more information).

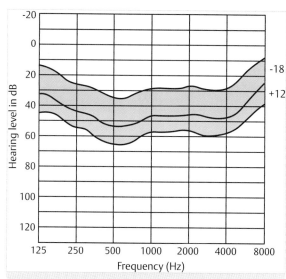

Fig. 14.8 Minimum audible field for combined male and female speech presented at 65-dB level. Note that although the measured level is reported as 65 dB from a sound-level meter, most of the speech information is between 30 and 40 dB and some of the high frequency cues are below 20 dB, requiring hearing levels of below 20 dB to accurately hear all the speech sounds.

the SII, is that greater importance is attributed to mid- and high-frequency components than to low-frequency components because mid- and high-frequency speech sounds (e.g., t, p, k, s, sh) carry more meaning than low-frequency speech sounds (e.g., u, ee, oh, m) in spoken language. For example, if a child has high-frequency hearing loss, he/she may have an SII score of only 45 (i.e., only 45% of the information in speech is audible), and yet to the parents the child appears to respond well to sounds and talking around him/her. This is because the child hears that someone is talking from hearing vowel sounds, voice quality, and intonation but cannot recognize and understand the words that were said through hearing alone.

Tips and Tricks

In general, reporting hearing levels as a percentage equivalent to the extent of hearing loss is misleading and should be avoided, for example, saying that 60-dB hearing loss is the same as 60% hearing loss. This under-represents the huge functional impact of the hearing loss on a child's speech understanding.

The important point about the speech spectrum (sometimes called the speech banana), which is used to derive

14.3.3 Measuring Middle Ear Function

A test battery approach is used to assess middle ear function and hearing threshold levels. Tympanometry is used to assess middle ear function and the mobility of the eardrum. This objective test confirms the presence of middle ear effusion when tympanometry shows a flat compliance trace (▶ Fig. 14.9). OAEs also make a helpful contribution to the test battery results to define the type of hearing loss for any individual case.

Type A: normal finding

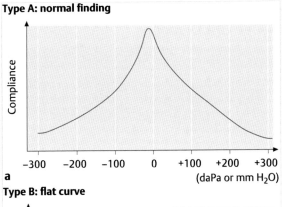

Type B: flat curve

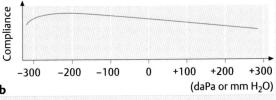

Fig. 14.9 Tympanogram. (a) Normal. There is a prominent, sharp peak between + 100 and –100 daPa. (b) Flat compliance trace of middle ear effusion, indicating immobility of the tympanic membrane. (Reproduced from Probst R, Grevers G, Iro H. Basic Otorhinolaryngology: A Step-by-Step Learning Guide. Stuttgart/New York; Thieme: 2006, with permission.)

Tips and Tricks

It is important that ENT practitioners occasionally observe the types of testing used in their departments to appraise the quality, competence, and reliability of the testing performed and thereby to be aware of potential errors in threshold measurements and appropriateness of referrals to audiology. Systems of peer review are commonly arranged between pediatric audiology teams to share new techniques and encourage reflective practice.

14.4 Types of Hearing Loss

14.4.1 Conductive Hearing Loss

A difference of more than 10 dB between air-conduction and bone-conduction thresholds at any frequency is indicative of a conductive hearing loss. Conductive hearing loss causes reduction in hearing sensitivity, but the ability to perceive increased loudness and resolution between different pitches is normal as long as the signal is fully audible. This means that conductive hearing loss can be well compensated for by hearing aid amplification and often may be correctable with surgery. The maximum possible extent of conductive hearing loss is 60 dB HL. However, all sounds are attenuated (reduced) equally by the extent of the hearing loss, so overall auditory deprivation from conductive hearing loss is greater than for an equivalent level of SNHL with recruitment.

The fluctuating nature of conductive hearing loss means that the child has inconsistent perception of sound patterns and consequently reduced opportunities for recognizing familiar patterns of sound.[23] With the relatively high incidence of middle ear pathology in children, conductive hearing losses are very common and can overlie cochlear-based SNHL, giving rise to a "mixed loss."

14.4.2 Sensorineural Hearing Loss

SNHL refers to impairment in the cochlea and/or the immediate (primary) nerve connections. The extent of SNHL can range from minimal to total and is usually permanent. Options for medical or surgical interventions are very limited in cochlear-based impairment. The inclusion of "neural" in sensorineural only refers to the level of the nerve connections from the inner hair cells to the auditory nerve (cranial nerve VIII). This is therefore different to *auditory neuropathy spectrum disorder* (ANSD) in which neural firing may be diminished or out of synchrony across nerve fibers, causing fluctuations and distortion in speech information.

> **i**
>
> SNHL is shown on the audiogram by both air- and bone-conduction thresholds being within 10 dB of each other.

There is a recognized artifact in the standards for bone-conduction thresholds at 4,000 Hz, which means that a discrepancy of 15 dB between air- and bone-conduction thresholds is often seen, but does not indicate a conductive hearing loss. A purely sensory loss is due to the cochlea failing to transduce vibrations arriving from the middle ear into neural impulses in the auditory nerve. Be aware that in moderate-to-profound hearing loss, some low frequency bone-conduction signals may be felt as vibration by the child, implying that there is a mixed hearing loss in the low frequencies. The thresholds at which children can *feel* the bone-conduction vibration can be as low as 25 dB at 250 Hz, 55 dB at 500 Hz, and 70 dB at 1,000 Hz (BSA-recommended PTA procedure).[18]

Cochlear hearing loss results in loss of sensitivity in hearing detection and also causes distortion in perception from a reduced dynamic range of hearing. This is shown on the audiogram as a reduced range of decibels between the threshold (the level at which the tone is just detected) and the uncomfortable loudness level (the tone is bordering on being unpleasantly loud). This is called "recruitment" and is a typical feature of cochlear hearing loss. Additionally, the hearing mechanism is less able to distinguish between sounds of different frequencies, and timing

14

cues may be smeared, both of which degrade speech understanding, particularly in the presence of competing noise. The synchrony of the firing of action potentials in the auditory nerve needs to be exact to encode very precise timing information in speech. For example, the cue that makes "pin" distinct from "bin" relies on perceiving a period of silence of approximately 60 ms between the /p/ and the /in/. If the timing information is blurred on the auditory nerve, as seen in ANSD and in adults with acoustic neuroma, speech understanding is disproportionally degraded, even though the audiogram may show only a marginal hearing loss.

Sources of Distortion In Cochlear Hearing Impairment

The normal-hearing cochlea may be envisaged as being made up of a set of overlying filters, each of which responds to its own narrow range of frequencies. In the impaired cochlea, there are fewer of these filters, and each one is wider. Therefore, an increased number of frequencies may fall into the same filter and therefore be perceived as the same pitch. Although most SNHLs are thought to be sensory (in the cochlea hair cells) and not neural (pathology located in the cochlea nerve), the distinction is not easy to determine without extensive hearing test batteries, so both are covered by the term *sensorineural hearing loss*. The neural component may have holes in hearing or "dead regions" (DR), which are not obvious on the audiogram, but which may mean a sound is perceived by neurons tuned to a different frequency within the cochlea rather than as a specific pitch of sound.[24] The ability to hear and understand speech within a cochlear DR, especially in noisy conditions, is greatly impaired, even when the audiogram shows a margin of useable hearing. These inherent sources of distortion in SNHL require careful hearing aid amplification with signal-processing strategies that help to preserve as many of the important acoustic characteristics of speech as possible within the narrower range of hearing capacity. Hearing aids can never restore normal hearing but can improve audibility of speech in many listening environments.

An infant with hearing loss from early life has already had deprivation of hearing in utero or following birth and therefore, in addition to fitting of hearing aids around the type and degree of loss, the child is helped by enhanced listening and communication experiences to derive meaning from hearing sound and vocalizations.[25]

14.4.3 Auditory Neuropathy Spectrum Disorder

The term *auditory neuropathy spectrum disorder* (ANSD) is used to describe hearing losses with functioning cochlear responses but impairment in the neural function of hearing.[26]

The hearing screening technique used for well babies is the OAE test that represents the hearing pathway up to, and including, the outer hair cells in the cochlea, thus identifying babies with conductive or sensory (cochlear-based) impairment. Approximately 10% of cases of early PCHI are due to auditory neuropathy in which the OAE is present but the ABR is absent or abnormal. The majority of this population are premature or sick babies, though there are also some genetic conditions that fall into this category. One example is Otoferlin deafness, which affects the neurotransmitters carrying information across the synapses between the inner hair cells in the cochlea and the primary neurons of the auditory nerve. Babies who have been in special care units are therefore screened using automated ABRs as well as OAEs as there is a higher prevalence of ANSD in this population. The perceptual effects of ANSD are very difficult to predict and can range from mild to profound loss and affected children may have disproportionate difficulty deriving meaning through audition. The use of hearing aids is only partially beneficial for some children with ANSD, though CI is more effective for some cases.

14.4.4 Mixed Hearing Loss

Though hearing deficits are classified as conductive, sensorineural, and auditory neuropathy types of hearing loss, each with different perceptual effects on hearing, it is often the case that a child may have two or even three of these co-occurring. Thus, for example, a premature baby may have SNHL secondary to lack of oxygen at birth, middle ear effusion due to having had a nasogastric tube for feeding, and delayed auditory maturation of the neural pathways arising from the prematurity. A child with a genetic hearing loss is just as likely to have episodes of middle ear effusion as a child with normal-hearing status.

The job of the ENT practitioner and audiologist is to optimize the infant's overall hearing potential and function at the earliest opportunity.

If there is an asymmetry in hearing levels between the two ears, masking is needed in testing. Masking is feasible in all audiology test techniques carried out by a skilled pediatric audiologist. Masking is required when a signal is sufficiently intense, when presented to the test ear, that it is perceived in the other (nontest) ear. In order to prevent this cross-hearing in asymmetric losses, masking noise is applied to the nontest ear (the better ear in cases of unilateral hearing loss [UHL]). The use of inserts is preferred over traditional headphones for ear-specific testing as the interaural attenuation of inserts is 55 dB, as opposed to 40 dB with headphones for air-conduction testing. In bone-conduction testing, the signal is transmitted equally to both cochleas, and without masking, it is impossible to determine which cochlea has responded. Therefore, masking is always needed to define ear-specific bone-conduction hearing thresholds.

14.4.5 Unilateral Hearing Loss: A Special Case

Cases of UHL are not specifically targeted by NHSP, but cases of UHL or *single-sided deafness* are inevitably picked up through the screen. The incidence of UHL is approximately half that for bilateral hearing loss in the newborn period, that is, approximately 0.5 per 1,000. The impact of early identification of UHL can be just as devastating for families as for cases of bilateral hearing loss.

Traditionally, UHL was thought to have little impact on the developmental profile of a child, and the management strategy was often for no active intervention and no etiology investigations. However, there are important factors in advice and management. All children with UHL at birth are at risk for speech delay and listening difficulties in the classroom with subsequent academic underachievement and potential for social isolation.

> The immediate priority is for full definition of hearing levels in the better hearing ear and investigations into the etiology of deafness.

This is important because for some etiologies, there is a risk of later deterioration in hearing in the better ear and progression to bilateral hearing loss, particularly from widened vestibular aqueduct syndrome or congenital infection, for example, congenital CMV. In these cases, there is a more pressing case for considering hearing aid amplification for the unilateral impairment to maintain the neural potential for hearing potential and to allow benefit from amplification when there is deterioration in the better hearing ear at a later date.

On a case-by-case basis, families may choose to have further investigations and possibly intervention as part of family-centered hearing management. Once the cause and extent of a UHL has been fully defined, options for management can be discussed around the wishes of the family.

Management Options for Unilateral Hearing Loss

If there is some residual hearing in the poorer ear, it may be helpful to discuss hearing aid fitting on that side. The earlier the intervention is initiated, the better for maintaining neural potential in that ear. This will depend on the degree and configuration of loss, and the views of parents. Binaural hearing improves speech understanding and ease of listening, particularly in noisy and reverberant conditions, and allows spatial separation of competing signals. Once the child starts school, the benefits of better spatial hearing may demonstrate improved auditory attention and listening ability in groups.

> The child with UHL is disadvantaged in all real-world listening environments.

Most group situations have challenging signal-to-noise ratios, reverberation, and classroom acoustics for children who need better listening conditions than adults to hear and understand speech. In each case, the individual circumstances should give rise to an appropriate plan, with close monitoring and evaluation of achievement. Techniques for improving the acoustic conditions in the home, school, and social environments include classroom sound field systems, personal radio aid systems, and sound absorption to reduce room reverberation.

> **Tips and Tricks**
>
> The traditional advice in UHL that "one ear is good enough" is not supported by the literature. A message conveying lack of urgency or negative impact from UHL is likely to result in parents deciding to defer management options and adopting instead a "watch and wait" approach. Use of simulations of the impact of mild or UHL on speech understanding is more insightful.

14.4.6 Nonorganic Hearing Loss

> Just as with adults, children may either feign a hearing loss or find it difficult to respond at their true auditory threshold at times. This is termed *nonorganic hearing loss* (NOHL).

14

The typical audiometric configuration is for a flat hearing loss with consistently raised thresholds across frequencies, usually (though not always) in both ears (see ▶ Fig. 2.7). The child is typically using a loudness matching technique by thinking "I will respond when the sound is a set loudness (of X) to me." Thus, the hearing configuration may show a moderate or severe flat hearing loss, or slightly better in the very low and very high frequencies (saucer-shaped). Asking the child a question about another topic using a conversational or low voice level when he/she cannot see your face may demonstrate disparity between the audiogram hearing levels and functional speech understanding.

Although feigned or exaggerated hearing loss may be tiresome to the clinician, it is very important not to dismiss the hearing loss or reprimand the child, or indeed to assume that a nonorganic overlay implies normal-hearing thresholds. Children may demonstrate NOHL as a method of getting professional attention for something that is causing them anxiety. Causes may range from bullying or underachievement in school to domestic abuse within the family. It is therefore crucial not to dismiss the reality of the hearing deficit, but to arrange for further testing or referral to other agencies for more focused assessment of the child's needs as appropriate on a case-by-case basis. The UK Health Department[27] initiative "Every Child Matters" puts a clear responsibility on all health and education professionals to identify and act for children in difficulty, regardless of the area of their specialization. NOHL may on occasion be used by children to try and communicate wider needs in cases of abuse or distress. A useful phrase in describing NOHL results to parents and carers, which is not judgmental, is that the child has "lost confidence" in their hearing or the test technique and that further tests are indicated. Speech testing is often very helpful alongside objective test methods of OAEs and ABR testing, where indicated.

> **Tips and Tricks** 👈
>
> In cases where there appears to be a nonorganic component to a hearing loss, all professionals have responsibility for considering an onward referral for more focused investigation of a child's needs.

14.4.7 Auditory Oversensitivity or Hyperacusis and Tinnitus

Reports of oversensitivity or aversion to high sound levels and noisy environments can also provide important indications for hearing and communication disorders. It is important to be aware that tinnitus is common for children with hearing deficits, but that they may not report it as they are unaware that other people do not have it. It may show up as difficulty sleeping, child humming or vocalizing to mask the sound, or tapping ears and head-shaking.

14.5 Fitting of Hearing Aids

As soon as a child has been identified as having a hearing loss, the options for improving hearing for sound around the child need to be considered. Early intervention is the rationale for hearing screening in the newborn period.

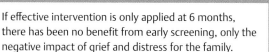

> ℹ
>
> If effective intervention is only applied at 6 months, there has been no benefit from early screening, only the negative impact of grief and distress for the family.

If the child is in the early months of life, the aim is to provide acoustic stimulation to prevent atrophy and pruning of neural networks that are not being stimulated by meaningful sound. In older infants and children, amplification aims to reduce the impact of poor hearing on many aspects of their development, including speech delay, social difficulties, educational underachievement, and frustration and anxiety.

14.5.1 Principles of Amplification with Hearing Aids

A hearing aid provides a method for amplifying sound so that it becomes audible to the wearer. The amount of additional amplification is called "hearing aid gain" and can be adjusted to match the extent of hearing loss at different frequencies. With an SNHL with a limited dynamic range of hearing due to recruitment (Chapter 14.4.2), the gain is typically about half of the total extent of hearing loss. This means that speech sounds are made audible, but other lower level sounds may not be. Low-level sounds need to be amplified more than moderately intense levels of sound. Sounds that are already loud may not need any additional amplification. In this way,, the spectrum of amplified sounds is compressed so that quiet sounds are made audible, moderate sounds are comfortable, and loud sounds are tolerable, within the narrow dynamic range of hearing between threshold and loud. There is also a maximum sound level of output (maximum power output or MPO) that can be adjusted on the hearing aid to prevent discomfort and distortion from loud sounds.

- There are surgical options for some types of conductive hearing loss, but well-fitted hearing aid amplification gives good access and clarity for speech, as there is little inherent distortion in conductive hearing loss.
- For sensorineural or mixed hearing loss, the most appropriate option for intervention is through hearing aid amplification.

For decades, there has been a negative social stigma implied by use of hearing aids, partly because hearing aids are associated with aging or reduced cognitive function. It is also because hearing aids were simple linear amplifiers that were not very effective in compensating for the sources of distortion that occur in the impaired cochlea and consequently limited improvement in speech understanding, especially in noisy situations. As described earlier, the impaired cochlear mechanism is unable to separate sounds as effectively as in normal hearing, the loudness of a sound grows abnormally fast with increasing intensity, and different frequencies are heard as the same pitch by someone with SNHL. A linear hearing aid was unable to help with any of these features of impaired hearing and therefore had limited benefit in most listening situations. It is hardly surprising that hearing aids have a negative image as the wearer still could not easily join the conversation. Over the last 10 years, there have been transformational improvements in hearing aids that are now high-technology devices incorporating innovative new signal-processing features. These aim to compensate more effectively for the degraded basilar membrane dynamics and neural encoding function of impaired hearing.

Hearing aids cannot restore normal hearing, but modern hearing aids can meet more of the challenges of impaired speech understanding in the real world than was possible for previous generations. They are also available in many different styles and cosmetic options and have compatibility with mobile phone and computer Bluetooth streaming to improve reception of speech in noise. There are published protocols for hearing aid fitting that require techniques for verifying the hearing aid output, having comfortable and secure earmolds for the child's ear, and use of a published prescription formula to set appropriate amplification in the hearing aids (e.g., Seewald et al[28]). The onus of responsibility for applying all of this intervention on a daily basis lies with the parents, which is why the focus of need is always around the family rather than around the professionals.

Tips and Tricks

Conductive hearing loss can be well matched by amplification, depending on fluctuations in hearing level. With the current move away from grommets for conductive hearing loss, temporary hearing aids can be an effective management intervention for noninfective OME.

14.5.2 Hearing Aids for Conductive Hearing Loss

In conductive hearing loss, the distortions in the cochlea that characterize SNHL with amplification are not present. Thus, hearing aids can effectively restore much of the sound quality of normal hearing if carefully fitted on the basis of the audiogram. The challenge for hearing aids with conductive hearing losses, particularly from middle ear effusion, is that the hearing levels tend to fluctuate depending on the effusion characteristics. This means that the hearing aid amplification needs to be adjustable, perhaps with a volume control or different programs, so that amplification is set for current hearing configurations. It is also recognized that more amplification per decibel of hearing loss is required for a conductive than for an SNHL, even if the audiogram air-conduction thresholds look the same.

Tips and Tricks

There are major improvements in hearing aids. Technology is key. Hearing aids now are advanced signal-processing systems, not the simple linear amplifiers that were used 10 years ago. Professionals need to have higher expectations for benefit from well-fitted hearing aid amplification from the outset.

The SPL-o-Gram

The initial fitting of hearing aid amplification aims to make the speech spectrum audible within the dynamic range of useable hearing. A helpful method for considering the principles behind amplification is the SPL-o-gram. This is configured as an upside-down audiogram, with the y-axis scaled in decibel sound pressure level (SPL), which is used to measure hearing aid output, rather than decibels hearing level, which is calibrated with reference to normal-hearing detection levels.

An SPL-o-gram (▶ Fig. 14.10) represents hearing aid amplification for an individual child on a graph orientated as an upside-down audiogram.

14

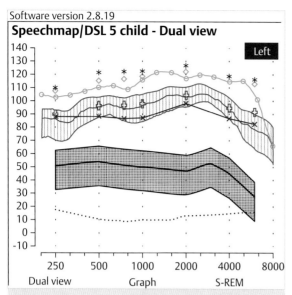

Software version 2.8.19

Speechmap/DSL 5 child - Dual view

Left

Dual view   Graph   S-REM

Fig. 14.10 An SPL-o-gram showing the hearing levels for a left ear (blue crosses). The line at the bottom represents normal-hearing thresholds. The gray-shaded area is unamplified speech. The pink-shaded area is amplified speech. The pink plus (+) signs are the targets for the amplification for the hearing aid gain for a prescription formula called desired sensation level version V, which has been developed to calculate the gain required for different levels of hearing loss.[28] Any of the amplified speech that comes above the blue left ear hearing line is now potentially audible to the listener. The asterisks at the top of the chart show predicted levels for sounds becoming uncomfortably loud, and the light blue circles indicate the targets for the MPO of the hearing aid. The software can calculate the proportion of information in speech that is now audible through the hearing aid as speech intelligibility index (SSI) compared to the unaided SSI for the hearing loss without a hearing aid (but is not shown here). This is the same concept that was introduced earlier in the section on Speech Intelligibility Index.

All hearing aid fittings should be verified with the hearing aid on the wearer's ear and a thin tube microphone in the ear to confirm the sound levels being delivered by the hearing aid in the wearer's ear.

Earmolds and Open Ear Fittings

The hearing aid needs to be coupled to the child's ear usually with a soft flexible earmold. The earmold is a piece of precision engineering that needs to be comfortable and secure and to have appropriate acoustic characteristics so that the child can hear his/her own voice well without reverberation effects. The acoustic effects of the earmold in the ear is measured using a procedure called "real ear to coupler difference" (discussed later) and the appropriate gain from the hearing aid is fed into the ear to match the child's exact hearing needs. There are many types and styles of hearing aids, earmolds, or open ear fittings available, though most children have behind-the-ear hearing aids with soft shell molds. When high levels of amplification are provided, the earmold needs to prevent leakage of sound from the ear, which could otherwise be picked up by the hearing aid microphone and give rise to acoustic feedback or whistling (▶ Fig. 14.11). Acoustic feedback can be controlled for much more effectively by signal-processing strategies in the hearing aid.

It is crucial that the child does not have feedback, as it degrades the experience and benefit from hearing amplified sound for both the child and the family. As the infant grows, new earmolds are needed on a regular basis to prevent sound leakage between the earmold and the growing concha and ear canal.

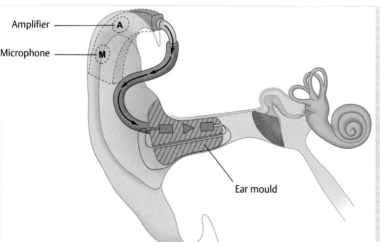

Amplifier — A

Microphone — M

Ear mould

Fig. 14.11 Source of acoustic feedback or hearing aid whistling. The amplified sound from the hearing aid is fed down the ear canal. If the amplified sound leaks back around the loosely fitting earmold, it can be picked up by the hearing aid microphone and the gain is increased again by the hearing aid. This causes a feedback loop, just as seen when a microphone is positioned too close to the loudspeakers at a conference or music venue, or piercing whistling. More closely fitting earmolds or active feedback cancellation in the hearing device can be used to reduce this very unpleasant effect. A child with whistling hearing aids not only has no benefit, but the hearing aids are also actively aversive.

Another cause of feedback for an infant with hearing aids is a buildup of wax in the ear canal or middle ear effusion reducing the transmission of amplified sound across the eardrum. It is always helpful to have an ENT opinion on removal of wax or insertion of grommets. However, it is important that the trust and confidence of the child is maintained with any examination or procedure as this is important for the regular taking of earmold impressions. It is very difficult to take closely fitting earmold impressions from a child who has had a traumatic experience with ear care.

> **Tips and Tricks**
>
> It is important that the trust and confidence of the child is maintained with any examination or procedure on the ears as the child needs to be settled and comfortable for taking earmold impressions and measuring the earmold effects on hearing aid fitting on a regular basis.

For young children, there is a method of measuring the effect of the earmold in the ear and recording this, rather than requiring the child to sit still and quietly with a microphone tube in the ear while hearing aid outputs are measured. This is called the real ear to coupler difference and is important as the actual sound levels in a baby's small ear will be much higher than for an adult-sized ear.

On closely scrutinizing the proportion of speech that is audible for a conversational voice level, for a child with moderately severe hearing loss, a difference of approximately 20 dB is the difference between hearing speech at all and hearing it fully. Thus, the small adjustments of even a few decibels are crucial in optimizing aided hearing in children.[29]

14.5.3 Constraints of Hearing Aids

> **i**
>
> If a child has profound hearing loss of > 90 dB, the likelihood of them being able to hear full speech information is very limited even through well-fitted hearing aids. In these situations, a child may have better access to speech through CI.

The advent of CIs has transformed the options for families with children with severe and profound hearing loss. Typical listening performance for children with CI inserted in early life, following an appropriate trial with hearing aids over the first 6 to 9 months, is equivalent to children with moderate or severe SNHL who are fitted with hearing aids. It is important that a full hearing aid trial is undertaken prior to assessment for CI, as some babies may show a spontaneous improvement in hearing levels over the first year of life, especially if they have ANSD. CI (see Chapter 15) is an area of innovation and extraordinary progress that could not have been predicted 20 years ago.

14.5.4 Assistive Listening Device Options for Children

Even with well-fitted hearing aids or CI, children are helped to hear the speech of one person (parent or teacher) over background noise or when at a distance by the use of a remote microphone worn by the talker and transmitting the signal directly to the hearing aids (or CI) through radio aid or more recently through Bluetooth technology. There is no doubt that listening in the classroom is more tiring for children with hearing loss, who need to apply high levels of attention and cognition to make sense of the degraded speech signals than their peers with normal hearing. Successful outcomes for HI children depend not only on the appropriate type/style of hearing aid, but also on technology selection, appropriate earmolds, the engagement of the parents in the process from the outset, and the communication choices of the family.

There are new technologies for improving access to speech in the classroom, watching television with family or music on i-pods and phones, using radio aid technology, or more recently Bluetooth connectivity to remote microphones or direct input leads.

In most countries with NHSP, there is a key habilitation professional designated to support the family and child with hearing loss. This may be a teacher of the deaf (ToD), speech and language therapist (SALT), or auditory verbal therapist (AVT). The role of these professionals is to support the family choice of communication mode, including use of sign language if requested, around the child's hearing and development needs. The most effective approaches coach families and build their competence and confidence through interaction so that the child is immersed in meaningful communication through the waking day.

14.5.5 Family-Centered Management

In order for the ENT and audiology team to be able to provide and use technology to improve a child's hearing potential for life, their first role is to support the family in the time of adjustment to hearing loss so that parents are able to be active in their child's use of amplification and communication. This has given rise to the concept of "family-centered management" for hearing loss for all practical early intervention. Recent studies have shown that families who have earlier adjustment to loss have better outcomes for their children.[30,31]

14

Hearing aid fitting from NHSP is typically undertaken from 6 weeks to 5 months of age, depending on individual circumstances. For the later identified cases of hearing loss, the pediatric audiology team helps to engage parents into effective use of communication dynamics and amplification by showing access to improved hearing through hearing aids and helping parents to observe their child's improving responses to sound and speech.

Supporting Parents in Feeling Competent and Confident in Use of Technology

In addition to supporting parents of newly diagnosed children through their grief by demonstrating residual hearing ability, the role of the audiologist is to help parents to feel competent and confident in managing the technology. The hearing aids are fundamental to improving outcomes for the HI child, and for families who choose talking and listening as the communication mode for their child, the parents are key to using the technology.

In order to understand the immediate needs of the parent and family in use of amplification, the ENT/audiology professional needs to listen carefully and nonjudgmentally to what parents say and specifically focus on the issues that are the current priority for the family. A family-centered approach aims to give the parent a sense of equal value and collaboration within the hearing intervention team. This is not the same dynamic that has typically existed between professionals and families, which facilitated the "expert" or "medical model," as historically practiced in ENT and pediatric audiology. In making a devastating diagnosis of hearing loss for a family around the time of birth of their baby, medical teams have a responsibility to engage with families on their own terms and not with a preconceived time line for progress around professionally centered care. The job is to manage the family's needs, and the baby's progress may be seen as the product of the intervention.

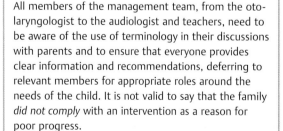

Tips and Tricks

All members of the management team, from the otolaryngologist to the audiologist and teachers, need to be aware of the use of terminology in their discussions with parents and to ensure that everyone provides clear information and recommendations, deferring to relevant members for appropriate roles around the needs of the child. It is not valid to say that the family *did not comply* with an intervention as a reason for poor progress.

14.6 Hyperacusis and Tinnitus

One of the common features of hearing loss that is recognized in adults, but much less in children, is the association of tinnitus with ear problems.[32] Children do not tend to bring this up, as they do not know that other people do not have tinnitus. They may get out of bed to ask what a sound is or talk about a virtual insect or animal. It is important to remember to ask a child whether he/she has a perception of sound when it is all quiet around them. This may be by saying "Do your ears make noises?" and then asking "Is it annoying for you?" Parents may be unaware of tinnitus and may be skeptical or shocked by the realization. It is important to stress that children normalize their sensory environment, especially if it has been present from early life, and that it is not necessarily traumatic to them, though they may benefit from an explanation as to what it is. To separate physiological sounds such as a pulse or from the crack of a Eustachian tube opening, one can ask if it sounds like a heartbeat or can ask them to make the same sound as they hear. Some children may be helped in their management of bothersome tinnitus by being asked to draw their tinnitus.

Another debilitating auditory symptom that is seen in children is termed *hyperacusis*, an abnormal aversion to sounds in the environment that are tolerated by most people. This oversensitivity is not associated with audiometric thresholds that are better than the normal-hearing line on the audiogram. Hyperacusis can be a very disruptive symptom for many children, including children with autistic spectrum disorders. There are programs for proactively managing the sound aversion using different techniques including the wearing of white noise maskers. It is important that prolonged use of earmuffs or sound protection is avoided as this will exacerbate the hyperacusis sensitivity in the long term.

Tips and Tricks

Children with oversensitivity to sounds or "hyperacusis" can be helped by enhanced but controlled exposure to sounds. They should not be advised to use earplugs or ear defenders as this exacerbates the sensitivity.

14.7 Outcomes for Hearing-Impaired Children

Testing speech perception in quiet with hearing aids or CI is an important component in evaluating the effectiveness of intervention for a child. However, this type of testing in the clinic gives very limited information on how well a child copes in a classroom or other social environment.

It is more appropriate to use test material that represents the complexity of language in the classroom and to perform the speech test in noise, for example, a sentence test presented in speech babble. The results obtained both with and without hearing aids can support decision-making on use and benefits of amplification, as well as fine-tuning the sound quality around the listener's preference in different places. As with adult hearing aids, there is an acclimatization period for the new hearing user to perceive benefit for speech understanding with amplification. It is important to listen very carefully to the comments and feedback of the wearer and not to assume that a hearing aid fitting that matches targets on the prescription formula is necessarily optimal for the wearer. Small adjustments around listening preferences, different programs for specific situations, or the use of assistive listening technology may be of greater benefit to the user.

Functional performance in real-life situations is more insightful than speech tests done in optimal listening conditions in the clinic for mild and moderate extents of hearing loss. Crandell[33] reviewed the available evidence of children with minimal hearing loss and UHL and showed significantly greater difficulties in speech recognition than their normal-hearing peers in the presence of noise or reverberation in a classroom.

Functional auditory outcome measures for infants and preschool children use auditory behaviors, hearing aid use, and vocalization information to evaluate functional benefit from amplification. These include the Infant-Toddler Meaningful Auditory Integration Scale,[34] Parent's Evaluation of Aural/Oral Performance of Children,[35] and Little Ears Auditory Questionnaire.[36]

The child using hearing aids or CIs will have a team of professionals to support his/her listening and language needs. These may include a SALT, ToD, classroom support assistant, social services, and educational psychologist. It is important that medical agencies recognize the parallel roles of multidisciplinary team members and avoid making comments or predictions that run counter to closer assessment or evaluation. Without looking holistically at a child's function in the classroom, including language and literacy skills, it is not possible to predict the impact of hearing loss from the audiogram alone.

Tips and Tricks ☞

Children with risk for educational underachievement need more active intervention, for example, for language delay, poor social skills, other sensory impairment, or learning disability than their peers.

There is widespread misconception that management of the child or adult with hearing loss rests on the selection and fitting of hearing aids, or CI, alone. The opportunity for enhanced auditory learning from the time of identification of hearing loss and hearing aid fitting is the cement that makes the technology most effective. For this reason, most HI children have a dedicated hearing support teacher, AVT, or SALT. The role of the parents is fundamental to the auditory learning and ultimate speech and language achievement of the child. Professionals who are able to coach families in skills for providing an acoustically and language-rich environment are applying their skills to the child throughout the waking day.

Children with permanent hearing loss have a wider range of options and opportunities for developing talking and listening than ever before due to early identification of hearing loss, new innovations in hearing aid and CI technology, and holistic communication support around the needs of the family. The expectations for these children are appropriately high, allowing families and children to make choices for themselves over the life ahead.

14.8 Key Points

- PHCI occurs in approximately 1 case per 1,000 live births in most populations.
- Congenital hearing losses with onset in childhood, rather than at birth, arise from genetic susceptibility to deterioration in cochlear hearing levels over time. The onset of a hearing loss may be the first indication of a wider genetic condition.
- When a parent or teacher expresses concern about their child's hearing, there is almost always a hearing or communication impairment. The child needs full and accurate assessment of hearing in each ear.
- Reports of oversensitivity or aversion to high sound levels and noisy environments can also provide important indications for hearing and communication disorders.
- The techniques used for hearing assessment depend upon the age and developmental status of the child.
  ○ Up to approximately 4 months of age, ABR testing is usually used. ASSRs, CERA, and acoustic reflex thresholds may also be used to give additional diagnostic information.
  ○ From approximately 6 months of age, behavioral tests are used to measure hearing levels. These include VRA, CPA, and PTA, which defines the quietest level at which a pure-tone signal is detected, in each ear.
  ○ The use of speech recognition testing and SII is a more holistic measure of the functional impact of hearing loss on the child.
  ○ Tympanometry is used to assess middle ear function and the mobility of the eardrum.
- Hearing loss can be classified as:
  ○ Conductive (a difference of > 10 dB between air- and bone-conduction thresholds at any frequency).
  ○ Sensorineural (impairment in the cochlea and/or the primary nerve connections).
  ○ ANSD (hearing losses with functioning cochlear responses but impairment in the neural function of hearing).

14

○ Mixed.

○ Unilateral.

○ Nonorganic.

- As soon as a child has been identified as having a hearing loss, the options for improving hearing for sound around the child need to be considered.
- In conductive hearing loss, hearing aids can effectively restore much of the sound quality of normal hearing.
- The initial fitting of hearing aid amplification aims to make as much of the speech spectrum audible within the dynamic range of useable hearing.
- The hearing aid needs to be coupled to the child's ear usually with a soft flexible earmold.
- Children with oversensitivity to sounds or "hyperacusis" can be helped by enhanced but controlled exposure to sounds.

References

[1] Fortnum H, Davis A. Epidemiology of permanent childhood hearing impairment in Trent Region, 1985–1993. Br J Audiol. 1997; 31(6): 409–446

[2] Kral A, Eggermont JJ. What's to lose and what's to learn: development under auditory deprivation, cochlear implants and limits of cortical plasticity. Brain Res Brain Res Rev. 2007; 56(1):259–269

[3] Wood SA, Sutton GJ, Davis AC. Performance and characteristics of the Newborn Hearing Screening Programme in England: the first seven years. Int J Audiol. 2015; 54(6):353–358

[4] Fortnum HM, Summerfield AQ, Marshall DH, Davis AC, Bamford JM. Prevalence of permanent childhood hearing impairment in the United Kingdom and implications for universal neonatal hearing screening: questionnaire based ascertainment study. BMJ. 2001; 323 (7312):536–540

[5] Martin F, Clark J, eds. Hearing Care for Children. Boston, MA: Allyn and Bacon; 1996

[6] Seewald R, Tharpe A. Comprehensive Handbook of Pediatric Audiology. San Diego, CA: Plural Publishing; 2010

[7] Courtmans I, Mancilla V, Ligny C, Le Bon SD, Naessens A, Foulon I. Incidence of congenital CMV in children at a hearing rehabilitation center. B-ENT. 2015; 11(4):303–308

[8] Cole EB, Flexer CA. Children with Hearing Loss: Developing Listening and Talking, Birth to Six. San Diego, CA: Plural Publishing; 2011

[9] Hogan SC, Moore DR. Impaired binaural hearing in children produced by a threshold level of middle ear disease. J Assoc Res Otolaryngol. 2003; 4(2):123–129

[10] Marulis LM, Neuman SB. The effects of vocabulary intervention on young children's word learning: a meta-analysis. Rev Educ Res. 2010; 80(3):300–335

[11] Moeller MP, Hoover B, Putman C, et al. Vocalizations of infants with hearing loss compared with infants with normal hearing: part I—phonetic development. Ear Hear. 2007; 28(5):605–627

[12] Dockrell JE, Shield B. Acoustical barriers in classrooms: the impact of noise on performance in the classroom. Br Educ Res J. 2006; 32(3): 509–525

[13] Goberis D, Beams D, Dalpes M, Abrisch A, Baca R, Yoshinaga-Itano C. The missing link in language development of deaf and hard of hearing children: pragmatic language development. Semin Speech Lang. 2012; 33(4):297–309

[14] Purdy S, Katsch R, Dillon H, Storey L, Sharma M, Agung K. Aided cortical auditory evoked potentials for hearing instrument evaluation in infants. In: A Sound Foundation through Early Amplification. Chicago, IL: Phonak AG; 2005:115–127

[15] Foerst A, Beutner D, Lang-Roth R, Huttenbrink KB, von Wedel H, Walger M. Prevalence of auditory neuropathy/synaptopathy in a population of children with profound hearing loss. Int J Pediatr Otorhinolaryngol. 2006; 70(8):1415–1422

[16] Madell JR, Flexer CA. Pediatric Audiology: Diagnosis, Technology, and Management. Stuttgart: Thieme; 2008

[17] Sutton G, Wood S, Feirn R, Minchom S, Parker G, Sirimanna T. Newborn Hearing Screening and Assessment: Guidelines for Surveillance and Audiological Referral of Infants and Children Following the Newborn Hearing Screen. NHS Newborn Hearing Screening Programme; 2012. Available at http://abrpeerreview.co.uk/onewebmedia/NHSP%20Surveillance%20guidelines%20v5-1%20290612.pdf

[18] British Society of Audiology. Recommended Procedure: Pure-tone air-conduction and bone-conduction threshold audiometry with and without masking. 2011. Available at http://www.thebsa.org.uk/wp-content/uploads/2014/04/BSA_RP_PTA_FINAL_24Sept11_Minor-Amend06Feb12.pdf

[19] The American Speech-Language-Hearing Association. Clinical Practice Guideline: Report of the Recommendations. Hearing Loss, Assessment and Intervention for Young Children (Age 0–3 years). New York State Department of Health; 2007. Available at http://www.asha.org/articlesummary.aspx?id=8589961117

[20] Stahl SA, Nagy WE. Teaching Word Meanings. Mahwah, NJ: Lawrence Erlbaum Associates; 2006

[21] Moeller MP, Tomblin JB, Yoshinaga-Itano C, Connor CM, Jerger S. Current state of knowledge: language and literacy of children with hearing impairment. Ear Hear. 2007; 28(6):740–753

[22] Taylor B. Speech-in-noise tests: how and why to include them in your basic test battery. Hearing J. 2003; 56(1):40–42

[23] Boothroyd A, Gatty J. The deaf child. In: A Hearing Family: Nurturing Development. San Diego, CA: Plural Publishing; 2012

[24] Moore B, Huss M, Vickers D, Baer T. Psychoacoustics of dead regions. In: Physiological and Psychophysical Bases of Auditory Function. Maastricht, The Netherlands: Shaker; 2000

[25] Yoshinaga-Itano C. From screening to early identification and intervention: discovering predictors to successful outcomes for children with significant hearing loss. J Deaf Stud Deaf Educ. 2003; 8(1):11–30

[26] Boudewyns A, Declau F, van den Ende J, Hofkens A, Dirckx S, Van de Heyning P. Auditory neuropathy spectrum disorder (ANSD) in referrals from neonatal hearing screening at a well-baby clinic. Eur J Pediatr. 2016; 175(7):993–1000

[27] Department for Children, Schools and Families. Every Child Matters (2003). Available at www.everychildmatters.co.uk. Accessed March 16, 2016

[28] Seewald R, Moodie S, Scollie S, Bagatto M. The DSL method for pediatric hearing instrument fitting: historical perspective and current issues. Trends Amplif. 2005; 9(4):145–157

[29] Walker EA, McCreery RW, Spratford M, et al. Trends and predictors of longitudinal hearing aid use for children who are hard of hearing. Ear Hear. 2015; 36 Suppl 1:38S–47S

[30] Watkin P, McCann D, Law C, et al. Language ability in children with permanent hearing impairment: the influence of early management and family participation. Pediatrics. 2007; 120(3):e694–e701

[31] Yoshinaga-Itano C. The social-emotional ramifications of universal newborn hearing screening, early identification and intervention of children who are deaf or hard of hearing. Proceedings of the Second International Pediatric Conference: A Sound Foundation through Early Amplification, November 8–10, 2001, Chicago, I

[32] Rosing SN, Schmidt JH, Wedderkopp N, Baguley DM. Prevalence of tinnitus and hyperacusis in children and adolescents: a systematic review. BMJ Open. 2016; 6(6):e010596

[33] Crandell CC. Speech recognition in noise by children with minimal degrees of sensorineural hearing loss. Ear Hear. 1993; 14(3):210–216

[34] Zimmerman-Phillips S, Osberger MF, Robbins AM. Infant-Toddler Meaningful Auditory Integration Scale (IT-MAIS). Sylmar, CA: Advanced Bionics Corp; 1997

[35] Ching TC, Hill M, Psarros C. Strategies for evaluation of hearing aid fitting for children. Paper presented at the International Hearing Aid Research Conference, August 23, 2000, Lake Tahoe, CA

[36] Kühn-Inacker H, Weichbold V, Tsiakpini L, Coninx S, D'Haese P. Little Ears: Auditory Questionnaire. Innsbruck, Austria: MED-EL; 2003

III

15 Surgical Management of the Hearing-Impaired Child

Christopher H. Raine and Jane M. Martin

15.1 Introduction

Deafness has a profound impact on children and their families. Hearing loss in infancy or childhood is often due to genetic causes and syndromic pathologies, sometimes with malformation of the ear as well as defective cochlear function. The effects on communication skills, educational achievement, and quality of life make for a very significant impact on the family and cost to society.

Early detection of permanent childhood hearing impairment (PCHI) through universal newborn hearing screening programs (NHSPs) has reduced the age at which impairment is confirmed,[1] enabling earlier intervention and rehabilitation (see Chapter 13).

Approximately half of PCHI is caused by genetic factors. Not all childhood hearing impairment is evident at birth; some children with progressive loss will only be detected with continuing surveillance. Amplification in the form of acoustic hearing aids can address the majority of cases of PCHI (see Chapter 13 and Chapter 14). Amplification should be provided as early as possible and certainly within the first 6 months of age to maximize language acquisition, but the supply and fitting of hearing aids in young children is demanding and requires skilled audiologists and the cooperation of parents, carers, and teachers to ensure optimum benefit. For bilateral hearing impairment, bilateral aids should be routinely fitted unless there are specific contraindications. Binaural hearing has numerous benefits, some of which include better sound localization, improved speech recognition in quiet and noise, and a general ease of listening.

> **i**
>
> Unilateral hearing loss has an increasingly recognized negative impact on speech and language development and on academic achievement and should now be identified and actively managed (see Chapter 14).

Conductive hearing losses caused by secretory otitis media with effusion and by middle ear pathology are frequently dealt with by surgery. This includes tympanoplasty and reconstructive ossicular surgery to restore hearing. These conditions are addressed in Chapter 8 and Chapter 9. This chapter looks at both readily available and emerging surgical implant technologies for children and adolescents with conductive, mixed, and sensorineural hearing loss (SNHL). This is a rapidly developing field with new techniques becoming increasingly accepted. ▶ Table 15.1 classifies the options currently available.

Table 15.1 Classification of otological implants

Conductive/mixed/sensorineural hearing loss	Bone conduction hearing devices:
	• Percutaneous
	• Transcutaneous (active/passive)
	Active middle ear implants:
	• Semi-implantable
	• Totally implantable
Severe-to-profound sensorineural hearing loss	Cochlear implant
	Auditory brainstem implant

15.2 Bone Conduction Hearing Devices

15.2.1 Physiology of Hearing through Bone Conduction

Conventional hearing by air conduction (AC) requires sound collection into the ear canal, where the sound produces vibrations of the tympanic membrane. The mechanical vibrations are, in turn, transmitted across the middle ear by the ossicular chain, producing sound pressure changes within the cochlea. These sound pressure changes move the basilar membrane and excite the sensory cells within the organ of Corti. Bone conduction (BC) sound transmission involves multiple pathways, which ultimately results in similar changes in the cochlea.[2]

> **i**
>
> BC hearing devices (BCHDs) should be considered when there is good cochlea function but failure to gain benefit from appropriately fitted acoustic hearing devices, or when these devices cannot be fitted, for example, for anatomical reasons such as microtia or atresia of the external ear canal.

There are currently two broad categories of BCHDs:
- *Percutaneous*: these involve penetration of the skin by a titanium abutment, which is anchored to the skull by an osseointegrated implant. An audio processor (AP) is fitted to the abutment as an ear level or body-worn device. Bone-anchored hearing aids (BAHAs) are in this category.
- *Transcutaneous*: by definition, the processors are not directly attached to the bone. Passive systems rely on implanted magnets which attract the external

15

III

processor. This is termed as "skin drive." Active systems involve the implantation of a transducer fixed to the bone, giving a "direct drive" to the cochlea. The external processor is again held in place by a magnet.

15.2.2 Clinical Indications for Bone Conduction Hearing Device

Congenital Conductive, Mixed, or Sensorineural Hearing Losses

Typically, these are children with congenital microtia and aural atresia (CAA) where reconstructive surgery is not feasible. Jahrsdoerfer et al[3] developed a grading scheme based on the preoperative temporal bone computed tomography (CT) scan and the appearance of the external ear in an effort to select those with the greatest chance of surgical success. They recognized that surgery for congenital aural atresia was difficult and unpredictable. Bouhabel et al concluded that BAHAs were a safe and efficient therapeutic option, with significantly better audiological outcomes when compared to unaided external auditory canal reconstruction for patients with CAA.[4]

Acquired Conductive, Mixed, or Sensorineural Hearing Losses

Acquired indications would commonly include chronic otitis externa, some cases of persistent and recalcitrant otitis media with effusion, chronic suppurative otitis media, and the effects of trauma to the external ear.

Unilateral Hearing Loss

> ⓘ
>
> It is now recognized that even a mild unilateral loss in children should not be disregarded as it can have an adverse impact on development and on educational achievement.

Conventional amplification with hearing aids, and in some circumstances BCHD, may be offered under the supervision of an experienced pediatric audiologist. BCHD may be indicated in children following a trial period of a Softband (Oticon Medical; ► Fig. 15.1) with their active participation.

Children with Special Needs

A number of children have congenital ear abnormalities as part of a syndrome or within the context of significant comorbidity (see Chapter 5). These children may have complex medical, social, and educational needs. Conventional aiding can be challenging, with problems around

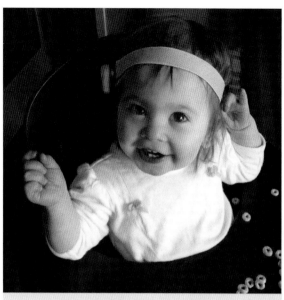

Fig. 15.1 Child wearing a Softband with a bone conduction hearing device. (Reproduced with permission from Oticon.)

fitting and compliance. Children with Down's syndrome are at particular risk for some degree of hearing impairment and many will benefit from early use of BCHDs.

15.2.3 Selection of Children

There are many issues to consider before performing surgery. Selection should be addressed on a case-by-case basis by a multidisciplinary team (MDT). It would be accepted practice in most European countries to consider surgery from a minimum of approximately 4 years of age, following trialing of children with Softbands (► Fig. 15.1) or BC headbands. In the United States and Canada, regulatory indications suggest this type of surgery for children 5 years and older. The main reason for this delay is to allow appropriate assessment and skull growth. Currently, there is no convincing evidence for earlier surgical intervention in children with such congenital hearing loss,[5] but amplification using more conventional aids is, of course, still used in the interim period.

Audiological Criteria

The audiological parameters for fitment must always be fulfilled as appropriate for the device selected. Selection is typically based on BC thresholds at 500 Hz, 1 kHz, 2 kHz, and 3 kHz. Some ear level devices (► Fig. 15.2) can be worn to levels equal to or better than 55 dB.

Body-worn processors such as the BAHA Cordelle (Cochlear; ► Fig. 15.3) increase the fitting range thresholds to ≤ 65 dB.

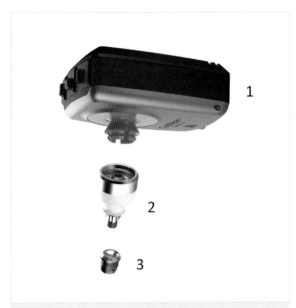

Fig. 15.2 Main components of a percutaneous bone conduction hearing device. 1, Ear level processor; 2, abutment; 3, bone implant. (Reproduced with permission from Cochlear.)

There are continued developments with these devices, so it is always advisable to look at up-to-date fitting data and shifting audiological selection criteria.

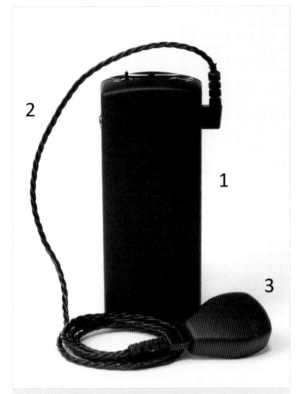

Fig. 15.3 Cordelle body-worn bone conduction. 1, Body-worn unit housing the microphone; 2, lead; 3, coupling/transducer to abutment. (Reproduced with permission from Cochlear.)

The preliminary assessment of audiological performance using a headband is very helpful. Transcutaneous devices tend to reflect what is obtained using the headbands, but allow up to 15 dB in BC, especially in the higher frequencies, when fitting the processor on a percutaneous abutment.

Looking into the benefit of bilateral implants, improvements in hearing thresholds, sound localization, and speech perception have been reported.[6] Binaural fitting is preferred for bilateral conductive loss when the BC thresholds do not vary by more than 10 dB in the higher frequencies of 3 and 4 kHz.

In cases of unilateral hearing loss (single-sided deafness [SSD]), the contralateral ear should have a BC average of ≤ 20 dB HL to reduce the head shadow effects. Reports show good improvement in hearing in noise and even with mild-to-moderate losses in the contralateral ear.[7,8]

15.2.4 Percutaneous Devices

There are currently two devices: the Baha (Cochlear) and the Ponto bone-anchored hearing system (Oticon Medical/Neurelec). Both are semi-implantable, with a titanium osseointegrated fixation into the skull and a skin-penetrating abutment to facilitate attachment for the sound processor aid (▶ Fig. 15.4).

Baha has been commercially available from 1984 and Oticon devices since 2009. Both systems can be trialed with the processor worn on a latex-free Softband (▶ Fig. 15.1) or headband.[9] This allows early amplification for children considered too young for surgical fitment of the implant/abutment. Softbands are also available for binaural fitting.

Surgery

There are two main goals of surgery:
- To optimize osseointegration.
- To prepare the implant site to minimize the occurrence of soft-tissue reactions. Recently, there has been a significant change from previous tissue reduction procedures to a simpler nontissue reduction using a "punch" technique with or without a minimal incision parallel or extension of the "punch" site (▶ Fig. 15.5). Measuring skin thickness aids selection of the use of the most appropriate length of abutment.

15

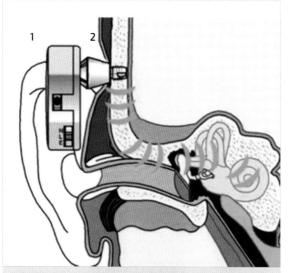

Fig. 15.4 Percutaneous abutment with direct sound transmission to the cochlea. 1, External processor; 2, abutment and implant. (Reproduced with permission from Cochlear.)

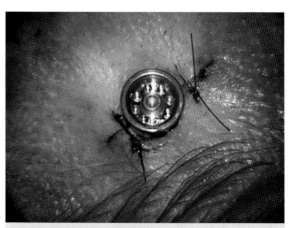

Fig. 15.5 Abutment in position using minimal approach.

Two-stage surgery has been recommended for children up to approximately 10 years of age, with 3 or more months between stages to allow for osseointegration.[10] Some centers advocate insertion of a second or "sleeper" fixation. However, with newer designs in abutment technology, single-stage surgery is now commonly performed. Early results indicate higher stability and faster osseointegration with newer implants both in adults and children.[11] With reduction in integration time, there is earlier loading with a processor.

Outcomes

The audiological outcomes should reflect the preoperative assessments with a slight improvement due to the direct coupling, and a lack of attenuation due to the skin, which can account for approximately 10 to 15 dB.

The main recognized drawbacks of the percutaneous abutment relate to varying degrees of soft-tissue reactions (▶ Table 15.2). These can occur in approximately a third of patients.

With improved implant design, using a curved abutment and tight connections between the implant components, such reactions are becoming less common.[13,14] Similarly, hydroxyapatite coating of the abutment to allow soft-tissue integration and reduced pocket formation around the skin penetrating abutment show promising results in preclinical studies.[15]

Loss of implants due to failure of integration and trauma are more common in the pediatric population as compared with adults. In children, the figures vary depending on the age at initial implantation and the group of medical conditions involved. Kraai et al[16] reported that

Table 15.2 Grading of soft-tissue reactions and their management[12]

Grade	Description
0	No irritation and slightly red, < 1 mm from the implant: epithelial debris removed if present
1	Red 1 mm or more from the implant: temporary local treatment indicated
2	Red and moist: no granulation tissue present
3	Red and moist with granulation tissue, skin overgrowth, or scar formation: local treatment indicated
4	Extensive soft-tissue reaction: could require implant removal

obesity and adverse socioeconomic factors appeared to contribute to a higher risk for complications. Frequent follow-up and meticulous care of the implant site may minimize complications.

15.2.5 Transcutaneous Devices

Transcutaneous devices can be classified into those with either passive or active internal transducer systems. Passive systems rely on the processor sending vibrations through the skin to an internal magnet system, which, in turn, keeps the processor in place. This has been termed *skin drive*. Conversely, active devices induce the surgically implanted system, which is fixed directly to the bone, to vibrate. The external processor does not produce any movements.

Two passive systems are available for use with children: Sophono (Medtronic PLC) and the more recently introduced Baha Attract (Cochlear). Such systems are known as "skin drive."

The Bonebridge is an active semi-implantable internal device produced by MED-EL (Vibrant Bonebridge).

Transcutaneous "Passive" Systems

Sophono

The Sophono Alpha 2 MPO bone-anchored hearing system comprises a surgically implanted internal plate that houses two magnets hermetically sealed in a titanium case. This internal component is attached to the mastoid bone behind the ear. It is completely passive and placed under the skin in a simple single-stage procedure. The external digital sound processor houses a bone oscillator and uses a metal disc and spacer (a "shim") to magnetically couple to the internal component and deliver auditory stimulation through the closed skin. Siegert[17] has reported on 100 patients whom he had implanted. The additional benefits of such a system are reduced risks of injury or inflammation and less of the psychological problems associated with the more prominent percutaneous abutments.[18]

Audiological Criteria

The Sophono is approved by the U.S. Food and Drug Administration and in Europe by Conformité Européenne (CE) Mark, for any type of conductive and mixed hearing loss with BC thresholds of ≤ 45 dB. The system is designed for patients 5 years of age and older. Criteria for SSD include patients with pure-tone average of ≤ 20 dB in the contralateral ear measured at 0.5, 1, 2, and 3 kHz.

Surgery

The principle involves fixing twin rare earth magnets encapsulated in titanium to the skull (▶ Fig. 15.6). To reduce attenuation, the skin flap should not be thicker than 4 mm. This is not usually a problem in children.

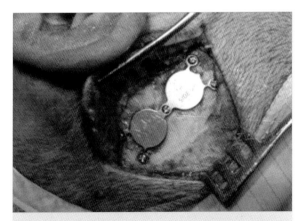

Fig. 15.6 Sophono magnets secured in position.

The external Alpha auditory processor is held in position by twin magnets of similar geometry to those implanted.

Outcomes

The external processor is typically fitted at 4 weeks postoperatively, allowing the tissues to settle. To minimize any skin reaction or discomfort, close attention to the magnetic coupling needs to be taken into consideration. The audiological outcomes by the nature of the device are similar to levels gained when using the processor on a soft headband. Case series have shown improvement in hearing over unaided conditions.[19,20]

Baha 4 Attract

This is a BC implant system that uses magnet retention to connect the Baha sound processor with the osseointegrated Baha BI300 implant. The same implant is used for Cochlear's percutaneous system. The BI300 implant and the implant magnet are placed entirely under the skin, providing a more cosmetically appealing design. The sound processor is attached with a single external sound processor magnet. By wearing a SoftWare pad, the force of the sound processor magnet allows the distribution of contact pressure evenly on the skin.

Audiological Criteria

The Baha 4 Attract System is approved for adults and children. In the United States and Canada, the system is not currently approved for children below the age of 5 years.

The audiological indications for the Baha Attract System are conductive, mild mixed hearing loss, and SSD with a pure-tone average of ≤ 20 dB in the contralateral ear. The fitting range is based on the performance of the selected sound processor. When evaluating candidates for the Baha Attract System, the outcomes are similar or better than using the same processor on a Softband.[21]

Surgery

The surgical steps have the same principles of fitting as the BI300 implant, but with the principle of raising a flap under which will be positioned the internal magnet. Particular care is required to ensure perpendicular placement (▶ Fig. 15.7) of the implant so that the magnet when fitted does not contact bone. The tissue over the magnet should not exceed 6 mm. The final position should make appropriate allowances for skull curvature and proximity of the pinna (▶ Fig. 15.8).

Outcomes

Simulation of an Attract processor on patients with established percutaneous systems introduced an attenuation starting from approximately 5 dB at 1,000 Hz, increasing to 20 to 25 dB above 6,000 Hz. However, aided sound field threshold shows smaller differences, and aided speech

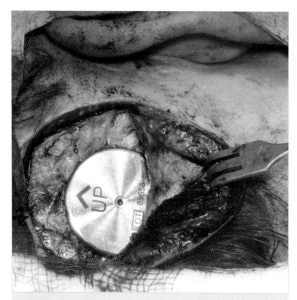

Fig. 15.7 Surgical placement of a right Baha Attract. (Courtesy of Iain Bruce.)

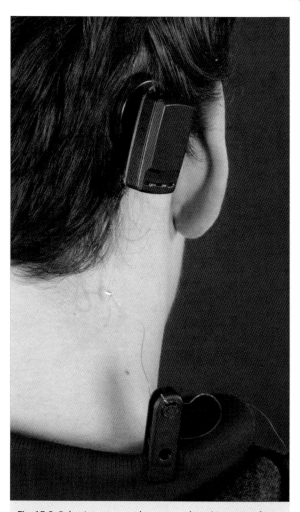

Fig. 15.8 Baha Attract worn by a young boy. (Courtesy of Iain Bruce.)

understanding in quiet and in noise does not differ significantly between the two transmission paths.[22] Transcutaneous systems offer good improvement in pure-tone thresholds and speech reception thresholds. Also, early studies have lower complication rate compared to those featuring the percutaneous.[23]

Transcutaneous "Active" Semi-Implantable System

Bonebridge

The Bonebridge (MED-EL) was clinically introduced within Europe in 2011. It is a semi-implantable system. The internal components are a receiving coil linked to the BC floating mass transducer (BC-FMT) that sends sound transmissions direct to the inner ear. The externally worn AP, held in place by magnetic attraction, transfers signals across the skin to the implant. The technology of the Bonebridge draws upon established technology developed for the Vibrant Soundbridge (VSB) system (▶ Fig. 15.9).

Audiological Criteria

The Bonebridge is intended for patients with either a BC loss up to 45 dB or 20 dB for unilateral sensorineural deafness as shown in the graphs in ▶ Fig. 15.10.

There should be stable thresholds with no evidence of auditory neuropathy and no retrocochlear or central hearing impairment.

Surgery

The aim of surgery is to place the BC-FMT either within a healthy mastoid or in the retrosigmoid/temporal position. Because of its size, surgery is reserved until there has been sufficient skull growth to accommodate it. Careful planning of the appropriate placement can be obtained using CT imaging and specialized software. Spacers or BCI Lifts can be used to help reduce the need to depress dura or the sigmoid sinus. The device is held in place by titanium osseointegrated screws.

Outcomes

Fitment of the external processor can be immediate, as the device does not require osseointegration to function. Additionally, immediate functionality is possible as there is no requirement for soft tissues to heal, as the processor

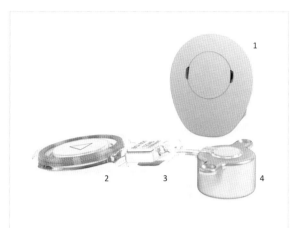

Fig. 15.9 Complete Bonebridge system with audio processor (SAMBA BB). 1, External audio processor; 2, internal receiver coil; 3, internal electronics (demodulator); 4, internal bone-conduction floating mass transducer. (Reproduced with permission from MED-EL.)

is not seated over the implant. Early outcome studies have reported minimal complications with good audiological outcomes.[24,25]

15.3 Active Middle Ear Implants

There is currently one commercial, semi-implantable active middle ear implant available for use in children in Europe and the United Kingdom. This is the VSB produced by MED-EL.

The fully implantable Carina (Cochlear) has just been released but is only available for children aged over 14 years.

15.3.1 Vibrant Soundbridge

The VSB is a semi-implantable electromagnetic hearing device consisting of an external AP, held in place by magnetic attraction. This converts sound into electromagnetic

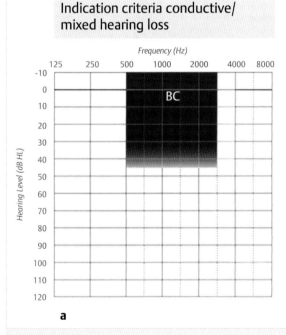

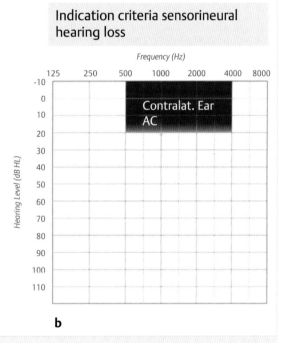

Fig. 15.10 Audiological indications for Bonebridge. **(a)** Bone-conduction loss. **(b)** Unilateral sensorineural hearing loss. (Reproduced with permission from MED-EL.)

15

waves and transmits them through the skin to the internal receiver package or vibrating ossicular prosthesis. This consists of the FMT, a conductor link, and an internal coil (▶ Fig. 15.11). The FMT is classically clipped onto the incus.

An assortment of couplers has been designed for the FMT to attach it to the incus, stapes, and into the round window.

Audiological Criteria

The VSB was originally intended for patients with moderate-to-severe SNHL. Pure-tone AC threshold levels at or within the levels shown in ▶ Fig. 15.12 would be considered suitable. There should be stable hearing thresholds with no evidence of auditory neuropathy, retrocochlear loss, or central hearing impairment.

For patients with conductive or mixed hearing loss, pure-tone BC threshold levels at or within the levels listed below are optimum (▶ Fig. 15.13).

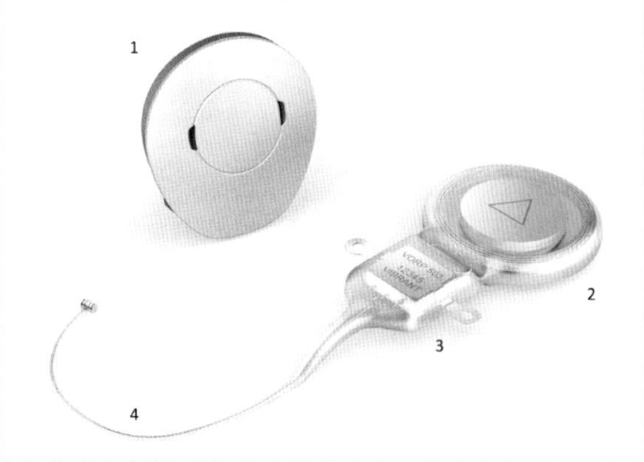

Surgery

Detailed preoperative imaging is required to evaluate ear anatomy and to facilitate positioning of the FMT in contact with a suitable vibratory structure of the ear. The main contraindication for surgery is the presence of active chronic suppurative middle ear disease.

The single-point attachment surgery as well as the reversibility of the treatment, make the VSB the only

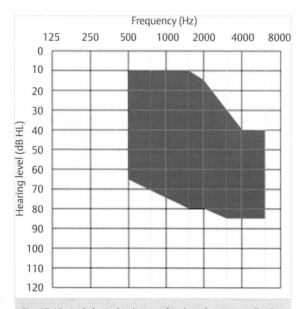

middle ear implant suitable for the younger hearing-impaired population. As it was reported in the consensus meeting,[26] even if the middle ear structures are fully developed at the time of birth, the middle ear cleft expands to some extent up to the age of 5 years. However, because the VSB uses a single-point attachment, it is not adversely affected by middle ear growth. As long as the

Fig. 15.11 Internal vibrating ossicular prosthesis (VORP) and external audio processor of the Vibrant Soundbridge system. 1, SAMBA external audio processor; 2, internal VORP receiver coil; 3, internal VORP electronics; 4, internal VORP conductor lead with floating mass transducer (FMT). (Reproduced with permission from MED-EL.)

Fig. 15.12 Audiological indication for the Vibrant Soundbridge in sensorineural hearing loss patients; shadows of air-conduction thresholds. (Reproduced with permission from MED-EL.)

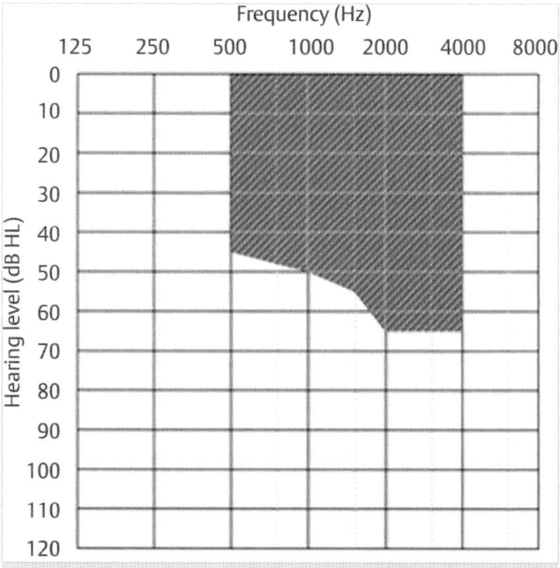

Fig. 15.13 Audiological indication for the Vibrant Soundbridge in mixed/conductive hearing loss (M/CHL) patients; shadows of bone conduction thresholds. (Reproduced with permission from MED-EL.)

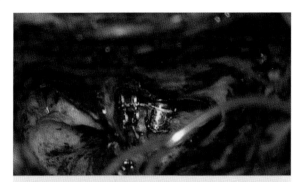

Fig. 15.14 Surgical view of floating mass transducer on the incus.

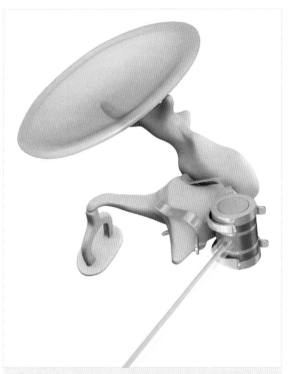

Fig. 15.15 Illustration of floating mass transducer in position on the body of the incus. (Reproduced with permission from MED-EL.)

middle ear cleft is large enough to accommodate the FMT, later cleft growth does not impede positioning and implant function.

Classically, the FMT is attached to the incus through a posterior tympanotomy approach (▶ Fig. 15.14, ▶ Fig. 15.15).

In 2006, Colletti et al introduced a new positioning by placing the FMT directly onto the round window membrane, therefore also providing treatment for patients with mixed and conductive hearing losses. They found that patients with a mixed loss of 30 to 60 dB HL of sensorineural component and 30 to 40 dB of air-bone gap could greatly benefit from the implant.[27]

Since then, various vibroplasty methods of coupling of the FMT to the ossicular chain remnants and oval window have been described with encouraging results.

Outcomes

The VSB has good reliability. According to the manufacturer, after 9 years, more than 98% of all implanted devices are still functional. Fitting and programming of the processor usually commences 6 to 12 weeks after the implant surgery, dependent on the type of surgery.

Frenzel et al reported[28] that surgery to place the VSB in children does not involve a higher risk or require further special procedures when compared with the "vibroplasty" treatment in adults. The VSB can be successfully used in combination with auricle reconstruction.[29] In fact, the vibroplasty does not affect the tissue, which is important for later ear reconstructive surgery.

The majority of children implanted with this device are syndromic, with ear malformations. The small number of VSBs implanted in children with SNHL is not well reported in the literature so far, but ongoing studies show clear benefit in these cases.

Evidence of VSB efficacy in children is well documented for patients with mixed and conductive hearing losses. On average, a functional gain of over 40 dB HL with complete restoration of speech understanding is achievable.[30,31] BC levels pre- and postoperatively should not change, showing complete hearing preservation.

15.3.2 Magnetic Resonance Imaging Compatibility

There is always a concern about implanting children as there is the probability they will require a magnetic resonance imaging (MRI) scan during their lifetime.

> In the case of the standard titanium percutaneous abutments, provided the external processor is removed, there is no contraindication to MRI. For even better reduction of artifact, the abutment can be unscrewed from the fixture.

Baha 4 Attract, Bonebridge, and VSB are conditional to 1.5 T, and Sophono has been tested up to 3.0 T.

When imaging the head, there will be a variable void and an area of distortion. Each manufacturer offers guidance notes and they should always be consulted.

The field of otological implants is rapidly expanding. Even though the existing solutions work well for the majority of children today, a wider selection of products will benefit them and make it easier for the professional to find the best solution for each child.

15

15.4 Severe-to-Profound Sensorineural Hearing Loss

15.4.1 Cochlear Implants

Approximately 1 in 1,000 children is born with a PCHI (≥ 40 dB HL in the better ear). The incidence doubles until 16 years of age.[32] It is important that children diagnosed at birth with a severe-to-profound hearing loss are assessed by a multidisciplinary cochlear implant team at a dedicated center.

> Those found suitable for implantation should receive their implants at an early age.

Experience in the United Kingdom and elsewhere has established that the most positive outcomes can be achieved if the child is implanted following a sudden or progressive hearing loss and if the congenitally profound deaf child is implanted at a very young age.

15.4.2 Cochlear Implantation

Rationale and General Principles

A CI is an electronic device designed to provide useful auditory sensations to people who are severely or profoundly hearing-impaired and who gain little or no benefit from acoustic hearing aids. CIs bypass dysfunctioning parts of the peripheral auditory system and directly stimulate the nerve of hearing with electrical signals.

The aim is to create the capacity to understand speech and to be understood when speaking.

An implant consists of two main components:

- The external component, which is worn outside the body, consists of a microphone, speech processor, and transmitter coil. These convert sound waves received by the microphone into radio waves that are transmitted to the receiver–stimulator package in the internal component.
- The internal component, which is surgically implanted, consists of a receiver–stimulator package and an electrode array inserted into the cochlea. The signals are decoded by the receiver–stimulator package, which generate electrical impulses to stimulate the auditory nerve (▶ Fig. 15.16)

There are currently four manufacturers supplying CIs in the United Kingdom: Advanced Bionics (www.advanced-bionics.com), Cochlear (www.cochlear.com), MED-EL (www.medel.com), and Oticon Medical (www.oticon-medical.com).

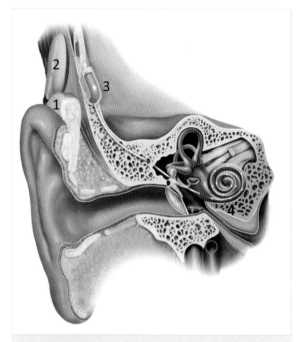

Fig. 15.16 External and internal parts of the SYNCHRONY Cochlear Implant System. 1, SONNET behind-the-ear audio processor; 2, transmitter coil; 3, receiver/stimulator; 4, electrode array. (Reproduced with permission from MED-EL.)

Referral Criteria

Typically, children with a severe-to-profound SNHL who do not receive adequate benefit from acoustic hearing aids should be referred for CI assessment.

> While there are many causes of acquired hearing loss, meningitis is of especially urgent concern because of the risks of ossification within the cochlea.

This may adversely affect the outcome of implantation. All patients who suffer with meningitis should have their hearing assessed, and if there are any concerns, an urgent referral should be "fast tracked" to their local CI center.

Assessment

A multidisciplinary CI team assesses the child. This includes thorough audiological assessment by experienced pediatric audiologists (see Chapter 13); a functional listening assessment, and detailed information exchange by a teacher of the deaf; a speech, language, and communication assessment by an experienced speech and language therapist; and a consultation with the senior ear, nose, and throat (ENT) surgeon who will carry out the surgery.

Tests carried out take into account the child's developmental age and any known disabilities. Information regarding general progress and development is also sought from the family and local professionals, for example, pediatricians, working with the child.

Detailed hearing tests and a hearing aid trial are undertaken to assess potential benefit. Further objective testing may include cortical and auditory brainstem responses, and measures of vestibular function.

As part of the overall medical examination of their ears, children will have imaging (MRI and/or CT) to evaluate any structural anomalies that could pose difficulties in inserting the electrode array into the cochlea. It is also important to confirm the presence of the auditory nerve. For the younger child, scans are performed either under general anesthetic or sedation.

To focus on the assessment, the Children's Implant Profile, devised by Hellman et al[33] and modified over time, is used by many teams.

The profile includes the following key areas:
- Chronological age at implant.
- Duration of profound loss.
- Radiology.
- Audiological factors.
- Speech and language development.
- Communication style.
- Additional needs (cognitive and noncognitive).
- Educational environment.
- Nature of support services.
- Family structure and support.
- Expectations of the family and child, if appropriate.

Surgery

> Prior to surgery the parents or carers, and in the case of the older child, the child him/herself will require full and detailed advice and information from the team who will be responsible not only for surgery but for subsequent care.

Issues discussed are expectations, surgery and its associated risks, need for ongoing rehabilitation, as well as issues related to the device itself.

ENT surgeons who have specialized training and ongoing experience, carry out implantation surgery. CIs are typically inserted through a transmastoid approach, but other routes are described as well. Soft surgical techniques are used to insert the electrode array into the cochlea either by the round window or through a separate cochleostomy. Preservation of residual hearing is possible. This is of importance when considering the use of dual electroacoustic stimulation.

> Complications of surgery are infrequent.

The receiver–stimulator package and array are very reliable, but experience from the CI centers indicates an average reimplantation rate of approximately 0.5 to 1.0% per year of the caseload. Causes include device trauma, infection, extrusion, and either sudden or progressive technical failure.

Magnetic Resonance Imaging

> MRI represents a significant risk to CIs. The magnet produces a void and distortion. Demagnetization may occur. In some designs, the magnet in the receiver–stimulator package may be removable prior to imaging. In all cases where an MRI is contemplated, liaise with the CI center and the implant manufacturers.

Rehabilitation/Habilitation

The rehabilitation service following implantation is provided to ensure that parents or carers and the child's local professionals are fully informed and involved in supporting the child postimplant. It aims to ensure optimal outcomes relating to the development of listening and communication skills. This service encompasses programming, assessment, clinic-based support, outreach work, and training.

The key needs of the postimplant child are as follows:
- Encouragement to wear the device all waking hours.
- The device to be in good working order.
- Opportunities to experience good listening conditions.
- Opportunities for nonlinguistic experiences such as music.
- Opportunities to develop spoken language and other appropriate communication skills.
- Experience of success in developing listening and communication skills.
- Cooperation and consistency from all involved.
- Opportunities to meet other CI users.
- An increasing understanding of his/her CI as he/she mature.

Outcomes

Research and experience shows that the long-term outcomes for profoundly hearing-impaired children are excellent and include the following:

15

Table 15.3 Category of auditory performance: typical progress for an early implanted child

Grade	Category	Pre	3 m	6 m	12 m	24 m	36 m
7	Uses telephone						■
6	Understands conversation						■
5	Understands common phrases					■	
4	Discriminates some speech sounds				■		
3	Identify environmental sounds			■			
2	Responds to speech sounds			■			
1	Aware of environmental sounds		■				
0	Unaware of environmental sounds	■					

Abbreviation: m, months post implant.
Note: Additional subdivisions of categories 6/7 have been developed.

- Children with no other significant additional needs are able to acquire intelligible spoken language supported by the use of hearing through a CI.
- Many children understand conversation without lipreading.
- Some children are able to use the telephone.
- Increasing numbers attend mainstream schools.
- Many show high academic attainment.

Profoundly hearing-impaired children who receive CIs at a very young age or those with the greater levels of residual hearing preimplantation tend to make better progress.

A variety of objective measures are used to record outcomes in children who have had undergone CI. These include "categories of auditory performance," which is a measure used to show progress over time and to record levels of achievement.[34] The assessment is linked to hierarchal functional listening skills. ▶ Table 15.3 shows the typical progress over time in months of an early implanted child who has no other significant complex needs.

Speech intelligibility rating is another tool used to evaluate a typical child's oral communication development over time (▶ Table 15.4).

Questionnaires such as Meaningful Auditory Integration Scale (MAIS) and Meaningful Use of Speech Scale (MUSS) are regularly used to assess the child's functional benefits in different environments such as at school and at home.

15.4.3 Bilateral Cochlear Implantation

In 2009, the UK National Institute for Health and Care Excellence concluded that it was both clinically appropriate and cost-effective to implant children with simultaneous bilateral CIs.[35] Additional benefits include the following:
- Better auditory performance in quiet and in background noise.
- Better sound localization.
- Better speech intelligibility.
- Improved music appreciation.
- Better parent attachment.
- Less social–emotional problems.
- Higher reading level at the age of 10 years.
- Stimulation of both auditory pathways.
- A guarantee that the better performing ear has been implanted.
- In the event that one device fails, the patient is not left without sound.

15.4.4 Unilateral Cochlear Implantation

Studies in adults have shown that unilateral CI can enhance auditory performance.

Table 15.4 Anticipated SIR of an implanted child

Criteria	SIR cat	Pre	6 m	12 m	24 m	36 m	48 m
Connected speech intelligible to all listeners	5					■	■
Connected speech to listener who has little experience of a hearing-impaired person's speech	4				■	■	
Connected speech intelligible to someone who concentrates and lip-reads	3			■	■		
Connected speech unintelligible	2			■			
Prerecognizable words in spoken language	1	■	■				

Abbreviation: m, months post implant; SIR, speech intelligibility rating.

15.4.5 Children with Complex Needs

CI programs are increasingly assessing hearing-impaired children who have multiple comorbid conditions including brain injury. This process requires a careful assessment by an MDT, including input from pediatric neurologists and child development specialists.

> ℹ
>
> Two key factors must be considered during the assessment process: the confirmation of a profound hearing loss and the child's ability to participate in the programming process postimplant.

Outcomes for a child with additional needs are difficult to predict. The rehabilitation process can be challenging and generally may take longer, and needs to be flexible as the child's additional needs may change over time. Greater consideration may need to be given to subjective benefits such as improved quality of life and family relationships.

15.4.6 Auditory Brainstem Implants

Auditory brainstem implantation (ABI) is similar in principle to a CI except that the electrode array or paddle is placed in the fourth ventricle over the cochlear nucleus. The principle use of an ABI is when there is no function or absence of the auditory nerve (VIII). Conditions of VIII that might warrant consideration of ABI include nerve aplasia, severe trauma following temporal bone fracture, and neuronal pathologies such as neurofibromatosis 2. Cochlear conditions include severe ossification or maldevelopment of the cochlea. ABIs are very rarely used in children and experience is very limited. Tonotopic placement is lost in the brainstem, so results are not nearly as good as with conventional CIs.

> ℹ
>
> CIs have revolutionized the management of severe-to-profound hearing loss. Outcomes have significantly improved over the years as technology and criteria have improved. Simultaneous bilateral surgery has been shown to be safe and efficacious in children, and binaural hearing has many advantages.

Unilateral CI surgery is now offered in some European centers to remediate unilateral profound hearing loss, so clinical indications are extending.

15.5 Key Points

- Newborn hearing screening is important for the early detection of permanent hearing loss.
- Adequate amplification should be provided as early as possible.
- Consider the use of otological implants when acoustic hearing aids are no longer appropriate.
- All implantable devices should be assessed through an MDT.

References

[1] Dalzell L, Orlando M, MacDonald M, et al. The New York State universal newborn hearing screening demonstration project: ages of hearing loss identification, hearing aid fitting, and enrollment in early intervention. Ear Hear. 2000; 21(2):118–130

[2] Stenfelt S. Acoustic and physiologic aspects of bone conduction hearing. Adv Otorhinolaryngol. 2011; 71:10–21

[3] Jahrsdoerfer RA, Yeakley JW, Aguilar EA, Cole RR, Gray LC. Grading system for the selection of patients with congenital aural atresia. Am J Otol. 1992; 13(1):6–12

[4] Bouhabel S, Arcand P, Saliba I. Congenital aural atresia: bone-anchored hearing aid vs. external auditory canal reconstruction. Int J Pediatr Otorhinolaryngol. 2012; 76(2):272–277

[5] Snik A, Leijendeckers J, Hol M, Mylanus E, Cremers C. The bone-anchored hearing aid for children: recent developments. Int J Audiol. 2008; 47(9):554–559

[6] Dun CA, de Wolf MJ, Mylanus EA, Snik AF, Hol MK, Cremers CW. Bilateral bone-anchored hearing aid application in children: the Nijmegen experience from 1996 to 2008. Otol Neurotol. 2010; 31(4):615–623

[7] Christensen L, Richter GT, Dornhoffer JL. Update on bone-anchored hearing aids in pediatric patients with profound unilateral sensorineural hearing loss. Arch Otolaryngol Head Neck Surg. 2010; 136(2):175–177

[8] Wazen JJ, Van Ess MJ, Alameda J, Ortega C, Modisett M, Pinsky K. The Baha system in patients with single-sided deafness and contralateral hearing loss. Otolaryngol Head Neck Surg. 2010; 142(4):554–559

[9] Zarowski AJ, Verstraeten N, Somers T, Riff D, Offeciers EF. Headbands, testbands and softbands in preoperative testing and application of bone-anchored devices in adults and children. Adv Otorhinolaryngol. 2011; 71:124–131

[10] McDermott AL, Williams J, Kuo M, Reid A, Proops D. The Birmingham pediatric bone-anchored hearing aid program: a 15-year experience. Otol Neurotol. 2009; 30(2):178–183

[11] Marsella P, Scorpecci A, D'Eredità R, Della Volpe A, Malerba P. Stability of osseointegrated bone conduction systems in children: a pilot study. Otol Neurotol. 2012; 33(5):797–803

[12] Holgers KM. Characteristics of the inflammatory process around skin-penetrating titanium implants for aural rehabilitation. Audiology. 2000; 39(5):253–259

[13] Dun CA, de Wolf MJ, Hol MK, et al. Stability, survival, and tolerability of a novel baha implant system: six-month data from a multicenter clinical investigation. Otol Neurotol. 2011; 32(6):1001–1007

[14] Faber HT, Dun CA, Nelissen RC, Mylanus EA, Cremers CW, Hol MK. Bone-anchored hearing implant loading at 3 weeks: stability and tolerability after 6 months. Otol Neurotol. 2013; 34(1):104–110

[15] Larsson A, Wigren S, Andersson M, Ekeroth G, Flynn M, Nannmark U. Histologic evaluation of soft tissue integration of experimental abutments for bone anchored hearing implants using surgery without soft tissue reduction. Otol Neurotol. 2012; 33(8):1445–1451

[16] Kraai T, Brown C, Neeff M, Fisher K. Complications of bone-anchored hearing aids in pediatric patients. Int J Pediatr Otorhinolaryngol. 2011; 75(6):749–753

15

[17] Siegert R. Partially implantable bone conduction hearing aids without a percutaneous abutment (Otomag): technique and preliminary clinical results. Adv Otorhinolaryngol. 2011; 71:41–46

[18] Zeitoun H, De R, Thompson SD, Proops DW. Osseointegrated implants in the management of childhood ear abnormalities: with particular emphasis on complications. J Laryngol Otol. 2002; 116(2): 87–91

[19] Denoyelle F, Leboulanger N, Coudert C, et al. New closed skin bone-anchored implant: preliminary results in 6 children with ear atresia. Otol Neurotol. 2013; 34(2):275–281

[20] Ihler F, Volbers L, Blum J, Matthias C, Canis M. Preliminary functional results and quality of life after implantation of a new bone conduction hearing device in patients with conductive and mixed hearing loss. Otol Neurotol. 2014; 35(2):211–215

[21] Briggs R, Van Hasselt A, Luntz M, et al. Clinical performance of a new magnetic bone conduction hearing implant system: results from a prospective, multicenter, clinical investigation. Otol Neurotol. 2015; 36(5):834–841

[22] Kurz A, Flynn M, Caversaccio M, Kompis M. Speech understanding with a new implant technology: a comparative study with a new nonskin penetrating Baha system. Biomed Res Int. 2014; 2014: 416205

[23] Baker S, Centric A, Chennupati SK. Innovation in abutment-free bone-anchored hearing devices in children: updated results and experience. Int J Pediatr Otorhinolaryngol. 2015; 79(10):1667–1672

[24] Sprinzl G, Lenarz T, Ernst A, et al. First European multicenter results with a new transcutaneous bone conduction hearing implant system: short-term safety and efficacy. Otol Neurotol. 2013; 34(6): 1076–1083

[25] Riss D, Arnoldner C, Baumgartner WD, et al. Indication criteria and outcomes with the Bonebridge transcutaneous bone-conduction implant. Laryngoscope. 2014; 124(12):2802–2806

[26] Cremers CW, O'Connor AF, Helms J, et al. International consensus on Vibrant Soundbridge® implantation in children and adolescents. Int J Pediatr Otorhinolaryngol. 2010; 74(11):1267–1269

[27] Colletti V, Soli SD, Carner M, Colletti L. Treatment of mixed hearing losses via implantation of a vibratory transducer on the round window. Int J Audiol. 2006; 45(10):600–608

[28] Frenzel H, Hanke F, Beltrame M, Steffen A, Schönweiler R, Wollenberg B. Application of the Vibrant Soundbridge to unilateral osseous atresia cases. Laryngoscope. 2009; 119(1):67–74

[29] Frenzel H, Hanke F, Beltrame M, Wollenberg B. Application of the Vibrant Soundbridge in bilateral congenital atresia in toddlers. Acta Otolaryngol. 2010; 130(8):966–970

[30] Mandalà M, Colletti L, Colletti V. Treatment of the atretic ear with round window vibrant soundbridge implantation in infants and children: electrocochleography and audiologic outcomes. Otol Neurotol. 2011; 32(8):1250–1255

[31] Roman S, Denoyelle F, Farinetti A, Garabedian E-N, Triglia J-M. Middle ear implant in conductive and mixed congenital hearing loss in children. Int J Pediatr Otorhinolaryngol. 2012; 76(12):1775–1778

[32] Fortnum HM, Summerfield AQ, Marshall DH, Davis AC, Bamford JM. Prevalence of permanent childhood hearing impairment in the United Kingdom and implications for universal neonatal hearing screening: questionnaire based ascertainment study. BMJ. 2001; 323 (7312):536–540

[33] Hellman SA, Chute PM, Kretschmer RE, Nevins ME, Parisier SC. Thurston LC. The development of a Children's Implant Profile. Am Ann Deaf. 1991; 136(2):77–81

[34] Archbold S, Lutman ME, Nikolopoulos T. Categories of auditory performance: inter-user reliability. Br J Audiol. 1998; 32(1):7–12

[35] National Institute for Health and Care Excellence. Cochlear implants for children and adults with severe to profound deafness. NICE technology appraisal guidance TA166. NICE. 2009, Available at https://www.nice.org.uk/guidance/ta166

Part IV

The Nose and Sinus

IV

16 Nasal Obstruction in Children

Michelle Wyatt

16.1 Introduction

Nasal obstruction in children is common and has a vast range of possible causes. The impact on the individual depends on his/her age and the severity of the blockage. A neonate, for example, is an obligate nasal breather for the first few months of life. If there is complete bilateral nasal blockage at birth, the neonate will have significant breathing issues and classically present with cyclical cyanosis (desaturations relieved by crying). Older children may be able to tolerate the obstruction more easily, and attention can be drawn to the problem by associated symptoms. These vary depending on the etiology but include rhinorrhea, stertor, mouth breathing, and sneezing. Sleep disruption and feeding issues, particularly if there is failure to thrive, raise levels of concern and a requirement for treatment.

16.2 Etiology of Pediatric Nasal Obstruction

The major causes of nasal obstruction in children are listed in ▶ Table 16.1. Some are dealt with in more detail in Chapter 17 but are included here for the sake of completeness.

16.3 Congenital Anomalies

16.3.1 Skeletal

Arhinia

Arhinia or complete nasal agenesis is extremely rare, with only 43 cases reported in the literature. It can be associated with other craniofacial anomalies due to a common embryological origin affecting the development of the nose and other structures. Partial arhinia is more common and is seen most often in facial clefting disorders (see Chapter 27).

The development of the nose occurs between the third and eighth week in utero and involves the superior frontal process and bilateral maxillary processes in the formation of the midface. The nasal placodes themselves develop in the fifth week and consist of medial and lateral nasal swellings with nasal pits between. The medial swellings fuse to form the septum, and cells within the pits migrate backward to form the nasal cavities. It is not entirely clear how arhinia arises. There may be a failure of development of the medial nasal swelling or even an overgrowth and premature fusion of this same structure resulting in an atretic plate. Most cases have normal chromosomal analysis, but there is a single case report of

Table 16.1 The major causes of nasal obstruction in children

Congenital anomalies	Acquired disorders
Skeletal: • Arhinia • Choanal atresia • Pyriform aperture stenosis • Midnasal stenosis Nasal masses: • Cysts • Glioma/encephalocele/ glial heterotopia • Vascular malformations	Inflammatory/infective: • Rhinosinusitis • Adenoidal pathology • Nasal polyps Traumatic: • Osseocartilaginous deformity • Foreign body Neoplastic: • Fibrous dysplasia • Ossifying fibroma • Olfactory neuroblastoma • Juvenile angiofibroma • Nasopharyngeal carcinoma • Teratoma Vascular Metabolic Autoimmune Idiopathic

familial arhinia and three individuals around the world have shown some abnormal karyotyping.

> **i**
>
> Complete arhinia presents as an airway emergency at birth, which can be alleviated with a Guedel oral airway or by oral endotracheal intubation if required. Partial arhinia can also cause severe airway obstruction and feeding difficulties that may require intervention in the first few weeks or months of life. A tracheostomy may need to be considered in either situation.

Reconstruction of the nose is remarkably difficult; multiple challenges include securing a stable skeletal structure with a functional mucosa and the appropriate skin cover. A bone-anchored prosthesis can be considered and gives an excellent cosmetic result.

Choanal Atresia

Blockage of the posterior choanae can be unilateral or bilateral and is generally of a mixed bony/membranous type. It is rare, with an incidence of approximately 1 in 7,000 live births. The condition can be an isolated lesion or occur in association with other congenital anomalies. One or more features of the CHARGE syndrome (coloboma, *h*eart defects, *a*tresia choanae, *r*etardation of growth, *g*enital anomalies, and *e*ar abnormalities) may be present. Some children have the full CHARGE syndrome due to mutations in the *CHD7* gene on chromosome 8.

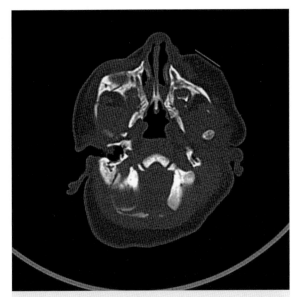

Fig. 16.1 Computed tomography scan (axial view) showing bilateral choanal atresia (mixed bony/membranous).

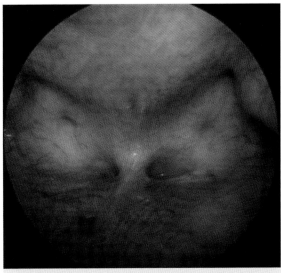

Fig. 16.2 Bilateral choanal atresia as viewed from postnasal space with a 120-degree endoscope.

A cardiac echo, renal ultrasound, audiology, and ophthalmology review are recommended.

> Bilateral obstruction presents as an acute airway emergency at birth with cyclical cyanosis (blue spells relieved by crying).

If the diagnosis is suspected, the midwife or the attending pediatrician will find that a nasal catheter will not pass into the nasopharynx as it is held up by the atretic plate. A useful confirmatory test is to place a cold steel spatula under the baby's nose and check for misting. If no air is exhaled through the nose, there is no misting; conversely, if there is misting, the nasal airway is patent, although it can still be partly obstructed. Flexible endoscopy can demonstrate the atretic plate. The correct placement of an oral airway can alleviate symptoms, although endotracheal intubation may be required.

If there is a strong suspicion of choanal atresia, the baby should be transferred to an appropriate center. Computed tomography (CT) scanning with 1-mm cuts (following nasal suction and the application of topical decongestant drops) aids surgical planning (▶ Fig. 16.1. The diagnosis is confirmed by rigid endoscopy. A 120-degree Hopkins rod provides an excellent view and facilitates surgical correction (▶ Fig. 16.2). Early surgery is important, and although the baby's airway can be safely managed with a Guedel oral airway and with careful observation in a neonatal unit, it proves impossible to establish oral feeding until the atresia is corrected.

Unilateral pathology does not usually cause issues until the child is older. There is persistent mucopurulent discharge in the absence of a foreign body. Occasionally, there can be airway or feeding difficulties in an affected baby, and earlier correction is indicated.

Management of Choanal Atresia

Different operative approaches for repair are described as follows[1,2]:

- Transpalatal surgery is less common now, although it may be useful in those with significant craniofacial anomalies such as Treacher Collins' syndrome where the dimensions of the nostrils and postnasal space provide extremely limited access.
- Transnasal repairs can either involve the use of a 120-degree endoscope in the oropharynx to look back at the postnasal space with the instruments and drill being introduced through the nostrils, or the repair can be carried out with the endoscope and instruments in the nasal cavities directly.

The factors affecting successful repair have been debated in the literature. Nasal stenting post bilateral repair in the neonate is reported as standard in a series of patients,[3] whereas Teissier et al[4] who reviewed 80 cases over a 9-year period feel it is only required for 2 days in this group and not at all in unilateral cases. Ibrahim et al[5] reported on 21 cases, an equal division of unilateral and bilateral, without stents and found similar success rates to the series quoted previously. If stents are used, soft tubes (Ivory Portex, Smiths Medical) are recommended. Treatment of associated gastroesophageal reflux disease and daily washing with sodium chloride solution were shown to positively affect outcome.[4] Regular suction to clear secretions is important. Wide surgical excision with resection of the posterior aspect of the vomer and early (1 week postrepair) removal of crusting/granulation tissue under general anesthesia (GA), if required, are reported as beneficial.[4]

Mitomycin C has been proposed as useful to reduce granulation tissue formation and hence fibrosis. Kubba et al[3] in a retrospective study found no difference in the outcome when 22 patients treated with mitomycin C were compared with 24 control patients. They suggested that the use of mitomycin C might just be a marker of refractory disease since it seems to be used in cases of children with poorer overall outcome.

A specific review of refractory cases[6] found an incidence of almost 10% of cases requiring repeated procedures. Risk factors for restenosis were found to be male gender, bilateral disease, associated congenital anomalies, low birth weight, and small stent size. There was no obvious relationship between the duration of stent placement and restenosis. Restenosis tended to occur early on, and so generally if the choanae were patent after the initial treatment pathway was completed, then routine outpatient follow-up was not required and the child can be reviewed as symptoms dictate.

The complications reported tend to relate to issues related to the stents, if used. Local irritation and infection are common while there are reports of injury to the nasal alar margins resulting in cosmetic deformity and even stenosis of the anterior nares.

Pyriform Aperture Stenosis

This is a very rare cause of nasal obstruction seen in the newborn and is related to bony overgrowth of the nasal process of the maxilla. Diagnosis is suggested clinically and by the inability to pass a narrow gauge nasogastric tube or 2.2-mm endoscope through the anterior part of the nose. Confirmation is through a CT scan with an aperture width of < 11 mm (measured on an axial CT at the level of the inferior meatus) in a term neonate (▶ Fig. 16.3).

There is a link between this condition and holoprosencephaly (a defect in development of brain and midline structures) and so affected individuals should have a formal review for other midline anomalies, including an assessment of function of the hypothalamic–pituitary axis and consideration of a brain magnetic resonance imaging (MRI). The solitary median maxillary central incisor syndrome is the least severe form of holoprosencephaly and three series have reported incidence rates of this condition with pyriform aperture stenosis (PAS) of 28, 50, and 60%, respectively.[7,8,9]

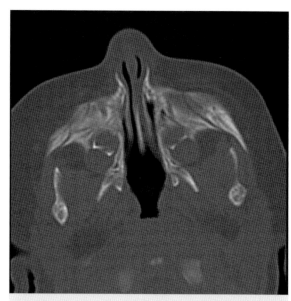

Fig. 16.3 Computed tomography scan (axial view) showing pyriform aperture stenosis.

This anomaly will not be seen at birth but is evident on CT scan and is suggested on examination by a single central maxillary alveolus, absent upper labial frenulum, and arch-shaped lower lip. Associated urogenital and cardiac anomalies have been described.

Management of Pyriform Aperture Stenosis

Initial treatment for PAS involves medical therapy in the form of saline irrigation and the short-term use of decongestants or nasal steroid drops. The maximum duration for such treatment is suggested to be 2 weeks.[9] A nasopharyngeal airway can also be considered, although dilation under GA may be required to allow satisfactory placement, and softer tubes can easily be kinked by the bony deformity.

If there is significant respiratory distress or failure to thrive, then surgical repair may be necessary. A recent review has found that those with an aperture of less than 5 mm required surgical intervention.[8]

- A sublabial approach is recommended with a gingivobuccal sulcus incision and elevation of the soft tissue and periosteum to expose the pyriform aperture.
- The bony narrowing is drilled away (diamond bur), with care being taken posterolaterally to avoid the nasolacrimal ducts and inferiorly to avoid the tooth buds. The mucoperiosteal flap is then replaced.

- As with choanal atresia, the use of nasal stenting post-operatively can be considered, with a period of 7 days to 4 weeks being reported.[7,8]

Satisfactory outcomes are reported in the three largest series reported, although small numbers are involved due to the rarity of the condition.

Complications including adhesions, septal ulceration, and septal perforation are described. Careful postoperative care with nasal irrigation, avoidance of aggressive suction, and management of gastroesophageal reflux are recommended to minimize such issues.[7]

16.3.2 Nasal Masses

Cysts

> ℹ️
>
> The most common form of nasal cyst is a dermoid. This is the most common midline nasal mass.

There are other rarer types of cyst are as follows:
- *Nasolacrimal duct cysts* can cause nasal obstruction or related eye symptomatology, and if so, endoscopic removal is recommended.
- *Nasolaveolar cysts* are developmental nonodontogenic maxillary cysts that usually present with due to aesthetic concerns but can result in obstruction. Excision through a sublabial approach or transnasal endoscopic marsupialization has been described.
- *Dentigenerous cysts* can present in the nose if they arise from the crown of an unerupted tooth in the upper jaw. Treatment involves liason with the dental team.
- *Tornwaldt's cyst* arises in the pharyngeal recess in the midline of the posterior wall of the nasopharynx. This recess ends adjacent to the adenoids and is usually lined with normal pharyngeal mucosa. Cystic transformation of this forms the lesions that bear the name of the individual who initially described it.

The *hairy polyp* sometimes seen in neonates and originally thought to be a cyst has been shown to contain mature ectodermal and mesodermal tissue and is therefore more correctly described as a *bigerminal choristoma*.

Dermoid Cysts

These originate from ectoderm and mesoderm and so can contain all the structures of normal skin. There is debate as to how they develop. In the embryo, there are two areas that are potential candidates: the fonticulus frontalis space, which is between the developing frontal and nasal bones, and the prenasal space, which is between the nasal bones and the developing septum (▶ Fig. 16.4). It is unclear as to whether dermoids occur due to inclusion of dermal tissue at the fonticulus frontalis or from

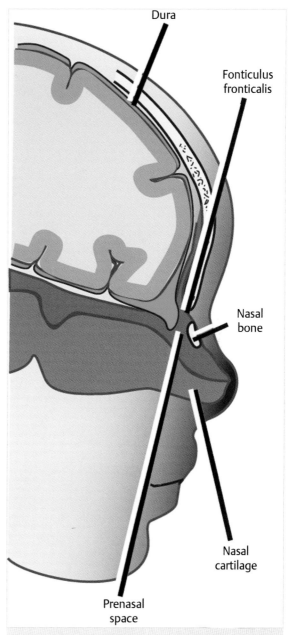

Fig. 16.4 Diagram to illustrate possible embryological sites of origin of dermoid cysts. (Reproduced from Alberstone CD, Benzel EC, Najm EM, Steinmetz MP. Anatomic Basis of Neurologic Diagnosis. Stuttgart/New York: Thieme; 2009, with permission.)

persistent dura in the prenasal space, which then makes contact with the skin and forms a cyst.

Clinical presentation is either as a mass in the midline, which gradually enlarges, or as a small pit on the skin surface, which can be anywhere from the glabella to the philtrum. The pit represents a sinus tract and so can intermittently discharge. Hair can also be present in the pit (▶ Fig. 16.5).

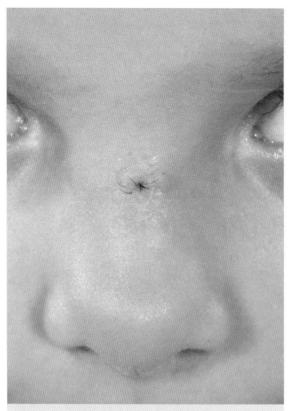

Fig. 16.5 Image of external pit of intranasal dermoid cyst.

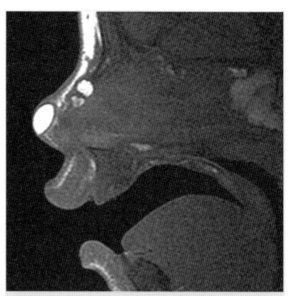

Fig. 16.6 Magnetic resonance imaging scan (sagittal view) showing multiple cystic dilations along the tract of an intranasal dermoid.

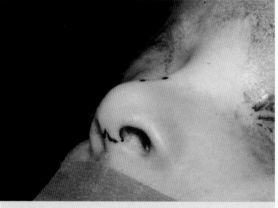

Fig. 16.7 Image of surgical incisions for external rhinoplasty approach.

The investigation of choice is an MRI scan to assess for single or multiple cysts and also to delineate any intracranial component (▶ Fig. 16.6). A CT scan can be useful to demonstrate the bony anatomy.

> ⓘ
>
> The cyst can become infected and early surgical excision is recommended:

- The external rhinoplasty approach (▶ Fig. 16.7) has been favored historically for lesions in the lower half of the nose, whereas others feel it is an excellent technique for all midline nasal masses.[10]
- A brow incision has been described for lesions higher up with intracranial extension.[11]
- More recently, endoscopic techniques have been successfully described.[12,13]

Encephalocele/Meningocele/Glioma/Glial Heterotopia

These congenital anomalies present as midline nasal masses causing varying levels of obstruction and deformity of the nose.

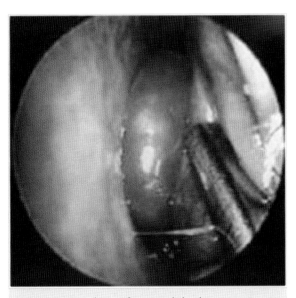

Fig. 16.8 Intranasal view of an encephalocele.

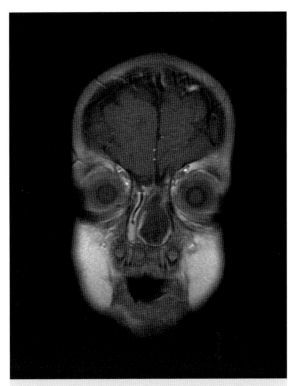

Fig. 16.9 Magnetic resonance imaging scan (T1-weighted sagittal view) showing an intranasal encephalocele.

A nasal *encephalocele* or *meningocele* is a herniation of intracranial contents into the nose, the former containing brain tissue and meninges and the latter containing meninges and cerebrospinal fluid (CSF) only (▶ Fig. 16.8). Their combined incidence is approximately 1 in 4,000 live births and they have an equal male/female distribution.

A classification of encephaloceles defines them as frontoethmoidal or basal.[14] The former arise between the frontal and ethmoid bones either at or anterior to the foramen caecum and so are seen at various exit points on the face and are more likely to be associated with craniofacial deformity. Basal types present intranasally through defects in the skull base causing nasal obstruction and broadening of the nasal bridge, so the otolaryngologist encounters these more frequently.

Gliomas are midline masses containing glial cells, fibrous and vascular tissue. They are similar to encephaloceles but have become separated from the intracranial structures. However, approximately 15% remain attached to the brain through a fibrous stalk. There is generally no associated abnormality of the child's brain. A mass of glial tissue in the nasal cavity or the nasopharynx is sometimes referred to as "glial heterotopia" to distinguish it from a neoplastic condition.

Gliomas are usually reddish in color, firm, and noncompressible as opposed to encephalocoles and meningoceles which tend to be bluish, pulsatile, and compressible.

A probe should pass laterally but not medially to an intranasal encephalocele. Compression of the internal jugular vein usually causes an encephalocele to enlarge but not a glioma (Furstenberg's test).

> Diagnosis can be suggested clinically but imaging is mandatory for all midline nasal masses in children.

MRI is the most effective modality (▶ Fig. 16.9) due to its improved soft-tissue resolution and also because the anterior skull base consists of unossified cartilage and so can appear as a bony dehiscence on CT. CT scan can also be useful though, particularly if excision under image guidance is planned.

Management of Encephalocele/Meningocele/Glioma/Glial Heterotopia

> Once the diagnosis is confirmed, surgical excision is recommended.

Gliomas in the lower part of the nose can be removed by the external rhinoplasty approach but increasingly endoscopic excision is recommended. A review of 15 patients aged between 0 and 14 years has shown successful outcomes with this approach under image guidance.[15] These lesions are generally removed when they present either because they are symptomatic or to ensure the correct diagnosis histologically.

Glial heterotopic tissue is excised as required.[16] This can be endoscopically from the postnasal space using a 0- or 120-degree telescope.

Joint care with a neurosurgical team is advisable for encephalocele and meningocele to allow for planning of the appropriate surgical route and repair of the defect created. Issues such as raised intracranial pressure can occur, and ventriculoperitineal shunting may be required preoperatively.

- A bicoronal flap with a frontal craniotomy has classically been used to access the intracranial portion with an intranasal approach for the extracranial part.
- A transcranial approach is associated with risks such as loss of the sense of smell, intracerebral hemorrhage, cerebral edema, epilepsy, and frontal lobe dysfunction. There is also the obvious postoperative scar.
- With the increasing experience of endoscopic skull base surgery under image guidance, safe excision can be achieved in some cases without the need for a formal craniotomy.[17,18] The lesion is ablated and the neck of the sac resected at the level of the skull base with the surrounding mucosa preserved as much as possible. The defect created must be closed to prevent CSF leak and possible meningitis. If small, then temporalis fascia, mucosa, or a composite graft from the interior turbinate may suffice with Gelfoam and nasal packing for support. Larger defects may warrant more extensive reconstruction with fascia lata and possibly bone from the septum or the mastoid cortex.

The role of antibiotic prophylaxis is debated.

Vascular Malformations

These lesions are described in more detail in Chapter 21. The most common type affecting the nose is a hemangioma. The natural history for these benign lesions involves a period of rapid growth at approximately 6 weeks of age, progressing to resolution by the age of 6 years. Ultrasound and MRI are the recommended modes of imaging, and treatment depends on the extent of involvement of surrounding structures or airway issues. Treatment has been transformed with the finding of the therapeutic effect of propranolol. In cases where there is immediate risk to the orbit, more aggressive chemotherapy has been used.

16.4 Acquired Disorders

16.4.1 Infective/Inflammatory

> **i**
>
> Nasal obstruction in babies and children most commonly has an infective and/or inflammatory etiology.

Neonatal rhinitis can cause airway and feeding issues from birth and adenoid pathology is responsible for sleep-disordered breathing in many young children. These topics are covered in Chapter 17 and Chapter 18.

> **i**
>
> Nasal polyps are rare and must not be confused with enlarged inferior turbinates. If polyps are truly present, then cystic fibrosis must be excluded.

16.4.2 Traumatic

Osseocartilaginous Deformity

Neonatal

Babies can present at birth with obvious nasal deformity. This can affect the septum only or also involve the bony pyramid. Etiology can be from passage through the birth canal or secondary to positioning in the uterus. There is debate as to appropriate management. Closed reduction at diagnosis is described if there are significant symptoms, whereas complete resolution without intervention is also recognized.

Pediatric

There has been debate for some time on the role of septoplasty in children due to concerns over adverse effects on nasal and facial growth. A recent review of the literature[19] has identified three long-term follow-up studies using anthropometric measurements that showed no evidence of interference with normal nasal or facial development from septoplasty. It also commented on a study on the role of external septoplasty though and did suggest a possible negative effect on growth of just the nasal dorsum. Interestingly, one study described a group of children with symptomatic uncorrected septal deformity who had an increased incidence of facial and dental anomalies. It is impossible to say whether the latter were as a result of the nasal problem or simply reflect a process that has affected overall midface development.

If symptoms of nasal obstruction are especially troublesome, then in children over the age of 6 years, there is increasing recognition that judicious surgery may be indicated. Limited surgery with the preservation of cartilage is now more generally accepted.

16.4.3 Neoplastic

Fibrous Dysplasia

Fibrous dysplasia (FD) is an uncommon, benign fibroosseous dysplastic lesion, which can present in monostotic (one site) or polyostotic (multiple sites) form.[20]
- The monostotic type is responsible for approximately 75% of all cases, with the craniofacial bones being the most common site in which it is found. Presentation is usually as pain and facial deformity between 10 and 30 years of age.
- Polyostotic disease occurs in 20 to 30% of presentations, most frequently in the femur and tibia followed by the skull and facial bones. In approximately 60% of individuals affected with polyostotic disease, there are symptoms below the age of 10 years.

Nasal obstruction with a mass noted on endoscopy or facial deformity due to growth of a lesion in the nose or sinus is the usual presenting feature. There can be loosening of the teeth or visual disturbance also related to local expansion.

There is a classical appearance radiologically with normal healthy bone being replaced with a more radiolucent "ground-glass" appearance. There can be endosteal scalloping of the inner cortex with a smooth nonreactive periosteal surface. Lesions have diffusely blending margins (▶ Fig. 16.10).

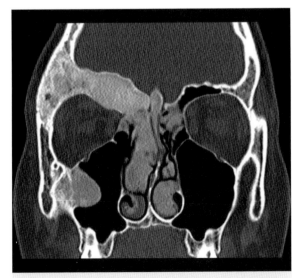

Fig. 16.10 Computed tomography scan (coronal view) showing polyostotic fibrous dysplasia in McCune–Albright's syndrome.

A subgroup of patients (~3%) with polyostotic FD has associated endocrine abnormalities such as hyperthyroidism, adrenal disorders, diabetes, hyperpituitarism, and hypercalcemia with café au lait spots. This is termed *McCune–Albright syndrome* after the two physicians who first described it in 1937.

> ℹ️
>
> FD usually becomes dormant by adulthood but there is a 1% risk of malignant transformation. This risk is increased in the polyostotic form. Sudden increased pain with radiological changes in mineralization is suggestive.

CT scanning is helpful in the diagnosis of possible malignancy and to assess its extent. Osteosarcoma is the most common associated malignancy (70%), with fibrosarcoma (20%) and chondrosarcoma (10%) next.

Management of Fibrous Dysplasia

Once the diagnosis of FD has been made, annual X-ray is suggested for follow-up, although some clinicians prefer monitoring with CT scanning.

Surgical excision is recommended with the aim of preserving function and limiting disability. The midfacial degloving approach has been shown to achieve good results with minimal cosmetic defect.[21]

Medical treatment involves medication to increase bone density such as bisphosphonates along with dietary modifications and exercise.

Juvenile Ossifying Fibroma

Juvenile ossifying fibroma (JOF) is a true neoplasm that is defined radiologically as a radiolucent, expansile, welldefined lesion with variable calcification. It can be unilocular or multilocular with cortical thinning and possible perforation. Pain is usually a rare symptom.

There are two subtypes, trabecular and psammomatoid, which have different histopathological appearances.
- In the trabecular form, the mean age of presentation is 8.5 to 12 years and is most commonly seen to affect the maxilla and mandible. Disease in the maxilla presents as nasal obstruction and epistaxis.
- Psammomatoid JOF more commonly affects the periorbital, frontal, and ethmoid bones. The age of presentation is a little older, usually late teens to early adulthood. Sinonasal tumors can extend orbitally and result in proptosis and disturbed eye movements along with nasal obstruction.

Surgical excision is recommended and this may need to be radical as recurrence rates are high (30–50%) probably due to the propensity of this disease to perforate cortical bone. Malignant change has not been reported.

Juvenile Nasopharyngeal Angiofibroma

Juvenile nasopharyngeal angiofibroma (JNA) is a rare, benign vascular tumor that is locally aggressive. It develops in young males; hence, a hormonal link has been suggested for its etiology. Other theories as to its origin do exist, though, including that it arises from paraganglionic cells in the terminal branches of the maxillary artery or results from a desmoplastic change in the nasopharyngeal periosteum or embryonic fibrocartilage between the basioccipital and basisphenoid bones.

Clinically, it develops from the sphenopalatine foramen and extends into the nose and nasopharynx and then to the deep spaces of the face and skull base through the foramina of the skull. It usually presents with nasal obstruction or severe epistaxis, though headache and facial swelling are also noted. Differential diagnoses include other nasal masses such as nasal tumors, encephalocele, antrochoanal polyp, or other causes of epistaxis, either systemic or local.

Imaging involves both CT and MRI. CT scan will demonstrate the extent of the bony erosion due to the tumor and MRI is useful to delineate the margins of the tumor particularly when there is intracranial extension.

Fisch has classified JNA as follows:
- Stage I: tumors limited to the nasal cavity and nasopharynx with no bony destruction.
- Stage II: tumors invading the pterygomaxillary fossa and paranasal sinuses with bony destruction.
- Stage III: tumors invading the infratemporal fossa, orbit, and/or the parasellar region but remaining lateral to the cavernous sinus.
- Stage IV: tumors invading the cavernous sinus, optic chiasmal area, and/or the pituitary fossa.

Angiography shows the vascular anatomy with the main feeding vessel being the internal maxillary artery. Bilateral vascular supply is well recognized and so angiography of bilateral carotid systems is recommended preoperatively.

Management of Juvenile Nasopharyngeal Angiofibroma

> i
>
> Embolization preoperatively is recommended to limit blood loss during surgery.

Classically, excision has been through external approaches such as lateral rhinotomy and midfacial degloving. The development of endoscopic skull base surgery and navigation systems has allowed this method to be a management options in appropriate cases. Benefits are well recognized for cosmesis and function. A recent review has supported this evolution in practice but points out that an external approach should still be considered for larger lesions and if there is extensive intracranial involvement or encasement of the optic nerve or internal carotid artery.[22]

Olfactory Neuroblastoma

This is a rare malignant neoplasm of olfactory epithelium, also known as esthesineuroblastoma. The incidence in children is extremely low, being approximately 0.1 per 100,000 up to the age of 15 years. Presentation tends to be more aggressive in younger patients with more cases presenting as advanced disease. Treatment is with a combination of craniofacial resection with radiotherapy and/ or chemotherapy.

Nasopharyngeal Carcinoma

The incidence of this lesion varies with ethnic and geographical factors. It is more common in males. In the Mediterranean locality, there is a bimodal age distribution, occurring at 10 to 20 and 50 to 60 years. It has an increased incidence in adults in Asia. It is rare, being responsible for less than 1% of childhood malignancies, but is one of the most frequent neoplasms of the nasopharyngeal and respiratory tracts. There is a close association with Epstein–Barr virus infection.

Unfortunately, at the time of presentation, there is often advanced local disease with metastases. Treatment involves combined radio- and chemotherapy, and adjuvant therapy involving interferon beta appears to have benefit. A recent review of 95 patients has shown a 15-year overall survival rate of 42.5% but there are often treatment-related morbidities such as xerostomia, dental and bone problems, thyroid disorders, and secondary cancers.[23]

Teratoma

A teratoma is a true neoplasm consisting of tissue from all three embryonic germ layers. The incidence of head and neck teratomas is approximately 1 in 4,000 live births with cervical forms being the most common and nasopharyngeal lesions being seen most frequently after that.

They are therefore uncommon causes of nasal obstruction but will present as a firm swelling in the neonate, which can result in significant airway difficulties. They can be sessile or pedunculated and can be associated with polyhydramnios due to impaired swallowing. Maternal serum alpha fetoprotein levels may be raised. Investigation is through CT and MRI scanning, with surgical excision being the treatment of choice. This can be done through an endoscopic or open approach, depending on the size of the lesion.

16.5 Key Points

- Nasal obstruction in children can be caused by a wide range of pathologies.
- Specialist imaging has greatly improved diagnosis of nasal disease in children.
- Improved endoscopic techniques have led to much better outcomes in many of the disorders described in this chapter.

References

[1] Eladl HM, Khafagy YW. Endoscopic bilateral congenital choanal atresia repair of 112 cases, evolving concept and technical experience. Int J Pediatr Otorhinolaryngol. 2016; 85:40–45

[2] Wormald PJ, Zhao YC, Valdes CJ, et al. The endoscopic transseptal approach for choanal atresia repair. Int Forum Allergy Rhinol. 2016; 6 (6):654–660

[3] Kubba H, Bennett A, Bailey CM. An update on choanal atresia surgery at Great Ormond Street Hospital for Children: preliminary results with Mitomycin C and the KTP laser. Int J Pediatr Otorhinolaryngol. 2004; 68(7):939–945

[4] Teissier N, Kaguelidou F, Couloigner V, François M, Van Den Abbeele T. Predictive factors for success after transnasal endoscopic treatment of choanal atresia. Arch Otolaryngol Head Neck Surg. 2008; 134(1): 57–61

[5] Ibrahim AA, Magdy EA, Hassab MH. Endoscopic choanoplasty without stenting for congenital choanal atresia repair. Int J Pediatr Otorhinolaryngol. 2010; 74(2):144–150

[6] Elloy MD, Cochrane LA, Albert DM. Refractory choanal atresia: what makes a child susceptible? The great Ormond Street Hospital experience. J Otolaryngol Head Neck Surg. 2008; 37(6):813–820

[7] Devambez M, Delattre A, Fayoux P. Congenital nasal pyriform aperture stenosis: diagnosis and management. Cleft Palate Craniofac J. 2009; 46(3):262–267

[8] Visvanathan V, Wynne DM. Congenital nasal pyriform aperture stenosis: a report of 10 cases and literature review. Int J Pediatr Otorhinolaryngol. 2012; 76(1):28–30

[9] Van Den Abbeele T, Triglia JM, François M, Narcy P. Congenital nasal pyriform aperture stenosis: diagnosis and management of 20 cases. Ann Otol Rhinol Laryngol. 2001; 110(1):70–75

[10] Locke R, Kubba H. The external rhinoplasty approach for congenital nasal lesions in children. Int J Pediatr Otorhinolaryngol. 2011; 75(3): 337–341

[11] Heywood RL, Lyons MJ, Cochrane LA, Hayward R, Hartley BE. Excision of nasal dermoids with intracranial extension - anterior small window craniotomy approach. Int J Pediatr Otorhinolaryngol. 2007; 71 (8):1193–1196

[12] Pinheiro-Neto CD, Snyderman CH, Fernandez-Miranda J, Gardner PA. Endoscopic endonasal surgery for nasal dermoids. Otolaryngol Clin North Am. 2011; 44(4):981–987, ix

[13] Schuster D, Riley KO, Cure JK, Woodworth BA. Endoscopic resection of intracranial dermoid cysts. J Laryngol Otol. 2011; 125(4):423–427

[14] Suwanwela C, Suwanwela N. A morphological classification of sincipital encephalomeningoceles. J Neurosurg. 1972; 36(2):201–211

[15] Bonne NX, Zago S, Hosana G, Vinchon M, Van den Abbeele T, Fayoux P. Endonasal endoscopic approach for removal of intranasal nasal glial heterotopias. Rhinology. 2012; 50(2):211–217

[16] Haloob N, Pepper C, Hartley B. A series of parapharyngeal glial heterotopia mimicking lymphatic malformation. Int J Pediatr Otorhinolaryngol. 2015; 79(12):1975–1979

[17] Woodworth BA, Schlosser RJ, Faust RA, Bolger WE. Evolutions in the management of congenital intranasal skull base defects. Arch Otolaryngol Head Neck Surg. 2004; 130(11):1283–1288

[18] Abdel-Aziz M, El-Bosraty H, Qotb M, et al. Nasal encephalocoele: endoscopic excision with anaesthetic consideration. Int J Pediatr Otorhinolaryngol. 2010; 74(8):869–873

[19] Lawrence R. Pediatric septoplasty: a review of the literature. Int J Pediatr Otorhinolaryngol. 2012; 76(8):1078–1081

[20] Riddle ND, Bui MM. Fibrous dysplasia. Arch Pathol Lab Med. 2013; 137(1):134–138

[21] Eze NN, Wyatt ME, Bray D, Bailey CM, Hartley BE. The midfacial degloving approach to sinonasal tumours in children. Rhinology. 2006; 44(1):36–38

[22] Cloutier T, Pons Y, Blancal JP, et al. Juvenile nasopharyngeal angiofibroma: does the external approach still make sense? Otolaryngol Head Neck Surg. 2012; 147(5):958–963

[23] Hu S, Xu X, Xu J, Xu Q, Liu S. Prognostic factors and long-term outcomes of nasopharyngeal carcinoma in children and adolescents. Pediatr Blood Cancer. 2013; 60(7):1122–1127

17 Pediatric Rhinitis and Rhinosinusitis

Wytske J. Fokkens and Fuad M. Baroody

17.1 Introduction

The mucosa of the nose and sinuses are contiguous, which accounts for the frequent involvement of the paranasal sinuses in diseases that cause inflammation of the nasal mucosa. Rhinitis and sinusitis usually coexist and are concurrent in most individuals; thus, the correct terminology is now "rhinosinusitis". Rhinosinusitis is a relatively common problem in children and is often underdiagnosed. In particular, viral upper respiratory tract infections (URTIs) are very frequently associated with disease in the sinus cavities. Recognition of history and symptoms are important to establish a diagnosis of rhinosinusitis.

17.2 Development of the Paranasal Sinuses

The pediatric nasal cavity and paranasal sinuses, when compared to those in adults, differ not only in size but also in proportions. Knowledge of the unique anatomy and pneumatization pattern of children's sinuses is an important prerequisite to understanding the pathogenesis of sinusitis and its complications. It is also important in the evaluation of radiographs and in planning surgical interventions.

17.2.1 Ethmoid Sinus

At birth, the ethmoid sinuses are the only sinuses that are large enough to be clinically significant as a cause of rhinosinusitis. Ethmoidal cells are present at birth and the ethmoid sinus rapidly expands until the age of 5 years due to pneumatization, whereas there is only little expansion in bone width. The final size of the ethmoid is reached by the age of 13 years.

17.2.2 Maxillary Sinus

The maxillary sinuses are present at birth but the volume is extremely small, less than 0.5 mL. The anteroposterior growth of the maxillary sinus increases rapidly during the early years of life, and the volume in patients at 2 years of age is approximately 2 mL (▶ Fig. 17.1). At the age of 4 years, the floor of the maxillary sinus is at the level of the hard palate. The lateral walls have advanced two-thirds of the way across the orbital floor past the infraorbital nerve. The maxillary sinus grows rapidly reaching approximately 10 mL in volume around 9 years of age with a variable final adult volume of 13 to 40 mL. Much of the growth that occurs after the 12th year is in

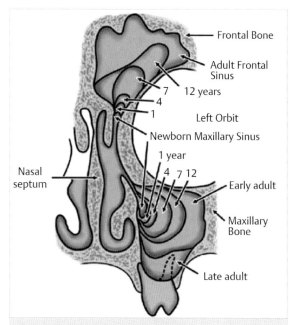

Fig. 17.1 Development of the frontal and maxillary sinuses with age. (Reproduced from Fatu C, Puisoru M, Rotaru M, Truta AM. Morphometric evaluation of the frontal sinus in relation to age. Ann Anat 2006;188:275–280, with permission.)

the inferior direction with pneumatization of the alveolar process after eruption of the secondary dentition. By adulthood, the floor of the maxillary sinus is usually 4 to 5 mm inferior to the floor of the nasal cavity.

17.2.3 The Frontal and Sphenoid Sinuses

The frontal sinus is absent at birth and is the last sinus to develop (▶ Fig. 17.1). Very often, frontal sinuses cannot be found before the age of 10 years. Their size continues to increase into the late teens, and more than 85% of children will show pneumatized frontal sinuses on computed tomography (CT) scanning at the age of 12 years.[1] The final volume is very variable between 2 and 17 mL. The sphenoid sinus starts to develop in the first year of life but the volume is negligible under the age of 6 years.

17.3 Definition and Classification of Disease

The diagnosis of rhinosinusitis is made by a wide variety of practitioners, including allergologists, otolaryngologists, pulmonologists, primary care physicians, pediatricians, and many others.[2] Therefore, an accurate, efficient, and accessible definition and classification of rhinosinusitis is required. The European position paper on rhinosinusitis and nasal polyps (EPOS) is now widely accepted.[3]

In the EPOS guidelines, pediatric rhinosinusitis is defined as follows[3]:

An inflammation of the nose and the paranasal sinuses characterized by two or more symptoms one of which should be either nasal blockage/obstruction/congestion or nasal discharge (anterior/posterior nasal drip):

± facial pain/pressure

± cough

and either

- endoscopic signs of:
  ○ nasal polyps, and/or
  ○ mucopurulent discharge primarily from middle meatus
  ○ and/or
- edema/mucosal obstruction primarily in middle meatus and/or
- CT changes:
  ○ mucosal changes within the ostiomeatal complex and/or sinuses

---

The disease can be divided into *acute rhinosinusitis* (ARS), which has an acute onset, lasts less than 12 weeks, and shows a complete resolution of symptoms, and *chronic rhinosinusitis* (CRS), which lasts more than 12 weeks without complete resolution of symptoms. CRS may also be subject to exacerbations. Many etiological factors contribute to ARS and CRS including viral and bacterial infections, genetic defects (such as in cystic fibrosis [CF]), and fungal infections, typically allergic fungal sinusitis [AFS] in the older child). Similar symptoms can occur in patients with allergic inflammation.

17.4 Acute Rhinosinusitis

ARS in children is common and usually occurs in the course of an upper respiratory viral illness. The diagnosis is mostly based on the type and duration of the aforementioned symptoms. The diagnosis is most frequently made in the primary care setting without recourse to endoscopy or imaging, so the clinical findings are of paramount importance. In most cases, this is a self-limited process but treatment with antibiotics seems to slightly accelerate resolution. Whether this benefit outweighs the risks associated with frequent antibiotic prescriptions remains to be clarified. Intranasal steroids might be useful adjuncts to antibiotics in the treatment of ARS, and very limited evidence in older children suggests that they

may be useful as a single agent. Ancillary therapy in the form of nasal irrigations, antihistamines, decongestants, or mucolytics has not been shown to be helpful. ARS can lead to serious orbital, intracranial, and osseous complications. Management of ARS complications is always multidisciplinary, and the advice of an ophthalmologist in cases of orbital involvement and of neurologist/neurosurgeon in intracranial involvement is mandatory (see Chapter 4).

17.4.1 Incidence of Acute Rhinosinusitis in Children

The incidence of acute sinusitis or ARS is high. It has been estimated that children may suffer 7 to 10 colds per year. Approximately 0.5 to 2% of viral URTIs are complicated by bacterial infection.

17.4.2 Definition and Diagnosis of Acute Rhinosinusitis in Children

The clinical diagnosis of ARS in children is challenging due to the overlap of symptoms with other common childhood nasal diseases such as viral URTIs and allergic rhinitis (AR) as well as the due to the challenges related to physical examination. The symptoms are often subtle and the history is limited to the observations and subjective evaluation by the child's parent. Because some younger children might not tolerate nasal endoscopy, clinicians are sometimes hindered in their physical examination and have to rely on history and or imaging studies for appropriate diagnosis.

Symptom profiles of ARS in children include the following:

- Fever (50–60%).
- Rhinorrhea (71–80%).
- Cough (50–80%).
- Pain (29–33%).

In children, ARS most often presents as either a severe upper respiratory tract illness with fever > 39°C, purulent rhinorrhea, and facial pain or, more commonly, as a prolonged URTI with chronic cough and nasal discharge.

In a study of the relationship between symptoms of acute respiratory infection and objective changes within the sinuses using magnetic resonance imaging (MRI) scans, 60 children (mean age = 5.7 years) were investigated who had symptoms for an average of 6 days before scanning.[4] Approximately 60% of the children had abnormalities in their maxillary and ethmoid sinuses, 35% in the sphenoid sinuses, and 18% in the frontal sinuses. In 26 children with major abnormalities, a follow-up MRI scan taken 2 weeks later showed a significant reduction in the extent of abnormalities irrespective of resolution of clinical symptoms. This study reinforces the notion that, like in adults, every URTI is essentially an episode of

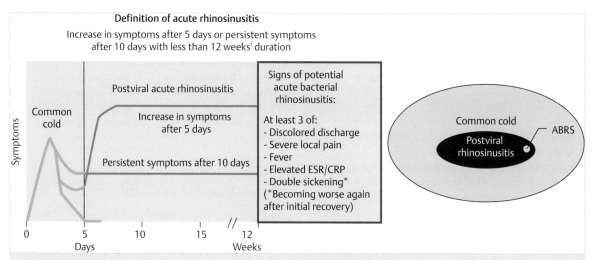

Fig. 17.2 Schematic representation of the timing of the symptoms during episodes of acute rhinosinusitis (left panel) and the relative proportions of upper respiratory tract infections, postviral rhinosinusitis, and acute bacterial rhinosinusitis (right panel). (Reproduced from Fokkens WJ, Lund VJ, Mullol J, et al. European position paper on rhinosinusitis and nasal polyps 2012. Rhinology 2012;50(Suppl 23), with permission.)

rhinosinusitis with common involvement of the paranasal sinuses by the viral process.

> ℹ
>
> ARS in children is characterized by the sudden onset of two or more of the defining symptoms (discolored nasal discharge, nasal blockage/obstruction/ congestion, cough at daytime and nighttime) for less than 12 weeks, with validation by telephone or interview.[3]

Symptom-free intervals may exist if the problem is recurrent. Questions on allergic symptoms (i.e., sneezing, watery rhinorrhea, nasal itching, and itchy watery eyes) should be included. As in adults, the "common cold"/ acute viral rhinosinusitis is defined by a duration of symptoms of less than 10 days. Acute postviral rhinosinusitis is characterized by an increase of symptoms after 5 days or persistent symptoms after 10 days. The more severe acute bacterial rhinosinusitis (ABRS; ▶ Fig. 17.2) should be considered in the presence of at least three of the following clinical features:
- Discolored discharge (with unilateral predominance) and purulent nasal secretions.
- Severe local pain (with unilateral predominance).
- Fever (> 38°C).
- Elevated erythrocyte sedimentation rate (ESR) and C-reactive protein (CRP).

- "Double sickening" (i.e., deterioration after an initial milder phase of illness).

17.4.3 Differential Diagnosis

When a child presents with the aforementioned symptoms of ARS, the differential diagnosis includes intranasal foreign body (▶ Fig. 17.3) and unilateral choanal stenosis or atresia. In these entities, the symptoms are usually unilateral and can be relatively easily differentiated clinically from ARS by history and physical examination, including nasal endoscopy.

Adenoiditis can have a very similar clinical presentation including anterior and posterior purulent drainage and cough and is very relevant in the differential diagnosis in the pediatric age group, although more in CRS than in ARS. AR will usually not manifest with purulent drainage as part of the clinical presentation. Migraine and tension type headaches also occur in children and should be differentiated from (recurrent) ARS.

17.4.4 Pathogenesis of Acute Rhinosinusitis

Predisposing Factors

Knowledge of the pathogenesis of ARS in children is very limited. However, we might consider it to be quite the same as in adults.

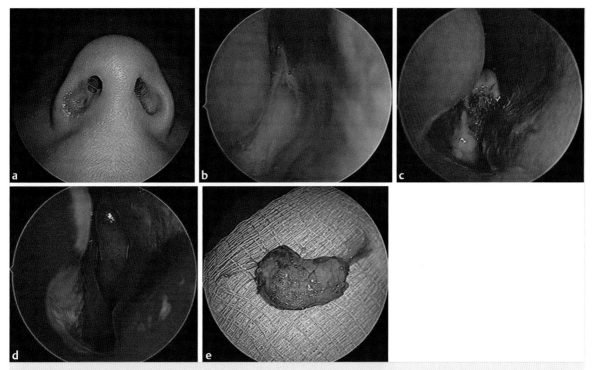

Fig. 17.3 **(a)** A child with unilateral right-sided nasal discharge. Endoscopy showed mucus in the right nasal cavity **(b)** and a foreign object **(c)**, which was removed successfully. The nose shows mild irritation **(d)** at the site of the removed foreign object **(e)**, which turned out to be foam from the mattress. Unilateral foul smelling nasal drainage is the typical presentation of a child with a nasal foreign body.

Factors that predispose children toward ARS are as follows:
- Winter months.
- Exposure to individuals with viral URTIs.
- AR.
- Passive smoking.
- Ciliary dyskinesia.
- Anatomical abnormalities.

The most significant predisposing factor is likely to be URTIs or the common cold. Children have on average six to eight colds per year, with 0.5 to 2% developing acute sinus infections.

There seems to be an association between ARS and atopy and AR, and an association between ARS and smoking. As in adults the relationship between anatomical abnormalities and ARS is very unclear and most likely unimportant.

Microbiology of Viral (Common Cold), Postviral, and Acute Bacterial Rhinosinusitis

Viral, postviral, and bacterial ARS show a considerable overlap both in their inflammatory mechanisms and their clinical presentation. Viral infection of the nose and sinuses induces multiple changes including postviral inflammation, which increases the risk of bacterial superinfection. These changes include epithelial damage and alteration of mechanical, humoral, and cellular defenses. The most common viruses isolated in pediatric viral rhinitis and rhinosinusitis are adenovirus and rhinovirus. Other viruses found are enterovirus, coronavirus, (para)influenza virus, and respiratory syncytial virus (RSV). The microbiology of ABRS, as documented in early maxillary antral puncture studies, is mainly as follows:
- *Streptococcus pneumoniae.*
- *Haemophilus influenzae.*
- *Moraxella catarrhalis.*

Inflammatory Mechanisms

Viral infection of the nose and sinuses induces multiple changes that increase the risk of bacterial superinfection. Viral infection induces epithelial disruption, increases the number of goblet cells, and decreases the number of ciliated cells. Eventually, these changes contribute to the obstruction of the sinus ostia in the nasal cavity. A transient increase in pressure develops in the sinus cavity due to mucus accumulation. This is quickly followed by the development of negative pressure in the sinus cavity due to impaired sinus aeration with rapid absorption of the oxygen that is left. This worsens local congestion, promotes further mucus retention, impairs normal gas exchange within the integrated airspace, decreases both the oxygen and pH content, impedes clearance of infectious material and inflammatory debris, and increases the risk of secondary bacterial infection. All these local changes in the nasal and paranasal space form an ideal environment for pathological bacterial colonization and growth.

17.4.5 The Diagnostic Work-Up

> The most important aspect of the diagnosis is the history.

- Most frequently, children present with symptoms of URTI that have persisted for more than 10 days or there is a worsening of symptoms after an initial improvement.
- The rhinorrhea is usually mucoid or purulent.
- The cough, which may be wet or dry, occurs in the daytime but is often worse at night.
- The child is mild to moderately ill and usually does not have high fever.
- The mother is worried about the persistence or increase of the symptoms.

A totally different presentation is the severely ill child with high fever that already persists for 3 to 4 days, much longer than expected with a common cold. The fever is accompanied by thick purulent rhinorrhea that is usually unilateral.

The nasal examination in children should begin with anterior rhinoscopy examining the middle meatus, inferior turbinates, mucosal character, and presence of purulent drainage. This is often accomplished easily using the largest speculum of an otoscope or, alternatively, a headlight and nasal speculum. Topical decongestion may be used to improve visualization.

Nasal endoscopy that will allow a good view of the middle meatus, adenoid bed, and nasopharynx is strongly recommended in children who are able to tolerate the examination. An oral cavity examination may reveal purulent postnasal drainage, cobblestoning of the posterior pharyngeal wall, or tonsillar hypertrophy. Obtaining a culture is usually not necessary in the context of uncomplicated ARS. The diagnosis of ARS in children is generally made on clinical grounds, and radiology (CT or MRI) should be reserved for patients with suspected complications.

17.4.6 Treatment of Acute Rhinosinusitis in Children

Medical Treatment of Acute Rhinosinusitis

Refer to ▶ Table 17.1 and ▶ Fig. 17.4.

Antibiotics

Antibiotics are the most frequently used therapeutic agents in ARS. Published trials in children and adults were reviewed in a recent meta-analysis of randomized controlled trials (RCTs) evaluating antibiotic treatment for ARS in which 3 of the 17 evaluated studies were performed in the pediatric age group.[5] In total, 3,291 outpatients (2,915 adults and 376 children) were treated in the trials included in the meta-analysis. The diagnosis of ARS in the trials was based on clinical criteria in most studies and radiological and other laboratory criteria in the rest. In most studies, inclusion of patients with viral URTIs was avoided by enrolling patients whose symptoms were more than 7 to 10 days in duration. The results suggest that compared with placebo, antibiotics were associated

Table 17.1 Treatment evidence and recommendations for children with acute rhinosinusitis

Therapy	Level	Grade of recommendation	Relevance
Antibiotic	Ia	A	Yes in ABRS
Topical steroid	Ia	A	Yes mainly in postviral ARS studies only done in children 12 y and older
Addition of topical steroid to antibiotic	Ia	A	Yes in ABRS
Mucolytics (erdosteine)	1b[a]	A[b]	No
Saline irrigation	IV	D	Yes
Oral antihistamine	IV	D	No
Decongestion	IV	D	No

Abbreviations: ABRS, acute bacterial rhinosinusitis; ARS, acute rhinosinusitis.
Source: Reproduced from Fokkens WJ, Lund VJ, Mullol J, et al. European position paper on rhinosinusitis and nasal polyps 2012. Rhinology 2012;50(Suppl 23):1–12, with permission.
[a]Study with negative outcome. [b]Grade A recommendation not to use.

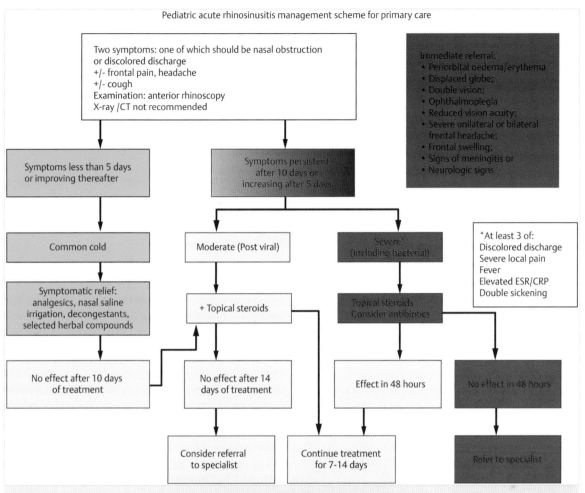

Fig. 17.4 Management scheme for acute pediatric rhinosinusitis. (Modified after Fokkens WJ, Lund VJ, Mullol J, et al. European position paper on rhinosinusitis and nasal polyps 2012. Rhinology 2012;50(Suppl 23), with permission.)

with a higher rate of cure or improvement within 7 to 15 days, with the rate of resolution of symptoms being faster with antibiotics in most RCTs. The overall positive effect in favor of antibiotics was significant but very modest. The results suggest that most cases of uncomplicated acute sinusitis will improve irrespective of treatment used but will do so a little faster if given antibiotics.

> **i**
>
> Based on this evidence, it would seem reasonable to recommend only symptomatic treatment for uncomplicated episodes of ARS in children. Antibiotic therapy would be reserved to children with complications (strength of recommendation: A).

When considering antibiotic choices, uncomplicated ARS in a child who has not received multiple previous courses of antibiotics can still be treated with amoxicillin (40 or

80 mg/kg/day). Other reasonable and safe choices are amoxicillin–clavulanate and cephalosporins that provide good coverage of typical organisms, especially those producing β-lactamase. If hypersensitivity to any of the aforementioned antimicrobials is suspected, alternative choices include trimethoprim/sulfamethoxazole, azithromycin, or clarithromycin.

Intranasal Steroids

In a pediatric trial, 89 children with ARS received amoxicillin–clavulanate and were randomized to additionally receive either budesonide or placebo nasal sprays for 3 weeks.[6] There were significant improvements in the scores of cough and nasal discharge at the end of the second week in the steroid group compared to placebo, suggesting a benefit of adding intranasal steroids to antibiotics in the treatment of ARS. Several trials in mixed adult and pediatric populations (usually 12–14 years and older) have demonstrated similar benefits of using an intranasal steroid along with an antibiotic for the treatment of ARS.[3]

> ℹ︎
>
> There is reasonable evidence to support the addition of an intranasal steroid to antibiotics if antibiotics are needed in the treatment of ARS (strength of recommendation: A).

Finally, in a randomized, placebo controlled trial in patients older than 12 years with ARS, mometasone, 200 μg twice daily (twice the AR dose), was more effective in controlling symptoms than placebo and amoxicillin.[7] Thus, there is also some evidence that a high dose of intranasal steroids in older children might be effective as monotherapy for ARS. Although studies in AR have shown that intranasal corticosteroids are safe in younger children, we do not have good data to support their efficacy for ARS in this age group; thus, individual clinical decision-making should be exercised relating to the administration of these medications for ARS in younger children.

Ancillary Treatment

A systematic review of the literature was undertaken to evaluate the efficacy of decongestants (oral or intranasal), antihistamines, and nasal irrigation in children with clinically diagnosed acute sinusitis.[8] RCTs or quasi-RCTs that evaluated children between 0 and 18 years of age with ARS defined as 10 to 30 days of rhinorrhea, congestion, or daytime cough were included. The authors conclude that there is no evidence to determine whether the use of the aforementioned agents is efficacious in children with ARS. In another publication, erdosteine, a mucolytic agent, was investigated in a randomized, placebo controlled trial.[9] In total, 81 patients completed the study, and their average age was 8.5 years and all had symptoms consistent with ARS. They were randomized to receive either erdosteine or placebo for 14 days and their symptoms recorded. Both treatment groups had an improvement in symptoms on day 14, but there were no statistically significant differences between the active and placebo groups.

> ℹ︎
>
> There is no good evidence to support the use of ancillary therapies in the treatment of ARS in children (strength of recommendation: A–, negative recommendation).[10]

17.4.7 Complications of Acute Rhinosinusitis

In the preantibiotic era, complications of rhinosinusitis represented common and dangerous clinical events. Today, thanks to more reliable diagnostic methods (CT and MRI), improved surgical techniques, and the wide range of available antibiotics, their incidence and related mortality have dramatically decreased. However, despite antibiotics, serious complications of rhinosinusitis do occur.

Complications of rhinosinusitis are classically defined as follows:
- Orbital (60–75%).
- Intracranial (15–20%).
- Osseous (5–10%).

Combinations often occur.

The incidence of complication of ARS in children is 3 to 10 cases per million of population per year (or approximately 1 per 12,000 ARS episodes).[3] There is a clear seasonal pattern of complications, mirroring the incidence of URTIs and appearing more often during winter months. In almost all studies, males are significantly more frequently affected than females. While orbital complications tend to occur primarily in small children, intracranial complications can occur at any age. Orbital complications, including pre- and postseptal cellulitis and subperiosteal and orbital abscess, are the most frequent, and children with acute ethmoiditis are especially prone to them (▶ Fig. 17.5, ▶ Fig. 17.6, ▶ Fig. 17.7, ▶ Fig. 17.8, ▶ Fig. 17.9, ▶ Fig. 17.10). Endocranial complications include epidural

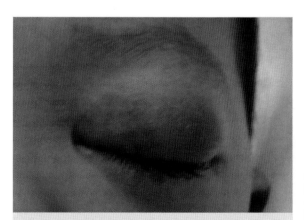

Fig. 17.5 Periorbital cellulitis, a typical clinical sign of an impending complication associated with acute bacterial sinusitis. This clinical picture should raise the suspicion of a subperiosteal orbital abscess.

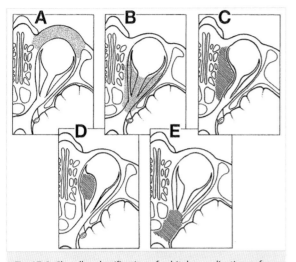

Fig. 17.6 Chandler classification of orbital complications of acute sinusitis. Schematics A to E depict increasing severity of such infections as they progress through the orbit to reach the cavernous sinus. A, Inflammatory edema (preseptal cellulitis); B, orbital cellulitis; C, subperiosteal abscess; D, orbital abscess; E, cavernous sinus thrombosis. (Reproduced from Chandler JR, Langenbrunner DJ, Stevens ER. The pathogenesis of orbital complications in acute sinusitis. Laryngoscope 1970;80 (9):1414–1128, with permission.)

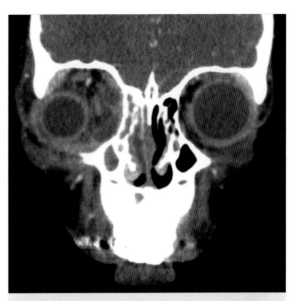

Fig. 17.7 Coronal computed tomography scan with contrast (soft-tissue windows) of a patient with a right-sided subperiosteal orbital abscess. Note pan-opacification of the visualized portions of the anterior ethmoid and maxillary sinuses. Also note lateral and inferior displacement of the right eye and rim enhancing abscess cavities on the medial aspect of the orbit alongside the lamina papyracea.

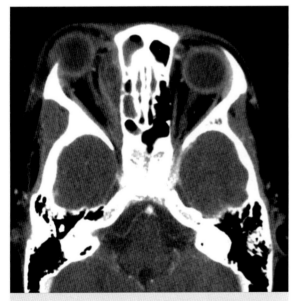

Fig. 17.8 Axial computed tomography scan with contrast (soft-tissue windows) of the same patient. Note proptosis of the right eye (left of the picture) and rim enhancing abscess cavity along the superior aspect of the lamina papyracea. The medial rectus muscle and the optic nerve are displaced laterally by the abscess.

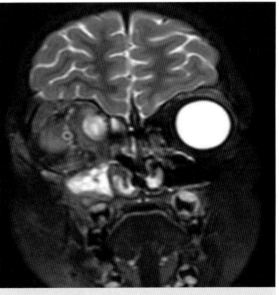

Fig. 17.9 Magnetic resonance imaging (MRI) appearance of a subperiosteal orbital abscess. Coronal T2-weighted MRI. Please note the fluid filled abscess in the right eye (left side of the picture) with lateral displacement of orbital contents. Ipsilateral maxillary sinus is seen filled with fluid on this view.

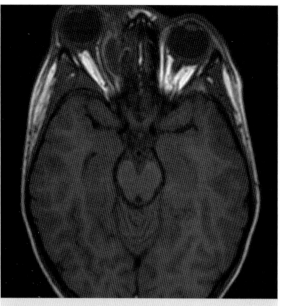

Fig. 17.10 Axial T1-weighted magnetic resonance image of the same abscess. Note proptosis of the right eye (left of the picture) and rim enhancing abscess cavity along the superior aspect of the lamina papyracea. The medial rectus muscle and the optic nerve are displaced laterally by the abscess.

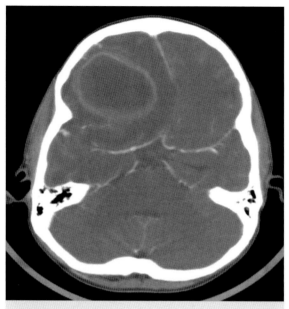

Fig. 17.11 Axial computed tomography image with contrast of a brain abscess secondary to an episode of acute rhinosinusitis. Note the rim enhanced abscess cavity in the right frontal area (left of the picture) with significant shift of the intracranial structures.

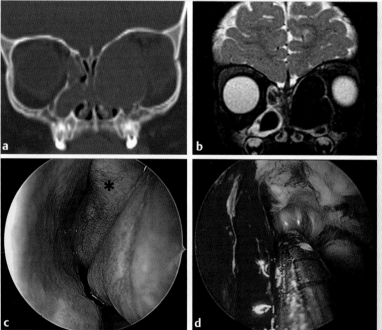

Fig. 17.12 Radiological and intraoperative pictures of a 15-month-old male with cystic fibrosis who presented with left eye proptosis. **(a)** Coronal computed tomography scan shows a large ethmoid mucocele, which is pushing the left orbital contents laterally. **(b)** T2-weighted magnetic resonance imaging shows the same mucocele with inflammation of the membrane and low signal intensity in the middle of the mucocele, which corresponds to inspissated mucus. **(c)** Intraoperative endoscopy of the left nasal cavity shows bulging of the lateral nasal wall medially (*asterisk*) and complete obliteration of the middle meatal area. After unroofing the mucocele, it was filled with **(d)** inspissated thick mucus, which after evacuation resulted in return of the eye to normal position.

or subdural abscesses, brain abscess (► Fig. 17.11), meningitis, cerebritis, and superior sagittal and cavernous sinus thrombosis. Osseous complications include steomyelitis and "Pott's puffy tumor" of the frontal sinus. Obstruction of the ethmoid sinus can result in an ethmoidal mucocele (► Fig. 17.12).

17.5 Chronic Rhinosinusitis in Children

17.5.1 Classification and Diagnosis

> ⓘ
>
> CRS is defined as the presence of the symptoms of discolored nasal discharge and/or nasal blockage/obstruction/congestion, combined with cough at daytime and nighttime, or facial pain for at least 12 weeks.

CRS is primarily due to infection, allergy, or, in some cases, a combination of the two. Although some of the aforementioned symptoms could also apply to AR, facial pain, cough, and discolored nasal drainage are not prominent in allergic disease, and sneezing and itching are not common in CRS. Because of the close association of the two entities, questions on allergic symptoms (i.e., sneezing, watery rhinorrhea, nasal itching, and itchy watery eyes) should therefore be included when taking a history. The adenoids are a prominent contributor to CRS in the pediatric age group.

CRS in children is not as well studied as the same entity in adults. Multiple factors contribute to the disease, including bacteriological and inflammatory factors. The mainstay of therapy is medical with surgery reserved for the minority of patients who do not respond to medical treatment.

17.5.2 Prevalence of Chronic Rhinosinusitis in Children

The exact prevalence of CRS in children is difficult to determine as only a small percentage of cases present to the physician's office. Many studies that address prevalence have been performed in select populations, typically in children, who have upper respiratory complaints. In one such study, CT scans were obtained in 196 children between 3 and 14 years of age presenting with chronic rhinorrhea, nasal congestion, and cough.[11] Maxillary involvement was noted in 63%, ethmoid involvement in 58%, and sphenoidal sinus involvement in 29% of the children of the youngest age groups. This contrasts with 10% of the ethmoids, 0% of sphenoids, and 65% of the maxillaries being involved in the older 13 to 14-year-old age group. There are few studies that follow the prevalence over time and suggest a decrease in the prevalence of rhinosinusitis after 6 to 8 years of age.

17.5.3 Pediatric Chronic Rhinosinusitis and Quality of Life

CRS has a marked impact on quality of life. Children with CRS have significantly lower quality-of-life scores when compared to healthy children and children with other common chronic childhood diseases such as asthma, attention deficit hyperactivity disorder, juvenile rheumatoid arthritis, and epilepsy.[12] The differences were most marked in the physical domains of the quality-of-life questionnaires, such as bodily pain and limitation in physical activity. There is also limited evidence showing improvement of quality of life using a validated sinus and nasal quality of life measure (the SN-5 tool) in patients with CRS after surgical intervention, for example, adenoidectomy or endoscopic sinus surgery.[13]

17.5.4 Pathogenesis of Chronic Rhinosinusitis in Children

Predisposing Factors for Chronic Rhinosinusitis in Children

Day Care

Although day care, that is, where several children congregate and spread of infection might be facilitated, is often thought to have a negative influence on URTIs and thus potentially on CRS, the available data suggest the opposite.[14,15]

There is evidence to suggest that children with a family history of atopy or asthma who attend day-care centers (crèches) in the first year of life have 2.2 times higher odds of having doctor-diagnosed sinusitis than children who do not attend day care.

Parental Lifestyle

Cigarette smoking and exposure to second-hand smoke is common and significantly independently associated with CRS. Other lifestyle-related factors are involved in the chronic inflammatory processes of CRS. For instance, low income was associated with a higher prevalence of CRS. The role of environmental factors in the development of CRS is unclear.

Anatomical Factors

Similar to adults, the osteomeatal complex is believed to be the critical anatomical structure in rhinosinusitis and is entirely present, though not at full size, in newborns. Studies in children and adults suggest that despite the common occurrence of anatomical variations such as pneumatized middle turbinate, Haller's cell, and the agger nasi cell, these do not seem to correlate with the degree and existence of CRS and most likely do not play a role in the pathophysiology of CRS.

Comorbidity

A number of pathological conditions may predispose to CRS in children (▸ Table 17.2).

Table 17.2 Pathological conditions that may predispose to CRS in children

AR	AR is a common coexisting disease in pediatric patients with CRS. The data about the association between the two diseases in children are variable. The causal relationship between allergies and CRS in children is still controversial and probably nonexistent.
Asthma	Asthma is another disease that is commonly associated with CRS in the pediatric age group. There are some studies supporting the concept that clinical control of CRS may be important in optimizing the control of difficult-to-treat asthma. However, the limitations of most available studies include the lack of good controls and randomization to different treatment modalities; therefore, the relationship between CRS and asthma in children remains largely descriptive.
GERD	GERD has been associated with rhinosinusitis in several studies. In a large case–control study, at Texas Children's hospital, 1,980 children with GERD and 7,920 controls (ages 2–18 y) were identified based on ICD-9 codes.[16] The number of cases with a concomitant diagnosis of sinusitis was significantly higher in the children with GERD (4.19%) compared to the control group (1.35%). The differential diagnosis between GERD and postnasal drip can be difficult. Although some evidence supports an association between GERD and CRS, more controlled studies are required to confirm this association and validate it. Routine antireflux treatment of children with CRS is not warranted based on current evidence.
Immunodeficiency	Abnormalities in immunity are frequently described in children with recurrent/chronic rhinosinusitis with IgG subclass deficiency and poor response to pneumococcal antigen being the most often reported. Therefore, it seems prudent to evaluate immune function in the child with recurrent/chronic rhinosinusitis with a total and subclass immunoglobulin quantitation, and titers to tetanus, diphtheria, and pneumococci. We usually measure titers for 23 common streptococcal serotypes. If responses are abnormal, a repeat set of titers 6 wk postpneumococcal vaccination is appropriate. We do not routinely evaluate immune function in every child with CRS and reserve this work-up for children with frequent infections in other organs such as otitis media and pneumonia, as well as children who have disease severe enough to consider surgical intervention. If abnormalities in humoral immunity are detected, the patient is managed jointly with colleagues from allergy/clinical immunology. Intravenous immunoglobulin therapy, usually administered monthly, has been used with success in some patients with documented immunodeficiencies. Another option is to consider prophylactic antibiotics.
Cystic fibrosis	Cystic fibrosis is a genetic disease with autosomal recessive inheritance that affects approximately 1 in 3,500 newborns. It is caused by a mutation in the *CFTR* gene on chromosome 7, which leads to disruption in cAMP-mediated chloride secretion in epithelial cells and exocrine glands. This leads to increased viscosity of secretions resulting in bronchiectasis, pancreatic insufficiency, CRS, and nasal polyposis. The prevalence of chronic sinusitis is very high and nasal polyps occur in 7–50% of affected patients.
PCD	The normal movement of mucus by mucociliary transport toward the natural ostia of the sinuses and eventually to the nasopharynx can be disrupted by any ciliary dysfunction or mucosal inflammation. The most common cause of severe ciliary dysfunction is PCD, an autosomal recessive disorder involving dysfunction of cilia and present in 1 of 15,000 of the population.[17] Half of the children with PCD also have situs inversus, bronchiectasis, CRS, and Kartagener's syndrome. The diagnosis should be suspected in a child with atypical asthma, bronchiectasis, chronic wet cough and mucus production, rhinosinusitis, and chronic and severe otitis media (especially with chronic drainage in children with ear tubes). Typically, the child already has these symptoms before the age of 6 mo. Screening tests for PCD include measuring nasal nitric oxide (very low levels). Specific diagnosis requires examination of cilia by light and electron microscopy, which is usually available only in specialized centers. The most commonly described structural abnormality involves lack of cilial outer dynein arms or a combined lack of both inner and outer dynein arms. Data on the prevalence of nasal polyps in patients with PCD are variable from none[18] to 25%.

Abbreviations: AR, allergic rhinitis; cAMP, cyclic adenosine monophosphate; CRS,chronic rhinosinusitis; GERD, gastroesophageal reflux disease; ICD-9, International Classification of Diseases, Ninth Revision; IgG, immunoglobulin G; PCD, primary ciliary dyskinesia; SNOT, Sino-Nasal Outcome Test.

Pathophysiology of Chronic Rhinosinusitis

Flora

The pathogens in CRS are difficult to identify due to low bacterial concentration rates and inconsistent data and because most cultures are obtained at the time of surgery after patients have had antibiotic therapy.

The most common bacterial species recovered during surgery are as follows:

- Alpha hemolytic streptococci.
- *S. pneumoniae.*
- *H. influenzae.*
- *M. catarrhalis.*
- *Staphylococcus aureus.*

Anaerobic organisms are grown from < 10% of specimens. The incidence of anaerobic organisms recovered increases with chronic infections.

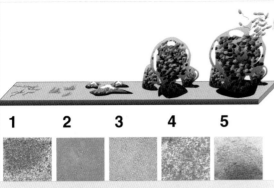

Fig. 17.13 Biofilm maturation is a complex developmental process involving five stages: stage 1, initial attachment; stage 2, irreversible attachment; stage 3, maturation I; stage 4, maturation II; stage 5, dispersion. Each stage of development in the diagram is paired with a photomicrograph of a developing *Pseudomonas aeruginosa* biofilm. All photomicrographs are shown to same scale. (Image credit D Davis. Reproduced from Monroe D. Looking for chinks in the armor of bacterial biofilms. PLoS Biol 2007;5(11):e307, with permission.)

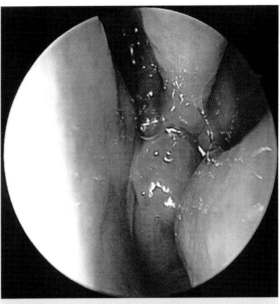

Fig. 17.14 Endoscopic picture of large adenoids blocking the left posterior choana and protruding into the nasal cavity.

Biofilms

The role of "biofilms" is now well documented in adults with rhinosinusitis, but more research is needed to clearly characterize their contribution to the pathophysiology of CRS in children.

Biofilms are complex aggregations of bacteria distinguished by a protective and adhesive matrix and have recently been implicated in CRS (▶ Fig. 17.13). They form when planktonic bacteria adhere and coalesce to various surfaces through glycoconjugate moieties and form well-organized ecosystems within the human host. Biofilms are also characterized by surface attachment, structural heterogeneity, genetic diversity, complex community interactions, and an extracellular matrix of polymeric substances, which all contribute to their resistance to antibiotic treatment. Intermittently, planktonic bacteria shed from the biofilm, migrate, and colonize other surfaces. It is therefore hypothesized that biofilms may provide a chronic reservoir for bacteria and may be responsible for the resistance to antibiotics seen in pediatric patients with CRS.

The Role of Adenoids

The adenoids are in close proximity to the paranasal sinuses. Adenoidectomy has been shown to be effective in resolving the symptoms in a proportion of children with CRS (see section on Adenoidectomy) (▶ Fig. 17.14). Data related to the role of adenoids in CRS are emerging but the studies are small and mostly evaluate the adenoids after their removal from the site. They do suggest a role for the adenoids in patients with CRS, both

from a bacteriological perspective and from an immunological perspective. Most of these studies, however, do not really shed light on the relative contribution of adenoiditis proper versus CRS in chronic nasal symptomatology in children.

When comparing middle meatal swabs and adenoid core cultures in children with hypertrophied adenoids and chronic or recurrent sinusitis, very similar bacteria can be found in both locations, suggesting that the bacterial reservoir in the adenoids mirrors the bacteriology isolated close to the paranasal sinuses in children. However, in children with nasal discharge who had a CT scan of the sinuses and underwent adenoidectomy, the results showed no correlation between the size of the adenoids and the severity of disease on CT scan. This suggests that the nasal discharge could be due to adenoiditis alone and that the bacterial reservoir of the adenoids more than their size was important in the relationship between CRS and the adenoids.

17.5.5 Diagnostic Work-Up for Chronic Rhinosinusitis

Clinical Evaluation

A complete physical examination should follow a careful medical and family history. The nasal examination in children should begin with anterior rhinoscopy and examination of the middle meatus and the inferior turbinates, noting the mucosal character and the presence of purulent drainage. This is often feasible in younger children using the otoscope fitted with the largest speculum.

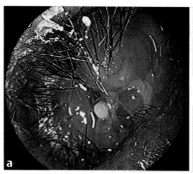
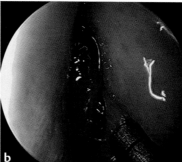

Fig. 17.15 (a) Adolescent female with nasal polyps protruding through the right nostril. (b) Endoscopic view of the left nostril shows polyps further back into the nasal cavity.

Topical decongestion may improve the view but may not always be tolerated in younger children.

Nasal endoscopy, which will allow superior visualization of the middle meatus, adenoid bed, and nasopharynx, is strongly recommended in children who are able to tolerate the examination. An oral cavity examination may reveal purulent drainage, cobblestoning of the posterior pharyngeal wall, or tonsillar hypertrophy.

> The finding of nasal polyps in children is unusual and, if seen upon examination (▶ Fig. 17.15), should raise suspicion for CF, PCD, or AFS.

Obviously, antrochoanal polyps occur in children, but those are usually unilateral and the rest of the sinuses are clear, which would help differentiate it from bilateral nasal polyposis (NP) with or without CF.

Allergy and Immunology Testing

Following the history and physical examination, appropriate diagnostic tests should be considered. Allergy skin testing or serological testing should be considered in children with CRS, particularly if there is evidence of AR.

Sensitization can be evaluated by measuring specific immunoglobulin E (IgE) in the serum or by skin prick tests. Both tests are equally reliable but measurement of serum-specific IgE is better tolerated in young children (involves only one blood draw) and is not affected by medication intake or skin conditions. Results of in vitro testing are usually available with 1 to 2 weeks, whereas skin test results are apparent within 15 minutes. Total IgE levels are elevated in 30 to 40% of individuals with AR but can also be elevated in other diseases such as worm infection, so total IgE alone cannot confirm or exclude allergy. It is important to realize that not all patients who have positive skin tests or elevated serum-specific IgE levels are considered to have AR.

> To make the diagnosis of AR, it is necessary to have both sensitization and a relevant clinical history.

Immunodeficiency testing should be pursued in children with recurrent or chronic disease, poor response to medical treatment, history of other infectious diseases (such as recurrent pneumonia or otitis media), or when unusual organisms are cultured from the sinus contents.

Imaging

> While the diagnosis of CRS in the pediatric population is generally made on clinical grounds, if imaging is necessary, CT is the modality of choice.

Findings on plain radiographs have been shown not to correlate well with those from CT scans in the context of chronic/recurrent sinus disease. In uncomplicated CRS, scanning is reserved to evaluate for residual disease and anatomical abnormalities after maximal medical therapy. Abnormalities in the CT scan are assessed in the context of their severity and correlation with the clinical picture and guide the plan for further management, which might include surgical intervention. In children with the clinical diagnosis of rhinosinusitis, the most commonly involved sinus is the maxillary sinus (99%) followed by the ethmoid sinus (91%).

Using the Lund–Mackay system (a commonly used CT staging system that quantitates sinus disease based on opacification of the sinuses and occlusion of the osteomeatal units and generates a score range from 0 for normal paranasal sinuses to 24 for pansinus opacification and occlusion of the osteomeatal units),[19] a cutoff score of 5 for diseased versus nondiseased patients offers a sensitivity and specificity of 86 and 85%, respectively, in making an appropriate diagnosis. Lund scores of 2 or less have an excellent negative predictive value, whereas scores of 5 or more have an excellent positive predictive value.

CT scans provide an anatomical road map for surgical treatment and are also useful for identifying areas of bony erosion or attenuation. Two examples of sinonasal diseases with characteristic radiological appearances are AFS and CF.

- In AFS, expansile disease may attenuate the bony skull base or orbital wall on CT scan. In addition, a speckled pattern of high attenuation (starry sky) on both soft-tissue and bone window settings correlates with the presence of thick allergic mucin and associated calcifications that may be noted intra-operatively (▶ Fig. 17.16, ▶ Fig. 17.17) MRI T1 images show low signal in areas of fungal mucin, and T2 images show central signal void in areas of fungal mucin with high signal in peripheral inflamed mucosa.
- In patients with CF, CT scans characteristically demon-strate pan-opacification of the sinuses and medial dis-placement of the lateral nasal wall, which may obstruct the nasal passages (▶ Fig. 17.18).

MRI of the sinuses, orbits, and brain should be performed whenever complications of rhinosinusitis are suspected.

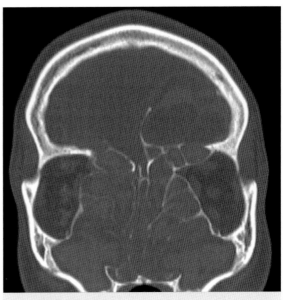

Fig. 17.16 Coronal computed tomography scan (bone win-dows) of a patient with allergic fungal rhinosinusitis. Note the complete opacification of the sinuses seen in this cut (ethmoid and maxillary) as well as bilateral nasal cavities that were completely filled with polyps. Also note extension of the process into the left frontal lobe area of the brain (right side of picture).

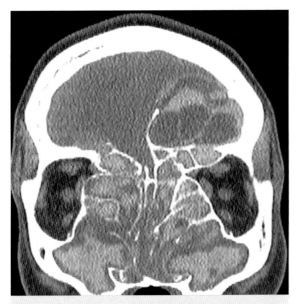

Fig. 17.17 Coronal computed tomography scan of the same patient showing the soft-tissue windows at the same level. Note the same extensive opacification of the sinuses and the typical speckled pattern of high attenuation that correlates with the presence of thick allergic mucin and associated calcifications. Again, extension of the process into the left frontal lobe area of the brain (right side of picture) is clear.

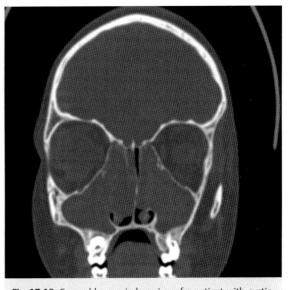

Fig. 17.18 Coronal bone window view of a patient with cystic fibrosis. Note the complete opacification of the maxillary and ethmoid sinuses and lack of any high attenuation. The osteomeatal bony anatomy is unrecognizable and the medial walls of the maxillary sinuses are bulging into the nasal cavities as a result of mucoceles within those sinuses from the inspissated secretions typical of patients with cystic fibrosis.

Physical examination and history alone do not help in differentiating between adenoiditis and CRS, especially in the younger child. As detailed previously, a high Lund–Mackay score (> 5) on the CT scan might be more suggestive of CRS than adenoiditis, but further studies are clearly required to help distinguish these two entities.

17.5.6 Management of Pediatric Chronic Rhinosinusitis

Medical Treatment of Chronic Rhinosinusitis in Children

Nasal Corticosteroids

There are no RCTs evaluating the effect of intranasal corticosteroids in children with CRS. However, the combination of proven efficacy of intranasal corticosteroids in CRS with and without nasal polyps in adults[20,21] and proven efficacy and safety of intranasal corticosteroids in AR in children makes intranasal corticosteroid the first line of treatment in CRS with or without nasal polyps (▶ Table 17.3; ▶ Fig. 17.19).[22,23]

Antibiotics

Short-Term Antibiotics

There is no good evidence in the literature to support the use of antibiotics in CRS in children.

Otten et al investigated 141 children between 3 and 10 years of age with CRS as defined by purulent nasal drainage lasting at least 3 months, signs of purulent rhinitis on rhinoscopy, and unilateral or bilateral abnormalities of the maxillary sinus on plain films.[24,25] The patients were

assigned nonselectively to receive one of the following four treatments for 10 days:
- Saline nose drops (placebo).
- Xylometazoline 0.5% nose drops with amoxicillin, 250 mg, orally, three times a day.
- Drainage of the maxillary sinus under anesthesia and irrigation through indwelling catheter for at least 5 days.
- A combination of drainage and irrigation with xylometazoline and amoxicillin.

They followed the patients for up to 26 weeks after treatment and there were no significant differences in cure rate among the treatments based on history, physical examination, or maxillary sinus films. In the total group, the cure rate was approximately 69%.

In a later study, the same group performed a randomized, double-blind study of cefaclor (20 mg/kg/day) versus placebo in 79 healthy children between the 2 and 12 years of age with chronic sinusitis defined essentially as in the first study. All patients had a tap and washout and were then randomized to cefaclor or placebo orally for 1 week and were followed at 6 weeks. After 6 weeks, there was no significant difference in resolution rate between the children on cefaclor (64.8%) and those on placebo (52.5%).

Despite the lack of good evidence to support the use of antibiotics for any length of time in children with CRS, in practice, these children are often treated with the same antibiotics listed in Chapter 17.4 but typically for longer periods of time that vary between 3 and 6 weeks. Because of the lack of data to support this practice, its usefulness must be weighed against the increasing risks of inducing antimicrobial resistance.

It is also difficult to ascertain whether what is actually being treated is CRS or acute exacerbations on top of pre-existing chronic disease. The exact type of antibiotics used is usually dependent on local resistance patterns that might be different in different countries. Furthermore, it is advisable to always treat with as narrow a spectrum of antibiotics as will likely cover the bacteria that are prevalent in a specific geographic locale.

Table 17.3 Treatment evidence and recommendations for children with chronic rhinosinusitis

Therapy	Level	Grade of recommendation	Relevance
Nasal saline irrigation	Ia	A	Yes
Therapy for gastroesophageal reflux	III	C	No
Topical corticosteroid	IV	D	Yes
Long-term oral antibiotic	No data	D	Unclear
Short-term oral antibiotic (< 4 wk)	Ib[a]	A[b]	No
Intravenous antibiotics	II[c]	C[d]	No

Source: Reproduced from Fokkens WJ, Lund VJ, Mullol J, et al. European position paper on rhinosinusitis and nasal polyps 2012. Rhinology 2012;50(Suppl 23):1–12, with permission.
[a]Study with negative outcome. [b]Grade A recommendation not to use. [c]Level III study with negative outcome. [d]Grade C recommendation not to use.

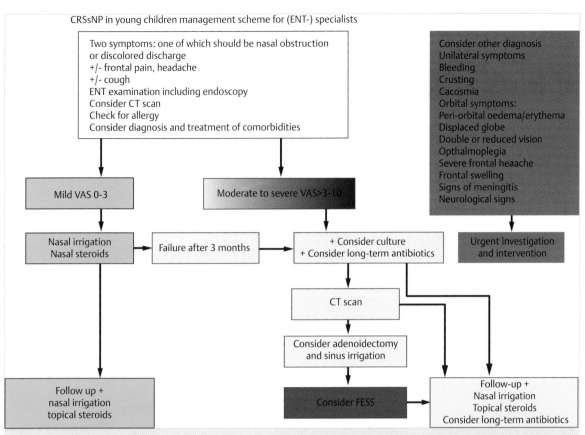

CRSsNP in young children management scheme for (ENT-) specialists

Two symptoms: one of which should be nasal obstruction
or discolored discharge
+/- frontal pain, headache
+/- cough
ENT examination including endoscopy
Consider CT scan
Check for allergy
Consider diagnosis and treatment of comorbidities

Consider other diagnosis
Unilateral symptoms
Bleeding
Crusting
Cacosmia
Orbital symptoms:
Peri-orbital oedema/erythema
Displaced globe
Double or reduced vision
Opthalmoplegia
Severe frontal heaache
Frontal swelling
Signs of meningitis
Neurological signs

Mild VAS 0-3

Moderate to severe VAS>3-10

Nasal irrigation
Nasal steroids

Failure after 3 months

+ Consider culture
+ Consider long-term antibiotics

Urgent investigation
and intervention

CT scan

Consider adenoidectomy
and sinus irrigation

Follow up +
nasal irrigation
topical steroids

Consider FESS

Follow-up +
Nasal irrigation
Topical steroids
Consider long-term antibiotics

Fig. 17.19 Management scheme for children with chronic rhinosinusitis without nasal polyposis. (Reproduced from Fokkens WJ, Lund VJ, Mullol J, et al. European position paper on rhinosinusitis and nasal polyps 2012. Rhinology 2012;50(Suppl 23), with permission.)

Available data do not justify the use of short-term oral antibiotics for the treatment of CRS in children (strength of recommendation: B).

Study design issues and the considerable side effects of this treatment do not justify the use of intravenous antibiotics alone for the treatment of CRS in children (strength of recommendation: C).

Long-Term Oral Antibiotic

There might a place for longer-term antibiotics for the treatment of CRS in children (equivalent to CRS in adults) (strength of recommendation: D). Possible antibiotics could be amoxicillin, macrolides, or cotrimoxazole.[26]

Intravenous Antibiotics

Intravenous antibiotic therapy for CRS resistant to maximal medical treatment has been studied as an alternative to endoscopic sinus surgery. In retrospective studies, intravenous antibiotics have been claimed to be successful in the treatment of CRS usually in combination with other treatments such as irrigation/aspiration of the sinus and adenoidectomy.

Nasal Saline Irrigation

A recent Cochrane review analyzed RCTs with a follow-up period of at least 3 months in which saline was evaluated in comparison with either no treatment, a placebo, or against other treatments.[27] Two trials satisfied inclusion criteria, both of which were conducted in adults. The review concluded that there is some benefit of daily, large volume saline irrigation with a hypertonic solution when compared with placebo, but no benefit of a low-volume nebulized saline spray over intranasal steroids. However, the quality of evidence was low.

A previous Cochrane review[28] included three trials that were conducted in children. The studies included a broad range of delivery techniques, tonicity of saline used, and comparator treatments.

Overall there was evidence that saline is beneficial in the treatment of the symptoms of CRS when used as the sole modality of treatment.

Evidence also exists in favor of saline as a treatment adjunct and saline was not as effective as an intranasal steroid. Various forms of administration of saline were well tolerated.

Unproven Treatments

Clinicians have certainly tried other treatments for CRS, including antihistamines and leukotriene modifiers, and antigastroesophageal reflux disease treatment. However, there are no good quality data about their potential efficacy in the context of CRS in children, and although widely used, particularly in primary care, they are of unproven benefit.

Pediatric Medical Evaluation

Interdisciplinary consultations are useful in evaluating the pediatric patient with medically refractory disease. Consultants may include those in the disciplines of allergy immunology, infectious disease, pulmonary disease, or genetics.

Treatment of Children with Cystic Fibrosis

In CF, CRS with and without nasal polyps is observed. The inflammatory profile of CRS in CF patients differs from CRS in patients without CF. Persistent colonization with *Pseudomonas aeruginosa* is a common finding. The paranasal sinuses often harbor distinct bacterial subpopulations, and in the early colonization phases, there seems to be a migration from the sinuses to the lower airways, suggesting that independent adaptation and evolution take place in the sinuses. The paranasal sinuses potentially constitute a protected niche of adapted clones of *P. aeruginosa*, which can intermittently seed the lungs and pave the way for subsequent chronic lung infections.

Due to a tendency to recur, repeated sinus surgery is often needed to achieve symptomatic relief. In CF patients, the paranasal sinuses may serve as a source for *P. aeruginosa* induced lung infections. Consequently, local antibiotic lavages after functional endoscopic sinus surgery (FESS) may help to prevent recurrent CRS and lung infection.

Surgery for Chronic Rhinosinusitis in Children

Surgical intervention for rhinosinusitis is usually considered for patients with CRS who have failed maximal medical therapy. This is hard to define but usually includes a course of antibiotics and intranasal and/or systemic steroids. Adenoidectomy, with or without antral irrigation and balloon sinus dilation, and FESS are the most commonly used modalities.

Adenoidectomy

The rationale behind removal of the adenoids in patients with CRS stems from the hypothesis that the adenoids are a nasopharyngeal bacterial reservoir and from the possibility that many of the symptoms might be related to adenoiditis proper. The benefit of adenoidectomy alone in the treatment of children with CRS was recently evaluated by a meta-analysis.[29]

All studies in the meta-analysis showed that sinusitis symptoms or outcomes improved in half or more patients after adenoidectomy.

The summary estimate of the proportion of patients who significantly improved after adenoidectomy was 69.3%.

Maxillary Antral Irrigation

Maxillary antral irrigation is frequently performed in conjunction with adenoidectomy. It has been suggested that antral irrigation adds to the efficacy of adenoidectomy.

Balloon sinuplasty was approved by the U.S. Food and Drug Administration for use in children in the United States in 2006, and a preliminary study in children has shown the procedure to be safe and feasible when addressing the maxillary sinus.

Whether or not balloon maxillary sinuplasty imparts additional benefit to irrigation alone, or in combination with adenoidectomy, cannot be established with available data to date (strength of recommendation: C).

Functional Endoscopic Sinus Surgery

A meta-analysis of FESS results in the pediatric population has shown that this surgical modality is effective in reducing symptoms with an 88% success rate and a low complication rate.[30] Initial concerns about possible adverse effects of FESS on facial growth have been allayed by a long-term follow-up study by Bothwell et al who showed no impact of FESS on qualitative and quantitative parameters of pediatric facial growth, evaluated up to 10 years postoperatively.[31] Many advocate a limited approach to FESS in children consisting of removal of any obvious obstruction (such as polyps and concha bullosa),

IV

as well as anterior bulla ethmoidectomy and maxillary antrostomy.

> ℹ
>
> This approach typically yields significant improvements in the following:
> - Nasal obstruction (91%).
> - Rhinorrhea (90%).
> - Postnasal drip (PND; 90%), headache (97%).
> - Hyposmia (89%).
> - Chronic cough (96%).

Whereas second-look procedures were common after FESS to clean the cavities, the advent of absorbable packing has made it possible to avoid a second-look procedure. There are a few reports on the causes of failure of ESS in children describing adhesions and maxillary sinus ostium stenosis or missed maxillary sinus ostium as the main issues. Sinonasal polyposis, history of AR, and male gender were significantly more frequently observed in the group that continued to have problems after ESS.

In children with CF, NP, antrochoanal polyposis, or AFS, FESS to decrease disease burden is the initial favored surgical option.

Surgical for Antrochoanal Polyp

Antrochoanal polyps are benign lesions that usually arise from the mucosa of the maxillary sinus, fill the sinus, and grow out of it into the nasal cavity, often reaching the posterior choana. Nasal obstruction is the main symptom. In comparison to NP, antrochoanal polyps are usually unilateral and appear in younger patients. Surgery is the indicated treatment for antrochoanal polyps, with endoscopic resection being the most recommended. Simple avulsion of the polyp has a high rate of recurrence, and full removal of the origin of the polyp in the maxillary sinus is necessary to prevent recurrence.

17.6 Allergic Rhinitis

AR is a common disease in children and has significant signs and symptoms that affect their quality of life as well as their ability to concentrate and learn effectively in school. It is a manifestation of the hypersensitivity of the nasal mucosa to foreign substances, mediated through IgE antibodies. It usually manifests with nasal and eye symptoms that include sneezing, runny nose, stuffy nose, and itching of the nose, throat, and ears, as well as eye tearing, redness, and itching. Because eye manifestations are often present, the disease is more commonly referred to as allergic rhinoconjunctivitis.

Available therapies are safe and effective and lead to an improvement in both symptoms and quality of life. These therapies include environmental controls, pharmacological therapy, and immunotherapy. AR is part of the allergic syndrome that also consists of conjunctivitis, asthma, atopic dermatitis, and food allergy. Moreover, AR is associated with a number of conditions in the upper airways such as adenoid hypertrophy (AH), tubal dysfunction, otitis media with effusion (OME), and rhinosinusitis. Clinical suspicion supplemented by specific diagnostic testing can identify the children who require allergy management.

17.6.1 Prevalence of Allergic Rhinitis

AR is the most common chronic condition in children and is most prevalent during school age. It is estimated to affect anywhere between 25 and 40% of the pediatric population in the western world. AR increases with age from early childhood to the beginning of adolescence. At the age of 13 years, almost half of all children with allergic parents and a quarter of those with nonallergic parents show symptoms of AR.

The prevalence of AR varies significantly throughout the world (► Table 17.4).

17.6.2 Quality of Life

> ℹ
>
> Although AR is not usually a severe disease, it alters the social life of patients and parents and affects school performance and sleep. Moreover, it is a major risk factor for developing asthma, and the costs incurred by rhinitis are substantial.

The Rhinoconjunctivitis Quality of Life Questionnaire for children and adolescents developed by Juniper et al is the most commonly used tool to measure quality of life in children.[32,33] A survey of 35,757 U.S. households, the "Pediatric Allergies in America" survey, focused on children with nasal allergy between 4 and 17 years of age. This showed a significantly lower percentage of allergic children being rated as having excellent health by their parents (43%) as compared to children without allergies (59%). Similarly, a lower proportions of children with allergies were described as "happy," "calm and peaceful," having "lots of energy," and being "full of life" as compared to children without allergies. Also, the proportion of children with diminished performance while at school as assessed by the parents was significantly higher in children with nasal allergies (40%) as compared to their nonallergic peers (11%).

Table 17.4 Reported rhinitis, hay fever, and rhinoconjunctivitis in 13- to 14-year-old children and change in reported symptoms in ISAAC Phase I and Phase III

Center	Phase III sample size	Hay fever ever		Rhinoconjunctivitis in the past year		Severe rhinoconjunctivitis in the past year	
		%	Change per year (%)	%	Change per year (%)	%	Change per year (%)
Africa (English speaking)	17,686	29.5	0.39	18.2	0.25	2.2	0.00
Africa (French speaking)	10,711	21.4	-0.26	21.7	1.07	3.2	0.31
China	7,044	5.9	0.19	10.4	0.33	0.3	0.04
Japan	2,520	30.6	0.99	17.6	0.34	1.0	0.02
South Korea	10,263	13.1	1.08	11.6	0.28	0.3	0.01
Iran	6,123	8.1	0.60	9.8	0.31	0.3	0.01
India	20,767	15.8	0.74	10.0	0.43	0.5	0.01
Brazil	15,681	24.9	0.61	15.8	-0.05	0.9	0.01
United States	4,920	33.3	-1.12	15.4	0.41	1.7	0.08
Finland	3,051	28.4	-0.10	15.5	0.04	0.4	-0.04
Georgia	2,650	3.8	-0.12	4.5	-0.01	0.5	0.04
Russia	3,769	3.2	0.08	11.7	0.65	0.9	0.05
New Zealand	13,317	39.8	0.48	18.0	-0.13	0.8	-0.01
Western Europe	82,844	21.2	0.31	14.5	0.02	0.5	0.00
Global total	304,679	22.1	0.3	15.1	0.18	1.0	0.01

Abbreviation: ISAAC, International Study of Asthma and Allergies in Childhood.
Source: Reproduced from Bjorksten B, Clayton T, Ellwood P, Stewart A, Strachan D. Worldwide time trends for symptoms of rhinitis and conjunctivitis: Phase III of the International Study of Asthma and Allergies in Childhood. Pediatr All Immunol 2008;19(2):110–124, with permission.

17.6.3 Classification

In the ARIA (Allergic Rhinitis and its Influence on Asthma, an international working group) guidelines,[34] AR is classified based on duration as follows:

- Intermittent (symptoms occurring less than 4 days a week *or* less than 4 weeks a year); or
- Persistent (symptoms occurring more than 4 days per week *and* for more than 4 weeks in a year).

Additionally, the rhinitis is classified based on the impact on quality of life as follows:

- Mild (the patient has normal sleep, daily activities, sport, leisure, work and school, and no troublesome symptoms); or
- Moderate to severe (the patient has abnormal sleep, impairment of daily activities, sport, and leisure, problems caused at work or school, and troublesome symptoms).

17.6.4 Pathogenesis of Allergic Rhinitis

Allergens

Allergic rhinoconjunctivitis in children is caused by indoor allergens (present throughout the year, such as house-dust mite and pet allergens) and outdoor allergens (seasonal, such as pollen from grass and trees). Food allergens in general do not cause allergic rhinoconjunctivitis.

Pathophysiology

The pathophysiological mechanisms in AR can be summarized in the following scenario:

- Sensitization of the nasal mucosa to a certain allergen entails multiple interactions among antigen-presenting cells, T lymphocytes, and B cells that lead to the production of antigen-specific IgE antibodies, which then localize to mast cells and basophils.
- Subsequent exposure leads to cross-linking of specific IgE receptors on mast cells and their resultant degranulation, with the release of a host of inflammatory mediators that are in large part responsible for allergic nasal symptoms.

Other proinflammatory substances are also generated after antigen exposure, the most prominent being eosinophil products and cytokines. Cytokines are thought to be generated in part by lymphocytes, which are abundant in resting and stimulated nasal mucosa, and also by mast cells, which have an important role in the storage, production, and secretion of cytokines. Cytokines upregulate adhesion molecules on the vascular endothelium, and possibly on marginating leukocytes, leading to the migration of these inflammatory cells into the site of tissue

IV

inflammation. Various cytokines also promote the chemotaxis and survival of these recruited inflammatory cells, leading to a secondary immune response by virtue of their capability to promote IgE synthesis by B cells.

Also important is the nervous system, which amplifies the allergic reaction by central and peripheral reflexes that result in changes at sites distant from those of antigen deposition, such as the eye, sinuses, and lower airway. These inflammatory changes lower the threshold of mucosal responsiveness to various specific and nonspecific stimuli, making allergic patients more responsive to stimuli to which they are exposed every day.

17.6.5 Diagnosis and Clinical Evaluation

History and Differential Diagnosis

> **i**
>
> The basis of the diagnosis of allergic rhinoconjunctivitis in children is the history.
>
> The most common symptoms of AR are recurrent episodes of sneezing, pruritus, rhinorrhea, nasal congestion, and watery and itchy eyes. Less common symptoms include itchy throat, itchy ears, and PND.

Children are often seen in the primary care doctor's office for a cough and malaise, and allergic rhinoconjunctivitis is only recognized when symptoms such as nasal congestion, discharge, and itch, and triggering factors are specifically queried for. The clinician should establish the pattern and timing of allergic symptoms as well as assess severity and interference with daily activities. Timing of symptoms during different seasons or after exposure to certain pets gives the physician an idea of the potential sensitizations of each particular patient. Perennial sensitization is a little more difficult to detect from history taking, but chronicity of symptoms may indicate perennial/persistent AR.

History should also be elicited about home and school environmental exposures, as well as the effectiveness of any prior allergy therapy. Allergic children have twice the likelihood of a history of asthma, eczema, chronic sinusitis, and OME compared to healthy children.

Children have 4 to 10 common colds per year. The typical duration of nasal symptoms during the common cold has been defined as < 10 days.[3]

> **i**
>
> Children whose nasal symptoms last longer than 10 days or those who seem to have colds all the time probably have allergic rhinoconjunctivitis.

Other causes of chronic nasal symptoms are AH (especially in the younger child) and CRS (more in the older child). In unilateral disease, uncommon causes such as unilateral choanal atresia, unnoticed foreign bodies, and tumors have to be taken into account.

Physical Examination

A complete ear, nose, and throat examination is required for children suspected of AR. Classic findings of AR in children include the following:
- Watery rhinorrhea.
- "Allergic shiners" (darkening of the lower eyelids as a result of suborbital edema).
- "Allergic salute" (the upward rubbing of the nose with the palm of the hand to relieve nasal itching).
- "Allergic crease" (a transverse white line across the nasal bridge caused by the allergic salute).
- Red watery eyes, a sign of conjunctivitis.

Anterior rhinoscopy using the largest speculum of the otoscope or a nasal speculum is very useful in evaluating the inferior and the middle turbinates. A pale nasal mucosal color is often very suggestive, though not pathognomonic, of AR, and children with allergies typically have clear, thin nasal drainage (▶ Fig. 17.20, ▶ Fig. 17.21). Nasal endoscopy can also be performed in the cooperative and willing child/adolescent. This examination allows

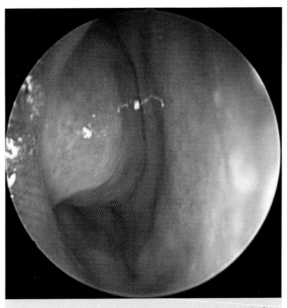

Fig. 17.20 View at anterior rhinoscopy of the right nostril of a patient with allergic rhinitis. The septum is seen on the right and the inferior turbinate on the left. Note significant obstruction of the nasal airway and thin clear secretions, and pale color of the nasal mucosa, which are common physical findings in patients with allergic rhinitis.

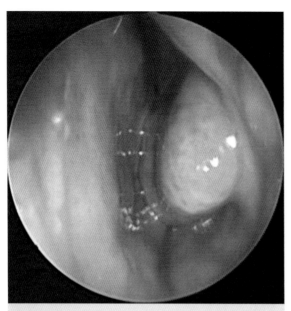

Fig. 17.21 View at anterior rhinoscopy of the left nostril of the same patient with allergic rhinitis. The septum is seen on the left and the inferior turbinate on the right. Typical findings similar to ▶ Fig. 17.19.

the appreciation of all the changes seen with anterior rhinoscopy and adds a thorough evaluation of the middle meatus for signs of sinusitis or NP, an appreciation of possible posterior septal abnormalities, and a good look at both posterior choanae and the adenoids. Mouth breathing is a common symptom, especially in children who also have concomitant AH. Investigations may include sensitivity testing as described previously. Imaging is rarely needed but may be dictated by the clinical findings, particularly if there is concomitant CRS with indication for surgery.

17.6.6 Comorbid Conditions and Allergic Rhinitis

AR is part of the allergic syndrome that also consists of conjunctivitis, asthma, atopic dermatitis, and food allergy. The sequential development of allergic disease manifestations during early childhood is often referred to as the atopic march. Children most often develop atopic dermatitis and food allergy first and asthma and rhinitis later.

Moreover, AR is associated with a number of conditions in the upper airways such as AH, Eustachian tubal dysfunction, OME, and rhinosinusitis.

Conjunctivitis

Most patients with AR also have conjunctivitis. Allergic conjunctivitis is more common with outdoor allergens than with indoor allergens. Patients complain of red,

itchy, and watery eyes. Eye problems are often overlooked by otorhinolaryngologists, but can affect daily life considerably; therefore, we always have to ask for them and treat them properly.

Oral Allergy Syndrome

Some pollen-sensitized individuals exhibit cross-reactivity to allergens present in pollen and foods, such as apples, nectarines, cherries, carrots, and celery. The symptoms are usually those of itching and swelling of the lips and tongue. Although the throat is sometimes affected, breathing is rarely compromised. This is the *oral allergy syndrome*. Cooking the food usually destroys allergenicity and prevents symptoms because the relevant proteins are heat-labile.

Patients will usually notice symptoms with some of these foods, but not all. A minority will experience more severe symptoms when exposed to certain foods, varying from generalized redness, itching and hives, gastrointestinal symptoms such as nausea, vomiting, and diarrhea, to respiratory symptoms, inability to swallow, and cardiovascular involvement, for example, low blood pressure and cardiac arrhythmias. Tree nuts and peanuts are best known for eliciting this potentially life-threatening response.

> **i**
>
> Avoidance is the only option until now; usually the help of a specialized dietician is mandatory, not only to instruct parents regarding how to avoid the involved foods but also to prevent unnecessary food avoidance and dietary shortcomings, especially in young children. Patients with a life-threatening response supported by evidence of elevated specific IgE to the offending allergen are counseled about avoidance and supplied with an epinephrine injection that they can use in case of emergencies to avoid severe airway compromise.

Otitis Media

> **i**
>
> The significant incidence of atopy associated with OME has suggested a role of allergy in the pathogenesis of OME.

Analysis of inflammatory mediators indicates that the mucosa of the middle ear can respond to antigen in the same way as does the mucosa of the lower respiratory tract. It remains difficult to interpret epidemiological data as we cannot estimate the extent to which the enhanced prevalence of allergy in otitis media patients reported by some authors represents a true finding or rather reflects a referral bias.

Adenoids

Little is known about the correlation between AR and AH in children. Children with AR appear to have a greater susceptibility to AH than nonallergic children. In view of the different therapeutic approach to these problems, it is important to recognize the possibility of AR in children prior to adenoidectomy to avoid parental dissatisfaction if complete control of symptoms is not achieved after surgery. Nasal corticosteroids are capable of reducing adenoid-related symptoms irrespective of atopic status in children, although the effect on symptoms is small. In these studies, the effects of nasal steroids on symptoms of allergic inflammation in the nose and adenoid cannot be dissociated from their anti-inflammatory effects on the adenoid itself.

Asthma

Asthma begins most often in infants as wheezing with respiratory infections. Most children with mild intermittent asthma will outgrow their condition or will have mild episodic asthma. The early commencement of an anti-inflammatory therapy, such as inhaled corticosteroids, may prevent progression of the disease. More severe disease and continued allergen exposure cause persistence.

In the *Pediatric Allergies in America* survey, children with AR were threefold more likely to have an asthma diagnosis and four times more likely to have had asthma in the last 12 months compared with their nonallergic counterparts.[35]

> According to the ARIA guideline,[34] all patients with AR, including children, should be evaluated for asthma through history, chest examination, and, if possible and when necessary, the assessment of airflow obstruction before and after a bronchodilator.

It is important not only to assess whether the patient has symptoms of lower airway disease but also to ascertain that the disease is well controlled in patients who are known to have asthma.

17.6.7 Treatment of Allergic Rhinoconjunctivitis in Children

Management includes *education* of the patient and parent(s), *avoidance of allergens* and *tobacco smoke*, and *pharmacotherapy*. A stepwise approach is recommended, which depends on the severity of the disorder, the patient's preferences and adherence to treatment, and the presence of comorbidities such as asthma.

Allergen Avoidance

Few studies are available on the effect of allergen avoidance in children with allergic rhinoconjunctivitis. A Cochrane review on house-dust mite avoidance measures for perennial AR in adults and children found that acaricides and extensive bedroom-based environmental control programs might reduce symptoms of AR for some people, but the evidence is not strong.[36] Only two small studies examined the effects of avoidance of pet allergens in children with allergic rhinoconjunctivitis. One found no effect, and the other showed some effect of a combined intervention for mites and pets.

It seems prudent to avoid owning a pet if the household includes a child with documented pet allergies. It is also reasonable and inexpensive to avoid upholstered furniture, curtains, and soft toys in the bedroom of an allergic child.

Medical Treatment of Allergic Rhinitis

Intranasal Glucocorticosteroids

> Intranasal glucocorticosteroids are the most effective treatment of allergic rhinoconjunctivitis in adults and children. They reduce nose and eye symptoms and the use of other drugs and improve overall daily functioning. They are more effective than antihistamines.

Most guidelines suggest the use of these agents as first line in moderate-to-severe disease and even in some cases of mild AR. Efficacy begins at 7 to 8 hours after administration, and starting these agents a few days before the start of the season has been recommended.

The most common local side effect is epistaxis. Application of a nasal cream usually solves the problem. Normal daily doses of most intranasal glucocorticosteroids have no systemic side effects in children. Growth retardation was not seen with 1 year of treatment with the newer corticosteroids such as fluticasone and mometasone. However, intranasal beclomethasone for 1 year was associated with a reduced growth rate, so this drug should be avoided in children.

> The authors prefer to use the agents that have been proven to have the least systemic absorption and the safety of which has been established in young children. These include mometasone furoate, fluticasone propionate, and fluticasone furoate. The duration of therapy depends on the symptoms. In seasonal disease, initiate intranasal steroids a week or so before the season and maintain it until the end of the season. In perennial/persistent disease, keep the patient on the agents all year long.

Antihistamines

- Second-generation H1 oral antihistamines such as (levo)cetirizine and (des)loratadine are effective and safe for treating allergic rhinoconjunctivitis in children. However, these agents have little or no effect on nasal congestion. They reduce malaise and may improve learning ability.
- First-generation oral H1 antihistamines should not be used because of their effects on the central nervous system.
- Intranasal antihistamines (azelastine and olopatadine) are also available for use in children for the treatment of AR. The efficacy of these agents is comparable to other antihistamines, and they might be more effective than oral antihistamines for nasal congestion. They are usually given twice daily and might cause somnolence. Taste alteration may occur immediately after use with an incidence as high as 20%.

Decongestants

Topical as well as systemic decongestants act to cause vascular constriction and reduce the nasal blood supply by alpha-adrenergic stimulation. Prolonged use of the intranasal agents can lead to rebound nasal congestion, also known as rhinitis medicamentosa.

> The use of local decongestants should be limited to situations where severe allergic nasal congestion precludes the administration of other intranasal medications, and not be given for more than a week.

In these cases, a short 3- to 5-day course of intranasal decongestants is used in conjunction with other intranasal agents (steroids, antihistamines) to facilitate access to the nasal mucosa. Systemic decongestants should not be used in children.

Immunotherapy in Children

> Subcutaneous allergen immunotherapy (SCIT) and sublingual allergen immunotherapy (SLIT) are effective for the treatment of AR in adults.[37] The levels of evidence of SCIT efficacy in children are low. In the last two decades, some evidence supporting the efficacy and safety of SLIT as an alternative treatment for seasonal allergic rhinoconjunctivitis in the pediatric population has been published, but the quality of the studies is low.[38]

The principle that underlies desensitization therapy is exposure to low doses of the offending allergen over a period of time either subcutaneously (SCIT) or sublingually (SLIT). This leads to changes in the immune system and eventual tolerance to the allergen in question with disappearance of symptoms after external exposure. Most practitioners administer such therapy for a 3- to 5-year period. Studies in adults, and some in children, support the concept that immunotherapy alters the natural history of allergic disease as demonstrated by the persistence of symptom control after discontinuation of a 3- to 5-year course of therapy.

Other Drugs

No other drugs are currently recommended.
- Disodium cromoglycate is available over the counter but is less effective than intranasal steroids or antihistamines. Another disadvantage is that it needs to be taken four to six times a day.
- The leukotriene receptor antagonist montelukast is more effective than placebo—it is as effective as oral H1 antihistamines but inferior to nasal steroids. Its use is not advocated in the treatment of AR alone because of the costs and the lack of data on long-term effects. It is used in the treatment of asthma in children.

17.7 Key Points

- ARS is most often viral in etiology and self-limited.
- Few viral ARS episodes progress to bacterial ARS.
- Most episodes of bacterial ARS are also self-limited and will resolve spontaneously.
- Antibiotic therapy seems to accelerate resolution of ARS, but whether an acceleration of improvement of the symptoms with antibiotics in these children is worth the increased risk of antimicrobial resistance remains to be determined.
- Intranasal steroids might have a beneficial ancillary role in the treatment of ARS.
- Other ancillary therapies have not been shown to be helpful in ARS.
- CRS has a negative impact on quality of life.
- A CT scan abnormality does not always correspond with clinical CRS in children.
- Biofilms and/or intracellular resident bacteria increase resistance to standard therapy.
- The inflammatory reaction in the sinus tissues of children with CRS is rich in lymphocytes and exhibits less eosinophilia and epithelial disruption compared to adults.
- Adenoidectomy is successful in improving CRS in 50% of operated children. Whether this is due to the fact that the symptoms were related to adenoiditis per se or to the elimination of the contribution of the adenoids to sinus disease is not clear.

IV

- In children with CF, NP, antrochoanal polyposis, or AFS, FESS to decrease disease burden is the initial favored surgical option.
- In CF patients, the paranasal sinuses may serve as a source for *P. aeruginosa* induced lung infections. Local antibiotic lavages after FESS may help to prevent recurrent CRS and lung infection.

References

[1] Spaeth J, Krügelstein U, Schlöndorff G. The paranasal sinuses in CT-imaging: development from birth to age 25. Int J Pediatr Otorhinolaryngol. 1997; 39(1):25–40

[2] Orlandi RR, Kingdom TT, Hwang PH, et al. International consensus statement on allergy and rhinology: rhinosinusitis. Int Forum Allergy Rhinol. 2016; 6 Suppl 1:S22–S209

[3] Fokkens WJ, Lund VJ, Mullol J, et al. EPOS 2012: European position paper on rhinosinusitis and nasal polyps 2012. A summary for otorhinolaryngologists. Rhinology. 2012; 50(1):1–12

[4] Kristo A, Uhari M, Luotonen J, et al. Paranasal sinus findings in children during respiratory infection evaluated with magnetic resonance imaging. Pediatrics. 2003; 111(5 Pt 1):e586–e589

[5] Falagas ME, Giannopoulou KP, Vardakas KZ, Dimopoulos G, Karageorgopoulos DE. Comparison of antibiotics with placebo for treatment of acute sinusitis: a meta-analysis of randomised controlled trials. Lancet Infect Dis. 2008; 8(9):543–552

[6] Barlan IB, Erkan E, Bakir M, Berrak S, Başaran MM. Intranasal budesonide spray as an adjunct to oral antibiotic therapy for acute sinusitis in children. Ann Allergy Asthma Immunol. 1997; 78(6):598–601

[7] Meltzer EO, Bachert C, Staudinger H. Treating acute rhinosinusitis: comparing efficacy and safety of mometasone furoate nasal spray, amoxicillin, and placebo. J Allergy Clin Immunol. 2005; 116(6):1289–1295

[8] Shaikh N, Wald ER. Decongestants, antihistamines and nasal irrigation for acute sinusitis in children. Cochrane Database Syst Rev. 2014 (10):CD007909

[9] Unuvar E, Tamay Z, Yildiz I, et al. Effectiveness of erdosteine, a second generation mucolytic agent, in children with acute rhinosinusitis: a randomized, placebo controlled, double-blinded clinical study. Acta Paediatr. 2010; 99(4):585–589

[10] Surda P, Fokkens WJ. Novel, alternative and controversial therapies of rhinitis. Immunol Allergy Clin North Am. 2016; 36(2):401–423

[11] van der Veken PJ, Clement PA, Buisseret T, Desprechins B, Kaufman L, Derde MP. CT-scan study of the incidence of sinus involvement and nasal anatomic variations in 196 children. Rhinology. 1990; 28(3):177–184

[12] Cunningham MJ, Chiu EJ, Landgraf JM, Gliklich RE. The health impact of chronic recurrent rhinosinusitis in children. Arch Otolaryngol Head Neck Surg. 2000; 126(11):1363–1368

[13] Rudnick EF, Mitchell RB. Long-term improvements in quality-of-life after surgical therapy for pediatric sinonasal disease. Otolaryngol Head Neck Surg. 2007; 137(6):873–877

[14] Biagini JM, LeMasters GK, Ryan PH, et al. Environmental risk factors of rhinitis in early infancy. Pediatr Allergy Immunol. 2006; 17(4):278–284

[15] Kvaerner KJ, Nafstad P, Jaakkola JJ. Otolaryngological surgery and upper respiratory tract infections in children: an epidemiological study. Ann Otol Rhinol Laryngol. 2002; 111(11):1034–1039

[16] El-Serag HB, Gilger M, Kuebeler M, Rabeneck L. Extraesophageal associations of gastroesophageal reflux disease in children without neurologic defects. Gastroenterology. 2001; 121(6):1294–1299

[17] Barbato A, Frischer T, Kuehni CE, et al. Primary ciliary dyskinesia: a consensus statement on diagnostic and treatment approaches in children. Eur Respir J. 2009; 34(6):1264–1276

[18] Alanin MC, Aanaes K, Høiby N. et al. Sinus surgery can improve quality of life, lung infections, and lung function in patients with primary ciliary dyskinesia. Int Forum Allergy Rhinol. 2016 [Epub ahead of print].

[19] Lund VJ, Mackay IS. Staging in rhinosinusitus. Rhinology. 1993; 31 (4):183–184

[20] Chong LY, Head K, Hopkins C, Philpott C, Schilder AGM, Burton MJ. Intranasal steroids versus placebo or no intervention for chronic rhinosinusitis. Cochrane Database Syst Rev. 2016; 4(4):CD011996

[21] Chong LY, Head K, Hopkins C, Philpott C, Burton MJ, Schilder AGM. Different types of intranasal steroids for chronic rhinosinusitis. Cochrane Database Syst Rev. 2016; 4(4):CD011993

[22] Meltzer EO, Tripathy I, Máspero JF, Wu W, Philpot E. Safety and tolerability of fluticasone furoate nasal spray once daily in paediatric patients aged 6–11 years with allergic rhinitis: subanalysis of three randomized, double-blind, placebo-controlled, multicentre studies. Clin Drug Investig. 2009; 29(2):79–86

[23] Schenkel EJ, Skoner DP, Bronsky EA, et al. Absence of growth retardation in children with perennial allergic rhinitis after one year of treatment with mometasone furoate aqueous nasal spray. Pediatrics. 2000; 105(2):E22

[24] Otten FW, Grote JJ. Treatment of chronic maxillary sinusitis in children. Int J Pediatr Otorhinolaryngol. 1988; 15(3):269–278

[25] Otten HW, Antvelink JB, Ruyter de Wildt H, Rietema SJ, Siemelink RJ, Hordijk GJ. Is antibiotic treatment of chronic sinusitis effective in children? Clin Otolaryngol Allied Sci. 1994; 19(3):215–217

[26] Delacourt C, Grimprel E, Cohen R. Antibiotic prophylaxis in pediatric pulmonology (excluding cystic fibrosis): which indications for rotating (or alternating) antibiotics and prolonged antibiotic therapy? [in French]. Arch Pediatr. 2013; 20 Suppl 3:S99–S103

[27] Chong LY, Head K, Hopkins C, et al. Saline irrigation for chronic rhinosinusitis. Cochrane Database Syst Rev. 2016; 4(4):CD011995

[28] Harvey R, Hannan SA, Badia L, Scadding G. Nasal saline irrigations for the symptoms of chronic rhinosinusitis. Cochrane Database Syst Rev. 2007(3):CD006394

[29] Brietzke SE, Brigger MT. Adenoidectomy outcomes in pediatric rhinosinusitis: a meta-analysis. Int J Pediatr Otorhinolaryngol. 2008; 72 (10):1541–1545

[30] Hebert RL, II, Bent JP, III. Meta-analysis of outcomes of pediatric functional endoscopic sinus surgery. Laryngoscope. 1998; 108(6):796–799

[31] Bothwell MR, Piccirillo JF, Lusk RP, Ridenour BD. Long-term outcome of facial growth after functional endoscopic sinus surgery. Otolaryngol Head Neck Surg. 2002; 126(6):628–634

[32] Juniper EF, Guyatt GH, Dolovich J. Assessment of quality of life in adolescents with allergic rhinoconjunctivitis: development and testing of a questionnaire for clinical trials. J Allergy Clin Immunol. 1994; 93(2):413–423

[33] Juniper EF, Howland WC, Roberts NB, Thompson AK, King DR. Measuring quality of life in children with rhinoconjunctivitis. J Allergy Clin Immunol. 1998; 101(2 Pt 1):163–170

[34] Brozek JL, Bousquet J, Baena-Cagnani CE, et al. Global Allergy and Asthma European Network, Grading of Recommendations Assessment, Development and Evaluation Working Group. Allergic Rhinitis and its Impact on Asthma (ARIA) guidelines: 2010 revision. J Allergy Clin Immunol. 2010; 126(3):466–476

[35] Meltzer EO, Blaiss MS, Derebery MJ, et al. Burden of allergic rhinitis: results from the Pediatric Allergies in America survey. J Allergy Clin Immunol. 2009; 124(3) Suppl:S43–S70

[36] Sheikh A, Hurwitz B, Nurmatov U, van Schayck CP. House dust mite avoidance measures for perennial allergic rhinitis. Cochrane Database Syst Rev. 2010(7):CD001563

[37] Calderon MA, Gerth van Wijk R, Eichler I, et al. European Academy of Allergy and Clinical Immunology. Perspectives on allergen-specific immunotherapy in childhood: an EAACI position statement. Pediatr Allergy Immunol. 2012; 23(4):300–306

[38] Calderon MA, Penagos M, Sheikh A, Canonica GW, Durham SR. Sublingual immunotherapy for allergic conjunctivitis: Cochrane systematic review and meta-analysis. Clin Exp Allergy. 2011; 41(9):1263–1272

18 Tongue, Floor of Mouth, Adenoids, and Tonsils

Sujata De

18.1 Introduction

This chapter provides a brief overview of some common pediatric oral and oropharyngeal conditions. It also describes the indications and principles of surgery for adenoids and tonsils.

18.2 Tongue-Tie (Ankyloglossia)

18.2.1 Definition and Prevalence

This is a congenital condition in which the lingual frenulum is abnormally short, resulting in reduced mobility of the tip of the tongue (▶ Fig. 18.1). The prevalence has been reported to be up to 11%, depending upon the definition and whether the finding is actively sought. It is commoner in males.[1] Diagnosis can be difficult particularly in an infant. The short frenulum restricts passive attempts to elevate the tongue. The parents or carer may have noticed a notch in the tongue or a heart shape to the tongue when the infant attempts to protrude it. In an older cooperative child, there is obvious restriction of protrusion and elevation. There have been some attempts to quantify or grade the degree of tongue-tie but there are obvious difficulties with this in an infant.

18.2.2 Effects

The symptoms of a tongue-tie relate to decreased mobility of the tongue tip. There is much controversy surrounding how much of an impact this has upon functions such as feeding and speech. Tongue tip mobility is required to produce lingual sounds (e.g., t, d, n) and sibilants (e.g., s, z). Children with ankyloglossia usually develop compensatory mechanisms to overcome the reduced mobility that allows them to produce these sounds. The overall effect of tongue-tie on speech is uncertain, and speech and language therapists seem to be divided upon whether or not there is a significant impact upon speech or on whether surgery for tongue-tie improves articulation.[2,3] There has certainly been an increased awareness of an effect upon breast-feeding in recent years,[4] with many reports of improved outcomes following release of the tight frenulum probably because the infant can then develop an improved "latch" to the breast during feeding.[5,6] Tongue-tie can also have an impact upon bottle-feeding. Other symptoms are mechanical and social and include the child not being able to clean his/her teeth with his/her tongue, a gap between the lower incisors, which can cause aesthetic concern, inability to protrude the tongue, difficulty playing wind instruments, and inability to "French kiss."

18.2.3 Management

> Treatment is only indicated if there are troublesome symptoms (including social ones). Many older children with tongue-tie, especially if the frenulum is only slightly shortened, need no treatment. Presumptive treatment in the newborn to avoid future symptoms is controversial.
>
> It is the author's practice to offer division in the outpatient setting to all infants with a tongue-tie below the age of 6 months, following a discussion with the parents concerning the current evidence base for treatment.
>
> The treatment is essentially division of the frenulum (*frenotomy*), which is more often than not a thin fibrous band.

Provided the surgeon is adequately trained and experienced, frenotomy can be performed safely in neonates (and infants) without the need for any local or general anesthesia. In an older child, general anesthesia is required. There have been some case reports of severe complications such as profuse bleeding and even infection leading to Ludwig's angina when the division was carried out by untrained personnel.[7] In some children, the frenulum can be very thick and a *frenuloplasty* (horizontal to vertical or Z-plasty) may be indicated.

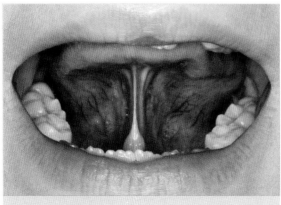

Fig. 18.1 Tongue-tie.

18.3 Macroglossia

18.3.1 Definition and Classification

> **i**
>
> Macroglossia is defined as protrusion of the tongue beyond the incisors in the resting state.

In *true macroglossia* (▶ Fig. 18.2) the tongue is enlarged, whereas in *pseudomacroglossia*, the tongue is of normal size but appears large as it protrudes beyond the incisors. True macroglossia can be:

- *Primary*, when there is hypertrophy or hyperplasia of the tongue musculature; or
- *Secondary*, where there is infiltration of normal tongue musculature with abnormal elements.

Causes of primary macroglossia include *Beckwith-Wiedemann's syndrome* and *hypothyroidism*, whereas secondary macroglossia is caused by *lymphatic malformations*, *hemangioma*, *neurofibroma*, metabolic disorders such as *mucopolysaccharidosis*, and *lipid storage diseases*.

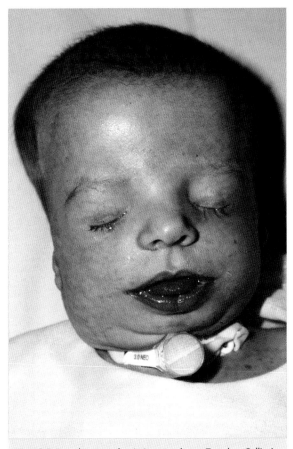

Fig. 18.2 Pseudomacroglossia in a newborn. Treacher Collins' syndrome.

Pseudomacroglossia may be due to *micrognathia* or poor muscle control as can occur in children with *hypotonia*. This is seen in Down's syndrome, some cases of cerebral palsy, and Pierre Robin sequence (see Chapter 27). It usually improves with age.

Symptoms of macroglossia in children include *drooling*, *speech* and *swallowing difficulties*, *anterior open bite*, *ulceration and necrosis of the exposed mucosa*, and *airway obstruction*. Moreover, the appearance can lead to social isolation, teasing, and bullying.

18.3.2 Management

> **i**
>
> Children who present with macroglossia may need investigations under the supervision of a pediatrician. The otolaryngologist may be asked to intervene if there is a significant functional issue such as airway obstruction or a disorder of speech articulation, or to address aesthetic concerns.

Children with airway obstruction due to macroglossia or pseudomacroglossia may require airway intervention such as an oropharyngeal (Guedel) airway, endotracheal intubation, or very occasionally tracheostomy particularly in the event of an acute deterioration, for example, during the course of a severe upper respiratory tract infection.

Surgical reduction of the tongue (partial glossectomy) under the care of an experienced team with appropriate support facilities is a safe procedure with relatively good results and low morbidity[8,9] This usually involves removing a wedge of tongue musculature from the anterior part of the tongue (▶ Fig. 18.3), often combined with dorsoventral reduction to reduce the thickness. There is a requirement for adjuvant speech and language therapy and also ongoing psychological support.

A variety of lesions can present as a swelling on the tongue and may need surgical excision (e.g., pyogenic granuloma; ▶ Fig. 18.4).

18.4 Ranula

18.4.1 Etiology and Presentation

A ranula is an extravasation mucocele that arises from the sublingual salivary gland either from a ruptured main duct or from ruptured acini following obstruction (▶ Fig. 18.5). The sublingual gland produces a steady flow of mucous even without stimulation. As the mucous extravasates, an inflammatory reaction takes place that creates a fibrotic pseudocapsule. When the extravasation is limited to the floor of the mouth, it leads to a painless swelling in the floor of the mouth. In some cases, the

V

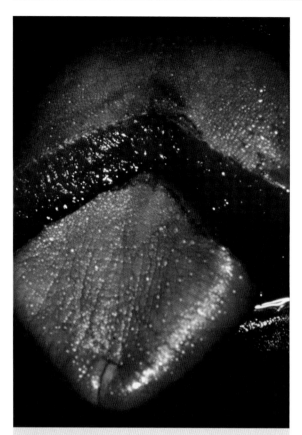

Fig. 18.3 Wedge excision of the tongue, a rarely needed treatment for macroglossia.

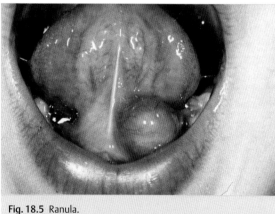

Fig. 18.5 Ranula.

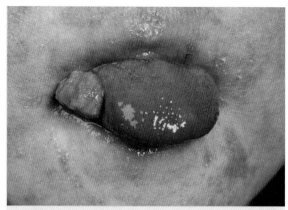

Fig. 18.4 Macroglossia in a child with Down's syndrome. A pyogenic granuloma has developed on the exposed tongue mucosa.

sound may help delineate the cyst and rule out rarer causes of intraoral swellings.

> **i**
>
> Treatment is surgical.

Incision and drainage alone has been shown to be successful in approximately 25% of neonates treated this way. It may be an acceptable treatment in this age group where more extensive surgery may result in complications associated with bleeding. Incision and drainage combined with marsupialization, that is, the incised edges of the cyst are sutured to adjacent tissue to minimize the risk of the cyst filling up again, gives a lower recurrence risk, but recurrence is least likely to occur when the ipsilateral sublingual gland is excised.[10,11,12] Success rates are approximately 95% if the sublingual gland is removed. Complications of this procedure are uncommon but include infection, bleeding, and rarely lingual nerve trauma leading to hypoesthesia of the anterior tongue.

18.5 Adenoids and Tonsils

18.5.1 Applied Physiology

Adenoids and tonsils form part of the Waldeyer's ring of lymphoid tissue in the oropharynx and nasopharynx. The function of these structures remains unclear but is thought to play a role in the development of B cells as part of the immune response. It is thought that this immune function peaks in early childhood and after that involution occurs associated with replacement of lymphoid tissue with fibrous tissue. There has been much discussion on the exact age at which the immune function declines without any real resolution.

extravasation extends through a hiatus in the mylohyoid muscle into the neck and forms a "plunging" ranula. This presents with a swelling in the neck.

18.4.2 Management

The diagnosis is clinical. Occasionally, a localized lymphatic malformation can cause confusion, and an ultra-

Biofilms are microbial communities that attach to surfaces and produce their own protective matrix. This enables the microbes to have increased resistance to environmental factors such as extremes of temperature, humidity, and light. This also confers increased resistance to antimicrobial therapy and to phagocytosis.[13] Biofilms have been demonstrated in up to 73% of enlarged tonsils removed from children for both recurrent tonsillitis and obstructive sleep apnea (OSA).[14] Biofilms may contribute to the development of tonsillar hyperplasia.

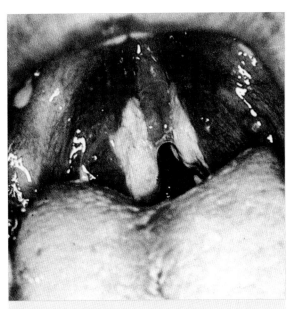

Fig. 18.6 Acute tonsillitis.

18.5.2 Acute Tonsillitis

Acute tonsillitis is a common infection of childhood and usually begins with a viral infection that may then lead to an acute bacterial infection. Acute infection causes obstruction or inflammation of the tonsillar crypts, leading to accumulation of debris and multiplication of bacterial flora leading to inflammation and pus exudates. *Streptococcus pyogenes* is the commonest bacterial organism associated with acute tonsillitis. However, up to 40% of children have positive cultures for this bacterium without evidence of active disease.

Symptoms and signs of acute bacterial tonsillitis include swelling, erythema, and exudate on the tonsils (▶ Fig. 18.6) in association with pain on swallowing, fever, and cervical lymphadenopathy. Penicillin V is the treatment of choice.

Viral tonsillitis can be caused by rhinovirus, adenovirus, enterovirus, and influenza virus. Infection caused by these organisms presents in much the same way as bacterial tonsillitis but usually is not associated with exudate.

Infection with Epstein–Barr virus causes enlarged tonsils with a coalescent exudate in association with posterior (often dramatic) cervical lymphadenopathy, fever, fatigue, and hepatosplenomegaly, a condition known as infectious mononucleosis. In this condition, amoxicillin can cause a generalized skin rash and should be avoided. There is a risk of airway obstruction.

18.5.3 Adenotonsillectomy

Adenotonsillectomy remains one of the commonest surgical procedures performed in children. An increasingly common indication for both adenoidectomy and tonsillectomy in children now is sleep-disordered breathing (see Chapter 19).

This chapter will focus primarily upon the other indications for tonsillectomy in children, surgical techniques, perioperative management, complications of surgery, and outcomes.

Indications for Adenotonsillectomy

Assessment of a child for (adeno)tonsillectomy begins with a history of one or more of the indications listed in Box 18.1 and Box 18.2.

Examination includes assessment of stertor, mouth breathing, and reduced nasal airflow, which are all indicators of nasal obstruction.

Some parents will bring videos of their child asleep demonstrating snoring and possible episodes of OSA. The adenoids themselves can only be viewed by using a postnasal mirror, something that is very rarely used and is not well tolerated by children, or nasendoscopy with a rigid or flexible nasendoscope. Tonsils can be assessed by asking the child to open his/her mouth and say "aah." This depresses the tongue and lifts the soft palate, allowing a view of the oropharynx without the need for a tongue depressor. Occasionally, a tongue depressor or wooden spatula is required to see the tonsils. Note the size and the nature of the uvula (a bifid uvula may be an indicator of a submucous cleft palate). A commonly used grading system for assessing the size of tonsils is the Brodsky Grading Scale.[15] The size of the tonsils are graded from 1 to 4 depending upon the percentage of the oropharyngeal airway that is occupied by the tonsils:

- Grade 1: ≤ 25%.
- Grade 2: 26 to 50%.
- Grade 3: 51 to 75%.
- Grade 4: > 75%.

This scale has been demonstrated to have good inter- and intraobserver reliability.[16]

Adenoid size has been a little more difficult to standardize given the difficulty in assessment in an outpatient setting. Attempts have been made using lateral skull X-rays, acoustic rhinometry, and assessment with flexible nasendoscopy intraoperatively. A recently proposed grading system by Parikh et al grades the adenoids as seen in outpatients with an endoscope and may be useful as a standard for reporting clinical outcome studies[17]:

- Grade 1: adenoid tissue not in contact with surrounding structures.
- Grade 2: adenoid tissue in contact with Eustachian tube cushions.
- Grade 3: adenoid tissue in contact with vomer.
- Grade 4: adenoid tissue in contact with soft palate.

Adenoidectomy and tonsillectomy are often undertaken together, but the indications for each may be different for each procedure. It is important to assess the need for each on its own merits rather than routinely combining the two, as each is associated with potential morbidity.

Box 18.1 Indications for Adenoidectomy

- Sleep-disordered breathing/OSA (see Chapter 19).
- Nasal obstruction: enlarged adenoids lead to physical impairment of the nasal airway causing nasal obstruction, nasal discharge, mouth breathing, hyponasal speech, and sleep-disordered breathing. There is some evidence that adenoidal hypertrophy is more likely in children with allergic rhinitis and that treatment with intranasal steroids reduces the size of the adenoids in this group.[18,19] There is also some evidence that intranasal steroids might benefit "adenoidal" children without allergic rhinitis, although the degree of improvement, the duration of required treatment, and persistence of benefit, and comparison with surgical removal have not yet been reported.[20,21]
- Otitis media with effusion (OME): adenoidectomy may have an important role in the management of some children with OME (see Chapter 8).
- Chronic rhinosinusitis (CRS) as considered in Chapter 17.

Box 18.2 Indications for Tonsillectomy

- Sleep-disordered breathing/OSA.
- Recurrent acute tonsillitis.
- Unilateral tonsillar enlargement.
- Peritonsillar abscess (quinsy).
- Pediatric autoimmune neuropsychiatric disorders associated with streptococcal infections (PANDAS).
- Periodic fever, aphthous stomatitis, pharyngitis, and cervical adenitis (PFAPA) syndrome.
- Halitosis secondary to tonsillar crypt debris/tonsilloliths.

Sleep-Disordered Breathing/Obstructive Sleep Apnea

Recurrent Acute Tonsillitis

Until the relatively recent increase in the acceptance of sleep-disordered breathing as an indication for tonsillectomy in children, recurrent tonsillitis was the most common reason for tonsillectomy in this age group. There have been numerous attempts to rationalize criteria for tonsillectomy for this indication in an effort to prevent unnecessary surgery and to ensure the desired outcome of an improvement in quality of life. There are large differences in the adenotonsillectomy rates internationally with low rates in Canada and the highest rates in Northern Ireland. It is unclear why these differences exist and also what the indications for adenotonsillectomy were in different studies.[22] In the United Kingdom, there have been increasing rates of hospital admissions recently with acute throat infections, whereas the tonsillectomy rates have decreased. It is felt that this increase in admissions with sore throats is unrelated to the decreasing adenotonsillectomy rate and is probably due to changing management protocols within the primary care setting.[22]

A recent Cochrane review concludes that tonsillectomy in children reduces the number of episodes of sore throat and the number of days with a sore throat.[23] This effect is most marked in severely affected children.[24] It has been shown that tonsillectomy is not an effective treatment for recurrent mild sore throat.[25] The potential benefit has to be weighed against the risks of surgery and against the fact that a significant number of patients with recurrent tonsillitis undergo spontaneous resolution of their symptoms.

There are currently multicenter projects underway studying the effect of tonsillectomy upon quality of life in children using the 14-item Paediatric Throat Disorders Outcome Test, which is an appropriate, disease-specific, parent-reported outcome measure for children with throat disorders.[26]

From a practical point of view, the following guidelines are used in the author's practice to determine whether tonsillectomy is indicated for recurrent tonsillitis. These are based on the Scottish Intercollegiate Guidelines Network guidelines and the ENTUK position paper on indications for tonsillectomy.[27]

- Sore throats are due to acute tonsillitis.
- The episodes of sore throat are disabling and prevent normal functioning, for example, missing school.
- Seven or more well-documented, clinically significant, adequately treated sore throats in the preceding year; or
- Five or more such episodes in each of the preceding 2 years; or
- Three or more such episodes in each of the preceding 3 years.

Unilateral Tonsillar Enlargement

This can cause a great deal of parental anxiety and is a common reason for referral to an otolaryngologist.

Unilateral tonsillar enlargement in children is commonly related to *Actinomyces* colonization and, in most cases, is entirely innocent.

Actinomyces are anaerobic, gram-positive, nonacid-fast, branched filamentous bacteria. There appears to be an association between *Actinomyces* colonization and tonsillar volume/hypertrophy.[28] It is extremely unlikely to be related to malignancy. However, malignancy cannot be excluded on clinical appearance alone, and tonsillar lymphoma is practically always associated with unilateral tonsillar enlargement at presentation.[29] Clinical judgment needs to be exercised and factors such as the length of the history and any recent changes are important, but given the implications of missed or late diagnosis in this situation, it is the author's practice to have a low threshold for performing tonsillectomy in the presence of gross asymmetry.

Peritonsillar Abscess (Quinsy)

Quinsy is an abscess in the peritonsillar space (see Chapter 4). A single episode of peritonsillar abscess in the absence of preexisting recurrent tonsillitis does not appear per se to be an indication for tonsillectomy. However, recurrent peritonsillar abscess does. The likelihood of having a tonsillectomy in the 5 years following an episode of peritonsillar abscess is approximately 40%.[30]

Pediatric Autoimmune Neuropsychiatric Disorders Associated with Streptococcal Infections

This is a condition in which repeated group A beta-hemolytic streptococcal infections are thought to trigger an autoimmune reaction that leads to or exacerbates neuropsychiatric disorders. Symptoms include tics, obsessive compulsive behavior, agitation, and hyperactivity. There are isolated case reports of (adeno)tonsillectomy leading to complete resolution of these symptoms.[31,32]

Periodic Fever, Aphthous Stomatitis, Pharyngitis, and Cervical Adenitis Syndrome

This is a condition that usually affects children around the age of 5 years and is associated with recurrent episodes of fever, aphthous ulcers, cervical lymphadenopathy, and cervical lymphadenopathy. The child is usually completely asymptomatic between episodes, and there is no effect upon growth and development. There is known to be a tendency toward spontaneous resolution. Treatment with corticosteroids has been shown to have some benefit, but tonsillectomy appears to be an efficacious treatment.[33] The exact mechanism of this treatment remains unclear.

Halitosis Secondary to Tonsillar Crypt Debris/Tonsilloliths

This is a problem particularly in adolescents with protuberant tonsils. Food debris gets trapped within the tonsillar crypts forming small "stones" that can cause symptoms such as a bad taste or bad breath, a choking sensation, or discomfort. The symptoms are usually alleviated by a tonsillectomy in these situations.

Surgical Techniques and Perioperative Care

There are a number of techniques for both adenoidectomy and tonsillectomy. The technique used is largely a personal preference, and there are numerous papers in the literature suggesting the superiority of one technique over another. Consideration has to be given to the greater impact of blood loss (both intraoperative and secondary) and dehydration (related to inadequate intake or vomiting) in children.

- In children, adenotonsillectomy is performed under general anesthesia. In recent years, with an emphasis on perioperative care and a desire to reduce postoperative hospital stay, a number of perioperative measures that have an impact upon subsequent outcomes have been introduced.
- Preoperative medication given to reduce postoperative pain, nausea, and vomiting include nonsteroidal analgesics and corticosteroids (▶ Table 18.1). There has been

Table 18.1 Perioperative management of children undergoing adenotonsillectomy

Preoperative	NSAIDs
	Paracetamol
At induction	Dexamethasone and ondansetron
	Opioids (morphine/fentanyl ± ketamine)
Postoperative	Paracetamol
	Ibuprofen
	Oral morphine
	Antibiotics (to prevent fetor)

Abbreviation: NSAIDs, nonsteroidal anti-inflammatory drugs.

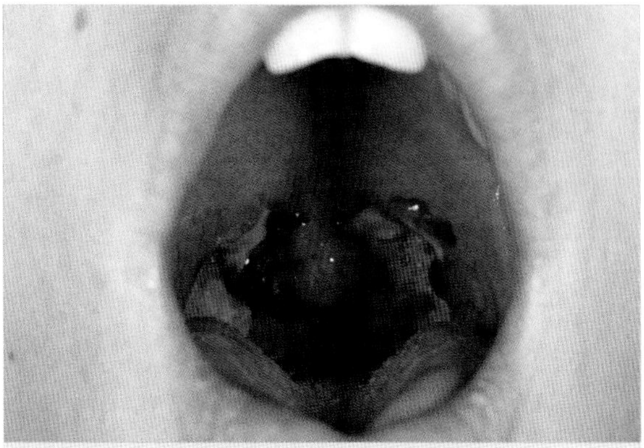

Fig. 18.7 Tonsil fossa 3 days postsurgery.

some anxiety that these might lead to an increased postoperative hemorrhage rate. A Cochrane review in 2005 concluded that nonsteroidal anti-inflammatory drugs do not increase the risk of postoperative hemorrhage and that they do have a positive effect of reducing postoperative nausea and vomiting.[34] A Cochrane review studying the effect of systemic dexamethasone concluded that although there is not an increased risk of postoperative hemorrhage, there is an increased risk of bleeding that requires operative intervention, suggesting that bleeds may be more serious in the group given steroids.[35] However, their meta-analysis did not include a recently published large multicenter randomised control trial that concluded no increased risk of postoperative bleeding requiring either hospital readmission or return to operating room when a single perioperative dose of dexamethasone (0.5 mg/kg) was administered.[36]

- The anesthetized patient is positioned supine with a roll beneath the shoulders and the head supported with or without a head ring. Care must be taken when extending the neck, particularly in children with Down's syndrome or other conditions associated with cervical instability. The tongue is retracted using a Boyle Davis gag (a Thackeray mouth gag is also useful in very small children), with the gag supported with Draffin rods.

Techniques for Tonsillectomy

The most common methods of tonsillectomy (▶ Fig. 18.7) in children are discussed next.

Cold Steel Dissection

Here, the tonsil is pulled medially, the mucosa over the lateral part of the tonsil in this position is incised, and dissection is carried out using a dissector or scissors until the lower pole is reached. The lower pole can then be snared or ligated. The tonsillar fossae are then packed and hemostasis secured using ties or diathermy.

Bipolar Diathermy Dissection

The tonsil is pulled medially to define the plane of dissection, and current between the tips of the bipolar forceps is used to simultaneously dissect and secure hemostasis. Dissection (like the cold steel technique) proceeds from the superior pole to the inferior pole. The inferior pole may then be ligated or dissected with diathermy.

Coblation Tonsillectomy

In this technique, the purpose-designed wand creates an ionized plasma that disrupts molecular bonds chemically rather than with heat. The tonsil is pulled medially and Coblation (Smith & Nephew) is carried out from anterior to posterior, starting either at the superior pole like in traditional tonsillectomy or at the inferior pole.

Tonsillotomy or Intracapsular Tonsillectomy

The principle here is to remove the tonsil tissue using a micrdebrider, Coblation, radiofrequency, monopolar or bipolar diathermy,[37] or laser, stopping just short of the tonsillar capsule so that the peritonsillar space is not entered. Reports seem to suggest a lower hemorrhage rate, less postoperative pain, and a faster return to normal activity.[38,39,40] Concerns remain about the potential for incomplete removal leading either to infection or to recurrence of symptoms, but the small risk of reoperation may be acceptable in light of the considerably lower secondary hemorrhage rate particularly in younger children.[41]

Other Techniques

Other techniques include monopolar diathermy dissection, harmonic scalpel, laser tonsillectomy, and the guillotine technique.

Techniques for Adenoidectomy

Prior to performing adenoidectomy, it is important that the palate is inspected and palpated for the presence of a submucous cleft. Its presence is suggested by the presence of a bifid uvula and confirmed by palpation of a midline notch in the hard palate (▶ Fig. 18.8). In this situation, "blind" adenoidectomy should be avoided altogether for fear of postoperative velopharyngeal incompetence, whereas if the adenoidectomy is carried out under vision, a "superior" or "limited" adenoidectomy can be performed.

Curettage and Packing

This is the traditional method of adenoidectomy. The adenoids are palpated with a finger placed into the postnasal space behind the soft palate. This gives an indication of the size of the adenoid pad and also enables the tissue to be swept medially away from the Eustachian tube cushions. A curette is then used to remove the adenoid tissue, and the postnasal space is packed with a swab to secure hemostasis. On rare occasions, hemostasis is not sufficient to enable pack removal and it then becomes necessary to insert an indwelling postnasal pack for 24 to 48 hours. In a child, the discomfort associated with this procedure means that the child is kept endotracheally intubated and sedated until the pack can be removed. For many years, most ENT surgeons have been very uncomfortable with using a technique that defies the basic surgical principle of exposure and visualization.

Techniques using Visualization

The surgeon can get a good view of the postnasal space by retraction of the soft palate using a suction catheter passed down the nostril and out through the mouth, combined with the use of a mirror (▶ Fig. 18.9) or even an angled endoscope (▶ Fig. 18.10). Thus, devices such as

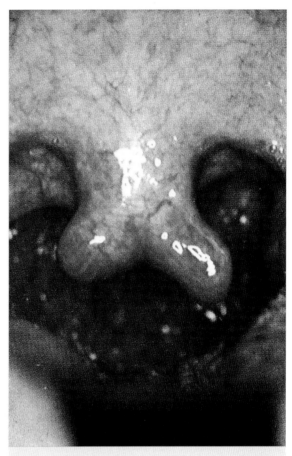

Fig. 18.8 Bifid uvula.

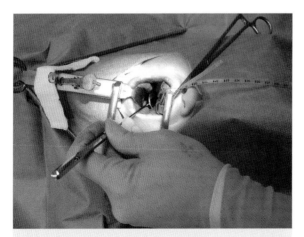

Fig. 18.9 Adenoids visualized with a mirror.

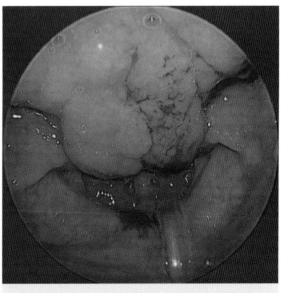

Fig. 18.10 Adenoids visualized with a 120-degree endoscope.

18

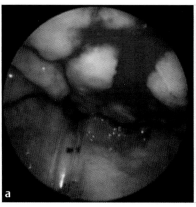
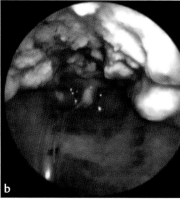

Fig. 18.11 Adenoids visualized with a 120-degree endoscope: **(a)** before and **(b)** after Coblation removal.

suction diathermy, microdebriders, and Coblation wands can be used to remove the adenoid tissue under vision. Suction diathermy and Coblation have the advantage of considerably reducing the intraoperative blood loss associated with this procedure (▸ Fig. 18.11). They do have the disadvantage of causing postoperative fetor presumably related to bacterial colonization of necrotic tissue and it is the author's preference to prescribe postoperative antibiotics to minimize this.

Postoperative Management for Adenotonsillar Surgery

Regular observations in the ward are carried out until it is deemed safe for the patient to be discharged home. Whether or not the procedure can be carried out as a day case is dependent upon a number of factors including age and weight, other comorbidities, and the indication for surgery (OSA). At the author's institution, children above the age of 2 years are discharged 2 hours following an adenoidectomy. For tonsillectomy, children above the age of 3 years, without a history of significant sleep-disordered breathing and without significant comorbidity, are discharged 3 hours postoperatively. Those with mild OSA or less than 3 years but without significant comorbidity are discharged 6 hours postoperatively, whereas all others are admitted overnight for observations. High dependency postoperative care and the availability of an intensive care facility is recommended for some children as detailed in Box 18.3.[42]

> ### Box 18.3 Indications for Postoperative High Dependency Care with Available Facility for Intensive Care
>
> - Age < 2 years.
> - Low weight (less than 15 kg) or failure to thrive.
> - Obesity.
> - Moderate or severely affected neuromuscular disorders such as cerebral palsy and uncontrolled epilepsy.

> - Mucopolysaccharidosis, significant craniofacial anomalies, and other syndromes associated with difficult airway.
> - Other significant comorbidity (e.g., congenital heart disease, chronic lung disease, ASA 3 or above).
> - Severe OSA.
>
> Modified after Robb PJ, Bew S, Kubba H, et al. Tonsillectomy and adenoidectomy in children with sleep-related breathing disorders: consensus statement of a UK multidisciplinary working party. Ann Royal Coll Surg England 2009;91(5):371–373.[42]

Regular postoperative analgesia is recommended. Paracetamol, ibuprofen, and oramorph are our favored analgesics. Codeine was previously a commonly used postoperative analgesic in this group but its use has recently been discontinued following guidance from the Medicines and Healthcare Products Regulatory Agency. (MHRA) This was a decision based upon reports in the United States of three young children who died following administration of codeine postoperatively after tonsillectomy for OSA.[43] The children were all found to be ultrarapid metabolizers of cytochrome P4502D6, resulting in greater production of morphine from the administered codeine. Early resumption of normal diet is encouraged.

Postoperative antibiotics are not routinely recommended as there is no robust evidence that they reduce the risk of postoperative secondary hemorrhage or have any beneficial effect upon postoperative pain.[44] However, they have been demonstrated to reduce postoperative fetor in the case of suction diathermy or Coblation adenoidectomy.

Complications of Surgery

Hemorrhage

Postoperative hemorrhage following tonsillectomy can be subdivided into primary hemorrhage, which occurs

V

within 24 hours of operation, and secondary hemorrhage, which occurs at any time after that usually between 5 and 10 days postoperatively.

> The risk of primary hemorrhage is between 0 and 4%. The risk of secondary hemorrhage is more difficult to ascertain because there is no standard definition, and levels of reporting and readmission criteria vary widely. Figures quoted in the literature are up to 30%.

A more consistent and therefore reliable measure of severe postoperative bleeding is the return to operating room rate. Significant secondary bleeding following a tonsillectomy usually settles spontaneously with observation and conservative management in the form of local pressure with or without gargles. Occasionally, a return to the operating room is required to either tie or diathermy a bleeding vessel in the tonsillar bed.

Hemorrhage can also occur following adenoidectomy. This is more likely to be primary hemorrhage; secondary hemorrhage is very rare. Bleeding can be controlled using coblation or suction diathermy under vision, packing with adrenaline, surgical, Kaltostat (ConvaTec), or failing that a postnasal pack.

> If a child needs a postnasal pack, he/she will usually require sedation and endotracheal intubation, with admission to a unit that can look after patients with an endotracheal tube in place, that is, an intensive care facility.

Infection

It is difficult to assess the incidence of post-tonsillectomy infection as diagnosis is hampered by the presence of postoperative pain, fever as a normal postoperative response, and the (white sloughy) appearance of the tonsillar fossa postoperatively. Nevertheless, up to 25% patients receive antibiotics from their general practitioners either for pain or bleeding.[45]

> Readmission criteria vary widely, but it is the author's practice to readmit patients with postoperative infection only if their oral intake is so compromised that they will not accept oral medication.

Velopharyngeal Incompetence

This is a very rare complication of adenoidectomy in children and can result in hypernasal speech and even nasal regurgitation of fluids. It is more likely to occur in children with a cleft palate, a submucous cleft palate or bifid uvula, 22q deletion syndromes, and neuromuscular conditions.[46] In most cases, there is some improvement in the months postoperatively, but there can be persistent hypernasality, reducing intelligibility of speech and requiring pharyngoplasty.

Atlantoaxial Subluxation (Grisel's Syndrome)

Atlantoaxial subluxation defined as increased mobility or laxity between the body of the first cervical vertebra (atlas) and the odontoid process of the second cervical vertebra resulting in impairment of rotation of the head has been described as a complication of adenotonsillectomy in children with Down's syndrome, but, in fact, it can occur in all children and as a result of any operative procedure that involves extension of the neck particularly with lateral rotation or with conditions such as infection that cause hyperemia of the transverse ligament of the atlantoaxial joint. It should be suspected if there is postoperative neck stiffness, torticollis, or paresthesia.[47] Management may be conservative or may involve cervical spine fusion.

18.6 Key Points

- Tongue-tie is a congenital condition in which the lingual frenulum is abnormally short, resulting in reduced mobility of the tip of the tongue. Treatment, that is, division of the frenulum, is only indicated if there are troublesome symptoms (including social ones).
- Macroglossia is protrusion of the tongue beyond the incisors. Children with macroglossia may require airway intervention or, exceptionally, surgical reduction of the tongue.
- A ranula is an extravasation mucocele that arises from the sublingual salivary gland. The diagnosis is clinical. Treatment is surgical.
- Adenoids and tonsils form part of the Waldeyer's ring of lymphoid tissue in the oropharynx and nasopharynx. They may harbor biofilms, which are microbial communities that attach to surfaces, and produce their own protective matrix. Biofilms may contribute to the development of tonsillar hyperplasia.
- Adenotonsillectomy is one of the commonest surgical procedures performed in children.
- Indications for adenoidectomy include sleep-disordered breathing/OSA, nasal obstruction, OME, and CRS.
- Indications for tonsillectomy include sleep-disordered breathing/OSA, recurrent acute tonsillitis, unilateral tonsillar enlargement, peritonsillar abscess (quinsy), (PANDAS), PFAPA syndrome, and halitosis secondary to tonsillar crypt debris/tonsilloliths.

18

References

[1] Messner AH, Lalakea ML, Aby J, Macmahon J, Bair E. Ankyloglossia: incidence and associated feeding difficulties. Arch Otolaryngol Head Neck Surg. 2000; 126(1):36–39

[2] Lalakea ML, Messner AH. Ankyloglossia: does it matter? Pediatr Clin North Am. 2003; 50(2):381–397

[3] Messner AH, Lalakea ML. The effect of ankyloglossia on speech in children. Otolaryngol Head Neck Surg. 2002; 127(6):539–545

[4] Power RF, Murphy JF. Tongue-tie and frenotomy in infants with breastfeeding difficulties: achieving a balance. Arch Dis Child. 2015; 100(5):489–494

[5] Mettias B, O'Brien R, Abo Khatwa MM, Nasrallah L, Doddi M. Division of tongue tie as an outpatient procedure. Technique, efficacy and safety. Int J Pediatr Otorhinolaryngol. 2013; 77(4):550–552

[6] Berry J, Griffiths M, Westcott C. A double-blind, randomized, controlled trial of tongue-tie division and its immediate effect on breastfeeding. Breastfeed Med. 2012; 7(3):189–193

[7] Opara PI, Gabriel-Job N, Opara KO. Neonates presenting with severe complications of frenotomy: a case series. J Med Case Reports. 2012; 6(1):77

[8] Kadouch DJ, Maas SM, Dubois L, van der Horst CM. Surgical treatment of macroglossia in patients with Beckwith-Wiedemann syndrome: a 20-year experience and review of the literature. Int J Oral Maxillofac Surg. 2012; 41(3):300–308

[9] Chau H, Soma M, Massey S, Hewitt R, Hartley B. Anterior tongue reduction surgery for paediatric macroglossia. J Laryngol Otol. 2011; 125(12):1247–1250

[10] Sigismund PE, Bozzato A, Schumann M, Koch M, Iro H, Zenk J. Management of ranula: 9 years' clinical experience in pediatric and adult patients. J Oral Maxillofac Surg. 2013; 71(3):538–544

[11] Patel MR, Deal AM, Shockley WW. Oral and plunging ranulas: what is the most effective treatment? Laryngoscope. 2009; 119(8):1501–1509

[12] Harrison JD. Modern management and pathophysiology of ranula: literature review. Head Neck. 2010; 32(10):1310–1320

[13] Macassey E, Dawes P. Biofilms and their role in otorhinolaryngological disease. J Laryngol Otol. 2008; 122(12):1273–1278

[14] Diaz RR, Picciafuoco S, Paraje MG, et al. Relevance of biofilms in pediatric tonsillar disease. Eur J Clin Microbiol Infect Dis. 2011; 30 (12):1503–1509

[15] Brodsky L. Modern assessment of tonsils and adenoids. Pediatr Clin North Am. 1989; 36(6):1551–1569

[16] Kumar DS, Valenzuela D, Kozak FK, et al. The reliability of clinical tonsil size grading in children. JAMA Otolaryngol Head Neck Surg. 2014; 140(11):1034–1037

[17] Parikh SR, Coronel M, Lee JJ, Brown SM. Validation of a new grading system for endoscopic examination of adenoid hypertrophy. Otolaryngol Head Neck Surg. 2006; 135(5):684–687

[18] Modrzynski M, Zawisza E. An analysis of the incidence of adenoid hypertrophy in allergic children. Int J Pediatr Otorhinolaryngol. 2007; 71(5):713–719

[19] Scadding G. Non-surgical treatment of adenoidal hypertrophy: the role of treating IgE-mediated inflammation. Pediatr Allergy Immunol. 2010; 21(8):1095–1106

[20] Bitar MA, Mahfoud L, Nassar J, Dana R. Exploring the characteristics of children with obstructive adenoid responding to mometasone fuorate monohydrate: preliminary results. Eur Arch Otorhinolaryngol. 2013; 270(3):931–937

[21] Chadha NK, Zhang L, Mendoza-Sassi RA, César JA. Using nasal steroids to treat nasal obstruction caused by adenoid hypertrophy: does it work? Otolaryngol Head Neck Surg. 2009; 140(2):139–147

[22] Koshy E, Murray J, Bottle A, et al. Significantly increasing hospital admissions for acute throat infections among children in England: is this related to tonsillectomy rates? Arch Dis Child. 2012; 97(12):1064–1068

[23] Burton MJ, Glasziou PP. Tonsillectomy or adeno-tonsillectomy versus non-surgical treatment for chronic/recurrent acute tonsillitis. Cochrane Database Syst Rev. 2009(1):CD001802

[24] Lock C, Wilson J, Steen N, et al. North of England and Scotland Study of Tonsillectomy and Adeno-tonsillectomy in Children (NESSTAC): a pragmatic randomised controlled trial with a parallel non-randomised preference study. Health Technol Assess. 2010; 14(13): 1–164, iii–iv

[25] van Staaij BK, van den Akker EH, Rovers MM, Hordijk GJ, Hoes AW, Schilder AG. Effectiveness of adenotonsillectomy in children with mild symptoms of throat infections or adenotonsillar hypertrophy: open, randomised controlled trial. Clin Otolaryngol. 2005; 30(1):60–63

[26] Hopkins C, Fairley J, Yung M, Hore I, Balasubramaniam S, Haggard M. The 14-item Paediatric Throat Disorders Outcome Test: a valid, sensitive, reliable, parent-reported outcome measure for paediatric throat disorders. J Laryngol Otol. 2010; 124(3):306–314

[27] Baugh RF, Archer SM, Mitchell RB, et al. American Academy of Otolaryngology-Head and Neck Surgery Foundation. Clinical practice guideline: tonsillectomy in children. Otolaryngol Head Neck Surg. 2011; 144(1) Suppl:S1–S30

[28] Kutluhan A, Salvız M, Yalçıner G, Kandemir O, Yeşil C. The role of the actinomyces in obstructive tonsillar hypertrophy and recurrent tonsillitis in pediatric population. Int J Pediatr Otorhinolaryngol. 2011; 75(3):391–394

[29] Dolev Y, Daniel SJ. The presence of unilateral tonsillar enlargement in patients diagnosed with palatine tonsil lymphoma: experience at a tertiary care pediatric hospital. Int J Pediatr Otorhinolaryngol. 2008; 72(1):9–12

[30] Wikstén J, Hytönen M, Pitkäranta A, Blomgren K. Who ends up having tonsillectomy after peritonsillar infection? Eur Arch Otorhinolaryngol. 2012; 269(4):1281–1284

[31] Alexander AA, Patel NJ, Southammakosane CA, Mortensen MM. Pediatric autoimmune neuropsychiatric disorders associated with streptococcal infections (PANDAS): an indication for tonsillectomy. Int J Pediatr Otorhinolaryngol. 2011; 75(6):872–873

[32] Heubi C, Shott SR, Sr. PANDAS: pediatric autoimmune neuropsychiatric disorders associated with streptococcal infections—an uncommon, but important indication for tonsillectomy. Int J Pediatr Otorhinolaryngol. 2003; 67(8):837–840

[33] Licameli G, Lawton M, Kenna M, Dedeoglu F. Long-term surgical outcomes of adenotonsillectomy for PFAPA syndrome. Arch Otolaryngol Head Neck Surg. 2012; 138(10):902–906

[34] Cardwell M, Siviter G, Smith A. Non-steroidal anti-inflammatory drugs and perioperative bleeding in paediatric tonsillectomy. Cochrane Database Syst Rev. 2005(2):CD003591

[35] Plante J, Turgeon AF, Zarychanski R, et al. Effect of systemic steroids on post-tonsillectomy bleeding and reinterventions: systematic review and meta-analysis of randomised controlled trials. BMJ. 2012; 345:e5389 (Clinical Res Ed)

[36] Gallagher TQ, Hill C, Ojha S, et al. Perioperative dexamethasone administration and risk of bleeding following tonsillectomy in children: a randomized controlled trial. JAMA. 2012; 308(12):1221–1226

[37] Shaul C, Attal PD, Schwarz Y, et al. Bipolar tonsillotomy: a novel and effective tonsillotomy technique. Int J Pediatr Otorhinolaryngol. 2016; 84:1–5

[38] Acevedo JL, Shah RK, Brietzke SE. Systematic review of complications of tonsillotomy versus tonsillectomy. Otolaryngol Head Neck Surg. 2012; 146(6):871–879

[39] Walton J, Ebner Y, Stewart MG, April MM. Systematic review of randomized controlled trials comparing intracapsular tonsillectomy with total tonsillectomy in a pediatric population. Arch Otolaryngol Head Neck Surg. 2012; 138(3):243–249

[40] Kiær EK, Bock T, Tingsgaard PK. Tonsillotomy in children with sleep-disordered breathing is safe and results in high parent satisfaction. Dan Med J. 2016; 63(5):A5228

V

[41] Zhang Q, Li D, Wang H. Long term outcome of tonsillar regrowth after partial tonsillectomy in children with obstructive sleep apnea. Auris Nasus Larynx. 2014; 41(3):299–302

[42] Robb PJ, Bew S, Kubba H, et al. Tonsillectomy and adenoidectomy in children with sleep-related breathing disorders: consensus statement of a UK multidisciplinary working party. Ann R Coll Surg Engl. 2009; 91(5):371–373

[43] Kelly LE, Rieder M, van den Anker J, et al. More codeine fatalities after tonsillectomy in North American children. Pediatrics. 2012; 129(5): e1343–e1347

[44] Dhiwakar M, Clement WA, Supriya M, McKerrow W. Antibiotics to reduce post-tonsillectomy morbidity. Cochrane Database Syst Rev. 2010(7):CD005607

[45] Doshi J, Damadora M, Gregory S, Anari S. Post-tonsillectomy morbidity statistics: are they underestimated? J Laryngol Otol. 2008; 122(4):374–377

[46] Milczuk HA. Effects of oropharyngeal surgery on velopharyngeal competence. Curr Opin Otolaryngol Head Neck Surg. 2012; 20(6):522–526

[47] Bocciolini C, Dall'Olio D, Cunsolo E, Cavazzuti PP, Laudadio P. Grisel's syndrome: a rare complication following adenoidectomy. Acta Otorhinolaryngol Ital. 2005; 25(4):245–249

18

19 Obstructive Sleep Apnea

Ari DeRowe

19.1 Introduction

A proposed definition for *obstructive sleep apnea* (OSA) is: "a disorder of breathing during sleep characterized by prolonged partial upper airway obstruction and/or intermittent complete obstruction (obstructive apnea) that disrupts normal ventilation during sleep and normal sleep patterns."[1] Some important terms used in the management of pediatric OSA are shown in ▶ Table 19.1.

OSA in children is part of a continuum of *sleep-disordered breathing* (SDB). The clinically mildest form of SDB is *primary snoring*. The child has episodes of stertorous breathing during sleep but no ventilation abnormalities. As the severity progresses, *upper airway resistance syndrome* (UARS) develops. In the UARS, there is increased respiratory effort during breathing with ventilation abnormalities but without apnea or hypopnea. OSA is the most severe form of SDB. The sleep disturbance has a profound negative impact on the child's growth and development. The correlation between severity of OSA and its consequences on the child are unpredictable. A mild OSA may have a profound impact, whereas a severe OSA may not. Other factors such as preexisting medical conditions, duration of the OSA, and the child's age seem to be important.

19.2 Epidemiology and Prevalence

Constant snoring is noticed by parents in approximately 10% of healthy children. It is usually self-limiting within 2 years in 50% of these children. OSA is observed in 2 to 3% of children.[2] Though some children with OSA may improve in time, the negative neurocognitive and developmental impact may be such that intervention is

Table 19.2 Adult versus pediatric OSA

Adults	Children
Obese	Failure to thrive
Not a mouth breather	Mouth breather
Male > female	Male = female
Daytime somnolence	Attention deficit hyperactivity disorder
Non REM	REM
No adenotonsillar hypertrophy	Adenotonsillar hypertrophy
Surgery usually not curative, requires CPAP	Surgery usually curative

Abbreviations: CPAP, continuous positive airway pressure; OSA, obstructive sleep apnea; REM, rapid eye movement.

warranted, and observing the child with overt OSA for possible improvement with natural history is inappropriate. This highlights the importance in differentiating simple snoring from OSA.

Pediatric OSA occurs mostly in infants and children below 6 years of age with a peak incidence at 3 to 4 years of age. This coincides with the physiological peak in adenotonsillar hypertrophy. There is another peak incidence in infants less than 1 year old due mostly to predisposing conditions such as craniofacial abnormalities, but early adenotonsillar hypertrophy causing OSA in infants has been described and should be considered.[3]

Pediatric OSA is a different pathophysiological entity from its adult counterpart. OSA has a very great impact on the child and family because developmental issues are of great importance (▶ Table 19.2).

19.3 Physiology of Normal Sleep

Normal sleep has five stages: stages 1 to 4 are increasing levels of sleep with increased slowing of brain activity as seen on electroencephalography (EEG) and a progressive decrease in muscular tone. Stage 5 is *rapid eye movement* (REM) sleep when the brain shows increased activity and dreaming takes place. Paradoxically, in REM sleep, there is a further decrease in muscular tone, possibly a failsafe mechanism to prevent running away from our dreams. Other sleep-induced physiological changes are increased upper airway resistance, decreased minute ventilation, and decreased ventilatory responses to hypoxia and hypercapnia. Thus, in the predisposed child during sleep, obstructive episodes lead to a marked impact on breathing and gas exchange. Because muscle tone decreases progressively from stage 1 through 4 sleep, reaching a

Table 19.1 Important OSA definitions

Obstructive apnea	Cessation of ventilation (i.e., no airflow), despite respiratory effort, for 10 s or two breath cycles in older children or 6 s or 1.5–2 breaths in younger children
Obstructive hypopnea	Decrease in airflow by 50%, despite respiratory effort, during the same time or breath cycles, associated with a desaturation or arousal
AHI	The total number of apneic events plus hypopneas per hour of sleep
RDI	Another term for the AHI
AI	Describes the number of arousals per hour of sleep

Abbreviations: AHI, apnea/hypopnea index; AI, arousal index; OSA, obstructive sleep apnea; RDI, respiratory disturbance index.

nadir during REM sleep, children are particularly vulnerable to airway obstruction during REM sleep. This vulnerability is especially prominent in children because a proportionally larger part of their sleep is in REM.

19.4 Pathophysiology of Obstructive Sleep Apnea

The upper airway is a collapsible tube. The collapsibility of the tube depends on diameter and compliance. The variables influencing diameter relate to skeletal and soft-tissue abnormalities. Compliance is influenced by muscle tone and central nervous system (CNS) drive. Upper airway obstruction in children with OSA is multifactorial. The three main predisposing factors are as follows:
- Hypertrophy of tonsils and adenoids or other tissue in the airway.
- Craniofacial anomalies.
- Oropharyngeal neuromuscular abnormalities.

Any one factor or a combination of these factors can cause OSA.

> William Osler wrote in "The Principles and Practice of Medicine," 1892: "Chronic enlargement of the tonsillar tissue is an affection of great importance, and may influence in extraordinary ways the mental and bodily development of children … At night, the child's sleep is greatly disturbed, the respirations are loud and snorting and there are sometimes prolonged pauses …"
> "The child responds slowly to questions…impossible to fix attention for long at a time … looks sullen … The influence upon mental development is striking."

OSA is to be differentiated from *central apnea* where the cause is related to a CNS lesion, and cessation of breathing is not due to obstruction. The pathophysiology of central apnea is related to lack of respiratory drive usually due to insensitivity to elevation of the partial pressure of carbon dioxide (CO_2) at the level of the brainstem. Central and obstructive apnea may coexist especially in neurologically impaired children. This is termed *mixed obstructive/central apnea.*

19.5 Effects of Obstructive Sleep Apnea

19.5.1 Metabolic

The intermittent ventilatory disturbance in OSA results in hypercarbia and hypoxia with an impact on the child's metabolism. This may result in endothelial dysfunction.

Many metabolic disturbances have been found including elevation in C-reactive protein, insulin resistance, hypercholesterolemia, elevated serum transaminase, decreased insulin-like growth factor (IGF), and decrease in growth hormone (GH) secretion. These metabolic sequelae present clinically as *failure to thrive* (FTT) in children but are also observed in obese children with OSA.[4]

19.5.2 Increased Health Care Utilization

A common misconception is that the tonsils and adenoids are important in protecting a child from illness and cause no adverse effects.

> Tonsillectomy and adenoidectomy (T + A) not only improves OSA but also results in a drastic reduction in health care utilization after surgery.

This was seen across all health care utilization measures including a reduction of visits to the emergency room (ER) and pediatrician, medications, and days of work missed by parents.[5]

19.5.3 Neurobehavioral Deficits

A hallmark of adult OSA is daytime somnolence. In children, the neurobehavioral sequelae are different. Most remarkable is attention deficit hyperactivity disorder most probably as a result of fragmented sleep in OSA. Other findings noted are reduced scholastic achievements and reduction in overall cognitive ability (intelligence quotient). Surgical intervention (T+A) has been shown to improve some of these deficits.[6] In a recent randomized study of adenotonsillectomy versus watchful waiting for OSA in school-aged children (Childhood Adenotonsillectomy Trial), surgery did not significantly improve attention or executive function as measured by neuropsychological testing but did reduce symptoms and improve secondary outcomes of behavior, and quality of life.[7]

19.5.4 Cardiovascular Dysfunction

Although now rarely seen, severe OSA over a prolonged period will result in pulmonary hypertension and cor pulmonale.

Early intervention has reduced these clinical findings. However, in a child with long-standing severe OSA, an echocardiogram should be considered with referral to a pediatric cardiologist for further assessment as needed. If pulmonary hypertension is found, there is an increased surgical and anesthetic risk, and postoperative management on a high dependency unit (HDU) or even a pediatric intensive care unit (PICU) may be required. OSA in children may also result in blood pressure dysregulation as a result of increased sympathetic tone.[4] There is recent evidence that pediatric OSA predisposes to long-term adult cardiovascular morbidity, which is presumably caused by chronic low-grade inflammation and endothelial dysfunction. However, it is a cofactor with obesity.[8]

19.5.5 Growth Retardation

FTT in children with OSA is now less commonly observed due to earlier diagnosis. The causes are GH–IGF axis dysregulation, poor food intake, and increased energy expenditure during sleep. In children with FTT, weight gain is observed following T + A probably as a result of decreased energy expenditure during sleep.[4]

19.5.6 Decreased Quality of Life

Studies using validated questionnaires reflecting quality of life in children with OSA have shown a decreased quality of life. Health-related quality of life as assessed by the OSA-18 questionnaire showed decreases in the domains of the following:

- Sleep disturbance.
- Physical symptoms.
- Emotional symptoms.
- Daytime functioning.
- Caregiver concerns.

These were greatly improved following surgery (T + A).[9]

19.6 Clinical Presentation

19.6.1 The History

OSA has a negative impact on the child's health, but the child who is seen in clinic may appear healthy and happy. It's during sleep that the drama occurs. Careful history is of the utmost importance.

> **i**
>
> Since most children with OSA are snorers, a key question to the child's parent or caregiver is: "Does your child snore?" This simple question is a good screening test for pediatric OSA.

Further questions regarding sleep should focus on restless sleep, effortful breathing, and cessation of breathing, all of which are helpful in defining the severity of OSA. Daytime symptoms such as behavioral problems, FTT, and chronic mouth breathing may also be elicited.

Table 19.3 Symptoms of OSA in children

Nighttime symptoms	Daytime symptoms
Noisy breath (snoring)	Hypersomnolence
Mouth breathing	Fatigue
Difficulty breathing	Hyperactivity
Paradoxical breathing	Delayed development
Breathing pauses	Learning problems
Sweating	"Adenoid facies"
Restless sleep	Pectus excavatum
Frequent movements	Failure to thrive
Unusual postures	
Frequent awakening	
Bed-wetting	
Abbreviation: OSA, obstructive sleep apnea.	

> **i**
>
> Most children with OSA are habitual snorers, whereas not all that snore have OSA.

Enquiry about snoring is an excellent question during history taking and can be used as a screening tool for OSA with high sensitivity but low specificity. Other questions related to sleep are as follows:

- Are there chest efforts while breathing?
- Are there episodes of cessation of breathing and gasping?
- Is the sleep restless?

Further questions are related to the sequelae of OSA: weight, growth curve, FTT, and behavioral and developmental issues especially attention deficit. Bed-wetting may also be a result of OSA. ▶ Table 19.3 summarizes daytime and nighttime symptoms of pediatric OSA.

19.6.2 Physical Examination

A full ENT examination must be performed when examining the child with a history of OSA. It's not only about tonsils and adenoids.

- Examine the nasal airway for masses, anatomical deviations, and the occasional foreign body.
- Palpate the neck for masses.
- Look for maxillofacial features such as dysplasia, micro- or retrognathia, macroglossia, etc.
- Examine for fluid in the middle ear; this can be due to nasopharyngeal obstruction.
- Examine the oral cavity.

The examination of the oral cavity is important but may be difficult in children who have a basic aversion to tongue depressors and will usually put up a fight. This can be avoided by establishing a rapport with the child

V

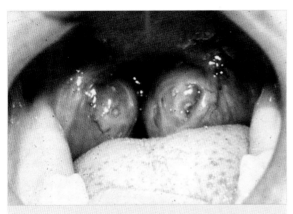

Fig. 19.1 Grade 4 + obstructing tonsils (kissing tonsils).

and even offering a bribe. But at times, the only way to achieve a good examination is to have the parent firmly but gently hold the child while gently opening the mouth and inserting the tongue depressor. Good lighting with a headlight will also help. The oral cavity can then be examined.

Tonsil size can be graded from 0 + to 4 +:

- 0 +: post-tonsillectomy.
- 1 +: tonsils inside the pillars.
- 2 +: tonsils outside the pillars.
- 3 +: tonsils reach the midpalate.
- 4 +: tonsils reach the uvula, also termed *kissing tonsils* (▶ Fig. 19.1).

Look at the palate for signs of a submucous cleft palate such as bifid uvula, maxillary notch, and zona pellucida (a clear strip of mucosa in the midline of the palate caused by the muscular diastasis of the tensor veli palatini). Children with submucous cleft palate are at particular risk of velopharyngeal insufficiency (VPI) after surgery.

Flexible nasopharyngolaryngoscopy is an integral part of the ENT examination in children. A small diameter pediatric scope is needed to reduce discomfort. In older children, cooperation can usually be attained by engaging the child in the examination. Younger children will require a strong hug by the parent. Spraying the nasal cavity with a combination of local anesthetic (lidocaine 1%) and decongestant (pseudoephedrine) can be helpful. With a combative child full of nasal discharge, the examination will lack value and may have to be deferred. In a child with OSA and small tonsils, the endoscopic examination is extremely important in order to elucidate the cause of obstruction.

19.7 Investigation and Diagnosis

Is history alone enough in the diagnosis of OSA? Obviously, in an otherwise healthy child with incessant snoring, observed cessation of breathing and extreme effort of breathing while asleep, especially when coinciding with FTT, is sufficient for diagnosis and prompt treatment. Most children are not in such an extreme category of OSA, making diagnosis more difficult. In multiple studies, history and physical examination were inadequate in diagnosing OSA when compared to full overnight sleep studies, polysomnography (PSG).[10] This cumulated data questions the physician's ability to make therapeutic decisions based on history alone.

19.7.1 Sleep Studies

The gold standard for diagnosis of OSA is considered to be a complete overnight PSG (or "full sleep study"). When asleep, recordings of the child's EEG, pulse rate, oxygen saturation, blood pressure, respiratory rate, apneic and hypopneic episodes, limb movements, and simultaneous video recording are obtained. The referring physician receives the data and summary, the bottom line being the respiratory disturbance index (RDI) or apnea/hypopnea index (AHI), representing the number of apneas and hypopneas per hour of sleep.[11]

> i
>
> There is no consensus on normative data, but in most centers, an RDI of 0 to 1.5 per hour is considered normal, RDI of 1.5 to 5 per hour is mild OSA and RDI of 5 to 10 per hour is moderate. Severe OSA with more than 10 episodes per hour requires prompt attention and intervention.

Many parents when asked say their child's sleep in the laboratory was not the same as at home. The environment is not always comfortable for the child and parent. The examination also entails a cost and, in many centers, a waiting list. This raises a question of necessity especially since the delay in attaining a sleep study may have an adverse effect on the child's health because of the delay in treatment. In many cases, the clinical diagnosis is sufficient and PSG has no added value.

> i
>
> PSG should be reserved for when the diagnosis is unclear or for more complex cases.

Although there are no clear guidelines, suggested indications for PSG are summarized in Box 19.1. This has led to increasing interest in looking at simpler reliable investigative techniques.

Box 19.1 Indications for PSG

- Neurologic disease.
- Age < 2 years.
- Increased surgical risk.
- Borderline cases.
- Craniofacial anomalies.
- Continued symptoms after surgery.

A UK multidisciplinary group looking at indications for adenotonsillar surgery for children with OSA suggested that "respiratory investigations" were appropriate in the following circumstances[12]:

- Diagnosis of OSA uncertain.
- Age less than 2 years.
- Weight less than 15 kg.
- Down's syndrome.
- Cerebral palsy.
- Hypotonia or neuromuscular disorder.
- Obesity (body mass index more than 2.5 or SDS more than 99th percentile for age and gender).
- Comorbidity, for example, congenital heart disease, lung disease, and mucopolysaccharidosis.
- Failure to respond to T + A surgery.

"Ambulatory" or "Home" Sleep Study

This is an appealing solution with the child sleeping in his/her natural environment and requiring fewer resources. The study is technically challenging since children tend to remove the leads and there is no technician to monitor and correct the deficient data, so an ambulatory PSG in children has no real advantage.

Overnight Pulse Oximetry

Pulse oximetry in sleep measures oxygen saturation but fails to show obstructive events that result in fragmentation of sleep and respiratory effort that do not result in decreased oxygen saturation. These events may have a profound negative effect on the child but are missed.

i

Pulse oximetry alone is inadequate for diagnosis of OSA in children.

Some suggest that oximetry can be used as screening for SDB and as a crude measure of severity. The McGill oximetry scoring system is a useful way to grade severity of OSA, as predicted from overnight pulse oximetry, on a 1 to 4 scale[13]:

- Score 1 (normal OSA/inconclusive): up to three drops in oxygen saturation between 85 and 90%.

- Score 2 (mild OSA): three or more drops in oxygen saturation below 90%, up to three of which are between 80 and 85%.
- Score 3 (moderate OSA): three or more drops in oxygen saturation below 85%, up to three of which are below 80%.
- Score 4 (moderate OSA): three or more drops in oxygen saturation below 80%.

The failure to be able to identify hypopneas and respiratory efforts that do not cause desaturations but can cause morbidity limits the usefulness of pulse oximetry.

Video Home Recording of Sleep

Known as "the poor man's sleep study" this is a reasonable compromise. It allows for the child to sleep in her home environment and for the physician to observe snoring, periods of apnea and respiratory effort. This is a *qualitative* and not a *quantitative* examination such as is seen in the sleep laboratory, and there are some limitations. It is impractical for the physician to observe the whole night, and the chosen segment may not be representative. The quality of the home recording is often suboptimal. To improve results, the parents should be guided on technical details of the recording, which should commence approximately 2 hours after sleep. A small night light should be on in the room so that the child's chest and face can be seen clearly. The video recorder should be placed on a tripod or stationary stand, not handheld. Usually, 30 minutes of recording is sufficient.[14]

i

With the widespread use of smartphones, we see more parents who present video clips of their child sleeping. Though helpful at times, we must remember the limitations.

19.7.2 Imaging for Obstructive Sleep Apnea

Imaging is not part of the routine work-up for children with OSA but may be needed in some circumstances. The diagnostic value of plain films (lateral neck imaging) of soft tissue is questionable. Getting the study in a small and combative child is challenging and the quality is often poor. There is no correlation between the findings of the lateral neck X-ray and the severity of OSA. The physical examination and endoscopy are far more informative. Some studies addressed cephalometric measurements as related to OSA. These studies do not appear to be of added value in the management of children and have been largely abandoned.

Computed tomography (CT)/magnetic resonance imaging (MRI) may be important when a tumor or other space-occupying lesion is the suspected cause of obstruction. Recently, cine MRI under sedation has been studied as a modality that can show site and mechanism of soft-tissue obstruction during drug-induced sleep. The clinical practicality of cine MRI in children with OSA requires further investigation.

19.7.3 Sleep Endoscopy

In most children with OSA, adenotonsillectomy brings about a dramatic improvement, but in a small percentage with persistent or relapsing OSA, the site of obstruction is elusive. The same problem occurs in children with craniofacial anomalies. Sleep can be simulated using intravenously induced sedation with flexible nasopharyngoscopy in an attempt to define the etiology of upper airway obstruction during sleep. The technique requires the support of a pediatric anesthetist and is not widely used other than in specialist centers.

There is a paucity of data in children regarding sleep endoscopy, but some studies have been able to show site of obstruction and the result of targeting the surgical approach to the findings.[15] In a child with OSA and small tonsils, or following adenotonsillectomy with residual or persistent symptoms, performing a drug-induced sleep endoscopy is important prior to further treatment such as lingual tonsillectomy for tongue base obstruction.

19.8 Treatment of Obstructive Sleep Apnea in Children

The management of OSA in children is primarily surgical, but nonsurgical interventions still have an important role.

19.8.1 Medical Treatment

Intranasal Steroids

Recent studies have shown some evidence that *intranasal steroids* may have a positive impact on obstructive symptoms,[16] but not all children respond. There is no consensus regarding which children have a potential to benefit from treatment, for how long should treatment be given, and what to do for relapse following treatment. In clinical practice, a trial of intranasal steroid spray can be an option in mild cases of OSA or snoring. Long-term compliance is difficult, and extended treatment with a nasal steroid spray may cause hormonal imbalance. Length of treatment and long-term results are unknown.

Oral Steroids

Oral steroids bring about an immediate and sometimes dramatic improvement in OSA. Long-term treatment with *systemic steroids* is devastating to the child's health and cannot be recommended. The results of short-term treatment with oral steroids are short-lived, with recurrence of OSA after a brief interval of improvement. This may be a short-term solution for the child with OSA until surgery is arranged.

Leukotriene Receptor Antagonists

Preliminary results of a study that examined the effect of leukotriene receptor antagonist montelukast on obstructive symptoms have also been promising.[17] This study only reported short term-effects related to adenoid size without considering tonsillar size.

> In general, medical therapy may be an option in borderline cases or when there are surgical or anesthetic contraindications. The treatment of severe OSA is not to be delayed.

19.8.2 Noninvasive Ventilation

Noninvasive ventilator modalities (continuous positive airway pressure [CPAP] and bilevel positive airway pressure [BiPAP]) that are the mainstay of treatment in adult OSA are less often suggested in children. This is first due to the high cure rate of adenotonsillar surgery. Second, the compliance is poor in children. In children who are not cured with conventional surgery, especially those with cranio facial anomalies or severe comorbidity, CPAP/BIPAP may be the only reasonable option.[18] Home ventilation programs for children have significant resource implications and availability varies across different health care systems. When considering CPAP/BiPAP in children, a multidisciplinary approach is needed, and home nursing to facilitate compliance may be necessary until the pattern is established. Long-term use of CPAP/BiPAP may result in facial bone deformities including maxillary hypoplasia.

> In severe and complicated cases of OSA, CPAP/BiPAP can be considered for children who have had failed surgical intervention (▶ Fig. 19.2, ▶ Fig. 19.3) or as a temporary treatment until surgery can be performed.

V

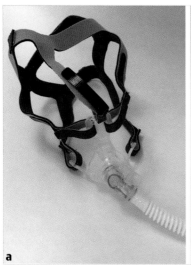

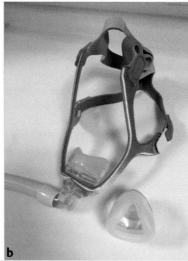

Fig. 19.2 Examples of continuous positive airway pressure and bilevel positive airway pressure masks.

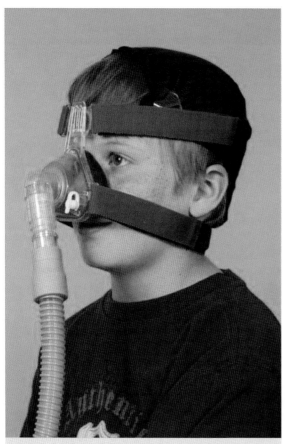

Fig. 19.3 Child undergoing noninvasive ventilation.

19.8.3 Oxygen Therapy

Nasal oxygen delivery during sleep appears to be a good idea to reduce desaturations during obstructive events, but it is no panacea for OSA. CO_2 retention has dire consequences and is not alleviated by oxygen. Oxygen may actually blunt the ventilatory drive of elevated partial pressure of carbon dioxide (pCO_2), resulting in worse apneas. Some children with OSA will also have severe parenchymal lung disease and so will need oxygen for this, but careful monitoring of the child on oxygen is essential.

19.8.4 Adenotonsillectomy

> i
>
> T + A is the first-line treatment in the majority of children with OSA and is usually considered to be curative.[19,20]

In the otherwise healthy child with OSA that is not part of a current upper respiratory illness, T + A is indicated. Some clinicians prefer to perform an adenoidectomy alone with the opinion that the adenoids are responsible for the obstruction and to avoid the complications of tonsillectomy. However, adenoidectomy alone is usually not enough for symptoms to resolve.[21] In mild cases, a period of observation with or without medical treatment may be appropriate since some cases are self-limiting. In more severe cases, waiting is unwarranted since there is a risk

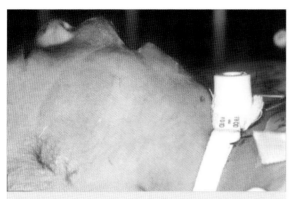

Fig. 19.4 Severe upper airway obstruction in Pierre Robin sequence requiring tracheostomy.

for neurodevelopmental and cardiovascular sequelae. In extreme cases, surgery should be performed as soon as possible.

Recent studies have led to some caution. In a study of 578 children, a reduction in the AHI following T + A was considerable from 18.2 ± 21.4 to 4.1 ± 6.4 ($p < 0.001$), but only 27% had complete resolution, that is, AHI less than 1.[19] The failure rate was more evident in obese children, children over 7 years of age, and children with severe OSA preoperatively. Children at higher risk for residual OSA may require postoperative sleep studies and may need further intervention, for example, CPAP or, in extreme cases such as severe cerebral palsy and craniofacial syndromes, even tracheotomy (▶ Fig. 19.4).

> ℹ
>
> Pediatric OSA is not only about adenotonsillectomy.

Surgical techniques of T + A have evolved over the years, but the operative technique seems to have little or no influence on the long-term outcome in OSA. The classic approach is termed *cold steel* where blunt and sharp dissection is used to separate the tonsil from the pharyngeal musculature, staying in the correct plain of dissection. The tonsil receives generous blood supply from the external carotid artery and these potential bleeders are addressed either by suture ligation or diathermy coagulation. Dissection may also be performed with a wire snare.[22] Various "hot" techniques[23] including diathermy and Coblation (Smith & Nephew) are now widely used (see Chapter 18 for more details).

Tonsillotomy or partial tonsillectomy techniques have been gaining popularity in the belief that they may cause less postoperative pain and less risk of postoperative bleeding. This may especially be suitable for very young children in whom the surgeon wishes to preserve some pharyngeal lymphoid tissue. Microdebrider intracapsular

tonsillar removal has been adopted in many U.S. pediatric centers where it is termed *powered intracapsular tonsillectomy and adenoidectomy* (PITA). Of concern in this procedure and other techniques of tonsillotomy is potential tonsillar regrowth and subsequent tonsillitis or peritonsillar abscess.[24]

In some children who were not cured of OSA following T + A, sleep endoscopy revealed tongue base obstruction due to lingual tonsil hypertrophy.[25] In these cases using radiofrequency ablation (Coblation) of the lingual tonsil, an improvement of the OSA was reported. Postoperative pain may be severe after lingual tonsillectomy and there is a risk of airway obstruction due to swelling and postoperative hemorrhage. These children should be looked after in a specialist center with appropriate facilities including PICU.

19.8.5 Mandibular/Maxillary Advancement

In children with craniofacial anomalies, these procedures are often undertaken for aesthetic reasons, and to permit skeletal growth but sometimes to alleviate obstruction. Techniques include the use of bone and soft-tissue grafts, prostheses, and a variety of distraction methods to the bone growth pattern (osteogenic distraction techniques). These children are best managed in a designated craniofacial center where a multidisciplinary team has developed the appropriate expertise. In Pierre Robin sequence (▶ Fig. 19.4), mandibular distraction increases the retrolingual airway. In some centers, it is performed in the neonate in severe cases, thus avoiding a tracheostomy. In the older tracheotomized child, mandibular distraction may allow deccanulation. Children with Apert's or Crouzon's syndrome may also require maxillary advancement in order to achieve deccanulation, but only after full dentition.

19.8.6 Intranasal Surgery

Septal and turbinate surgery is rarely indicated in children. Bilateral choanal atresia is rare but requires prompt intervention after birth. Unilateral choanal atresia is usually detected later in life and can cause OSA along with a unilateral nasal discharge. An endoscopic approach is currently popular in these cases (see Chapter 16).

19.8.7 Hyoid/Tongue Suspension

In cases of failed T + A, as seen, for example, in children with Down's syndrome, obstruction may be at the level of the hypopharynx with marked hypotonia and glossoptosis (tongue base prolapse). This can be demonstrated by sleep endoscopy. A series of patients using a minimally invasive technique was recently reported showing improvement in the RDI following surgery, but this is not available outside of specialist centers and its place in OSA management is still uncertain.[26]

19.8.8 Tracheostomy

Tracheostomy is a drastic measure but it should be remembered that severe hypoxic events during sleep can result in neurologic damage and even death. Tracheostomy may sometimes be the only option for a child with severe OSA. Many of these children will manage with a smaller canula that can be plugged during the day and unplugged during sleep. The parents and caregivers must be trained in all aspects of tracheostomy care.

19.9 Comorbidity and Specific Conditions in Pediatric OSA

There are many unique clinical presentations of children with OSA that require special consideration; they are discussed next.

19.9.1 Congenital Anatomical Anomalies

These include skeletal anomalies such as those that occur in a variety of craniofacial syndromes, as listed in Box 19.2. Maxillary and mandibular hypoplasia, dental malocclusion, a reduced nasal airway, and abnormalities of the palate and the nasopharynx all contribute to OSA in these conditions. In Pierre Robin sequence that includes micrognathia due to mandibular hypoplasia, glossoptosis (a tendency for the tongue to prolapse into the pharyngeal airway especially when the child lies supine), and cleft palate, severe OSA can cause respiratory failure. This can be life-threatening and may warrant immediate management of the airway by insertion of a nasopharyngeal tube or, in extreme cases, endotracheal intubation and eventual tracheotomy (▶ Fig. 19.4).

> **i**
>
> Children with craniofacial syndromes require a multidisciplinary approach and are best managed by a team in a specialist center where expertise and resources are available.[27]

Osseodistraction techniques using bone grafts or prostheses have improved greatly, and many centers now offer this type of surgery that can help address both aesthetic and functional concerns and has gained popularity in experienced centers.[28] In severe cases of mandibular hypoplasia, the child may be managed using a nasopharyngeal airway until the mandible develops and the airway improves. Primary mandibular distraction is very

rarely considered, but in extreme cases this may avoid the need for a tracheotomy.

> **Box 19.2 Differential Diagnosis of Congenital and Neonatal Upper Airway Obstruction and OSA**
>
> - Craniofacial anomalies:
>   - ◦ Apert's or Crouzon's syndrome.
>   - ◦ Treacher Collins' syndrome.
> - Achondroplasia.
> - Beckwith–Wiedemann's syndrome.
> - Down's syndrome.
> - Mucopolysaccharidosis.
> - Pierre Robin sequence (▶ Fig. 19.4).
> - Prader Willi's syndrome.
> - Choanal atresia/stenosis.
> - Pyriform aperture stenosis.
> - Meningoencephalocele, nasal glioma, and other rare tumors.

Soft-tissue abnormalities such as macroglossia, lymphangiomas, and hemangiomas may obstruct the airway and give rise to OSA in very young children (▶ Fig. 19.5).

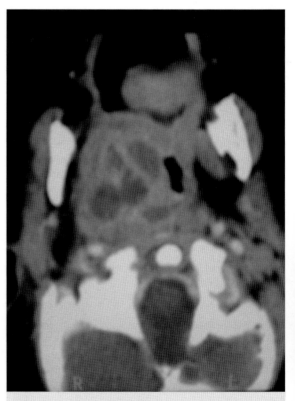

Fig. 19.5 Lymphatic malformation causing progressive obstructive sleep apnea in a 2-year-old.

19.9.2 Down's Syndrome

Children with Down's syndrome have multiple causes for sleep apnea including the following:
- Small midface and cranium.
- Narrow nasopharynx.
- Large tongue.
- Muscular hypotonia.
- Obesity.
- A small larynx.
- Midfacial dysmorphia.

Congenital heart disease and cor pulmonale may contribute to the severity of OSA. Liaison with the pediatric team, including the pediatric cardiologists is usually required. Children with Down's syndrome require special consideration and carefully planned perioperative care. Management may include pre- and postoperative PSG and postoperative HDU, or, in some situations, PICU observation.

> Children with Down's syndrome may have atlantoaxial instability, and extending the neck during surgical positioning may risk dislocation with catastrophic neurologic consequences. Position and move the head gently and carefully, and manipulate the neck as little as is practicable.

19.9.3 Head and Neck Neoplasm

This is a rare but important cause of OSA and needs to be considered as early diagnosis may be lifesaving. A history of recent onset or progressive OSA in an otherwise healthy child is a red light. When such a history coincides with unilateral tonsillar enlargement and lymphadenopathy, lymphoma is a consideration. ▶ Fig. 19.5 depicts an infant with progressive OSA and deviation of the tonsil without signs of infection. CT scan is suggestive of a lymphatic malformation and this was verified during surgery.

19.9.4 Obesity

This is a condition with increasing and alarming prevalence in children. Although children with OSA are usually underweight, obesity is an independent risk factor for OSA. Dietary management is essential and, if successful, may improve the OSA.[29] Long-term dietary management is difficult in children and requires a multidisciplinary approach and familial cooperation. Standard surgical treatment with T + A may reduce the severity of OSA

although not always resolve it. A meta-analysis showed that in approximately 80% of obese children, OSA persisted following T + A.[30] CPAP, if tolerated, may improve symptoms. Gastric bypass and sleeve operations have been suggested for extreme morbid obesity if conventional measures fail. In exceptional circumstances, tracheostomy may need to be considered.

19.9.5 Neonatal Nasal Obstruction

Due to anatomical and physiological attributes that are unique to the newborn, neonates are considered to be obligate nasal breathers. At birth, the larynx is in a cephalad position with the epiglottis reaching above the soft palate. This position allows the child to swallow and breathe simultaneously. Obstruction at the nasal/nasopharyngeal level will cause severe OSA and is life-threatening. The differential diagnosis is different than in older children, and OSA in the newborn must be treated immediately (Box 19.2).

19.9.6 Neurologic Conditions

Children with OSA and a neurologic condition are a challenge to treat. The upper airway obstruction can be caused by pharyngeal collapse due to the inherent hypotonia associated with the underlying neurologic disease. OSA in these children may improve after a T + A but is likely to persist. There may also be an element of CNS involvement causing central apnea or neuromuscular regulatory dysfunction. It may prudent to obtain a PSG as part of the preoperative evaluation and to liaise carefully with the pediatric neurologist. Occasionally, a child who is thought clinically to have OSA with episodes of apnea is in fact convulsing, and in many children with neurologic dysfunction, apneas are central or mixed rather than purely obstructive.

> OSA in a neurologically impaired child can have drastic effects on function and must be treated quickly.

In cases of brainstem compression such as seen in Arnold–Chiari malformation, surgical decompression may result in improvement of OSA. Perioperative treatment of children with neurologic disorders and OSA must be undertaken with great consideration and care. These children are at increased risk for postoperative complications and should be observed in the PICU following surgery. Box 19.3 shows a list of some neurologic diseases that are associated with risk for OSA.

> **Box 19.3 Neurologic Disease Contributing to OSA**
>
> - Generalized hypotonia: Down's syndrome, neuromuscular disease.
> - Diffuse brain injury: anoxic, traumatic.
> - Brainstem injury.
> - Tumor.
> - Brainstem compression: Arnold–Chiari, foramen magnum (achondroplasia).
> - Cerebral palsy.
> - Duchenne muscular dystrophy.

19.10 Perioperative Management of Children with OSA

Adenotonsillectomy is now almost exclusively undertaken under general anesthesia using a variety of techniques as described in Chapter 3 and 18. Anesthetic technique, minimizing excessive preoperative fasting, maintenance of adequate hydration, minimizing blood loss with its potentially irritant effect on the gastric mucosa, and judicious use of medications all help to reduce morbidity. The ideal is for the child to experience a smooth comfortable recovery with a return to normal diet and activity as soon as possible.

Postoperative nausea and vomiting has been reported in as many as 70% of children in some studies.[31] Serotonin antagonists (e.g., ondansetron) and a single dose of intraoperative steroid (e.g., dexamethasone 0.625 mg/kg) are now widely used and well supported by the available evidence (see Chapter 3).[32,33]

19.11 Complications of Adenotonsillectomy

19.11.1 Bleeding

Postoperative bleeding can be early (first 24 hours) or late (after 24 hours; see Chapter 18). The incidence of postoperative bleeding is considered to be approximately 2% and can be life-threatening. Death following tonsillectomy is extremely rare but clearly represents a catastrophic complication. It is caused by bleeding, airway obstruction, acute pulmonary edema, respiratory failure, or related problems and is reported in 1 per 10,000 to 20,000 cases.

Postoperative bleeding that requires further surgery usually occurs in the early postoperative period and before the child has been discharged. The child should be transferred to the operating room (OR) as soon as possible to secure the airway and control the bleeding.

> **i**
>
> If the child has gone home and has a bleed, the parents should seek help immediately.

If there is a profuse bleed, especially in the hours following surgery, the child should be taken to the nearest ER, where resuscitation is begun, blood tests are obtained, the child is typed and crossmatched for blood, and blood is ordered. The child may then need urgent transfer to the OR for exploration of the tonsil bed and arrest of bleeding. A skilled anesthetist should be on hand to manage the child's perioperative care and to ensure safe induction and maintenance of anesthesia in a situation where there may be a combination of a full stomach and hypovolemic shock. The child is likely to need a nasogastric tube to aspirate the contents of the stomach. Aspiration of blood filled gastric contents into the trachea can be catastrophic.

Access to the airway may also be a problem with blood clots obstructing the anesthesiologist's view making intubation difficult. The OR staff should be prepared for the very rare event that an emergency tracheotomy may be needed to manage the airway.

19.11.2 Infection

Postoperative infections are uncommon following T + A. *Grisel's syndrome* (atraumatic subluxation of the atlantoaxial joint) is rare but important to recognize. It should be suspected in a child presenting a few days after surgery with torticollis and fever. It is supposed that a local infection of the posterior pharyngeal wall causes laxity of the spinal ligaments with a risk for subluxation of the atlantoaxial joints. Treatment should include antibiotics, nonsteriodal anti-inflammatory drugs (NSAIDs), and neck stabilization or traction. Orthopaedic consultation should be obtained.

19.11.3 Dehydration

Postoperative pain and emesis may result in insufficient oral intake and dehydration. Postoperatively, the child should be encouraged to drink, and if not cooperative, analgesics should be given. Adequate hydration can be monitored by recording urine output. If signs of dehydration appear, intravenous (IV) fluids are warranted to avoid sequelae such as prerenal failure.

19.11.4 Postobstructive Pulmonary Edema

In children with severe and prolonged OSA, the operative removal of the obstruction may cause a dramatic shift in respiratory pathophysiology. Rapid and severe pulmonary edema can occur. This complication can also be seen when laryngospasm follows extubation. These children may require treatment in the PICU under the supervision of a pediatrician or intensivist (see Chapter 3).

19.11.5 Tonsil Regrowth

Following conventional tonsillectomy techniques, regrowth of tonsillar tissue is unlikely. When tonsillotomy techniques are used, regrowth can be an issue. This is of concern if obstructive symptoms recur. In a multicenter study reviewing experience with PITA, a recurrence rate of 0.1 to 0.3% was found. When choosing tonsillectomy technique, this should be discussed with the parents.[24]

There is more concern regarding adenoid regrowth. It is important to remove the adenoids under vision, using a mirror, and to check they have been completely removed. Suction cautery of the adenoid bed helps in this regard. When a sound technique of adenoidectomy is adhered to, the likelihood of regrowth is small.

19.11.6 Velopharyngeal Insufficiency

Many children following T + A have voice changes, mostly hypernasality. These changes resolve spontaneously in a short period of time. Rarely VPI persists, but if so, it can be of great concern to the child and parents due to incomprehensible speech (see Chapter 27). Children with craniofacial anomalies, submucous cleft palate, those who have had cleft palate repair, and those with neurologic impairment are especially at risk for VPI. It is important to advise parents of this potential risk especially in susceptible children.

19.12 Postoperative Monitoring and Treatment

In many centers in the United States and in much of Europe, T + A is a day-case procedure.

There is a subgroup of children that require hospitalization and includes the following:
- Neurologically impaired children.
- Children with severe OSA.
- Very young children.
- Low-weight children (e.g., < 15 kg).
- Children with blood disorders such as sickle cell syndrome.
- Children with significant comorbidities.

Some of these children should be observed in the HDU with intensive monitoring and a few may even require the full facilities of a PICU (Box 19.3). Guidelines have been suggested in many health care systems to determine the children that need inpatient postoperative follow-up. Most children with OSA can have safe surgery in a local hospital where staff are skilled and experienced in the care of children, for example, most District General Hospitals in the United Kingdom. A small number should be operated on in a regional/subregional center that is able to provide an additional tier of postoperative respiratory care.

> In general day-case surgery, is possible in the otherwise healthy child with mild-to-moderate OSA.[12]

19.13 Pain Management

Tonsillectomy is a painful procedure for the child, and pain management is of the greatest importance.

> In the immediate postoperative period, opioids can be considered if the child is closely monitored but this may delay discharge and make day surgery more difficult.

In infants with severe OSA, the use of opioids may blunt the respiratory drive and may result in apnea and hypoxia, so they should be avoided if at all possible in such cases.

> After discharge, the mainstay of analgesia is paracetamol and NSAIDs.

These should be administered based on recommended dosing schedules for the first few days and then as needed. Pain may persist for up to 3 weeks. There is some concern regarding an increased risk of bleeding with the use of NSAIDs. In a meta-analysis addressing this issue, the risk was found to be negligible.[34] When considering the suffering of the child, treatment with an NSAID may be the best option for pain relief.

Besides the discomfort, undertreating pain can result in poor fluid intake and even dehydration requiring hospitalization for IV fluids. A soft and cold diet may also be less painful for the child and should be offered. The management of post-tonsillectomy pain is discussed in Chapter 3 and 18.

19

19.14 Key Points

- OSA in children has a negative impact on the child's health and development and should be treated.
- In most cases, surgical treatment will resolve the disease but follow-up is important to verify resolution.
- Box 19.4 summarizes the current recommendations of the American Academy of Pediatrics regarding children with OSA.[10]

Box 19.4 Recommendations of the American Academy of Pediatrics Subcommittee on OSA Syndrome[10]

- All children/adolescents should be screened for snoring.
- PSG should be performed in children/adolescents with snoring and symptoms/signs of OSAS; if PSG is not available, then alternative diagnostic tests or referral to a specialist for more extensive evaluation may be considered.
- Adenotonsillectomy is recommended as the first-line treatment of patients with adenotonsillar hypertrophy.
- High-risk patients should be monitored as inpatients postoperatively.
- Patients should be reevaluated postoperatively to determine whether further treatment is required. Objective testing should be performed in patients who are at high risk or have persistent symptoms/signs of OSAS after therapy.
- CPAP is recommended as treatment if adenotonsillectomy is not performed or if OSAS persists postoperatively.
- Weight loss is recommended in addition to other therapy in patients who are overweight or obese.
- Intranasal corticosteroids are an option for children with mild OSAS in whom adenotonsillectomy is contraindicated or for mild postoperative OSAS.

References

[1] Tauman R, Gozal D. Obstructive sleep apnea syndrome in children. Expert Rev Respir Med. 2011; 5(3):425–440

[2] Lumeng JC, Chervin RD. Epidemiology of pediatric obstructive sleep apnea. Proc Am Thorac Soc. 2008; 5(2):242–252

[3] Greenfeld M, Tauman R, DeRowe A, Sivan Y. Obstructive sleep apnea syndrome due to adenotonsillar hypertrophy in infants. Int J Pediatr Otorhinolaryngol. 2003; 67(10):1055–1060

[4] Katz ES, D'Ambrosio CM. Pediatric obstructive sleep apnea syndrome. Clin Chest Med. 2010; 31(2):221–234

[5] Tarasiuk A, Simon T, Tal A, Reuveni H. Adenotonsillectomy in children with obstructive sleep apnea syndrome reduces health care utilization. Pediatrics. 2004; 113(2):351–356

[6] Landau YE, Bar-Yishay O, Greenberg-Dotan S, Goldbart AD, Tarasiuk A, Tal A. Impaired behavioral and neurocognitive function in pre-school children with obstructive sleep apnea. Pediatr Pulmonol. 2012; 47(2):180–188

[7] Marcus CL, Moore RH, Rosen CL, et al. Childhood Adenotonsillectomy Trial (CHAT). A randomized trial of adenotonsillectomy for childhood sleep apnea. N Engl J Med. 2013; 368(25):2366–2376

[8] Kaditis A. From obstructive sleep apnea in childhood to cardiovascular disease in adulthood: what is the evidence? Commentary Sleep. 2010; 33(10):1279–1280

[9] Baldassari CM, Mitchell RB, Schubert C, Rudnick EF. Pediatric obstructive sleep apnea and quality of life: a meta-analysis. Otolaryngol Head Neck Surg. 2008; 138(3):265–273

[10] Marcus CL, et al. Diagnosis of childhood obstructive sleep apnea. Pediatrics. 2012; 130(3):576–584

[11] Oliveira VX, Teng AY. The clinical usefulness of sleep studies in children. Paediatr Respir Rev. 2016; 17:53–56

[12] Robb PJ, Bew S, Kubba H, et al. Tonsillectomy and adenoidectomy in children with sleep-related breathing disorders: consensus statement of a UK multidisciplinary working party. Ann R Coll Surg Engl. 2009; 91(5):371–373

[13] Nixon GM, Kermack AS, Davis GM, Manoukian JJ, Brown KA, Brouillette RT. Planning adenotonsillectomy in children with obstructive sleep apnea: the role of overnight oximetry. Pediatrics. 2004; 113(1 Pt 1):e19–e25

[14] Sivan Y, Kornecki A, Schonfeld T. Screening obstructive sleep apnoea syndrome by home videotape recording in children. Eur Respir J. 1996; 9(10):2127–2131

[15] Durr ML, Meyer AK, Kezirian EJ, Rosbe KW. Drug-induced sleep endoscopy in persistent pediatric sleep-disordered breathing after adenotonsillectomy. Arch Otolaryngol Head Neck Surg. 2012; 138(7):638–643

[16] Brouillette RT, Manoukian JJ, Ducharme FM, et al. Efficacy of fluticasone nasal spray for pediatric obstructive sleep apnea. J Pediatr. 2001; 138(6):838–844

[17] Goldbart AD, Greenberg-Dotan S, Tal A. Montelukast for children with obstructive sleep apnea: a double-blind, placebo-controlled study. Pediatrics. 2012; 130(3):e575–e580

[18] Marcus CL, Beck SE, Traylor J, et al. Randomized, double-blind clinical trial of two different modes of positive airway pressure therapy on adherence and efficacy in children. J Clin Sleep Med. 2012; 8(1):37–42

[19] Bhattacharjee R, Kheirandish-Gozal L, Spruyt K, et al. Adenotonsillectomy outcomes in treatment of obstructive sleep apnea in children: a multicenter retrospective study. Am J Respir Crit Care Med. 2010; 182(5):676–683

[20] Brietzke SE, Gallagher D. The effectiveness of tonsillectomy and adenoidectomy in the treatment of pediatric obstructive sleep apnea/hypopnea syndrome: a meta-analysis. Otolaryngol Head Neck Surg. 2006; 134(6):979–984

[21] Brietzke SE, Kenna M, Katz ES, Mitchell E, Roberson D. Pediatric adenoidectomy: what is the effect of obstructive symptoms on the likelihood of future surgery? Int J Pediatr Otorhinolaryngol. 2006; 70(8):1467–1472

[22] Messner AH. Tonsillectomy. Operative Techniques Otolaryngol. 2005; 16:224–228

[23] Solares CA, Koempel JA, Hirose K, et al. Safety and efficacy of powered intracapsular tonsillectomy in children: a multi-center case series. Int J Pediatr Otorhinolaryngol. 2005; 69(1):21–26

[24] Lowe D, van der Meulen J, National Prospective Tonsillectomy Audit. Tonsillectomy technique as a risk factor for postoperative haemorrhage. Lancet. 2004; 364(9435):697–702

[25] Lin AC, Koltai PJ. Persistent pediatric obstructive sleep apnea and lingual tonsillectomy. Otolaryngol Head Neck Surg. 2009; 141(1):81–85

[26] Wootten CT, Shott SR. Evolving therapies to treat retroglossal and base-of-tongue obstruction in pediatric obstructive sleep apnea. Arch Otolaryngol Head Neck Surg. 2010; 136(10):983–987

[27] Cielo CM, Marcus CL. Obstructive sleep apnoea in children with craniofacial syndromes. Paediatr Respir Rev. 2015; 16(3):189–196

V

[28] Hong P. A clinical narrative review of mandibular distraction osteogenesis in neonates with Pierre Robin sequence. Int J Pediatr Otorhinolaryngol. 2011; 75(8):985–991

[29] Kassim R, Harris MA, Leong GM, Heussler H. Obstructive sleep apnoea in children with obesity. J Paediatr Child Health. 2016; 52(3):284–290

[30] Costa DJ, Mitchell R. Adenotonsillectomy for obstructive sleep apnea in obese children: a meta-analysis. Otolaryngol Head Neck Surg. 2009; 140(4):455–460

[31] Mukherjee K, Esuvaranathan V, Streets C, Johnson A, Carr AS. Adenotonsillectomy in children: a comparison of morphine and fentanyl for peri-operative analgesia. Anaesthesia. 2001; 56(12):1193–1197

[32] Plante J, Turgeon AF, Zarychanski R, et al. Effect of systemic steroids on post-tonsillectomy bleeding and reinterventions: systematic review and meta-analysis of randomised controlled trials. BMJ. 2012; 345:e5389

[33] Gallagher TQ, Hill C, Ojha S, et al. Perioperative dexamethasone administration and risk of bleeding following tonsillectomy in children: a randomized controlled trial. JAMA. 2012; 308(12):1221–1226

[34] Cardwell ME, Siviter G, Smith AF. Non-steroidal anti-inflammatory drugs and perioperative bleeding in paediatric tonsillectomy. Cochrane Database Syst Rev. 2005; 18(2):CD003591

19

20 Airway Obstruction in Children

Adam J. Donne and Michael P. Rothera

20.1 Introduction

Respiratory problems are relatively common in children attending emergency medical departments. Respiratory failure is the most common cause of cardiac arrest in children.

Children are not simply small adults. Their airways are indeed physically smaller but there are additional differences such as neonatal dependence on nasal patency and a funnel-shaped laryngeal profile compared to a more tubelike larynx in adults. Children have a higher breathing and heart rate, each of which changes according to age, a higher metabolic rate, and less respiratory reserve than adults.

> Complete airway obstruction is rapidly fatal. Incomplete and slowly progressing obstruction results in classical signs of increased work of breathing, hypoxemia, and respiratory failure.[1]

20.2 Physics of Airway Obstruction

20.2.1 Resistance to Airflow

Poiseuille's law (Box 20.1) explains changes that occur as fluid (liquid or gas) passes through a tube. It describes the relationship between pressure and flow rate when the diameter of the tube is varied. Even though the equation does not completely fit for the respiratory tract, the principles remain true.

> Minor reductions in airway diameter result in dramatic increases in airway resistance.

The law demonstrates this as the radius is altered to the power of 4. This principle is pivotal to understanding the effects of reducing the diameter of a tube.

Box 20.1 Poiseuille's Law

$$R = \frac{8\mu l}{\pi r^4}$$

where R is resistance, μ is viscosity, l is length of pipe, and r is radius.

20.2.2 Laminar and Turbulent Flow

In *laminar* flow, the fluid moves in parallel waves, in contrast with the irregular fluctuations that characterize *turbulent* flow (▶ Fig. 20.1). The healthy flow of air within the airway depends on *laminar flow* as the resistance is least in this situation.

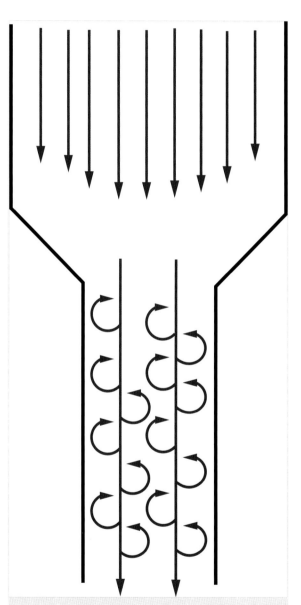

Fig. 20.1 Laminar versus turbulent flow.

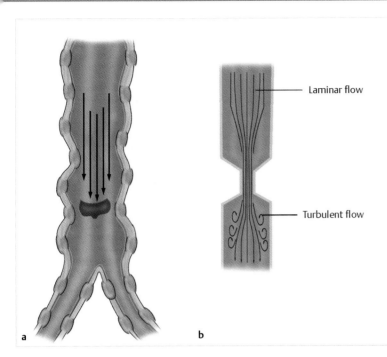

Fig. 20.2 Stridor in relation to the Reynold's number. **(a)** Normal caliber airway, laminar flow. **(b)** Narrowed airway. As air passes through the narrowed segment, laminar flow becomes turbulent, that is, the threshold for laminar flow (Reynold's number) is exceeded.

Laminar flow

Turbulent flow

a   b

20

> In the presence of a stricture, the diameter is reduced, so to maintain flow through that stricture, the flow rate at that point must increase and hence turbulence may occur.

Progressively reducing the airway radius eventually results in a critical radius that brings about turbulent flow. The critical point at which turbulent flow occurs is indicated by the Reynold's number (see Box 20.2). The use of heliox (helium 80% plus oxygen 20%) exploits knowledge of the Reynold's number. Heliox reduces stridor as its density is lower than that of air (nitrogen 79% plus oxygen 21%). Heliox improves the clinical condition because it reduces the work of breathing. The lower density of heliox means a lower Reynold's number and hence lower probability of turbulence/stridor.[2]

> **Box 20.2 Factors Affecting the Critical Point (Reynold's Number, Re) at which Airflow Becomes Turbulent**
>
> $$Re = \frac{\rho v d}{\mu}$$
>
> where Re is the Reynolds number, d is the diameter of the pipe, v is the mean velocity, μ is the dynamic viscosity, and ρ is the density.

20.2.3 The Bernoulli Principle

This indicates that in order for the fluid/gas to pass through a narrowed point in a tube, it must speed up. Consequently, the pressure at the point of narrowing drops. It is this reduction of pressure plus the increased flow rate that results in the vibration of the walls of the airway and column of air that we hear as a stridor.[1] The point at which stridor occurs within a given airway is at the change from laminar to turbulent flow (i.e., the Reynolds number; ► Fig. 20.2). What does this mean in real clinical terms?

> The resistance to airflow rises with a reduction in tracheal diameter. When the diameter reduces by approximately 70%, there is a significant change in resistance. This means that when a child has stridor, even at the onset and even if the stridor is very mild, a significant narrowing of the airway is present.

The Venturi effect is the name given to the phenomenon that results in a narrowed collapsible tube collapsing further as air passes through it. This is because the pressure exerted by a gas within a tube is equal in all directions except when there is flow in a forward linear direction. Linear flow results in a reduction of the vector of force exerted outward against the walls of the tube. This allows some collapse of the tube, as demonstrated in clinical practice with bilateral vocal cord palsy when the vocal cords (sitting within the flow of air) are seen to prolapse toward each other during inspiration. This is also the effect that causes supraglottic collapse and stridor in laryngomalacia.

The collapsible nature of the intrathoracic airway is additionally important as an obstruction at the bronchi (e.g., foreign body causing a ball valve effect) may mean the child requires considerable extra effort to exhale. The intrathoracic pressure has to be greater than atmospheric pressure to permit exhalation of air; hence, the airway diameter may reduce, thus increasing the difficulty of breathing. If there is an obstruction within the airway outside the thorax, then forced inspiration will result in an intrathoracic low pressure to generate a pressure gradient enough to "suck" air in. This may result in the extrathoracic trachea collapsing by the Venturi effect.

> Changes in intrathoracic pressure may be one of the factors that precipitates gastroesophageal reflux as the low pressure causes a pressure gradient across the gastroesophageal junction and stomach contents enter the thoracic esophagus.

20.3 Assessment of the Airway

The history and examination will direct the otolaryngologist's attention to particular anatomical regions of the airway. There may be synchronous pathology, for example, laryngomalacia plus bronchial stenosis. Understanding severity aids the management of the compromised child and dictates the urgency of intervention.

20.3.1 Clinical Assessment by History

> Stertor is a relatively low-pitched sound that originates at the level of the nasopharynx or oropharynx.

It is typically due to the partial collapse of pharyngeal wall structures into the airway. The most frequent causes of stertor include adenotonsillar hypertrophy. However, tongue position and placement are also important in children with relative macroglossia or with hypotonia due to neurologic conditions.

Stridor is upper airway noise arising from the large diameter airway, that is, the larynx and trachea. The noun "stridor" is derived from the Latin. The verb "stridere" means to make a harsh sound (squeak or screech). Stridor is a clinical term reserved characteristically for a noise generated from the large diameter airways. Smaller diameter airways give rise to wheeze, as with asthma (and this is expiratory). This chapter will concentrate on stridor.

Stridor can occur from birth. The commonest cause of congenital stridor is laryngomalacia, followed by congenital vocal cord palsy, which is a significantly less frequent second cause. Both these conditions will be present at birth but may take a couple of weeks to develop. Stridor that occurs 3 months after birth may be due to a subglottic hemangioma. A history of previous intubation (particularly with prematurity) is a risk for subglottic cyst formation.

A history of recurrent croup is often associated with subglottic stenosis. It is believed that many different virus types cause croup. These viruses cause some degree of subglottic edema. If the subglottis has a preexisting subglottic narrowing, the croup becomes more clinically important. The same viruses may cause subglottic edema in children without subglottic narrowing. However, they may not induce enough edema to reduce the tracheal diameter by the approximately 70% needed to result in a clinically audible stridor.

With a history of tracheoesophageal fistulas (TOFs), some element of tracheomalacia is to be expected as this condition is due to a defect in the development of the trachea and esophagus, and therefore weakness of the tracheal wall is present. If the stridor changes with a change in position of the infant, this indicates the site of pathology, for example, lying down on the left side may reduce the stridor caused by left-sided vocal cord palsy. This sign is not reliable.

In a stridulous child, fever, hoarseness, and a rapid onset may indicate an infective etiology. The history of airways symptoms is an important determinant of management.

> A rapid onset indicates infection or foreign body whereas a gradual history implies cysts, stenosis, hemangiomas, or recurrent papillomatosis.

A prodromal upper respiratory tract infection may signify croup, tracheitis, or the now rare epiglottitis. If previous endotracheal (ET) intubation has occurred, consider cysts or stenosis. With altered voice or hoarseness one should exclude respiratory papillomatosis, a glottic web and foreign body. "Singer's" or "Screamer's" nodules in children do not cause airway compromise. For children with feeding difficulty, coughing, choking, or cyanosis, TOF, a vascular ring, or an inhaled foreign body may be the cause.

> If a parent expresses concern about the work of breathing of their child, they are usually correct and there is a diagnosis that can be made.

20.3.2 Clinical Assessment by Examination

It is important to recognize that the airway starts at the nose and mouth and these must be included in any airway assessment. A cold spatula can identify a patent nasal airway bilaterally. It is not unusual to find a unilateral choanal atresia presenting in later childhood. Even with bilaterally patent posterior nasal apertures, a baby can still develop nasal airway obstruction, for example, if there is an intranasal mass, severe rhinitis, or the rare congenital nasal pyriform aperture stenosis (see Chapter 16). The size and position of the jaw is important as *retrognathia* can cause supraglottic crowding and obstructive symptoms. Typically, obstruction at this level will cause stertor rather than stridor, but parents and referring clinicians may be uncertain and the history cannot be relied upon completely.

Stridor has the following three basic forms that help determine the level of airway obstruction:

- Inspiratory.
- Expiratory.
- Biphasic.

Inspiratory stridor usually occurs when there is an obstruction *above the level of the vocal cords*, for example, laryngomalacia causes inspiratory stridor because the epiglottis or arytenoid mucosa prolapses into the laryngeal airway with inspiration but the inlet opens again with expiration. Be cautious as occasionally severe tracheomalacia can also result in inspiratory stridor.

> Biphasic stridor is always a significant clinical sign, as it signifies a severe obstruction and requires *early* airway endoscopy. Stridor can be biphasic in any severe laryngotracheal obstruction but is classically described in either vocal cord palsy or severe subglottic stenosis.

Expiratory stridor is relatively uncommon. It may occur in tracheomalacia, when the noise is largely expiratory due to tracheal collapse as the child breathes out, but can also arise due to a prolapsing subglottic mass. During inspiration, the mass is drawn in. On expiration, the mass may partially obstruct the inferior aspect of the vocal cords (this ball valve effect can be seen with respiratory papillomatosis; however, these children are additionally hoarse).

> Assessing the nature of the stridor is the first part of the assessment of a child's airway. It is normally this that alerts the parents to a problem.

Additional features of airway obstruction include poor feeding, and a distressed and unhappy child with the following:

- Tracheal tug.
- Sternal recession.
- Subcostal recession.

This order approximately indicates the increasing severity of the obstruction. Additional signs include the *use of accessory muscles of respiration*. A drooling child with quiet stridor and bracing him/herself holding the head upright is a classical image of acute epiglottitis. In an infant, the *extended head position, nasal flaring*, and *head bobbing* are also significant.

Rate of breathing is also a reliable and relatively objective sign that can be appreciated readily by parents, carers, nurses, and clinicians. *Tachypnea* is more likely with increased work of breathing. Perhaps unsurprisingly, as the child tires, breathing becomes less effective and the volume of breathing reduces.

> This reduced breath volume results in a quietening of stridor and is deceptively dangerous (Box 20.3).

The dusky color of a child may indicate poor oxygen saturation and is a valuable sign.

> True cyanosis is a very late sign and should indicate impending catastrophe unless there is a coexisting cardiac condition.

Transcutaneous oxygen saturation monitoring using *pulse oximetry* is also valuable. In addition to demonstrating severity, it indicates objectively the effect of treatment. Overreliance on such measures is not recommended as a child may have saturations remaining above 90% but can still have a significant airway obstruction particularly if the child is on high flow oxygen. Arterial blood gas analysis is seldom used in children as it is both painful and difficult. Capillary blood gas analysis is the norm for carbon dioxide (CO_2) assessment.

Transcutaneous CO_2 monitoring may have a place in the assessment of the more chronic airway problems as with central or obstructive sleep apnea where the CO_2 may rise as the night progresses. However, it can be difficult to achieve a good trace.

Box 20.3 Emergency Airway Management

When a child has stridor and is struggling to breathe, immediate management is required.

- Check that the child has a clear and patent airway, using suction as needed.
- Administering *high flow oxygen* is the first stage of management that can be applied in many varied situations. High flow can only be correctly achieved using a rebreathing bag.
- *Nebulized adrenalin* 2 mL (1 in 1,000) plus 2 mL of normal saline (to increase the volume enough to allow the solution to be nebulized) can be administered readily. If edema is contributing to the airway obstruction, there is typically an improvement in symptoms within minutes. In the emergency situation, this can be repeated as required until the airway is safe.
- *Steroids* have an early role in emergency airway management as proven in the treatment of croup.[3] Dexamethasone (0.3 mg/kg) will work quickly either orally or intravenously. Inhaled budesonide (2 mg) has been used increasingly and is of value.
- *Heliox* (as mentioned earlier) can be used to reduce the effort of breathing. It is easier to breathe but only contains 20% oxygen content. It does have not have a direct therapeutic benefit but may permit better airway oxygenation until definitive measures can be undertaken. However, caution should be applied as the need for heliox implies severe airflow obstruction. The use of heliox should therefore prompt emergency airway endoscopy and a securing of the airway (e.g., by ET intubation).
- In a baby or drowsy child, the application of a face mask and positive end-expiratory pressure (PEEP) may be beneficial. Introduction of an oral (Guedel) airway is not recommended for stridor—although it is useful in other forms of airway obstruction—unless the diagnosis is already known or the child is getting worse despite the aforementioned first-line measures.
- If the child's condition deteriorates due to progressive airway obstruction, then the only remaining strategy is to establish an alternative airway. This will usually take the form of ET intubation. If this is not possible due to abnormal anatomy at the level of the larynx, then a laryngeal mask can be very helpful. Ultimately, intubation may need to be performed endoscopically (discussed in the following). In an emergency situation, if there is no clinician sufficiently skilled at ET intubation or if there is a bolus such as an impacted foreign body obstructing the larynx, an emergency cricotracheal puncture as recommended in the Advanced Pediatric Life Support manual may be life-saving (▶ Fig. 20.3; see Chapter 23).
- Importantly, the child is more than his/her airway; heart monitoring should be employed throughout. Hypoxia if severe and prolonged enough will result in acidosis and bradycardia; this must be recognized early before it leads to cardiac arrest. Ideally, resuscitation is designed to prevent this.

20.3.3 Airway Endoscopic Assessment

Airway endoscopic assessment using Hopkins rigid telescopes is also called microlaryngotracheobronchoscopy (MLTB) and direct laryngotracheobronchoscopy (DLTB), but they are the same procedure. The prefix "micro" relates to the operating microscope, which some otolaryngologists use particularly to facilitate the use of microlaryngeal instruments. This form of assessment requires a high level of trust and coordination between the anesthetist and laryngologist as the airway is being "shared" between the two specialists. The fundamental requirement of this procedure is to ensure continuing ventilation of the airway during the examination. This usually means that the child is spontaneously breathing such that he/she does not need ET intubation before the origin of the stridor can be located. There are significant challenges for the anesthetist and the procedure is best undertaken in a specialist center, where both the surgeon and anesthetist have the appropriate experience, other than in an extreme emergency. If you do not have the requisite experience or anesthetic backup, the safest approach is to insert an ET tube, secure the airway, and arrange transfer of the child to a specialist unit.

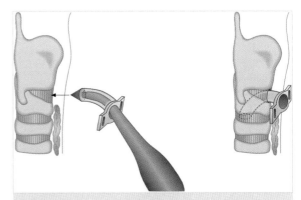

Fig. 20.3 Emergency cricothyrotomy. (Reproduced from Probst R, Grevers G, Iro H. Basic Otolaryngology: A Step-by-Step Learning Guide. Stuttgart/New York; Thieme: 2006, with permission.)

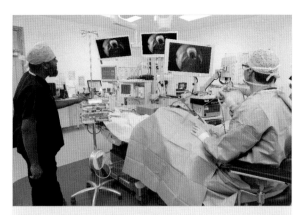

Fig. 20.4 Airway endoscopy under general anesthesia in a baby. The images are projected on the screens and the anesthetist (left) and the rest of the team can see them in "real time."

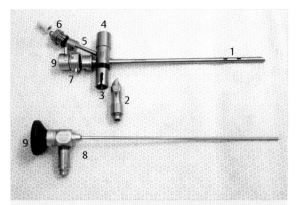

Fig. 20.5 Storz ventilating bronchoscope showing component parts. 1, Perforations for ventilation; 2, prism; 3, port for prism; 4, port for anesthetic gases; 5, suction channel; 6, metal and rubber caps for suction channel; 7, bridge to ensure snug fit for telescope; 8, Hopkins rod telescope; 9, eyepiece.

20

Before starting the procedure, it is important to check equipment. "White-balancing" and the ability to view the endoscopic findings on a large screen are important for the otolaryngologist and the view on the monitor gives important feedback to the anesthetist (▶ Fig. 20.4). A video recording and high-quality printouts can be invaluable as a clinical record, to explain findings to parents, and to plan future interventions.

Anesthesia and Perioperative Care

Intravenous access is established before any instrumentation is permitted. Techniques vary (see Chapter 3) but the author's preference is as follows:
- The child has sevoflurane gas administered through a face mask. The child slowly becomes anesthetized.
- The vocal cords are identified and seen by the anesthetist using an intubating laryngoscope (Macintosh) and topical local anesthetic spray (lidocaine 2%) is applied at a dose appropriate for the age of the child. Some element of laryngospasm always occurs at this point, but if the child is deep enough, this is very temporary.
- When the child is "deep" enough, a nasopharyngeal airway (NPA) is inserted, with the proximal end of the tube just above the level of the epiglottis.
- Sevoflurane is then administered through the NPA. (Laryngospasm can also occur if the NPA is inserted before the topical anesthetic is applied and the larynx is stimulated by a very long NPA.)
- The child then has a shoulder roll inserted to gently support and extend the neck.

Technique of Airway Endoscopy

- Before the laryngoscope is inserted, take care to protect the lips, gums, and teeth, if present, by using a damp gauze swab or gum guard.

- Inserted a laryngoscope (Lindholm) into the oropharynx and confirm that the lower end of the NPA tube is at the correct level just above the epiglottis.
- Insert the laryngoscope into the valleculae, then gently but firmly "lift" the laryngoscope anteriorly without pivoting it onto the upper alveolar margin. There should be no anatomical fulcrum. This significantly reduces risk of damage from the procedure. Make sure that the lips are well free of the laryngoscope, particularly if you reposition it. The lips can easily become trapped between the teeth/gums and the instrument, causing bruising.
- Insert a 4-mm Hopkins rod carefully through the laryngoscope.

In most circumstances, a 4-mm Hopkins rod can then be inserted through the laryngoscope to deliver the first clear view of the larynx. Open communication should be maintained with the anesthetist throughout the procedure as laryngospasm can still occur. Camera heads attached to Hopkins rods and large viewing screens allow the whole operating room team to witness the endoscopic findings. It is important that the team is aware of the level of severity of the stridor as swift action may be needed to have additional equipment at hand, for example, a smaller straight ET tube.

If the child is maintaining a good level of oxygen saturation the rest of the procedure can proceed with simply a 4-mm Hopkins rod through a laryngoscope. If there is an obstruction significant enough such that there is inadequate tidal volume, then keeping the child adequately anesthetized can be problematic. In this situation, Storz ventilating bronchoscopes are ideal (▶ Fig. 20.5, ▶ Fig. 20.6). If the light source is attached to the prism, the operator will still get a view of the tracheobronchial tree, and the ventilating bronchoscope effectively functions as a metal ET tube. The lumen of the bronchoscope

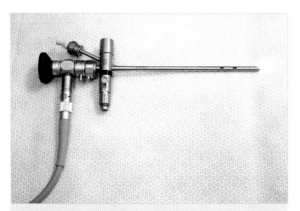

Fig. 20.6 Bronchoscope assembled and ready for use with telescope in position.

can be used to facilitate the use of rigid suction for thick secretions, or a forceps can be used for retrieval of a foreign body, although in this situation, the optical forceps with its integral telescope will give a much better view wherever practical (▶ Fig. 20.7). If a Hopkins rod is introduced, oxygen and anesthetic gas can pass alongside it yet within the hollow bronchoscope, albeit with a reduced caliber of the available air passage, making ventilation more difficult. The illumination provided by a telescope gives an immeasurably better view. This enables a high fidelity image to be seen on the screen and is nearly always preferred.

There are numerous sizes of ventilating bronchoscopes that correlate to a normal range of airway diameters according to age. The smallest of ventilating tubes can be prone to "stacking" of gases. This is a situation in which gases can be introduced into the lungs but the "exhalation" phase is less efficient, so CO_2 can build up.

The sizes of instruments inserted into the airway are gauged against known normal diameters of the airway (▶ Table 20.1). Essentially beyond 1 month of age, a

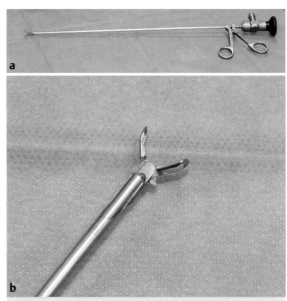

Fig. 20.7 (a) Optical (grasping) forceps with integral telescope for removal of bronchial foreign body. **(b)** The forceps is introduced through a ventilating bronchoscope. The distal end of the telescope provides excellent illumination, so the foreign body can be easily seen, engaged, and removed.

4-mm Hopkins rod can be inserted up to the carina without damage in a normal airway. This is not possible with even minor subglottic stenosis. However, if you are simply using a rigid Hopkins rod for the assessment of infants in which the size of the airway is only slightly bigger than the rod, there will be reduced opportunity for ventilation. The rod itself acts as an obstruction. In this situation, with spontaneous breathing, an exaggeration of airway collapse occurs and may produce an artificial "tracheomalacia." Fortunately, a small 2.7-mm endoscope reduces this risk significantly, but the view is less sharp and less bright than with a larger bore telescope. True tracheomalacia is a reduction of the tracheal diameter by 50% or more on expiration. A ventilating bronchoscope is also useful to allow the application of PEEP. This indicates whether continuous positive airway pressure would be effective in postoperative management.

At the start of the endoscopy, there will already be some indication from previous history and examination as to the patency of the nasal airway, the integrity of the palate, the presence of any retro- or micrognathia, and the size of the palatine tonsils. All these features must be documented.

Occasionally, the larynx appears to be in closer contact against the posterior tongue, resulting in difficulty accessing the valleculae. The additional outcome is that intubation is difficult and the epiglottis tends to project down over the laryngeal inlet.

Table 20.1 ET tube sizes for children under 2 years based on age and weight

Age	Tracheal diameter (mm)	ET tube size
Preterm	<4	2.5–3.0
0–1 mo	4–4.5	3–3.5
1–6 mo	4.5–5.5	3.5
6–12 mo	5.5–6	3.5–4
12–24 mo	6–6.5	4–4.5

Note: Size 2.5 tubes are available for very small babies but they are very easily obstructed by secretions. The tube size is based on the internal diameter, so a size 3 ET tube provides an airway that is only 3 mm wide. Have an age-appropriate sized tube and a size smaller for use in an emergency. These figures are typical, but the diameter of the individual child's trachea will of course vary.

Any movement of supraglottic structures should be assessed to rule out laryngomalacia. Within the larynx, active and passive vocal cord mobility is assessed to rule out vocal cord palsy and cricoarytenoid joint fixation. However, establishing the correct anesthetic balance to assess active vocal cord mobility can be difficult in the neonate and infants with chronic lung disease of prematurity.

> A thorough and complete airway endoscopy includes assessment of the posterior nasal apertures (choanae) and a dynamic assessment of vocal cord mobility.

20.3.4 Combined Flexible and Rigid Airway Endoscopy

> Flexible awake laryngoscopy should be considered complimentary to formal MLTB, and in most nonacute cases of stridor, this can be done as part of the initial consultation.

When performing awake flexible laryngoscopy, the infant should ideally be seated upright and on the mother's lap. Between 18 months and 4 years of age, it is difficult to perform an awake laryngoscopy as the child struggles, and although restraint is inappropriate, if the mother gently holds the child, it may be possible to get a good view provided neither the mother nor the child is distressed or upset. Over the age of 4 years, it is possible to negotiate with the child. A laryngeal cleft should be routinely excluded as a small cleft (type 1) can be easily missed with a relatively minor amount of posterior com-

missure edema. The size/diameter of the subglottis should be assessed under direct endoscopic view using straight ET tubes of known outer diameter and compared to known standards for the child's age. The shape and patency of the trachea should be noted as tracheomalacia is only significant if there is a reduction in the airway by at least 50%. The carina should be sharp and the primary (main stem) bronchi not malacic. The left main stem bronchus is often more difficult to access given its relatively horizontal position. Turning the head in the contralateral direction often improves access, that is, turn the head to the right to access the left main bronchus.

ET intubation may be required during routine MLTB or in an acute airway emergency situation. There is no better way to view the larynx than by endoscopy using a Hopkins rod. The light intensity of anesthetic intubating laryngoscopes is often poor.

> During the endoscopy, an ET tube can be easily guided into the trachea using a Hopkins rod. In a difficult intubation, place a Hopkins rod endoscope inside an appropriately sized ET tube to guide the ET tube into the trachea under direct vision.

For a baby, a 2.7-mm Hopkins rod sheathed with a size 3.0 ET tube is adequate (► Fig. 20.8). The blue connector should be removed during this procedure until the endoscope is withdrawn (► Fig. 20.9). For all other circumstances, a 4-mm Hopkins rod sheathed with a tube larger than 4.5 mm (internal diameter) is appropriate. The key is having an adequately long Hopkins rod sheathed with a straight ET tube that is at least 0.5 mm larger in diameter. A longer Hopkins rod is the best as it prevents the need to cut short the ET tube and will ensure the tube is inserted well into the trachea.

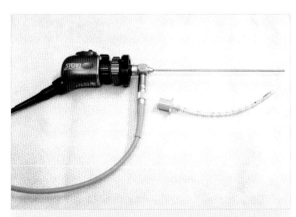

Fig. 20.8 A 2.7-mm Hopkins rod ready to be sheathed with a size 3.0 endotracheal tube.

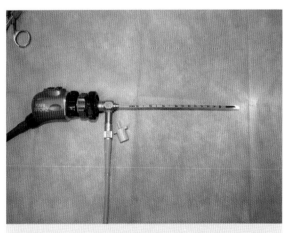

Fig. 20.9 An endotracheal tube mounted on a Hopkins rod. The blue ventilation connector has been removed.

20

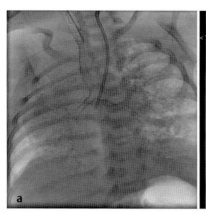
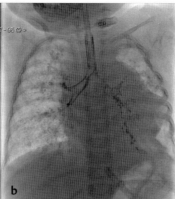

Fig. 20.10 Bronchograms. **(a)** Normal. **(b)** Bronchomalacia. The bronchi show filling defects on expiration. The caliber of the right main stem bronchus has greatly reduced. The left main stem has almost completely occluded.

20.3.5 Imaging the Airway

It is occasionally appropriate to perform radiological investigation to better understand hence manage the condition.[4] Chest radiographs may be beneficial in diagnosing a radio-opaque inhaled foreign body. If a ball-valve phenomenon is present, there will be hyperinflation of one lung field and collapse of the contralateral side. If severe enough, this may cause mediastinal shift and a compromise in cardiac output.

- Magnetic resonance imaging is helpful to confirm the diagnosis of subglottic hemangioma and to define the extent of the lesion.
- Computed tomography scanning is ideal for further investigating a child with tracheomalacia when vascular compression is suspected. The conditions of the scanning take the heartbeat into account and hold the ventilatory phase in expiration. This requires a degree of PEEP and hence the severity of tracheomalacia cannot be evaluated from such a scan. Additionally, the child will necessarily be intubated. The ET tube will to some degree stent open the malacic trachea.
- A bronchogram is useful in diagnosing bronchomalacia as this is more difficult to quantify by MLTB (▶ Fig. 20.10). Ultimately, the MLTB is the gold standard investigation of the tracheal lumen. The additional radiological investigation should be used for support and not exclusion.

20.4 Transfer of Acute Airway Child

With the development of specialist services and retrieval networks, children with a compromised airway will increasing be transferred to specialist centers. This allows these patients to have care from centers with the greatest expertise. This, of course, means transferring airway-compromised children safely. In most circumstances, this will result in intubations, often difficult, being carried out by transfer teams. There are limits to the equipment available at outside sites, and therefore a "difficult intubation kit" will be necessary as part of the team's stock of equipment. The use of endoscopic intubation in these circumstances will entirely depend upon the training and expertise of the retrieval team members. In many circumstances, a laryngeal mask is a good means of maintaining normal oxygen levels and it may be the safest option, although it is less secure than an ET tube (see ▶ Fig. 3.2, ▶ Fig. 3.3).

20.5 Tracheostomy

For details on tracheostomy, see Chapter 23.

20.6 Key Points

- A reduction in airway diameter of 70% precipitates the onset of stridor.
- History and examination indicates level of obstruction and severity.
- MLTB confirms diagnosis.
- Biphasic stridor is a serious finding and dictates compulsory and early MLTB.
- Nebulized adrenalin and steroids (oral or intravenous) are of proven benefit in the management of acute airway obstruction.
- Endoscopic intubation is an essential skill for the difficult airway.
- Tracheostomies block and require urgent airway management (suction and replacement).

References

[1] Ida JB, Thompson DM. Pediatric stridor. Otolaryngol Clin North Am. 2014; 47(5):795–819
[2] McGarvey JM, Pollack CV. Heliox in airway management. Emerg Med Clin North Am. 2008; 26(4):905–920, viii
[3] National Institute for Health and Care Excellence. Clinical Knowledge Summaries: Croup. September 2012
[4] Darras KE, Roston AT, Yewchuk LK. Imaging acute airway obstruction in infants and children. Radiographics. 2015; 35(7):2064–2079

21 Congenital Disorders of the Larynx, Trachea, and Bronchi

Daniel Tweedie and Benjamin Hartley

21.1 Introduction

Congenital disorders of the larynx, trachea, and bronchi are not uncommon. This is an important group of disorders. This chapter covers the embryology, anatomy, and clinical features of the principle conditions.

21.2 Applied Basic Science

The larynx is a complex, funnel-shaped organ (▶ Fig. 21.1). It comprises a cartilaginous framework that supports membranes and fascial layers to allow the attachment of a number of intrinsic and extrinsic muscles and has a luminal surface lined with epithelium and an intricate neurovascular supply. Negus was the first to prioritize laryngeal functions in evolutionary order as follows[1]:

- Protection of the airway.
- Respiration.
- Phonation.

Voluntary closure of the glottis occurs when straining to increase intra-abdominal pressure. The trachea and bronchi consist of a series of incomplete cartilaginous rings, completed posteriorly by a layer of muscle with a continuous internal mucosal lining of columnar epithelium. The tracheobronchial tree transmits respiratory gases to and from the lung parenchyma with minimal resistance (see Chapter 20) while also facilitating toilet of the terminal airways and alveoli.

These diverse and highly specialized functional requirements of the larynx and tracheobronchial airway are reflected in their complex embryology, anatomy, and physiology, anomalies of which can lead to life-threatening clinical sequelae.

21.3 Embryology

Development of the larynx, trachea, and bronchi begins in the fourth week of gestation. The respiratory (laryngotracheal) diverticulum arises from the ventral surface of the foregut, just distal to the fourth pharyngeal arch (▶ Fig. 21.2; see also Chapter 24). Its endodermal lining forms the pseudostratified columnar epithelium that lines the definitive airway. The enlarging diverticulum is then invaginated by splanchnic mesenchyme, the precursor of the cartilaginous and muscular structures of the lower respiratory organs. The caudal end of the diverticulum finally gives rise to primordial bronchopulmonary buds by the end of the fourth week of gestation, and the

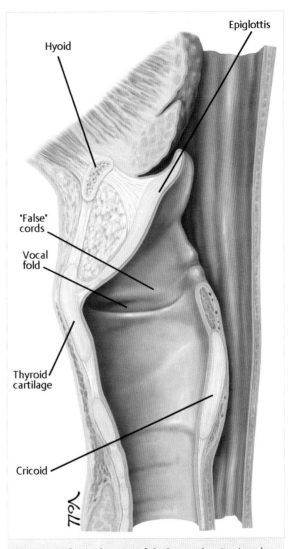

Fig. 21.1 Midsagittal section of the laryngeal cavity viewed from the left side. (Reproduced from Gilroy and MacPherson, Atlas of Anatomy, 3rd edition, © 2016, Thieme Publishers, New York. Illustration by Markus Voll.)

bronchi and primordial pleural cavities develop during the fifth week. In parallel with this, the esophagus develops as an outpouching of the ventral foregut—a ventrocaudal elongation of the respiratory diverticulum—reaching its full length by the seventh week.

The laryngeal cartilages and intrinsic muscles arise from fourth and sixth pharyngeal arch mesenchymal derivatives (▶ Fig. 21.2). The fourth arch gives rise to the thyroid and epiglottic cartilages and the cricothyroid muscle, receiving

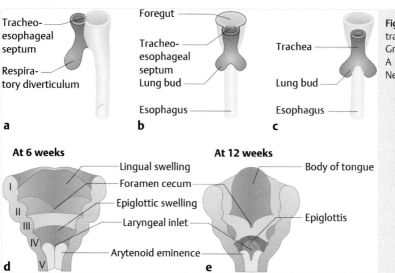

Fig. 21.2 Embryology of the larynx and trachea. (Reproduced from Probst R, Grevers G, Iro H. Basic Otorhinolaryngology: A Step-by-Step Learning Guide. Stuttgart/New York: Thieme; 2006, with permission.)

sensory and motor innervations from the superior laryngeal branch of the vagus nerve. The sixth arch produces the cricoid, arytenoid, and corniculate cartilages and all other intrinsic laryngeal muscles, innervated by the inferior (recurrent) laryngeal branch of the vagus nerve. The glottis itself forms from primordia in the floor of the primitive pharynx, at the origin of the respiratory diverticulum.

Importantly, in the context of congenital anomalies, the mesenchyme of the developing larynx proliferates very rapidly from the sixth week of gestation, which eventually leads to obliteration of the primordial pharyngolaryngeal lumen. Recanalization occurs in a dorsoventral direction from 10 weeks onward, with eventual formation of contiguous supra- and subglottic lumina and laryngeal ventricles on either side. Failure of this recanalization process is believed to be responsible for congenital laryngeal atresias.

21.4 Clinical Anatomy

The laryngeal framework consists of the thyroid and cricoid cartilages, which articulate at the cricothyroid joint and are connected anteriorly by the cricothyroid membrane (▶ Fig. 21.3). The thyroid cartilage comprises two laminae that meet in the midline, but are separate superiorly (the thyroid notch) and posteriorly. Superior and inferior cornua, and the oblique line of each lamina serve as sites of muscular and fascial attachment, allowing suspension from the hyoid superiorly and the sternum inferiorly.

> The cricoid cartilage is the only complete ring of cartilage in the airway and is shaped like a signet ring, with short anterior and longer posterior laminae.

The epiglottis (epiglottic cartilage and loosely adherent squamous mucosal coverings) is attached to the thyroid cartilage, folding down passively over the laryngeal inlet during food bolus ingestion. The arytenoid cartilages articulate with the superior border of the posterior cricoid lamina through synovial joints to allow rotation in the vertical axis and side-to-side gliding movements during phonation. Their vocal and muscular processes attach to the vocal folds and intrinsic laryngeal muscles, respectively.

Various fibroelastic membranes are suspended from the cartilaginous framework. The quadrangular membrane hangs down from the thyroid, epiglottic, and arytenoid cartilages. The upper free edges form the aryepiglottic folds at the laryngeal inlet, within which the corniculate and cuneiform cartilages are suspended. The lower free edges are the vestibular folds (false cords). The cricothyroid membrane completes the lateral gap between the cricoid and thyroid cartilages, and the upper free edges of this form the vocal ligaments within the vocal folds. The laryngeal ventricles are pouches on either side between the true and false cords. Each ventricle has a further outpouching beyond the quadrangular membrane (the saccule), lined with mucinous glands to lubricate the glottis.

> The vocal folds are the structures between the vocal processes of the arytenoids and the anterior commissure (▶ Fig. 21.4). They are covered by nonkeratinizing stratified squamous epithelium (in contrast to the pseudostratified columnar epithelium elsewhere), with three deep layers of lamina propria to this. The intermediate and deep layers of lamina propria are also termed the *vocal ligaments*, overlying the thyroarytenoid muscles, which form the *body* of each fold. The lower and deeper fibers of each thyroarytenoid muscle are also referred to as *vocalis*. The vocal cords comprise the vocal folds anteriorly and the bodies and vocal processes of the arytenoids posteriorly.

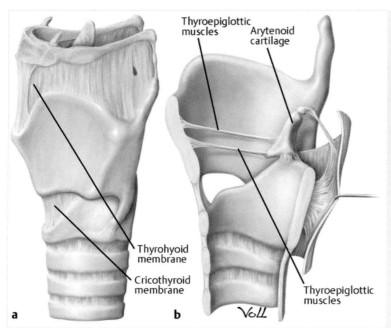

Fig. 21.3 Midsagittal section of the laryngeal cavity viewed from the left side. (Reproduced from Gilroy and MacPherson, Atlas of Anatomy, 3rd edition, © 2016, Thieme Publishers, New York. Illustration by Markus Voll.)

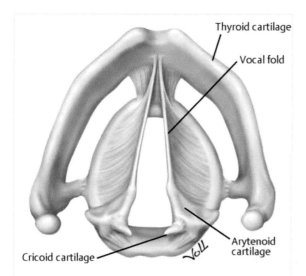

Fig. 21.4 Superior view of the structure of the larynx. (Reproduced from Gilroy and MacPherson, Atlas of Anatomy, 3rd edition, © 2016, Thieme Publishers, New York. Illustration by Markus Voll.)

This distinction has functional significance: the narrow anterior, membranous portion of the glottis (*glottis vocalis*) is involved primarily in phonation and airway protection, whereas the wider posterior cartilaginous portion (*glottis respiratoria*) is more relevant to respiration. The larynx is divided arbitrarily into the supraglottis (epiglottis, aryepiglottic folds, arytenoids, false cords, and ventricles), glottis (vocal cords), and subglottis (undersurface of vocal cords to lower border of cricoid).

In contrast to the extrinsic laryngeal muscles of the laryngohyoid complex that raise, lower, or stabilize the larynx, the intrinsic laryngeal muscles are restricted to the larynx itself (▶ Fig. 21.5). The cricothyroids are the largest of these, located externally and innervated by the superior laryngeal nerve. They tilt the thyroid cartilage forward, tensing the vocal folds to raise pitch. Fibers run in two bellies: the *pars recta* (running vertically) and *pars obliqua* (running obliquely). These muscles form a useful surgical landmark for the cricoid cartilage during pediatric laryngeal surgery, particularly when the area has undergone scarring as a result of pathology or previous procedures. The remainder of the intrinsic muscles are located posteriorly and/or internally, all supplied by the recurrent laryngeal nerve. The posterior cricoarytenoids are the sole abductors of the cords. The lateral cricoarytenoids are their main antagonists, adducting, elongating, and lowering the cords. The unpaired interarytenoid muscle acts to bring the arytenoid bodies together, thereby closing the posterior glottis (*glottis respiratoria*). Further extensions into the aryepiglottic folds on each side (aryepiglotticus) assist in closure of the laryngeal inlet during swallowing.

In line with its embryological origins, the supraglottis receives sensory supply from the superior laryngeal nerve; the glottis, the subglottis, and the proximal trachea are supplied by the recurrent laryngeal nerve.

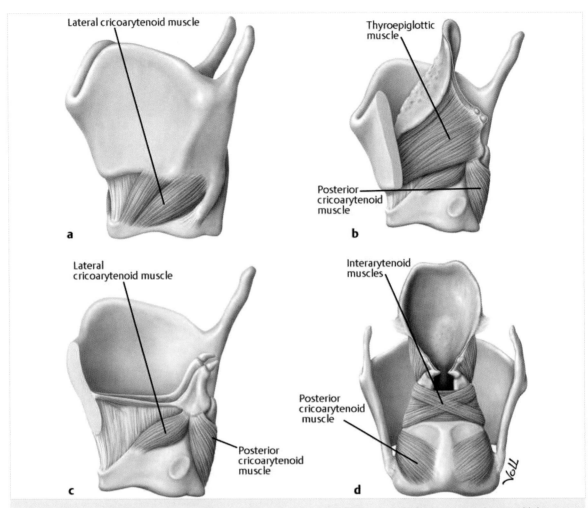

Fig. 21.5 Laryngeal muscles. (Reproduced from Gilroy and MacPherson, Atlas of Anatomy, 3rd edition, © 2016, Thieme Publishers, New York. Illustration by Markus Voll.)

Pediatric upper airways differ from those of adults in several ways:

- The infantile larynx is about a third the size of the adult equivalent, with vocal cords 6- to 8-mm-long and subglottic dimensions of 4.5 by 7 mm.
- In contrast to adults, where the glottis is the narrowest section of the upper airway, the subglottis is the narrowest point in children, hence the propensity of acquired pathology to affect this area. This explains the importance of routine assessment of the subglottic dimensions during microlaryngoscopy.
- The larynx is also situated higher (vertebral level C2–C4) and more anteriorly in the neck than in an adult (C4–C6), tucked right up to the hyoid. This is reflected in the obligate nasal breathing of infants, in whom the nasal passages account for 50% of total airways resistance.
- The epiglottis is rather more tightly Ω-shaped and softer than in the adult, tending to flop down over the laryngeal inlet more readily during swallowing.

These geometrical and anatomical differences adapt the infant well to a wholly liquid diet, facilitating nasal ventilation during milk feeds and reducing the risks of aspiration. Such a configuration is also seen in ruminant herbivores for the same reasons. A young child has a relatively large head, prominent occiput, short neck, and large tongue.

Together with the high anterior position of the larynx, these factors mean that the infant is most appropriately mask-ventilated in a neutral rather than the neck-flexed, head-extended position used for adults.

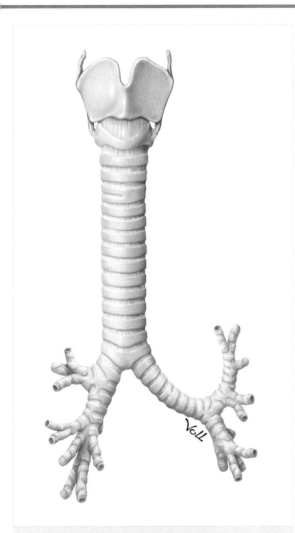

Fig. 21.6 The trachea and bronchial tree. (Reproduced from Schuenke, Schulte, and Schumacher, Atlas of Anatomy: Inner Organs [Volume II], © 2016, Thieme Publishers, New York. Illustration by Markus Voll.)

The trachea is a fibroelastic and muscular tube (▶ Fig. 21.6), comprising 16 to 20 C-shaped cartilaginous rings open posteriorly, spanned by smooth muscle, the trachealis. This runs from the lower border of the cricoid (level of C4 in the child) to its bifurcation at the carina (level of T3/T4 in the child). Importantly, variable tone of the trachealis allows its caliber to alter with the phase and level of respiration, adjusting the physiological dead space. Additionally, apart from being distensible, the trachea has a significantly larger cross-sectional area than the cricoid ring (subglottis) in infants.

> **i**
>
> An age-appropriate tracheostomy tube will therefore require a larger external diameter than the age-equivalent endotracheal tube to enable ventilation with minimal leak.

Innervation is primarily from the recurrent laryngeal nerves. Important anatomical relations include the esophagus posteriorly, and the left brachiocephalic (innominate) vein, aortic arch, and left brachiocephalic (innominate) artery anteriorly. These structures are important to consider during surgical approaches to the trachea, and abnormalities of them may consequently lead to tracheal anomalies and pathology.

The bronchi are similarly structured, with the right wider, slightly shorter, and more vertically oriented than the left, hence the propensity for inhaled foreign bodies to lodge on the right side (▶ Fig. 21.6). They divide into upper, middle, and lower lobe bronchioles on the right, and upper and lower lobe bronchioles on the left. Overall, the airway has 23 divisions from the larynx proximally to the alveoli terminally.

21.5 Clinical Manifestations of Airway Pathology

The precise presenting features of airway pathology, congenital or acquired, result from derangements of normal functions and vary with the subsite affected. Typical laryngeal sequelae are total or partial respiratory obstruction, inspiratory stridor, a weak or abnormal cry, dyspnea, tachypnea, aspiration, and eventually death from asphyxiation. Tracheobronchial pathology on the other hand tends to produce biphasic or expiratory stridor (wheeze), but many of the aforementioned features may also be seen. Laryngeal and tracheobronchial pathology not infrequently coexist (see Chapter 20).

The congenital anomalies affecting these areas, and their features and management options will be discussed according to anatomical level rather than in order of incidence. It is important from the outset to be mindful that such anomalies, while by definition present at the time of birth, may not be manifested in early life and should also be considered in older children presenting with suggestive symptoms and signs. Complete endoscopic examination of the airway (microlaryngobronchoscopy [MLB]) complemented by other modalities as appropriate remains the gold standard of investigation.

21.5.1 Supraglottis

Laryngomalacia

Laryngomalacia (congenital flaccid larynx) is a clinical entity characterized by collapse of the supraglottic structures during inspiration. Although it is by far the commonest congenital laryngeal anomaly,[2] its pathophysiology remains uncertain. The particular structures and mechanisms involved are likely to vary on an individual basis. Dynamic endoscopic assessment will demonstrate any of a number of possible findings: a tightly curled, Ω-shaped epiglottis (▶ Fig. 21.7) often particularly soft

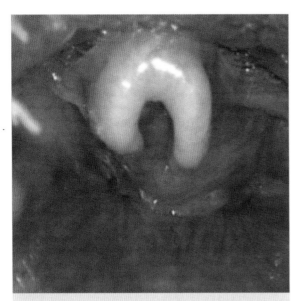

Fig. 21.7 Laryngomalacia. Tight aryepiglottic folds resulting in a Ω-shaped epiglottis.

and retroverted; tall and bulky aryepiglottic folds, which are tightly tethered to the epiglottis; and redundant arytenoid and supra-arytenoid mucosa, often with antero-medial prolapse of the mucosa/corniculate complex and the arytenoids themselves into the posterior glottis during inspiration.

> **i**
>
> Most cases of laryngomalacia present within the first few weeks of life; the majority resolve spontaneously within infancy, and almost all by 2 years of age. Importantly, other airway pathologies may coexist in a small proportion of cases.

Inspiratory stridor is the characteristic feature. This is often harsh in quality and tends to be more pronounced during periods of excitement, distress, or feeding, accentuated in the supine position, and improved when prone or when asleep. Most cases are mild, or even subclinical, but some children will experience significant respiratory distress, tracheal tug, sternal recession, and, very occasionally, cyanosis.[3] Feeding may be disrupted.[4] Gastroesophageal reflux often coexists, although no causative relationship has been confirmed. Long-term sequelae in more severe cases include sternal deformity (pectus excavatum) and failure to thrive due to disruption to feeding, coexisting reflux, and increased work of breathing (noting that respiratory effort accounts for 15% of the healthy infant's oxygen consumption and energy utilization).

Management of Laryngomalacia

> **i**
>
> - Mild cases are often managed in the primary care setting or by pediatricians, frequently without further investigations.[5] Regular reviews are required to ensure nonprogression and eventual resolution of symptoms, with careful monitoring of weight and height. Antireflux therapy (ranitidine or omeprazole plus domperidone) may or may not be indicated, and it is our preference to restrict medical treatment to those cases with obvious signs and symptoms of reflux.
> - Cases with sufficient symptoms to warrant otolaryngological referral should undergo flexible nasendoscopic assessment in clinic in the first instance. This allows an excellent dynamic view in most cases, demonstrating the aforementioned features. However, the subglottis and distal airway will not be seen in this way.
> - Severe cases, and certainly those with any suspicion of coexisting pathology, should undergo complete MLB under general anesthesia.[6] A full structural and dynamic assessment is always advisable, as milder forms of laryngomalacia are easily missed, particularly if the epiglottis is pulled forward strongly by the blade of the laryngoscope and/or if the child is too heavily anesthetized for adequate self-ventilation. It is usually possible to anesthetize children to allows spontaneous ventilation of sufficient intensity for a dynamic assessment, although this may be challenging in young infants, in whom awake flexible endoscopy may be more informative.

The cause of laryngomalacia is not certain.[7] Histological analysis has demonstrated edematous, redundant arytenoid mucosa, little or no aryepiglottic musculature, and loose mucosal lining of the epiglottis, findings that correlate well with macroscopic clinical assessment. Neuromotor immaturity leading to discoordinated activity of the vagal nuclei has also been suggested as a cause, accounting for arytenoid prolapse and the association with gastroesophageal reflux. It is certainly recognized that some children with underlying neurologic problems will also have problematic laryngomalacia that may persist for several years. Apart from the prolonged duration of symptoms, it should be borne in mind that these children generally have poorer outcomes with surgical treatment, highlighting the mixed structural and functional pathophysiology of this condition.[8]

Once coexisting pathology has been excluded, monitoring as mentioned previously, is sufficient for the great majority of children, typically under the care of pediatricians. Reflux may be treated medically, if required. Parents should be reassured that the condition will resolve spontaneously with time, albeit more slowly in neurologic cases, in whom surgery is typically best avoided.[8]

Surgery should be reserved for the most severe cases, and then only after serial clinical and/or endoscopic assessments have shown persistent problems, rather than at the first MLB.

Supraglottoplasty may take various forms and should be tailored to the individual findings.[9]
- Division of short aryepiglottic folds (aryepiglottoplasty; ▶ Fig. 21.8) and/or trimming of excessive arytenoid mucosa are typical options, although more unusual techniques have been described, including epiglottopexy.
- We prefer cold steel dissection rather than power-assisted or hot techniques, where lateral thermal injury and scarring may occur.

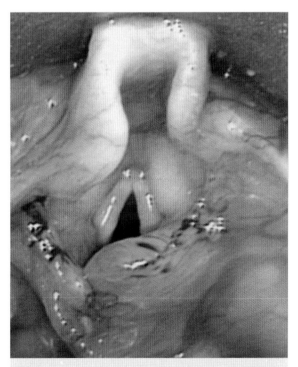

Fig. 21.8 Same patient as in ▶ Fig. 21.7 following division of the aryepiglottic folds (aryepiglottoplasty).

Parents should be fully aware that the child's stridor may persist despite surgery. Feeding may be disrupted, necessitating temporary nasogastric feeding and prolonged admission, and rarer complications such as bleeding, aspiration,[10] and even supraglottic stenosis may occasionally occur. Tracheostomy is virtually never required in cases of isolated laryngomalacia. Severe symptoms should alert the clinician to possible coexisting pathology.

Laryngoceles and Saccular Cysts

Both these anomalies are the results of dilatation of the saccule of the laryngeal ventricle. Congenital forms, which present in infancy, are much rarer than their acquired counterparts more typically seen in adults such as glass blowers who produce high intraluminal airway pressures. In the natural world, congenital saccular dilatation is most dramatically seen in howler monkeys, the loudest of all land animals. Laryngoceles communicate with the airway and typically have an air-filled lumen, whereas saccular cysts do not communicate with the airway and are fluid-filled.

Laryngoceles and saccular cysts may be difficult to diagnose and indeed to distinguish clinically, endoscopically, and even radiologically, particularly as laryngoceles may themselves become inflamed and fill with fluid or pus (laryngopyocele). Both may present with a rather variable history, most often with dysphonia and/or respiratory distress, made worse when crying, as a result of raised intraluminal pressure. The individual presentation will depend upon the size, site, and distensibility of the lesion.

Laryngoceles are classified as follows:
- Internal (completely within the laryngeal cartilage).
- External (piercing the thyrohyoid membrane).
- Combined (with internal and external components).

Internal lesions are usually visible endoscopically, although they may be missed after collapse under general anesthesia. External lesions are usually suggested by parental history, but are not obvious endoscopically. Computed tomography (CT) may be helpful, but may also miss a collapsed laryngocele or confuse a fluid-filled one with a saccular cyst.[11]

Saccular cysts (▶ Fig. 21.9) are thought to result from loss of patency between the laryngeal ventricle and saccule, resulting in a walled-off saccule that fills with fluid. They are classed as anterior (extending medially and posteriorly and protruding into the laryngeal airway between the true and false cords) or lateral (the commoner form in infants, which protrudes into the false cord and the aryepiglottic fold).

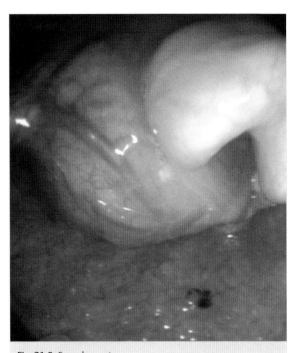

Fig. 21.9 Saccular cyst.

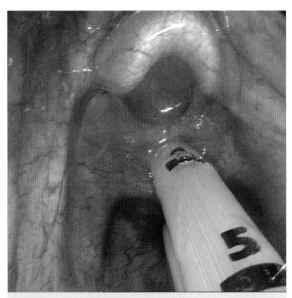

Fig. 21.10 Supraglottic atresia. This neonate was intubated with a size 2.5 tube. Note the absence of typical supraglottic anatomy. After initial tracheostomy, definitive reconstruction with laryngotracheal reconstruction and stents was undertaken at 6 months.

> Treatment of these anomalies should be tailored to individual presentation and symptoms. Conservative management is certainly reasonable for external laryngoceles, although the propensity of internal laryngoceles and saccular cysts to become infected, increase in size, and cause airway embarrassment usually necessitates preemptive surgery.

- Both types of lesion may be tackled endoscopically, particularly saccular cysts that can be widely marsupialized.
- An open approach (midline, with full laryngofissure or lateral cervical with a "window" through the thyrohyoid membrane and thyroid ala) is an alternative for more extensive or recurrent lesions and allows complete excision of all secretory epithelium.

Supraglottic Atresia

This is a rare cause of neonatal respiratory distress, which may or may not have been appreciated on antenatal scans (congenital high airway obstruction syndrome). It is seldom an isolated problem (▶ Fig. 21.10). Many cases will have associated glottic atresia and subglottic stenosis (SGS), as well as other congenital anomalies including esophageal atresia (OA), tracheoesophageal fistula (TOF), genitourinary, and skeletal anomalies.

> Where the diagnosis is made antenatally, the baby may be best delivered by elective caesarean section, allowing ex utero, intrapartum treatment (EXIT) in the form of a tracheostomy. Where the diagnosis is not made antenatally, the baby may tolerate initial mask ventilation as a result of airflow down the esophagus and through a TOF (see Chapter 28).[12] This affords some extra time to secure the airway, but it also offers a false sense of reassurance to the unwary, with little possibility of endotracheal intubation once the child inevitably deteriorates. A high index of suspicion and prompt tracheostomy are essential in these rare cases.

Supraglottic Webs

These are rare and are considered as part of the laryngeal atresia spectrum. They may be associated with systemic anomalies in approximately 10% of cases.[7] They may also be seen in the context of other laryngeal abnormalities, but sometimes occur in isolation (as opposed to the far commoner congenital glottic webs, which almost always involve concomitant SGS).

Management is tailored to individual circumstances. Tracheostomy may be required, but division of the web plus balloon dilatation is often effective. This technique uses an expandable balloon to radially dilate the web following an endoscopic incision. This is in contrast to glottic webs, where formal laryngotracheal reconstruction (LTR) is the surgical treatment of choice, allowing separation of the cords and simultaneous expansion of the subglottis.

Epiglottic Anomalies: Absent or Bifid Epiglottis

These anomalies are also very rare. The epiglottis develops from the third and fourth branchial arches, therefore epiglottic agenesis is almost always associated with other major laryngeal abnormalities including glottic stenosis. Neonatal respiratory distress is likely and urgent tracheostomy is usually required.

A bifid epiglottis (▶ Fig. 21.11) occurs as a consequence of failure of fusion in the midline, resulting in a cleft that extends to just above the epiglottic tubercle. Although few isolated cases are reported in the literature, it has been noted in Pallister–Hall's syndrome (polydactyly, hypothalamic hamartoma, laryngeal cleft, renal dysgenesis, imperforate anus). Presentation may be mistaken for that of laryngomalacia, with stridor and respiratory distress during feeds, although cyanotic spells and aspiration are also often seen, which should alert the clinician to an alternative diagnosis. Treatment will depend upon symptom severity. Tracheostomy may be necessary in the first instance. Amputation of the epiglottis may subsequently improve the airway, although chronic aspiration may result.

Vascular Anomalies: Hemangiomas, and Lymphatic and Venous Malformations

Supraglottic hemangiomas are much rarer than those of the subglottic airway. Presentation is similar to other forms of supraglottic pathology, but the onset is usually after 2 or 3 months of life and the symptoms are progressive. Diagnosis and treatment options are as for subglottic hemangiomas, as discussed in the following.

Lymphatic malformations are most commonly found in the head and neck. Upper aerodigestive tract disease should certainly be excluded in neonates presenting with gross cervical and/or facial disease: microcystic disease affecting the tongue and the floor of mouth is seen relatively often in these cases and this may extend down the tongue base to the epiglottis (▶ Fig. 21.12). Isolated supraglottic disease, by contrast, is rare. In any event, MLB is usually diagnostic.

Management will depend upon the extent of disease. Neonatal tracheostomy is often undertaken in the first instance for patients with gross disease, although this may be avoided with prompt intervention. It is our preference to excise the cervical disease in the first few days of life, which may avert the need for tracheostomy, leaving facial components to be managed with surgery and/or sclerotherapy after a few years, when the risks of facial nerve injury are reduced. Upper airway disease may be managed in a multimodality fashion. We now favor radiofrequency ablation (Coblation [Smith & Nephew])

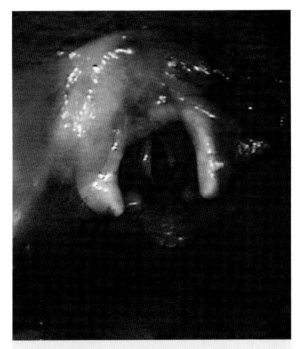

Fig. 21.11 Bifid epiglottis.

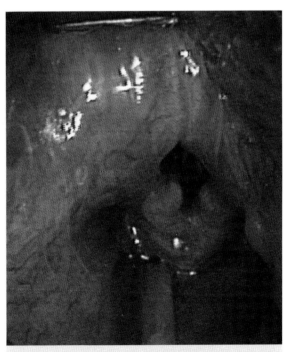

Fig. 21.12 Supraglottic lymphatic malformation in a child with gross cervicofacial disease and long-term tracheostomy.

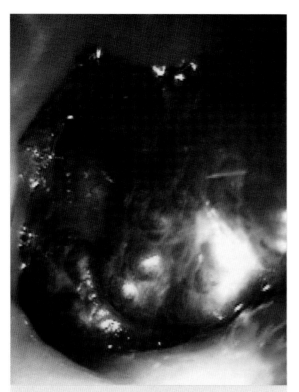

Fig. 21.13 Airway venous malformation in a teenager with blue rubber bleb nevus syndrome. Long-term tracheostomy in situ.

15% of cases of neonatal stridor. It may occur bilaterally or unilaterally, as a result of neurologic impairment anywhere from the vagal nuclei to the recurrent laryngeal nerves.

The history may offer some clues regarding the site of the lesion. Unilateral palsy may present after cardiothoracic surgery, as a result of (left) recurrent laryngeal nerve injury, but this may also be seen as a result of compression from cardiac and great vessel anomalies rather than the surgery itself. Unilateral palsy may be missed, as the airway is generally not severely compromised. The child will typically have a weak cry, perhaps an abnormal cough, and mild choking episodes during feeds and may have noticeable inspiratory stridor when distressed, but these are not invariably noticed. A high index of suspicion is therefore required.

Bilateral vocal cord paralysis is more typically the result of a central cause, although many cases are idiopathic. These children present with respiratory distress at birth or within the first few weeks of life. The paramedian position of the cords results in marked inspiratory stridor, weak cough, and aspiration. Some cases require immediate intubation and/or tracheostomy, although others may initially manage with more conservative measures including continuous positive airway pressure (CPAP).

> Diagnosis in these cases is one of the foremost challenges. MLB is mandatory, attempting to confirm the diagnosis and to exclude concomitant pathology, and should be performed before tracheostomy (▶ Fig. 21.14). However, it is difficult in neonates to achieve a plane of anesthesia, which allows both laryngoscopy without provoking spasm, and spontaneous ventilation of sufficient intensity for vocal cord abduction to be seen during inspiration. Only in this way can vocal cord movements be properly assessed. It is often necessary to continue direct laryngoscopy while the anesthesia is lightened until the baby is moving and almost awake to be sure that no spontaneous cord movements are seen.

for microcystic disease of the tongue dorsum, tongue base, and supraglottis.[13] This minimizes lateral thermal injury, edema, and scarring associated with high-temperature techniques (monopolar diathermy and laser) and also allows swift recovery for the child. Tongue reduction through a combination of anterior wedge resection and horizontal core excision (to reduced tongue length and thickness, respectively), and transoral clearance of floor of mouth disease are used as necessary.

Venous malformations also occasionally affect the larynx, occurring in isolation or in the context of other head and neck manifestations. Rarely, there may be an underlying syndromic cause, such as the blue rubber bleb nevus syndrome (▶ Fig. 21.13). Unlike hemangiomas and lymphatic malformations, venous malformations tend to present with later onset of laryngeal symptoms during late childhood or early adulthood. MLB and magnetic resonance imaging (MRI) will usually confirm the diagnosis. Treatment may include tracheostomy, sclerotherapy, and occasionally excisional surgery, although the risks of severe hemorrhage and airway compromise are often high.

21.5.2 Glottis

Vocal Cord Paralysis

This is the second commonest congenital laryngeal anomaly (after laryngomalacia) and accounts for 10 to

It should also be borne in mind that the right cord usually starts to move before the left cord during the wake-up period in the otherwise normal child. In the absence of obvious coordinated abduction, the cricoarytenoid joints should be probed to assess mobility, allowing distinction between cord palsy and cord fixation. Further investigation by awake flexible nasendoscopy and vocal cord ultrasound is often helpful in confirming the diagnosis of congenital vocal cord palsy. It cannot be overemphasized that this is often a difficult diagnosis to reach and requires experience on the part of otolaryngologist, anesthetist, and radiologist before perhaps committing the child to tracheostomy.

V

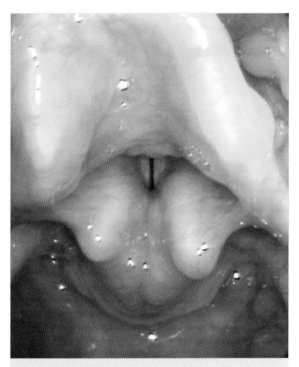

Fig. 21.14 Bilateral vocal cord palsy.

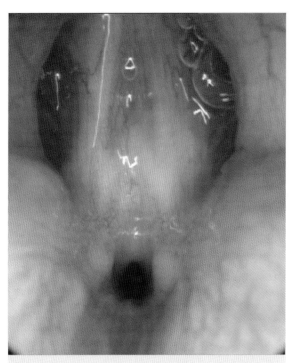

Fig. 21.15 Laryngeal web (glottic atresia).

21

Unilateral paralysis may require further investigation if the cause is in doubt, for example, chest radiography or CT and/or head and neck MRI to assess the course of the nerve in question. Most of these cases will manage without initial intervention, but it is important to have an early speech and language therapy assessment to exclude aspiration and commence vocal training. Nasogastric feeding may occasionally be necessary.

> **i**
>
> Bilateral cases are managed more aggressively. An urgent brain MRI should be undertaken to exclude hydrocephalus and the Arnold–Chiari malformation, which may stretch the vagus nerves over the lip of the foramen magnum. Urgent neurosurgical intervention and decompression in these cases may allow spontaneous resolution, but in many cases, no central abnormality is found.

Management of cases of bilateral paralysis is tailored to the individual, bearing in mind that spontaneous resolution is seen in almost two-thirds of cases. This usually occurs in the first few years of life, but may still be seen after 5 years of age; one case had even reported resolution aged 11 years.[14] Tracheostomy is necessary in early life in approximately half of cases, often in children with concomitant airway pathology, but every effort should be made to avoid this if it is safe to do so. In children with no evidence of spontaneous resolution, the timing and

extent of further interventions is controversial. Indications are to widen the posterior glottic airway (in the tracheostomized child to allow decannulation, or sometimes in the child with no tracheostomy to improve exercise tolerance). These interventions, mostly irreversible, must be balanced against the risks of aspiration and in the context of the ever-diminishing ongoing possibility of spontaneous resolution.

A multidisciplinary approach involving child, parents, speech therapist, and surgeon is essential. Options include the following:

- Excisional techniques (unilateral arytenoidectomy and/or partial cordotomy through cold steel dissection or laser, endoscopic or open laryngofissure approaches).
- Suture lateralization of one cord.
- Posterior expansion of the cricoid ring with cartilage to separate the cords (LTR, endoscopic or open, single-, or two-stage procedure).

Nocturnal CPAP is a further option for some children who manage by day but struggle at night, although this is not always tolerated and runs the risk of destabilizing the cricoarytenoid joints with long-term use.

Laryngeal Web (Atresia)

This is a result of failure of recanalization of the larynx during the first trimester, resulting in a variable degree of atresia. The glottis is affected in the great majority of cases, resulting in thick webbing at this level (▶ Fig. 21.15). This generally occurs anteriorly, with a concave opening of the posterior glottis. As previously stated, almost all cases are associated with a degree of SGS. A simple division of the thick web, particularly with laser, should be avoided at all costs; reformation of the web is almost invariable, with scarring affecting long-term voice outcome, and the narrow subglottis will not have been addressed at all. Only the very few exceptional cases of isolated gossamer-thin congenital glottic webs should be managed by endoscopic division alone.

Presentation will depend upon the degree of atresia. A history of stridor and a weak cry or aphonia is typical, but the diagnosis is easily missed; flexible nasendoscopy may overlook milder cases and therefore MLB remains mandatory. While some present as neonates, others may manage for several months prior to diagnosis, despite major glottic webbing; infants often tolerate congenital airway narrowing surprisingly well and so the authors have seen cases of 80 to 90% glottic webs being first diagnosed at 4 to 6 months of life.

All cases should be referred for genetic testing, as more than 50% are associated with chromosome 22q11.2 deletion syndrome (velocardiofacial syndrome).[15] Allied investigations, including echocardiography, will be undertaken in confirmed cases.

Management will vary according to severity:

- Those with major compromise should undergo urgent tracheostomy.
- Mild variants may require no intervention at all.

Timing of corrective surgery in more severe cases will depend on a number of factors including comorbidities, body weight, and existing voice production; a complete lack of voice will have to be addressed early in life, ideally within the first 2 years, if the child is to develop intelligible speech in the long term. Others may progress reasonably with or without tracheostomy and are considered for later intervention (when larger and the surgery is technically easier) prior to school entry.

---

i

Definitive surgery is challenging. The aims are to separate the atretic anterior glottis into two mobile vocal folds and at the same time to expand the subglottic airway. This is best achieved by a full laryngofissure, with meticulous attention to midline separation of the cords.

- This is often facilitated by initial endoscopic division in the midline in combination with open surgery of the laryngeal framework.
- Augmentation of the cricoid ring with an anterior rib cartilage graft is usually necessary.
- Some form of postoperative stent, for example, a cut segment of endotracheal tube left in situ for 6 weeks in a two-stage procedure or full nasal intubation for a

week in the case of a single-stage approach is required to avoid luminal restenosis.
- Silastic keel insertions have also been used in some cases to help preserve vocal fold separation.

In practice, a clear understanding of the pathology, careful primary surgery, and very regular initial follow-up MLB procedures (including granulation excision and balloon dilatation) are prerequisites for a successful outcome.

Cri-du-Chat Syndrome

This syndrome results from a partial deletion of the short arm of chromosome 5 (5p15:3). It is characterized by a catlike mewing cry during infancy, microcephaly, downsloping palpebral fissures, developmental delay, and hypotonia. Laryngoscopy demonstrates that the posterior glottis remains open during phonation, but there is no airway compromise. No treatment is required for the larynx, and the cry becomes more normal with age.

Other Rare Congenital Anomalies

A number of other extremely rare abnormalities of the larynx have been described. These include anterior laryngeal cleft, where the thyroid cartilage is not fused in the midline. Voice pitch may be altered, but no surgical treatment is required. Duplication of the vocal cord has also been seen, and again no problems were encountered and no treatment was required.

21.5.3 Subglottis

Congenital Subglottic Stenosis

As for laryngeal atresia, congenital SGS is believed to result from incomplete recanalization of the airway in the first trimester, affecting particularly the region of the cricoid cartilage (▶ Fig. 21.16). It may be encountered as an isolated anomaly, in combination with glottic web (as above) or in certain syndromes, particularly Down's syndrome.[16]

The characteristic abnormality is a thick anterior cricoid lamina in a child with no prior history of intubation or other trauma. Presentation is variable. Severe stenosis will typically present with neonatal respiratory distress and often requires tracheostomy. In milder cases, the child may have a history of persistent stridor, or alternatively episodic croup-like episodes with marked stridor that respond well to glucocorticoids and adrenaline nebulizers. It is not uncommon for children to have numerous general pediatric admissions with "croup" before a diagnosis of congenital SGS is considered, hence the importance of a high index of suspicion and early referral for diagnostic MLB. A further group of children will have congenital SGS diagnosed after an elective anesthetic

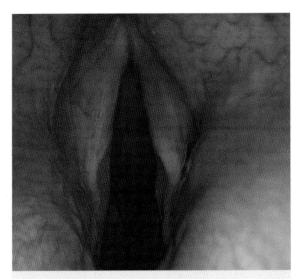

Fig. 21.16 Congenital subglottic stenosis. Note the thick anterior cricoid lamina and U-shaped subglottic cross-section.

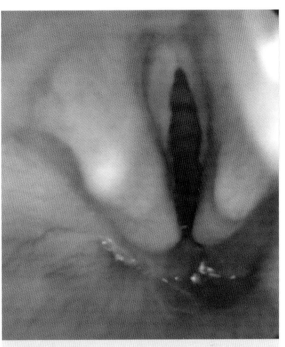

Fig. 21.17 Posterior laryngeal cleft (type III) with glottic involvement.

endotracheal intubation for an unrelated procedure, where an age-appropriate tube cannot be passed or is a very tight fit despite good laryngoscopic views.

The diagnosis is usually obvious on MLB. As for acquired SGS, attempts may be made to measure the subglottic airway using a series of endotracheal tubes. The Myer–Cotton grading system[17] that grades SGS 1 (mild) to 4 (complete) is best suited for circumferential SGS, typically acquired, rather than the U-shaped subglottic lumen in cases of congenital SGS (see Chapter 22).

Specific treatment options are also subtly different for congenital, as opposed to acquired SGS, and an appreciation of the different pathology is essential.

Before any surgery, an overriding consideration should be that the cricoid ring will usually grow commensurately with the child in congenital SGS: active monitoring is therefore reasonable in all but the most severely affected.

The endoscopic scar division and balloon expansion techniques described for acquired SGS tend to be ineffective in congenital cases, as the thick anterior cricoid lamina is not addressed. Such treatments, however tempting, may worsen the condition of a child with an already marginal airway, precipitating tracheostomy.

LTR,[18] as a single- or two-stage procedure, is our surgical management of choice in symptomatic cases of congenital SGS.

- Anterior division of the cricoid ring and augmentation with costal cartilage may be sufficient, although a posterior split, with or without augmentation, is often required in addition.
- Cricotracheal resection[19] (see Chapter 22) is reserved for the most severe stenoses or for salvage cases after failed primary surgery. This technique involves resection of the anterior cricoid arch and upper trachea but preserves the posterior cricoid and arytenoid cartilages. An end-to-end anastomosis is performed.

Symptomatic resolution and/or decannulation rates are inversely proportional to the initial degree of stenosis.

Posterior Laryngeal Cleft

This rare congenital anomaly results from failure of rostral extension of the tracheoesophageal septum in the fifth week of gestation. This leads to a posterior defect that may extend into or through the posterior lamina of the cricoid cartilage and, in severe cases, into the trachea itself (▶ Fig. 21.17, ▶ Fig. 21.18). Many patients will have associated congenital anomalies, particularly TOF. This is known to occur in 20 to 27% of children with laryngeal cleft; conversely, 6% of children with TOF will also

V

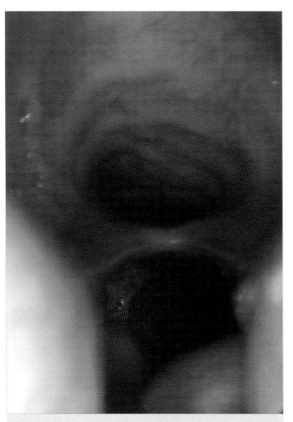

Fig. 21.18 Posterior laryngeal cleft (type III) with extension into the trachea. The esophagus is open posteriorly.

It is essential that the posterior glottis and supraglottis are probed as part of any MLB examination, regardless of the history, to ensure that the posterior cricoid lamina and interarytenoid tissues are intact. The diagnosis of small type I clefts may be difficult to establish even with careful endoscopy. Modified barium swallow (videofluoroscopy) assessment may be required to confirm posterior glottis aspiration.

The characteristic clinical picture for more severe cases includes feeding difficulties, respiratory distress with stridor and cyanosis, aspiration, and resulting recurrent lower respiratory tract infections. Severe type III and type IV clefts invariably present with neonatal respiratory distress requiring intubation, whereupon problems with tube positioning and a huge leak around the tube, together with gross reflux and aspiration, suggest the diagnosis.

The priorities in these patients are to secure the airway, confirm the diagnosis, and identify other airway and systemic pathology before planning treatment. Long-term management of these patients is challenging and requires considerable surgical experience.

have a laryngeal cleft. Syndromic associations are also recognized, including Pallister–Hall's syndrome (described above) and Opitz-Frias syndrome (hypertelorism, cleft lip and palate, hypospadias, and laryngeal cleft).

The Benjamin and Inglis classification[20] is widely used and correlates well with clinical severity and management options.

- Type I clefts extend between the arytenoids to the level of the vocal cords.
- Type II clefts extend into the posterior lamina of the cricoid cartilage.
- Type III clefts extend into the cervical trachea.
- Type IV clefts extend intrathoracically, affecting most or all of the posterior trachea and thus stopping short of, or involving, the carina itself.

As suggested, clinical presentation varies according to the extent of the cleft and the presence of other anomalies. The cleft itself may lead to initial presentation and diagnosis or it may be an incidental finding on airway endoscopy. Minor (type I) clefts may produce minimal symptoms and are easily missed on MLB, particularly as the local mucosa is usually edematous as a result of reflux.

- Short type I clefts may require no treatment at all if the child is not aspirating (confirmed by modified barium swallow).
- Longer type I and type II clefts, where aspiration is very likely, may be repaired endoscopically. The edges of the cleft, and the invariable associated redundant mucosa, are completely excised, and the defect is then closed from distal to proximal in two layers. Nasogastric feeding is usually required for a few weeks after the repair.
- Type III clefts require open repair through full laryngofissure, using similar principles. Some surgeons interpose a section of fascia between tracheal and esophageal layers, but this has no proven advantages. Many cases will have required a tracheostomy at initial presentation, given the high rates of tracheomalacia and/or other anomalies, although this is sometimes avoidable (thereby reducing local trauma, inflammation and infection and improving postoperative recovery). Postrepair swallowing problems and aspiration are inevitable and persistent, given the congenital absence of a large section of the anterior esophageal wall and associated neural plexuses. Long-term nasogastric feeding is not appropriate, as the delicate suture line will be compromised. Gastrostomy (and fundoplication if required) should therefore be performed at the outset.

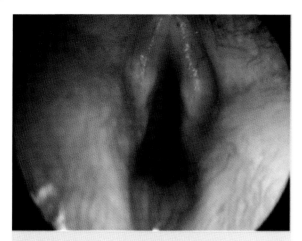

Fig. 21.19 Subglottic hemangioma at presentation.

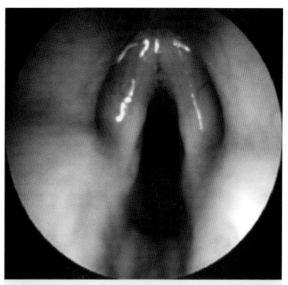

Fig. 21.20 Subglottic hemangioma after 6 months of treatment with propranolol.

21

• Type IV clefts have the poorest prognosis and highest mortality, particularly in the presence of comorbidities.[21] Any repair will require a cervicothoracic approach and then years of rehabilitation. The main distinction within this group is between those with an intact tracheal stump above the carina, in whom repair and survival is possible (albeit with high mortality), and those with a complete cleft, in whom mortality is inevitable. The importance of a coherent multidisciplinary approach to these patients cannot be overstated, particularly in the case of those children in whom medical treatment is eventually withdrawn.

Subglottic Hemangioma

Hemangiomas are the commonest tumors in white infants, present in approximately 10 to 12%. Two-thirds are found in the head and neck, with a female-to-male ratio of 3 to 5:1. Extremely premature infants (birth weight < 1,000 g) are at particular risk, with approximately 30% affected. They are less common in non-Caucasians. Most lesions are solitary, with multiple cutaneous lesions being associated with a higher risk of visceral involvement. Laryngeal hemangiomas are particularly associated with cutaneous hemangiomas in a beard distribution.

Hemangiomas have recently been subdivided according to presentation and behavior as follows:
• Congenital, by definition present and obvious at birth.
• Infantile, the commoner variants, which usually proliferate from original pink macules during the first 2 months of life.

Involution of hemangiomas tends to begin at approximately 1 year of age and continues for the next 5 to 7 years. An overlapping period of proliferation and involution may be seen.

Airway obstruction by hemangiomas may occur at several possible levels, and it should be noted that in up to 50% of cases, there may be no cutaneous manifestation to raise diagnostic suspicion. Subglottic hemangiomas (▶ Fig. 21.19, ▶ Fig. 21.20) typically present with progressively worsening stridor from 2 to 3 months, with eventual airway obstruction in the absence of other obvious precipitants or symptoms. MLB demonstrates a characteristic smooth subglottic swelling, typically arising posteriorly and just to the left of the midline, although posterolateral cushions may alternatively be seen bilaterally, just below the vocal cords.

Simple active monitoring is rarely practical on account of the high risk of airway compromise.

> **i**
>
> Medical treatment with propranolol is now the mainstay of our management of these cases, although tracheostomy and/or open excision through laryngofissure are occasionally still required.

Propranolol has revolutionized the management of these children (Box 21.1), largely replacing other medical treatments and, in most cases, surgery. Its efficacy was first described by Léauté-Labrèze et al from Bordeaux, France, who noted a dramatic reduction in size of a nasal hemangioma in a child receiving propranolol for cardiomyopathy.[22] The mechanisms of action are not entirely clear. Vasoconstriction, a direct beta-blocker effect, will allow the hemangioma to become softer and paler, often within 24 hours of treatment, with decreased expression of fibroblast growth factor (FGF) and vascular endothelial growth factor (VEGF) and promotion of apoptosis, perhaps accounting for accelerated resolution.

Our cases are managed jointly by the ear, nose, and throat, and dermatology departments, with additional input from other specialties as required.[23] A full clinical assessment is made prior to treatment, and a number of blood tests are organized to exclude anemia, coagulopathy, diabetes, renal, hepatic, and thyroid abnormalities. Baseline pulse and blood pressure assessments, electrocardiography, and echocardiography are also mandatory. Further radiological imaging and other investigations may be arranged in addition to the original diagnostic MLB.

Box 21.1 Propranolol for Subglottic Hemangioma

Propranolol is commenced at 1 mg/kg/day, in three divided oral doses. At this point, and at any time the dose is increased, pulse rate and blood pressure are checked every 30 minutes for the first 2 hours before allowing the child home. The dose is increased to 2 mg/kg/day after the first week of treatment, with further adjustments over the coming months to match the child's weight gain. Blood pressure is checked twice weekly for the first 2 weeks and then weekly thereafter. Side effects, typically minor (weakness, fatigue, altered sleep) or occasionally major (bronchospasm, hypotension, bradycardia, and hypoglycemia), are looked for, although these are more often seen in neonates than in older children. Propranolol should not be used in asthmatics or together with salbutamol and other selective β-2 agonists. Serial assessment (clinical and endoscopic, in the case of subglottic lesions) allows monitoring of initial response to propranolol. This is typically done at 6 weeks and then at 3 months for the first year, covering the proliferative phase of disease. Weaning from propranolol in stages may then be possible, usually over about 4 weeks.

In some cases, the response to propranolol is less dramatic. In these circumstances, other medical treatments may be considered, particularly corticosteroids. Historical treatments, including alpha interferon, are no longer recommended.

Surgical excision (open, through laryngofissure) remains a reasonable option in some cases, particularly those with poor response to propranolol and other medical treatments. Surgical excision has the potential for complete and immediate resolution from the outset in contrast to medical therapy, which requires a long period of treatment and regular follow-up and carries significant risks of its own. The relative benefits of surgery in this context should not be overlooked, and surgery must form part of the initial multidisciplinary discussion of treatment options. It is also very reasonable in some cases to employ a dual-modality approach, using propranolol to reduce proliferation, followed by excision as necessary. The authors caution against laser treatment for subglottic hemangiomas because of the risks of circumferential scarring and stenosis. As with other airway pathologies presenting in infancy, tracheostomy is an option, allowing time to organize further management, particularly in areas where specialist treatment is not available locally.

21.5.4 Trachea and Bronchi

Agenesis

Tracheal agenesis is rare, often associated with other major congenital anomalies, and not amenable to corrective surgery. It may be complete or partial and is thought to result from abnormal differentiation in the third and fourth week of gestation. Of the cases that have been missed on antenatal ultrasound, many will have immediate respiratory obstruction and the child will be stillborn. A small number may survive for a short period as long as there is communication between the esophagus and one of the bronchi, but this will not be sufficient for longer-term ventilation. Bronchial agenesis is also often incompatible with life. There are rare instances of partial bronchial agenesis that may be localized enough to allow ventilation.

Webs

Congenital webs of the trachea and bronchi are localized narrowings resulting from films of tissue lying across the airway, in the absence of underlying cartilage abnormalities. As such, they are distinguished from true cartilaginous stenoses and are therefore managed by simple endoscopic web division rather than airway framework surgery.

Congenital Tracheal Stenosis

> **i**
>
> Congenital stenosis of the trachea is far more common than the acquired form. The primary anomaly is the presence of complete tracheal rings, with an entirely cartilaginous circumference of the airway.

This may be localized (very-short segment; ▶ Fig. 21.21) or longer (medium length, long, and very long segment)—the distinction having a major influence on management and

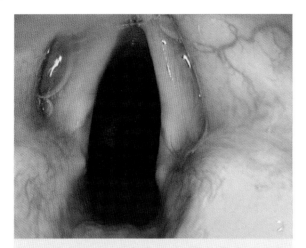

Fig. 21.21 Congenital tracheal stenosis. This proximal lesion presented in a 10-year-old boy, following recurrent respiratory tract infections but no previous intubation or trauma and normal histology. A tracheal resection was undertaken.

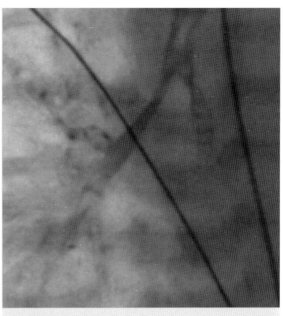

Fig. 21.22 Bronchogram. This infant has tracheobronchomalacia and a hypoplastic left lung, hence the absence of contrast on that side.

21

prognosis.[24] In general, the trachea may be generally hypoplastic (narrow along its entire length), funnel-shaped down to the stenotic segment, or segmentally hypoplastic (with normal anatomy and dimensions elsewhere).

The presentation of tracheal stenosis is surprisingly variable. Other major congenital anomalies (especially cardiac, pulmonary, anal, urogenital, and limb) are seen in 50% of cases; therefore, the airway abnormality may be initially overlooked. The minority will present with characteristic biphasic neonatal stridor and respiratory distress as primary symptoms and are diagnosed before the baby goes home. More will have the diagnosis initially missed. Many will deteriorate at home, representing *in extremis*, whereas others have prolonged histories of respiratory problems and resistant chest infections since birth. A few are also picked up after difficult intubations or failed extubations. It is worth bearing in mind that the stenotic segment may lie distal to the tip of the endotracheal tube and/or may have a diameter similar to that of the subglottis (as opposed to being larger in the normal child); therefore, intubation with an age-appropriate tube is still sometimes achieved without raising suspicion. A high index of suspicion is once again essential.

Investigations should confirm the diagnosis, assess the degree and length of stenosis, and exclude any distal tracheobronchial or other anomalies (including systemic disease), all of which have a major bearing on treatment options. MLB and chest CT with contrast (to examine the airways and great vessels in two or three dimensions) are a minimum. Contrast bronchography is also extremely useful in assessing the distal airways (▶ Fig. 21.22). Other modalities now include optical coherence tomography, which allows high-resolution imaging of the tracheal wall.

Management begins with stabilizing the child. Conventional intubation and satisfactory ventilation may be impossible; therefore, extracorporeal membrane oxygenation is sometimes necessary. Corrective surgery is tailored to the individual circumstances and may be combined with treatment of associated cardiac and vascular anomalies. Again, it should be borne in mind that congenital stenoses will tend to grow commensurately with the child. As for congenital SGS, an active monitoring policy is reasonable in milder cases.

- Very short segment stenoses are usually resected with end-to-end primary anastomosis. This is usually achievable with cross-field ventilation, but cardiopulmonary bypass (CPB) is occasionally required.
- Longer-segment stenoses are now predominantly managed by slide tracheoplasty (▶ Fig. 21.23) under CPB.[25] This involves extensive mobilization of the trachea and main bronchi before the stenotic segment is transected at its midpoint. The proximal and distal free ends are then incised vertically (distal end anteriorly, proximal end posteriorly) and the corners are trimmed to spatulate them, before sliding and suturing the ends together. Other procedures include patch tracheoplasty, where the stenotic segment is incised longitudinally anteriorly from above to below. A patch of autologous pericardium is usually used to close the defect, resulting in an expanded section of trachea.

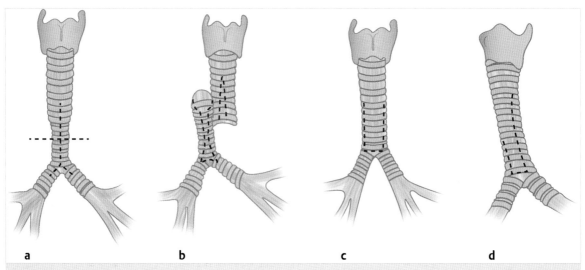

a b c d

Fig. 21.23 Slide tracheoplasty. **(a)** The stenotic segment is transected at its midpoint. **(b)** The cut ends are then incised longitudinally and the corners are spatulated. **(c)** The segments are then sutured to expand the stenotic segment. **(d)** Final result.

Complications of these procedures are not infrequently encountered, particularly given the complex nature of many patients. Granulation tissue at the anastomosis is anticipated, and in this center is usually managed with endoluminal balloon dilatation under fluoroscopic control. This has the benefit of limiting mucosal trauma and further granulation formation that accompanies cold steel excision. Incipient restenosis is managed similarly. Tracheobronchomalacia is a very common sequela, and the treatment options are outlined next.

Tracheoesophageal Fistula

This is a relatively common congenital anomaly, affecting 1 in 2,000 to 4,000 live births. It results from failed fusion of the tracheoesophageal ridges during the third week of gestation. It usually occurs in association with OA, and a number of configurations may be encountered. By far, the most common variant (87% of cases) involves proximal OA (esophagus continuous with the mouth ending in a blind loop superior to the sternal angle), with the distal esophagus arising from the trachea or a main bronchus (see also Chapter 28). Other possibilities are as follows:
- OA without a TOF (6%).
- OA and proximal TOF (2%).
- OA and both proximal and distal TOFs (1%).
- TOF without OA (H-type fistula, 4%).

Approximately 50% of all cases have additional congenital anomalies of the airway (tracheomalacia in 20% of all cases and laryngeal cleft in 6%) and other structures (VACTERL association: vertebral anomalies, anal atresia, cardiac anomalies, TOF, and renal, radial, and limb anomalies).

The diagnosis may be elusive, particularly for the H-type fistulas, where no upper esophageal hold up occurs, and the child may feed normally. Indeed, the authors have encountered a child with a history of recurrent chest infections who reached the age of 7 years before diagnosis.

Tube esophagography allows double-contrast examination of the esophagus under distension and remains the gold standard diagnostic technique. A satisfactory examination is not always possible; therefore, MLB may also be used, with the additional advantage of excluding concomitant anomalies. Typical findings are a V-shaped mucosal fold on the posterior tracheal wall just above the carina, but this is easily missed. Good conditions, with minimal secretions, and an experienced endoscopist are prerequisites. Instillation of methylene blue into the esophagus prior to the MLB may also help if the diagnosis is still in question.

Treatment involves ligation and division of the fistula. This tends to leave a characteristic posterior tracheal pouch, separated from the tracheal lumen by a bar of trachealis (▶ Fig. 21.24). While this does not produce symptoms, it may interfere with endotracheal intubation and use of tracheostomy tubes, as the tips of these may come to rest in the pouch, causing obstruction. Careful endoscopic assessment (particularly with a small flexible endoscope down the tube) is very useful at the time of tube insertion and at subsequent changes, particularly if tube length is increased.

Vascular Compression: Rings and Slings

Although approximately 3% of the population have anomalies of the great vessels, most do not produce

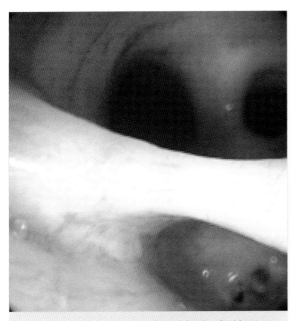

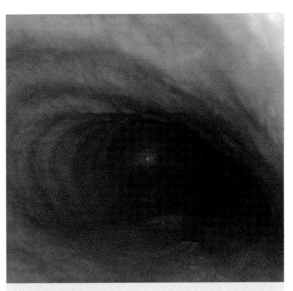

Fig. 21.25 Vascular ring. This pulsatile compression is caused by a double aortic arch.

21

Fig. 21.24 Repaired tracheoesophageal fistula. The blue Prolene (Ethicon) sutures are still visible in the posterior tracheal pit, in which the tip of an endotracheal or tracheostomy tube may lodge. Division of the anterior bar of tissue may resolve the problem.

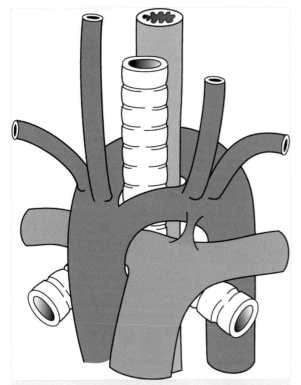

Fig. 21.26 Double aortic arch. (Reproduced from Haas NA, Kleideiter U. Pediatric Cardiology: Symptoms-Diagnosis-Treatment. Stuttgart/New York: Thieme; 2015, with permission.)

airway symptoms. Those that press on and compress the airway are as follows:

- Vascular rings (▶ Fig. 21.25), which encircle the trachea and esophagus.
- Vascular slings, which are not circumferential.

A double aortic arch is the commonest vascular ring (▶ Fig. 21.26). From a single ascending aorta, the aortic arch is duplicated into left (anterior) and right (posterior) arches. The left passes anterior to the trachea, whereas the right passes behind the esophagus, encircling these, before the two arches rejoin to form the descending aorta. The compressive effect results in biphasic stridor, respiratory distress, dysphagia, and a brassy cough.

A less common variety of ring involves a right-sided aortic arch, which loops behind the esophagus, as mentioned previously, together with an anomalous left subclavian artery that is connected to the pulmonary trunk by the ligamentum arteriosum, completing the loop anteriorly.

The commonest type of vascular sling is an aberrant innominate artery, which arises more posteriorly and more from the left side than normal, crossing the trachea anteriorly just above the carina.

The pulmonary artery sling, resulting from an anomalous left pulmonary artery, is less common (▶ Fig. 21.27). Rather than passing anterior to the trachea, this loops round from right to left in between the trachea and esophagus, causing compressive symptoms of both. This

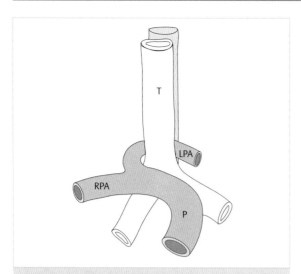

Fig. 21.27 Left pulmonary artery sling. (Reproduced from Statz G, Honnef D, Piroth W, Radkow T. Pediatric Imaging. Stuttgart/New York: Thieme; 2008, with permission.)

anomaly is associated with distal tracheal and right main bronchial stenosis.

Other vascular slings include an enlarged pulmonary artery (secondary to cardiac anomalies), causing anterior compression of the trachea and carina. An anomalous right or left subclavian artery may arise from the descending aorta, passing behind the esophagus. This causes characteristic *dysphagia lusoria* but no airway symptoms.

Cases of vascular rings tend to present earlier and with more pronounced airway symptoms, whereas vascular slings tend to produce less severe obstruction and a more protracted history of expiratory stridor, cough, and recurrent chest infections.

Diagnosis involves direct endoscopy (to assess the compressed section and exclude other pathology), echocardiography, CT with contrast, and other radiological examinations as necessary, including contrast swallow and contrast bronchography. These modalities allow assessment of tracheomalacia at the site of compression and distally, a common and refractive problem even after corrective cardiovascular surgery.

Although surgical correction of rings is usually necessary, some vascular slings may be actively monitored. Arteriopexy (e.g., aortopexy) procedures to suspend the offending vessels away from the trachea are sometimes required.

Tracheomalacia and Bronchomalacia

These are common end points of some of the conditions discussed previously and so are considered now. They are characterized by deficiencies in the supporting mechanisms of the tracheobronchial tree, resulting in partial or complete collapse during the respiratory cycle. Two synergistic problems underlie this phenomenon: weakness of the cartilaginous tracheal wall and hypotonia of the trachealis muscle posteriorly. These cause luminal collapse as the cartilages are drawn back and in during inspiration with forward ballooning of the trachealis during expiration, causing airway obstruction and characteristic biphasic stridor (see Chapter 20).

Clinical manifestations usually appear within the first year of life and in 60% of cases by 3 months of age. The precise presentation differs between cases and is influenced by the site and length of the malacic segment, as well as the state of the distal airways, lung parenchyma, and other comorbidities. Breathing difficulties with stridor or wheeze are typical, tending to be worse when the patient is supine, during distress or exertion, and at night. Indeed, some children will have the so-called death attacks with acute apnea and cyanosis as a result of airway collapse, sometimes requiring resuscitation. Recurrent lower respiratory tract infections, secondary to poor secretion clearance, and a brassy chronic cough are common.

Tracheomalacia may be classified as follows:
- *Primary* (resulting from inadequate tracheal ring development).
- *Secondary* (usually in the context of OA/TOF or after compression by a vascular sling/ring, an abnormal heart, or a mediastinal mass).

The underlying cause, comorbidities, and the length and severity of malacia will determine prognosis.

Investigations should allow both accurate assessment of the malacia and identify underlying causes and comorbidities. In practice, direct endoscopy (flexible tracheobronchoscopy or rigid MLB) is the first-line investigation; a collapsed trachea, apostrophe-shaped in cross-section, is characteristic (▶ Fig. 21.28). Associated pulsations may suggest vascular compression. It is important to note that endoscopy under general anesthesia, with the child breathing quietly, may not demonstrate the full extent of the malacia and does not allow easy measurement of airway caliber in the different phases of respiration. For these reasons, contrast bronchography is a very useful adjunct, usually combined with flexible bronchoscopy. This allows measurement of the caliber of the tracheobronchial tree at each phase and also enables measurement of closing pressures, helpful if CPAP is being considered. Chest CT enables airway assessment in inspiration and expiration and evaluation of the lung parenchyma, the heart, and relationships between the great vessels. MRI, esophagoscopy, and tube esophagography may also be appropriate. Management of these patients should be individualized and multidisciplinary, bearing in mind the etiology, severity, comorbidities, and likely natural history.

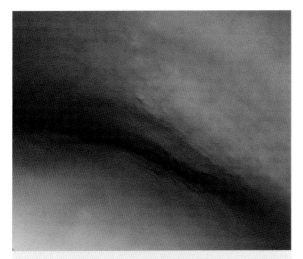

Fig. 21.28 Tracheomalacia in a child with tracheoesophageal fistula. This child also had a type II laryngeal cleft.

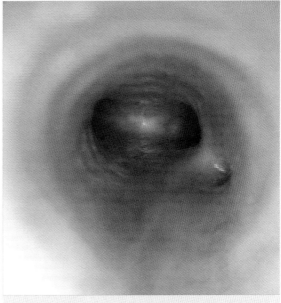

Fig. 21.29 Right upper lobe (pig) bronchus.

21

The etiology of primary tracheomalacia remains unclear, and indeed the absence of neonatal symptoms suggests that some cases may be acquired rather than truly congenital. An inherent cartilaginous deficiency may be responsible, particularly in syndromic cases.

Mild primary cases may be managed conservatively, bearing in mind that many will resolve spontaneously by 2 years of age. Treatment of any gastroesophageal reflux, chest physical therapy, and prophylactic antibiotic treatment may help.

More severe cases, particularly those with a history of "death attacks," should be managed more actively, as there is often a real risk of respiratory compromise and even death.

- Pressure support in the form of CPAP or bilevel positive airway pressure ventilation is often indicated, particularly for long-segment cases with bronchial and distal airways collapse. This is difficult to deliver long-term by face mask in a young child; therefore, tracheostomy may be required to facilitate this. Indeed, the tracheostomy tube may stent the airway sufficiently to avoid the need for pressure support.
- Aortopexy is indicated for severe, localized, and distal tracheomalacia. The aortic arch is suspended from the posterior surface of the sternum, relieving any airway compression.
- Endoluminal stents may also be used with the aim of increasing airway caliber until such a time that the trachea achieves natural rigidity. A variety of endoluminal stents are used: self- or balloon-expandable, nonabsorbable or absorbable. Migration, erosion, and blockage with granulations are possible complications, hence the need for managing these children in units with full intensive radiology, cardiothoracic, and critical care support.

Cases of secondary tracheomalacia are managed in much the same way, once the precipitating lesion has been corrected. Tracheomalacia is often a very resistant problem despite surgical management. Parents and clinicians should be prepared from the outset for a prolonged period of treatment.

Bifurcation Anomalies

Anomalies of the tracheal bifurcation and the distal bronchial branching pattern are relatively common. A right upper lobe bronchus (pig bronchus) is one of the commoner (► Fig. 21.29). No treatment is usually required for this and the other anomalies, but clinicians should be aware of the possibility of mistaking such as bifurcation for the true carina during endoscopic evaluation and when inserting endotracheal or tracheostomy tubes.

Congenital Tracheobronchial Cysts and Tumors

Congenital cysts of the lower airway are uncommon. They are believed to arise from outpouchings of the primitive tracheal bud (reduplication anomalies) and may be found anywhere along the tracheobronchial tree. They are mucus-filled, epithelium-lined true cysts, which may or may not open directly into the airway lumen. Larger cysts, particularly when tense with mucus, may compress the airway and result in symptoms, as in the case of vascular compression. Excision through thoracotomy is the treatment of choice in these cases.

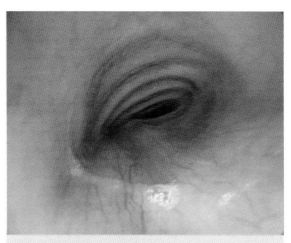

Fig. 21.30 Tracheal compression secondary to a mediastinal tumor in an infant

V

A variety of congenital mediastinal tumors (including teratomas and thymomas) may result in airway compression and symptoms (▶ Fig. 21.30). Chest CT with contrast and/or MRI will usually define the size and position and are often diagnostic.

21.6 Key Points

- A variety of congenital airway anomalies are described, the understanding of which is crucial to their correct treatment.
- Prompt diagnosis demands a high index of suspicion and appropriate investigations.
- Management should be multidisciplinary and tailored to the individual circumstances, bearing in mind the natural history of each anomaly, current symptoms, and presence of comorbidities.
- In many cases, active monitoring will suffice.
- Surgery and other forms of definitive treatment should be undertaken only after careful consideration.

References

[1] Negus VE. The comparative anatomy and physiology of the larynx. London: Heinemann; 1949

[2] Friedman EM, Vastola AP, McGill TJ, Healy GB. Chronic pediatric stridor: etiology and outcome. Laryngoscope. 1990; 100(3):277–280

[3] Jani P, Koltai P, Ochi JW, Bailey CM. Surgical treatment of laryngomalacia. J Laryngol Otol. 1991; 105(12):1040–1045

[4] Thottam PJ, Simons JP, Choi S, Maguire R, Mehta DK. Clinical relevance of quality of life in laryngomalacia. Laryngoscope. 2016; 126 (5):1232–1235

[5] Lane RW, Weider DJ, Steinem C, Marin-Padilla M. Laryngomalacia. A review and case report of surgical treatment with resolution of pectus excavatum. Arch Otolaryngol. 1984; 110(8):546–551

[6] Carter J, Rahbar R, Brigger M, et al. International Pediatric ORL Group (IPOG) laryngomalacia consensus recommendations. Int J Pediatr Otorhinolaryngol. 2016; 86:256–261

[7] Cotton RT, Reilly JS. Congenital malformations of the larynx. In: Bluestone CD, Stool SE, Kenna MA, eds. Pediatric Otolaryngology. 3rd ed. Philadelphia, PA: Saunders; 1996

[8] Toynton SC, Saunders MW, Bailey CM. Aryepiglottoplasty for laryngomalacia: 100 consecutive cases. J Laryngol Otol. 2001; 115(1):35–38

[9] Munson PD. Recurrent croup and persistent laryngomalacia: clinical resolution after supraglottoplasty. Int J Pediatr Otorhinolaryngol. 2016; 84:94–96

[10] Civantos FJ, Holinger LD. Laryngoceles and saccular cysts in infants and children. Arch Otolaryngol Head Neck Surg. 1992; 118(3):296–300

[11] Anderson de Moreno LC, Burgin SJ, Matt BH. The incidence of postoperative aspiration among children undergoing supraglottoplasty for laryngomalacia. Ear Nose Throat J. 2015; 94(8):320–328

[12] Gatti WM, MacDonald E, Orfei E. Congenital laryngeal atresia. Laryngoscope. 1987; 97(8 Pt 1):966–969

[13] Grimmer JF, Mulliken JB, Burrows PE, Rahbar R. Radiofrequency ablation of microcystic lymphatic malformation in the oral cavity. Arch Otolaryngol Head Neck Surg. 2006; 132(11):1251–1256

[14] Daya H, Hosni A, Bejar-Solar I, Evans JN, Bailey CM. Pediatric vocal fold paralysis: a long-term retrospective study. Arch Otolaryngol Head Neck Surg. 2000; 126(1):21–25

[15] Miyamoto RC, Cotton RT, Rope AF, et al. Association of anterior glottic webs with velocardiofacial syndrome (chromosome 22q11.2 deletion). Otolaryngol Head Neck Surg. 2004; 130(4):415–417

[16] Hamilton J, Yaneza MM, Clement WA, Kubba H. The prevalence of airway problems in children with Down's syndrome. Int J Pediatr Otorhinolaryngol. 2016; 81:1–4

[17] Myer CM, III, O'Connor DM, Cotton RT. Proposed grading system for subglottic stenosis based on endotracheal tube sizes. Ann Otol Rhinol Laryngol. 1994; 103(4 Pt 1):319–323

[18] Cotton RT, Evans JN. Laryngotracheal reconstruction in children. Five-year follow-up. Ann Otol Rhinol Laryngol. 1981; 90(5 Pt 1):516–520

[19] Monnier P, Savary M, Chapuis G. Partial cricoid resection with primary tracheal anastomosis for subglottic stenosis in infants and children. Laryngoscope. 1993; 103(11 Pt 1):1273–1283

[20] Benjamin B, Inglis A. Minor congenital laryngeal clefts: diagnosis and classification. Ann Otol Rhinol Laryngol. 1989; 98(6):417–420

[21] Shehab ZP, Bailey CM. Type IV laryngotracheoesophageal clefts — recent 5 year experience at Great Ormond Street Hospital for Children. Int J Pediatr Otorhinolaryngol. 2001; 60(1):1–9

[22] Léauté-Labrèze C, Dumas de la Roque E, Hubiche T, Boralevi F, Thambo JB, Taïeb A. Propranolol for severe hemangiomas of infancy. N Engl J Med. 2008; 358(24):2649–2651

[23] Jephson CG, Manunza F, Syed S, Mills NA, Harper J, Hartley BE. Successful treatment of isolated subglottic haemangioma with propranolol alone. Int J Pediatr Otorhinolaryngol. 2009; 73(12):1821–1823

[24] Cantrell JR, Guild HG. Congenital stenosis of the trachea. Am J Surg. 1964; 108:297–305

[25] Tsang V, Murday A, Gillbe C, Goldstraw P. Slide tracheoplasty for congenital funnel-shaped tracheal stenosis. Ann Thorac Surg. 1989; 48(5):632–635

22 Acquired Disorders of the Larynx, Trachea, and Bronchi

Michael Saunders and R. W. Clarke

22.1 Introduction

Laryngotracheobronchial disorders in children often present during the months and years after birth. Infection and trauma (including iatrogenic airway stenosis related to endotracheal intubation) are the commonest etiologies. This chapter considers the presentation and management of these conditions.

22.2 Infection

22.2.1 Historical Perspective

Historically acute airway infection was a major cause of morbidity and mortality in children. Airway obstruction due to upper respiratory infections was an important cause of child death even in well-to-do families during the preantibiotic era. Diphtheria was a major public health problem until well into the 20th century. Pediatric tracheostomy was largely developed for the treatment of severe diphtheria and was a well-established technique by the early 20th century, but it remained a treatment of last resort as the mortality in children undergoing tracheotomy was so high.[1] The decline in tracheostomy as a treatment for diphtheria was partly as a result of the availability of antitoxin but mainly because of the development of endotracheal intubation as a method of securing the airway. Childhood immunization has now almost eradicated diphtheria in western communities but it remains a significant disease in some parts of the world.

Tracheostomy remained in widespread use for epiglottitis until the 1970s when it was also replaced by endotracheal intubation (▶ Fig. 22.1), better medical treatment, and the improvements in pediatric intensive care unit (PICU) facilities that permit careful monitoring and early intervention for these children.[2,3]

Modern intensive care techniques, better training of health care staff, and the ability to safely intubate and ventilate children have completely revolutionized the management of children with acute infective airway obstruction. Instead of undergoing acute or emergency tracheostomy (with its not insignificant mortality), children with critical airway obstruction due to infection are now generally intubated to secure the airway and kept on

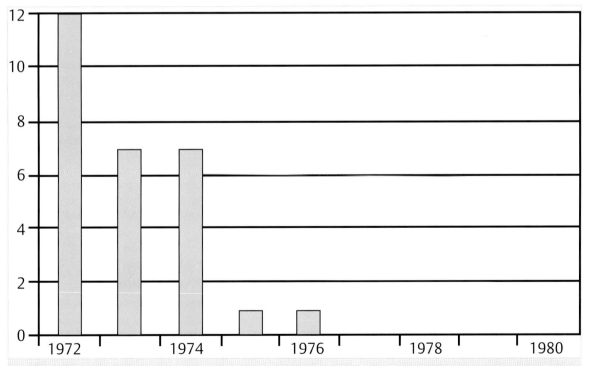

Fig. 22.1 Decline in tracheostomy for epiglottitis, even before the introduction of *Haemophilus Influenzae* B vaccine. (Modified after Carter P, Benjamin B. Ten-year review of pediatric tracheotomy. Ann Otol Rhinol Laryngol 1983;92(4 Pt 1):398–400, with permission.)

an intensive care unit until medical treatment such as systemic steroids or antibiotics lead to an improvement in the child's condition and extubation becomes practical.

The role of the otolaryngologist in the management of these conditions has also changed. Pediatric intensive care physicians (intensivists) or pediatricians now manage most of these children. An otolaryngologist will often be required at initial intubation to provide the option of an emergency tracheostomy or to facilitate intubation using rigid bronchoscopy. Operative surgical airway intervention is only considered if there is a failure of medical treatment resulting in failure to extubate.

22.2.2 Acute Epiglottitis

Acute epiglottitis is a condition characterized by rapidly progressive airway obstruction due to swelling of the supraglottic larynx, usually associated with severe systemic infective illness. Children—typically aged 2 to 7 years, although the condition can occur at any age—presenting with epiglottis are toxic and febrile. They tend to lean forward, keep still, drool, and demonstrate inspiratory stridor and marked features of airway obstruction.[4]

Presentation can be atypical, and because of the relative scarcity of the condition and concern about the airway, an otolaryngologist, as well as pediatric and intensive care or anesthetic staff, is best involved early in the sequence of care.

Since the *Haemophilus Influenzae* (B) vaccine was introduced in the early 1990s, epiglottitis has almost disappeared in children.[5] The vaccine is given in the first 6 months of life (see Chapter 2).

Acute epiglottitis still occurs in adults, and sporadic cases are reported in children, typically due to vaccine failure, which is rare, or in immunocompromised children. Children with immunosuppression—for example, those undergoing treatment with toxic chemotherapy agents—may also be at increased risk. Historically, more than 90% of cases were associated with infection with *H. influenzae*, but, especially in immunocompromised patients, epiglottitis is occasionally caused by a different organism.

Continued awareness of this potentially devastating condition remains important.

Management of Acute Epiglottitis

If epiglottitis is suspected, the child should be intubated under as controlled and safe conditions as are possible.[6]

The child should then be carefully monitored until his/her condition improves enough to permit extubation. Epiglottitis responds to intravenous antibiotics and extubation is normally possible after a few days. Further otolaryngological intervention is normally only required

if an epiglottic abscess develops, in which case the systemic response to antibiotics will be poor and the laryngoscopic appearance of the epiglottis on the intensive care unit will become increasingly abnormal. If the epiglottis is tense and bulging due to an abscess, then simple transoral drainage is normally adequate.

---

i

Key Points in the Care of a Child with Suspected Epiglottitis
- Avoid the use of a tongue depressor, a nasendoscope, and any form of instrumentation in the airway until the child is intubated.
- Do nothing that might trigger laryngospasm in an already critical airway.
- Secure the airway. The child may deteriorate very quickly.
- Admit for urgent inpatient supervision and monitoring.
- Avoid investigations such as blood tests or radiology that lead to delay.

22.2.3 Croup or Viral Acute Laryngotracheobronchitis

Although "croup" may be a general term used to describe stridor of infectious origin, historically including diphtheria and epiglottitis, the more common modern usage of the term is to describe viral acute laryngotracheobronchitis (ALTB).

ALTB is a respiratory infection that affects children of all ages but mostly in the 6-month to 3-year age group with a peak in the second year of life when 5% of children develop one or more episodes of ALTB. The commonest infective agents are parainfluenza virus types 1 to 3, but other organisms such as respiratory syncytial virus (RSV) can be implicated. There is a 1.4:1 male preponderance. The classic features include a pyrexial illness, stridor, and a characteristic barking cough. As the mucosa of the larynx and trachea become more edematous with progressive infection, airway obstruction leads to worsening inspiratory stridor with eventual fatigue and respiratory failure.

Management of Acute Laryngotracheobronchitis

Children with ALTB are mainly treated by pediatric general medical specialists or by emergency care doctors without involving the otolaryngologist. Most will respond quickly to corticosteroids (systemic and inhaled).[7] Oral dexamethasone at a dose of 0.4 mg/kg is very effective. Nebulized adrenaline can bring about dramatic symptom relief. Children with mild-to-moderate croup no longer

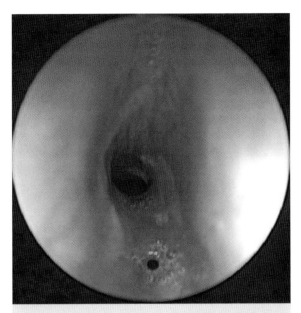

Fig. 22.2 Acute laryngotracheobronchitis. The mucosa is diffusely inflamed.

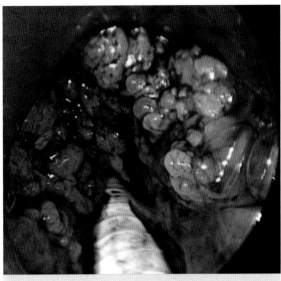

Fig. 22.3 Recurrent respiratory papillomatosis. (Reproduced from Sclafani AP. Total Otolaryngology–Head and Neck Surgery. Stuttgart/New York: Thieme: 2015, with permission.)

require admission to hospital if home circumstances are good and the parents can arrange rapid transport should the child deteriorate.

> A small number of children will not respond to medical treatment and will require endotracheal intubation. It is at this point that the otolaryngologist may become involved in the care.

Because most children with this condition do respond to medical treatment, the subset of children requiring intubation may have an alternative diagnosis (bacterial tracheitis, coexistent subglottic stenosis, foreign body). It is sensible to undertake the intubation in the operating room with an otolaryngologist present and with bronchoscopy and tracheostomy equipment available should an emergency airway be needed. The diagnosis is usually obvious at laryngoscopy (▶ Fig. 22.2). The child is intubated and the tube left in place for several days until the edema and inflammation resolve, allowing extubation. Ear, nose, and throat (ENT) follow-up is not required in cases of uncomplicated croup.

22.2.4 Bacterial Tracheitis (Pseudomembranous Croup)

Secondary bacterial infection of a larynx and trachea already affected with viral croup can lead to much more severe inflammation with the production of mucopus and the formation of inflammatory exudates and pseudo-

membranes within the tracheal lumen.[8] The causative agents include *Staphylococcus aureus*, *Streptococcus pneumonia*, and *Streptococcus pyogenes*. Although this is a much rarer disease than viral croup, 2% of children admitted to hospital with croup have bacterial tracheitis.[9] Bacterial tracheitis is now a commoner condition than acute epiglottitis.[10]

The clinical picture is generally worse than that associated with viral croup with pyrexia and increasing tracheal obstruction from the exudates.[11]

Patients will be toxic from bacterial infection with high white cell counts and a raised C-reactive protein.

Otolaryngological input may be required both at intubation and on occasion for therapeutic endoscopy to remove debris, sloughing, and necrotic mucosa from the airway.

> The long-term effects of bacterial tracheitis are significant. Affected children should be followed up to watch for signs of subglottic and tracheal stenosis developing in the weeks and months after discharge.

22.2.5 Recurrent Respiratory Papillomatosis

This is a viral condition in adults and children (juvenile onset recurrent respiratory papillomatosis [JORRP]) characterized by exophytic, usually multiple, lesions on the mucosal surface of the aerodigestive tract (▶ Fig. 22.3).

The larynx is mainly affected, with a particular predilection for squamocolumnar mucosal junctions.

Etiology of Juvenile Onset Recurrent Respiratory Papillomatosis

> ℹ
>
> The causative agent is the human papilloma virus (HPV), typically types 6 and 11. These are the HPV subtypes also associated with maternal genital warts.

The virus is thought to be transmitted at birth by direct contact with infected secretions in the birth canal. The mode of transmission is probably more complex than this[12] as babies born by Caesarian section can be affected, and there is almost certainly transplacental transmission of the virus as well. The traditionally quoted susceptibility factors for RRP are as follows:

- First-born children.
- Maternal genital warts.
- Young maternal age.
- Vaginal delivery.
- Low maternal socioeconomic status.

Often, however, none of these applies.

HPV contamination of the birth canal is common (25% of pregnant women) yet JORRP is rare, approximately 1 in 25,000 children, so host susceptibility factors must come into play. In the case of children born to mothers with genital warts, HPV deoxyribonucleic acid (DNA) has been found in one-third to one half of aerodigestive tract swabs of these babies but very few, 1 in 400, develop JORRP. At one time, particularly in the United States, caesarean section was recommended for expectant mothers with genital warts but current evidence does not support this as a protective measure against JORRP. Despite recent work on human leukocyte antigen polymorphisms that may help to identify pregnancies where the infant is at particular risk, this host susceptibility is currently unpredictable.[13,14]

The widespread availability and uptake of HPV vaccination in girls (and in some cases in boys) in many western countries is likely to bring about a big reduction in the incidence of JORRP as this cohort of girls enter their reproductive years.[15] Vaccination was introduced as a protective measure against the development of carcinoma of the uterine cervix, where HPV has a crucial etiological role, but a reduction in the prevalence of genital tract HPV contamination—especially with types 6 and 11 where the quadrivalent vaccine against subtypes 6, 11, 16, and 18 is used—may make JORRP a condition that ENT surgeons see even more rarely in years to come.

Clinical Presentation of Juvenile Onset Recurrent Respiratory Papillomatosis

Presentation is usually with hoarseness, typically in school-age children. A small number of children may present with stridor. Younger children can be affected, and in these cases, the course tends to be more aggressive with a poorer prognosis. It is thought that the virus remains dormant in the laryngeal epithelium for several years before giving rise to the typical warty lesions. Viral particles are widely distributed in the epithelial cells even after thorough removal of the excrescences, making for the characteristic tendency for multiple recurrences.

Treatment of Juvenile Onset Recurrent Respiratory Papillomatosis

> ℹ
>
> Treatment is surgical.
> - At laryngotracheoscopy, get a good view of the larynx, preferably without an endotracheal (ET) tube in place, and carefully remove the exophytic lesions.
> - Take particular care in the region of the anterior commissure as repeated trauma here will lead to scarring and web formation.

Various techniques are described, including a carbon dioxide (CO_2) laser, which for many years was the mainstay of treatment but has the disadvantages of causing heat damage to surrounding tissue, a tendency to scarring, the logistic difficulties of setting up the equipment and ensuring staff are appropriately trained, and the very small risk of airway fire.

Most units nowadays use the *microdebrider* (▶ Fig. 22.7). This is a suction device containing a high-speed rotating blade. The orifice of the hand-piece is swept along the free margin of the lesion in a "brushing" movement until normal tissue is exposed. If the papillomas are very extensive, it may be wise to do some initial débridement with an ET tube in place until the airway is safe. Careful liaison with a skilled pediatric anesthesiologist is essential.

Some surgeons favor the Coblator (ArthroCare), but it will cause thermal damage to adjacent tissue and is not widely used.

> ℹ
>
> Repeat surgery is the norm with a frequency depending on the severity and aggressiveness of the disease.

Some children manage with 6-monthly or even annual endoscopies, whereas some may need surgery as often as every few weeks. The course is variable and periods of rapid growth can be followed by periods of relative quiescence. It is the authors' practice to arrange a repeat surgery date at each endoscopy and to instruct parents to get in touch quickly should the child become hoarse, and urgently should the child develop stridor, so that earlier admission can be expedited.

> A very small proportion of children with JORRP will require tracheostomy, although this must be avoided if at all possible. It will be considered in children with rampant disease who do not respond to conventional measures including adjuvant treatments detailed next and in whom airway obstruction is already established or imminent, but tracheostomy facilitates tracheobronchial spread of disease and is a last resort.

Adjuvant Medical Treatment for Recurrent Respiratory Papillomatosis

Various adjuvant medical treatments have been suggested. The evidence base for most is poor. Cidofovir, interferon, acyclovir, ribavirin, mumps vaccine, and indole-3-carbinol have been used with varying enthusiasm.

- Photodynamic therapy works on the principle of making specific target tissues susceptible to therapeutic intervention by prior administration of a photosensitive drug and is now rarely used.
- Cidofovir is the most often used contemporary adjuvant therapy, and even though reviews of cidofovir efficacy appear to demonstrate an improvement in outcome in a significant proportion overall, a double-blind randomized controlled trial indicates that there is no benefit over normal saline.[16] The apparent benefit of cidofovir may result from the necessary frequent debulking at the time of injection. There is some evidence to question the safety of cidofovir, and as it acts by becoming incorporated in DNA, there is real worry about its potential to facilitate malignant tissue change.[17,18,19] There is increasing interest in the therapeutic potential of the HPV vaccine (Gardasil [Merck]) and many surgeons are now recommending it for children with established JORRP.[20,21]

Prognosis of Juvenile Onset Recurrent Respiratory Papillomatosis

JORRP is usually confined to the larynx but runs a variable course, and may become quiescent as the child progresses through adolescence.[22]

In particularly aggressive cases, the virus spreads to the tracheobronchial tree with the potential for fatal airway obstruction. These children need frequent and demanding surgery, including potassium titanyl phosphate (KTP)

laser excision if disease needs to be removed from hard-to-access sites in the tracheobronchial tree and may warrant adjuvant therapy. Extension to the small airways and ultimately the alveoli results in cavitating cystic lesions in the chest and may be fatal.

Squamous carcinoma of the bronchus has been reported and in this respect JORRP can be regarded as a premalignant condition, albeit the risk is very small.

22.3 Injury and Stenosis of the Larynx and Upper Trachea

Although major trauma to the larynx and trachea can result in immediate and dramatic loss of function, injury to the upper airway more usually results in a slower process of mucosal tearing, edema, or necrosis, with healing and the formation of fibrous repair tissue. This process of scarring in a hollow tube such as the trachea tends to narrow the lumen, "cicatrization" (▶ Fig. 22.4). This is the etiology of the majority of the cases of acquired airway stenosis that present to the pediatric otolaryngologist.

There are several potential causes, but by far the commonest etiology of trauma to the larynx and trachea that results in airway stenosis is intubation and the use of ET tubes, that is, iatrogenic laryngotracheal stenosis.

22.3.1 Mechanisms of Injury to the Larynx and Trachea

Chemical Injury

Caustic ingestion remains a significant problem in young children. Although generally the more significant effects

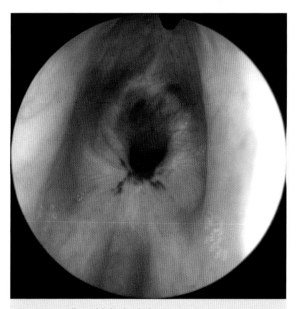

Fig. 22.4 Well-established subglottic stenosis.

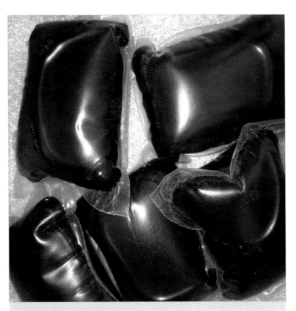

Fig. 22.5 Liquitabs

are seen in the pharynx and esophagus, mild chemical burns of the supraglottis are not uncommon in cases of caustic ingestion, and any child with a history of suspected caustic ingestion who is undergoing an endoscopy of the esophagus and stomach should have a careful assessment of the larynx and trachea under the same general anesthetic. Ingestion of cleaning agents was a significant public health problem in years gone by, but better product labeling, safer packaging, child-proof lids, and increased parental awareness have made for much less frequent admissions of children with caustic burns.

> **i**
>
> In recent years, "liquitabs" (▶ Fig. 22.5; see also Chapter 28) containing washing-up and dishwasher fluid have become more widely used. These are typically brightly colored, stored in ground-level cupboards, and attractive to toddlers who may mistake them for sweets or ice-lollies. They have been implicated in several esophageal and laryngotracheal mucosal injuries.[23]

Thermal Injury

Inhalational burns in the pediatric airway are thankfully rare but are potentially serious. With inhalation of steam from hot liquids, significant thermal energy can be transmitted to the soft tissue of the upper airway and this tends to cause more serious laryngeal injury than hot dry gases. Laryngospasm helps to prevent burns distal to the glottis, but the supraglottis is at risk and the resulting edema may cause life-threatening airway obstruction in the acute phase. Long-term stenosis of the pediatric airway after inhalational burns is relatively uncommon.

Laser Injury

Significant long-term iatrogenic injury may be caused to the developing larynx by therapeutic use of the laser in the pediatric airway. The most commonly used laser in airway surgery worldwide is the CO_2 laser.

- The major advantage of laser surgery is that it offers a relatively bloodless technique allowing endolaryngeal ablation of tissue (including stenosis, webs, granulations, subglottic cysts, hemangiomas) without immediate injury to surrounding tissues. The initial postoperative results can be impressive, and with judicious use, the CO_2 laser can be a very useful tool.
- The major disadvantage is that the tissue surrounding the operated area suffers a significant degree of submucosal thermal injury, not always apparent at the time of surgery. This can lead to long-term scarring, webbing, and stenosis. On occasions, the airway obstruction resulting from iatrogenic scarring can be more problematic than the original pathology.

Laser surgery carries the risk of airway fire, although this is extremely rare. Safety precautions such as the use of "laser safe" ET tubes, wet swabs, protection of tissues outside the operative field, eye-protection for staff, and appropriate training, including refresher courses for all operating room personnel, are essential.

In the last decade, laser airway surgery has become a far less popular treatment modality amongst pediatric otolaryngologists. The microdebrider (see below) is increasingly popular. Some surgeons now use the Coblator (see Chapter 18) with good effect in the larynx and trachea, although this is not without risk of causing mucosal burns.

> **Treatment of Airway Burns**   **i**
>
> The initial care of burns affecting the larynx is supportive. Treatment with systemic corticosteroids may be indicated if there is concern about the possibility of airway compromise, and in severe cases, endotracheal intubation and short-term ventilation should be considered. Long-term airway compromise is now uncommon after caustic ingestion, but occasional cases requiring tracheostomy have been reported. In severe cases, early tracheostomy is a better option than prolonged intubation, as this adds the risk of intubation trauma complicating the preexisting burn injury.
>
> Long-term treatment of burn-related scarring may require a similar approach to the treatment identified in the following for intubation-related injuries.

Blunt External Trauma

The infantile larynx lies at a higher level in the neck than the adult larynx, and blunt injuries are relatively less likely. The cartilaginous skeleton is softer, more elastic, and less likely to fracture as a result of a direct impact.[24]

Significant injury is generally associated with high velocity accidents, particularly a blow from the handlebars of a motorcycle or bicycle, or a horse-rider striking a fence. Although children are less likely to be involved in a high-speed accident than adults, neck injury associated with motorized vehicle including snowmobiles and quad bikes is becoming more common in children. Fortunately, significant injury is rare with very few blunt neck injuries involving the larynx.

Severity of injury can range from minor contusions to complete laryngotracheal disjunction, which can be fatal (Box 22.1[25]).

> ### Box 22.1 Severity of Acute Laryngeal Injuries[25]
>
> - Minor endolaryngeal hematoma or laceration without detectable fracture.
> - Edema, hematoma, and minor mucosal disruption without exposed cartilage.
> - Massive edema, mucosal tears, exposed cartilage, vocal cord immobility, and displaced fractures.
> - As above with more than two fracture lines or massive trauma to laryngeal mucosa.
> - Laryngotracheal separation.

Management of Blunt Laryngeal Injuries

The management of blunt laryngeal injuries[26,27,28] can thus be summarized as follows:
- Recognize the injury:
  - Suspect significant injury to the larynx and trachea with any of the following:
    - History of significant force of impact to the anterior neck.
    - Loss of voice, stridor, dysphagia or odynophagia.
    - Bruising around the neck or chest.
    - Loss of palpable laryngeal landmarks or obvious palpable fracture.
    - Surgical emphysema or free air on plain X-rays.
    - The airway may seem stable on initial presentation but can rapidly deteriorate with the onset of mucosal swelling.
- Investigate:
  - Flexible nasoendoscopy is extremely useful in cooperative children.
  - Plain X-rays are of limited use as children's cartilage is not calcified but you may identify free air and also injury to the adjacent cervical spine.
  - The best investigation of the injured larynx is computed tomography (CT) scanning. This may not be practical if there is significant concern about impending airway obstruction.
- Secure the airway:
  - Where there is airway obstruction or significant concern, make the airway safe with an ET tube or a tracheostomy.
  - Simple edema and submucosal hematoma can be treated by intubation, whereas major disruption of the laryngeal skeleton (such as cricotracheal separation) can be worsened by standard intubation techniques.
  - The best approach is to examine and secure the airway using rigid endoscopy and then decide on the need for tracheostomy and/or immediate laryngeal repair under the same anesthetic.

Intubation Trauma

History

Intubation trauma is a significant cause of laryngotracheal morbidity in children. Long-term ventilation for premature neonates, who earlier would almost certainly not have survived, started in the 1960s, and with it came a huge increase in intubation-related stenosis in the pediatric airway. At the time, permanent tracheostomy was the only effective available intervention. In the 1980s, pioneers including Cotton, Seid, and Zalzal started to report novel surgical techniques to treat subglottic stenosis so as to remove tracheostomies from affected children or to avoid tracheostomy altogether. At the same time, a greater understanding of the causes of intubation injury and of the dangers of prolonged, ill-fitting, and inappropriate tubes contributed to by pioneer workers such as Benjamin and Lindholm changed neonatal intensive care unit (NICU) practice. The risk of subglottic stenosis is now very much reduced, but the increasing number of extremely premature and medically complex neonates and children surviving NICUs means that more children are intubated and ventilated in large children's hospitals, and the laryngotracheal consequences of intubation injury continue to present to the pediatric otolaryngologist.[29]

Pathogenesis/ Mechanism of Injury

Mucosal injury can be caused by either of the following:
- The endotracheal intubation itself.
- The continued presence of a tube in the lumen of the airway.

Emergency or repeated intubation is more likely to result in airway trauma. The physical process of intubation may cause a breach in the mucosal surface, which leads to ulceration with the potential for scarring and cicatrization. On rare occasions, intubation can cause more significant acute injury including arytenoid dislocation or a tracheal tear.

22

The presence of the ET tube in the airway, particularly if it is too "snug" a fit, leads to edema and then ischemia of the mucosa. Modern tubes tend to be made of material that causes minimal tissue reaction. The early "red rubber" tubes were especially liable to cause stenosis, and there is some evidence that repeated contact between the tube and the mucosa during respiratory cycles may predispose to injury. Ischemia leads to mucosal ulceration and the formation of granulation tissue. The healing processes after ulceration then leads to fibrosis, deposition of scar tissue, and narrowing of the lumen of the airway.

Severe stenosis is becoming far less common as medical care of very sick babies improves, but pediatric otolaryngologists are increasingly seeing evidence of mucosal ischemia giving rise to vesicular "cobblestone" reactions in the subglottic mucosa (subglottic cysts; ▶ Fig. 22.6). These may be large enough to obstruct the airway when the child is extubated and probably represent an early stage in the evolution of subglottic stenosis. The larger cysts may need surgical debulking by marsupialization or using the microdebrider (▶ Fig. 22.7).

Trauma from the ET tube can also cause inflammatory swellings on the mucosal surface of the vocal cords (▶ Fig. 22.8, ▶ Fig. 22.9). A large solitary lesion can project into the lumen of the glottis: "intubation granuloma." These will usually settle when the tube is removed but may be large enough to warrant endoscopic removal.

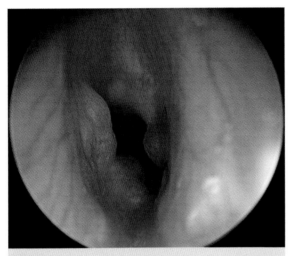

Fig. 22.6 Subglottic cysts.

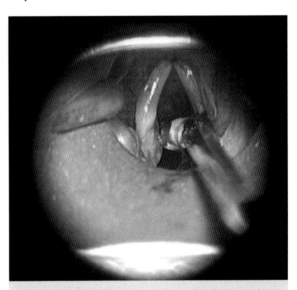

Fig. 22.7 Large subglottic cyst. The microdebrider is used to open the cyst and remove redundant tissue.

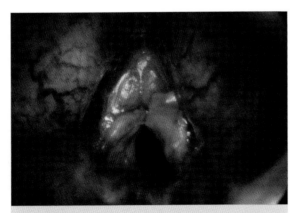

Fig. 22.8 Brisk inflammatory mucosal reaction to endotracheal tube. Granulations on the vocal cords.

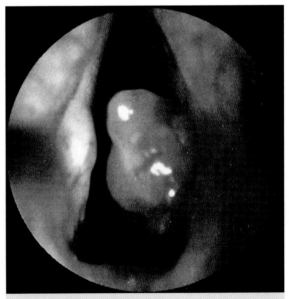

Fig. 22.9 Right arytenoid granulation.

Acquired Tracheal Stenosis

Tracheal stenosis in children can result from the following:

- *Intubation trauma*: as the cricoid is the narrowest part of the airway in children, it is the segment at greatest risk of injury with standard uncuffed tubes. There has been an increase in the use of cuffed tubes in intensive care units in the last few years, and unless care is taken to maintain a correct cuff pressure or to deflate the cuff from time to time, ischemic injury to the mucosa of the trachea can result leading to stenosis.
- *Tracheostomy*: after the removal of a tracheostomy tube (and particularly if a persistent tracheacutaneous fistula is closed surgically), the process of cicatrization can lead to a significant narrowing at the level of the stoma. Always avoid the removal of cartilage in the creation of a child's tracheostomy and make sure the trachea is incised well below the first tracheal ring.

  The anterior wall of the trachea immediately above the site of a tracheostomy is prone to softening and prolapses inward in a process known as suprastomal collapse. This can become so severe as to occlude the lumen of the airway so much that decannulation is impossible even if the original indication for the tracheostomy has resolved.
- *Infection*: bacterial tracheitis may lead to significant scarring and stenosis often at several levels in the trachea.

22.3.2 Site of Injury

The Subglottis

The narrowest part of the infant laryngotracheal airway is the complete cartilaginous ring of the cricoid cartilage. In the newborn, the internal diameter here is approximately 4 mm. Compared to the incomplete cartilaginous rings of the trachea, the cricoid ring is less distensible and the lumen is more vulnerable to injury. An overtight ET tube will lead to ischemia and subsequent edema or ulceration.

> **Grading of Subglottic Stenosis** ℹ
>
> The Meyer–Cotton classification has become widely used for the grading of subglottic stenosis[30]:
> - Grade 1: lumen obstructed by up to 50% of diameter.
> - Grade 2: lumen reduced by 50 to 90%.
> - Grade 3: lumen reduced by more than 90%.
> - Grade 4: complete obstruction.

> ℹ
>
> The size of the lumen is effectively estimated by identifying the largest ET tube that can be comfortably passed through the stenosis, that is, without using excessive force as the resulting mucosal trauma can itself lead to worsening of the stenosis.
>
> The Meyer–Cotton classification takes no account of whether the stenosis involves the glottis, which makes subsequent treatment more complicated, or of the nature of the stenosis, whether it is organized, soft, or active. The McCaffrey scale[31] focuses more on the site of the stenotic segment and may better predict the outcome of surgery, but the Meyer–Cotton scale is more widely used internationally.

The Glottis

The glottis is a triangular opening, and a circular ET tube tends to exert mucosal pressure unevenly. Areas at particular risk are the posterior commissure mucosa and the middle of the vocal cord on either side. The anterior commissure is relatively protected from intubation injury.

Pressure over the vocal process of the cord may lead to the formation of granulations, which, if large enough, may obstruct the airway. Pressure and ulceration over the posterior commissure will lead to scarring and webbing with reduced mobility of the vocal cords and what is now referred to as *posterior glottic stenosis* (▶ Fig. 22.10).

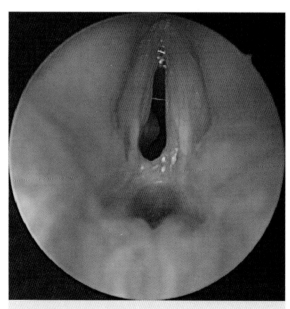

Fig. 22.10 Posterior glottic stenosis.

22

The Arytenoid Cartilage

The cricoarytenoid joint can be dislocated by significant direct trauma to the neck. This produces a tear in the capsule of the synovial joint and the arytenoid cartilage prolapses to an abnormally anteromedial position leading to airway obstruction. The joint rapidly ankyloses and becomes fixed. Attempts to reduce the dislocation are often unsuccessful because of the loss of integrity of the joint capsule.

Ulceration from direct pressure over the cricoarytenoid joint may lead to an inflammatory synovitis, with subsequent fibrosis and immobility. This usually results in the vocal cord being fixed in a median position and unable to abduct, causing a reduced airway. Less commonly the joint is fixed in abduction.

22.3.3 Clinical Problems in Acquired Stenosis of the Larynx and Trachea

Acquired stenosis and trauma to the larynx and trachea leads to the following three main problems:
- Airway obstruction.
- Dysphonia.
- Aspiration.

Airway Obstruction

The most significant problem related to laryngotracheal injury is airway obstruction. This tends to present to the otolaryngologist in one of the following three clinical scenarios:
- The intubated child who fails extubation.
- The child without a tracheostomy but with stridor or recurrent croup.
- The child with an existing tracheostomy and subglottic stenosis.

Dysphonia

Hoarseness or an abnormal cry is a common problem related to glottic injury and scarring, which can also result from surgical attempts to enlarge the airway. Generally, in smaller children, this is less of a clinical priority than establishing a secure airway, and interventions to improve the voice can be left until the child is older.

Aspiration

This results from failure of the sphincteric action of the supraglottis and glottis in preventing liquid or solids entering the subglottic airway. In practice, this is the least common of the problems encountered and usually a result of severe injury or a complication of surgery. It may be so severe that the child needs to be fed through a gastrostomy.

22.3.4 Assessment of Airway Stenosis

History

Apart from establishing a possible cause for the stenosis, consider a child's other medical problems before embarking on treatment. Many of these children have lung disease and other comorbidities that will adversely influence the chance of successful surgical treatment of subglottic stenosis.

> **i**
>
> Management is usually part of a multidisciplinary package of care involving respiratory pediatricians, anesthesiologists, and intensive care specialists.

Investigations

In the majority of cases, the only otolaryngological investigation needed is airway endoscopy. In a small number of older and cooperative children, lung function tests may be helpful in, first, determining the extent of airway obstruction by comparison with normal values and, second, in distinguishing between large airway and small airway disease in children with existing lung problems. This tends to be limited to older children, and many of the patients treated with subglottic stenosis will be under 5 years of age, and this is not really a practical test.

Endoscopy

Acquired laryngotracheal stenosis is very well demonstrated at endoscopy. This requires a general anesthetic— a reasonable view of the supraglottis and glottis is possible in an awake child using a flexible nasendoscope but characterization of the nature of subglottic stenosis is not practical (see Chapter 20).

Most otolaryngologists use rigid endoscopy to assess the larynx and trachea, although recent improvements in the optical quality of flexible endoscopes make them an attractive adjunct.

Endoscopic assessment should consider the whole of the airway, but the following are critically important:
- Active movement of the vocal cords and mobility of the cricoarytenoid joints.
- Location of scarring: is scarring limited to the glottis, the subglottis, or both?
- Nature of the stenosis: is it soft/edematous, or organized, or is it avascular?
- Condition of tracheostomy, if present, presence of granulation, or suprastomal collapse.
- State of the distal trachea.

V

Imaging

Radiology is generally not relied on in the evaluation of the caliber of the lumen of the larynx and subglottis. Cross-sectional imaging (CT or magnetic resonance imaging) is useful in the assessment of both intrinsic tracheal abnormalities and extraluminal compression of the trachea. Tracheobronchography using contrast may demonstrate bronchomalacia particularly in the distal segmental bronchi (see ▶ Fig. 20.10).

22.3.5 Treatment of Airway Stenosis

Conservative Treatment

If a stenosis is mild and not causing any airway problems, manage the child with outpatient follow-up and interval endoscopy as required.

If the laryngotracheal stenosis is sufficient to require a tracheostomy, it may be best to delay definitive treatment until other medical problems have been addressed; a common clinical example involves children born prematurely with lung disease who have a persisting oxygen requirement.

Medical Treatment

Corticosteroids

> ℹ️
>
> The anti-inflammatory action of corticosteroids is helpful in reducing edema.

In the scenario of a failed extubation in the premature neonate, where the stenosis is often edematous and reversible rather than organized, short-term administration of steroids is helpful to facilitate extubation. There is no evidence to suggest that longer-term administration of systemic corticosteroids prevents the formation of organized scar tissue, and the side effects resulting from a dose required to achieve this would be considerable. Steroids have no effect on established stenosis.

Antireflux Treatment

Gatroesophageal reflux is frequently present in children with subglottic stenosis. The exact relationship between the two conditions is unclear, specifically whether reflux is a causative or promoting factor in the development of stenosis and to what extent long-term reflux treatment can modify the course. Some children with reactive airway disease will improve on antireflux treatment.[32] Particularly in children with soft, inflammatory, or reactive stenosis, it reasonable to investigate reflux or consider a period of empirical long-term antireflux treatment. It is also reasonable to address reflux in the peri-operative period in children undergoing major airway surgery (see Chapter 28).

Other Medical Treatments

- Mitomycin C is an antifibroblast drug that is used in an attempt to reduce scar tissue formation after surgery. It is applied topically on pledgets to raw surfaces after division of scar tissue at a concentration of 0.1 to 0.4 mg/mL. There is some evidence of efficacy in animal models, but the evidence in humans use is uncertain[33] and the role of mitomycin C in this situation is unclear.[34]
- Azithromycin is a macrolide antibiotic with a significant anti-inflammatory action. There is recent interest in its use as an adjuvant medical treatment for the reactive or inflammatory phase of airway stenosis in children undergoing surgery or as a main treatment agent for inflammatory stenosis.

Surgical Treatment

Principles of Surgical Treatment

Laryngeal Stenosis: Cord Lateralization

Stenosis at the level of the glottis impairs the airway not only by the mechanical effect of the narrowing but also by limiting abduction of the vocal cords. This can be because of scarring around the posterior commissure or because the cricoarytenoid joints are fixed, or a combination of the two.

Occasionally, a well-defined synechia (▶ Fig. 22.11) between the arytenoids can simply be divided with microscissors, but this is unusual. Thicker webs tend to recur after simple division. Some surgeons advocate web

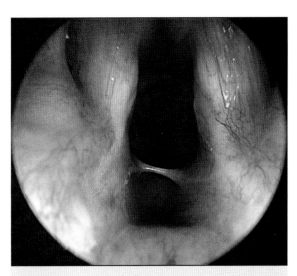

Fig. 22.11 Interarytenoid adhesion.

22

division with application of mitomycin C, and in larger larynxes, it is possible to rotate a mucosal flap into the posterior commissure to prevent rescarring.

> Most cases of symptomatic posterior glottic stenosis will require some form of cord lateralization procedure.

Subglottic Stenosis

The diameter of the airway can be increased (and the resistance decreased) by either of the following:
- Resection of obstructing scar tissue.
- Expansion of the laryngotracheal skeleton.

An endoscopic approach has traditionally been used for ablation/resection of scar tissue, whereas framework expansion is undertaken by an open approach. Recent developments have blurred this distinction, and a wide range of surgical options is currently available.

Subglottic stenosis is rare, and randomized controlled trials of one surgical procedure against another are impractical. The best evidence is from retrospective case series or cohort studies, and the surgical approach to airway surgery can vary significantly between centers.

The "Reactive" Larynx

The scar tissue should be mature and organized before surgical treatment is undertaken. In some cases, the mucosa of the larynx and trachea is prone to recurrent edema leading to variable degrees of airway obstruction. This makes the planning of surgical interventions difficult and the results unpredictable. A reactive larynx can be observed at laryngoscopy with significant erythema and visible worsening of glottis and subglottic edema over the course of the procedure caused by the irritation from the instrumentation and anesthetic gases (▶ Fig. 22.12).

Surgical intervention should be delayed in this instance and the stenosis be allowed to mature while contributory factors such as gastroesophageal reflux are investigated and treated.

Endoscopic Surgical Treatment

Microdebrider

The microdebrider allows precise endolaryngeal removal of tissue without significant trauma to surrounding structures and without the submucosal thermal injury associated with laser surgery. Although organized subglottic scar tissue is usually too firm for this technique, the microdebrider is useful in the removal of granulations and in the marsupialization of subglottic ductal retention cysts.

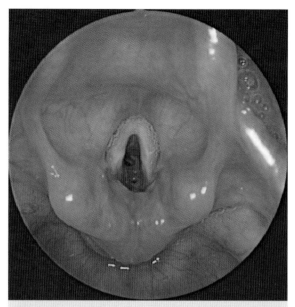

Fig. 22.12 A "reactive larynx" with contact bleeding. Surgery is best deferred until the scar has matured.

Balloon Dilatation

Dilation of the pediatric airway with bougies has had a limited role in the past. The trauma resulting to the free epithelial edge of the stenosis generally leads to restenosis. The recent development of highly specialized balloon catheters for the treatment of arterial occlusion has significantly changed the endoscopic treatment of laryngotracheal stenosis. Angioplasty balloons were initially used, but catheters specific to the pediatric airway are now available. A key feature is that the balloon cannot distend beyond a known diameter regardless of the inflation pressure. This allows control of the degree of dilatation. The risk of significant injury to the airway is now very low. The balloon is very effective in the treatment of short-segment organized stenosis in the subglottis and to a lesser degree in the posterior glottis (▶ Fig. 22.13).

It is less effective on long-segment stenosis and in the reactive phase as edema reaccumulates rapidly after dilation. The technique is occasionally effective in the management of failed extubation in the newborn as an alternative to tracheostomy or cricoid split. Some surgeons combine balloon dilatation with an endoscopic cricoid split.[35,36]

Endoscopic Anterior Cricoid Split

This is a full-thickness incision in the cricoid. The surgeon, usually with a sickle knife, incises the whole of the midportion of the cricoid from the luminal surface, separating the two halves and creating a midline defect. The subglottis can then be dilated with an airway balloon sufficient to allow the child to be intubated with a larger

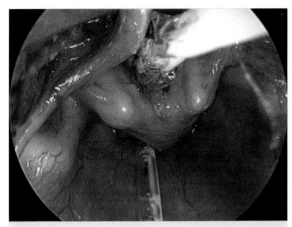

Fig. 22.13 Balloon dilatation of the subglottis.

tube postoperatively for several days. This is an alternative to open airway procedures for cases of failed extubation in the neonate.[37]

Endoscopic Posterior Cricoid Split and Graft

The placement of a graft into the posterior glottis has traditionally been a part of laryngotracheal reconstruction (LTR) using an anterior laryngofissure approach. Posterior glottic stenosis has been treated recently by splitting the posterior cricoid plate in the midline endoscopically and inserting a cartilage graft carved such that it sits securely in the defect created.

This allows expansion of the posterior glottic airway as an alternative to vocal cord lateralization techniques. It has been used to treat posterior laryngeal webbing, fixation of the cricoarytenoid joints, and congenital bilateral vocal cord palsy.

Laser Treatment of Stenosis

Laser resection of stenosis has the advantage of a relatively bloodless no-touch technique that offers immediate improvement in airway diameter and reduction of symptoms. The thermal injury to the surrounding tissue leads to longer term restenosis, and as a result and because of the success of other techniques, laser surgery has become less popular in recent years and is now rarely used.

Open Surgical Treatment

Cricoid Split

The cricoid split is the simplest open surgical procedure for the treatment of subglottic stenosis. It was first described in 1980 by Alan Seid and Robin Cotton. Its main use is the treatment of the neonate who has failed extubation because of subglottic stenosis. Children being considered for this technique do best if they have a good birth weight (> 1,500 g), low supplementary oxygen need, and good cardiorespiratory reserve, and are free of active infection.[38]

Technique

The approach and preparation is similar to a tracheostomy, using a horizontal skin incision over the cricoid cartilage. The cricoid, thyroid, and upper tracheal cartilages are exposed, and a vertical full thickness incision is made from the lower third of the thyroid cartilage, through the cricoid and into the first two tracheal rings (▶ Fig. 22.14). An age-appropriate ET tube is then inserted and the skin is closed over an open drain that is left in position for a few days to reduce the risk of surgical emphysema.

The split itself allows a modest amount of distraction of the cricoid cartilage such that the correct-sized ET tube can be admitted despite the presence of the mucosal

22

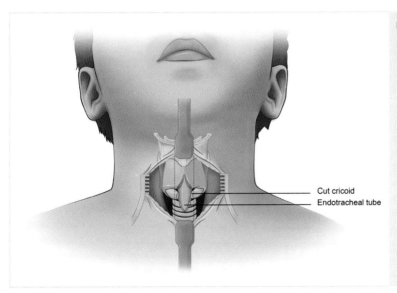

Fig. 22.14 Anterior cricoid split.

Cut cricoid
Endotracheal tube

edema. The child remains intubated for 7 to 10 days and the drains need to be left in situ for 2 to 5 days as there is likely to be a significant leak of air.

The child is treated with systemic corticosteroids prior to extubation (e.g., dexamethasone 0.4 mg/kg intravenous), and in the authors' practice, steroid treatment continues for 1 to 2 days after extubation to reduce edema.

The cricoid split is similar to the first part of a single-stage anterior LTR. The placement of a graft into the midline split effectively turns a cricoid split procedure into an LTR. Some authors feel that if a cricoid split is undertaken then the addition of a graft to fill the resulting defect confers little extra morbidity. Small grafts can be taken from the thyroid ala through the same incision or from the auricular cartilage with a low risk of donor site morbidity. The main extra risk is the presence of a non-vascularized graft in the airway, which itself is a potential source of infection or granulation.

Laryngotracheal Reconstruction

The following are the essential steps in LTR:
- Create a longitudinal incision in the laryngeal skeleton.
- Distract the edges of the incision to increase the diameter of the airway.
- Insert a graft to maintain the distraction and to achieve an airtight seal.
- Stabilize the graft until it heals.

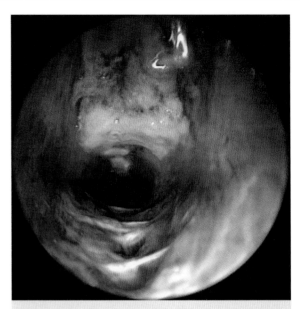

Fig. 22.15 An anterior costal cartilage graft, 7 days postoperative.

Single-Stage versus Two-Stage Reconstruction ⓘ

The term single-stage is used to describe a procedure in which the child is left without a tracheostomy at the end of the procedure. In a two-stage procedure, the child retains a tracheostomy temporarily after the first procedure, to then have it removed at a second stage. The graft is supported by a stent which is fixed into the subglottic lumen until it is removed at the second stage. In the single-stage procedure, the graft is supported in place by the presence of an ET tube, which is generally left in situ with the child intubated for 5 to 10 days after the procedure. Comparison of the relative merits of the two techniques is difficult as randomized trials are unfeasible, but most surgeons, and most parents, would prefer a single-stage technique where possible. The two-stage technique is best in children with poor respiratory function or in particularly severe and complex surgical cases where the risk of failure to extubate is significant. The single-stage technique also requires the use of a fully staffed PICU with the facility to ventilate patients for prolonged periods. The two-stage technique potentially allows reconstruction to be undertaken without PICU and may be safer in many health care settings depending on local facilities.

Single-Stage Laryngotracheal Reconstruction

This approach is similar to the cricoid split, with a vertical slit from the lower third of the cricoid cartilage, through the junction of the lamina of the thyroid cartilage in the midline and continuing through the upper two tracheal rings.[39] If this incision alone allows sufficient distraction of the cricoid ring to allow an age-appropriate tube into the lumen, then only an anterior graft will be needed (▶ Fig. 22.15). If more distraction than can be provided by an anterior split alone is required, then a posterior split is indicated. Access to the posterior split may require a complete anterior laryngofissure with division of the anterior commissure. This is a much more invasive approach with separation of the cords and a risk of long-term impairment of voice. The posterior lamina of the cricoid directly overlies the esophagus, and there is a risk of perforation. The recurrent laryngeal nerves lie behind the posterior lamina and are also at risk particularly if there if much dissection laterally behind the cartilage.

In most cases, the surgeon will have decided in advance if a posterior graft is necessary based on endoscopic findings (▶ Fig. 22.16).

Graft Material and Shape

Although thyroid alar cartilage and auricular cartilage are potential sources of grafts for small midline splits, the most widely used material is costal cartilage, which is easily harvested from the medial ends of the seventh and eighth ribs on the anterior chest wall. The right side is preferred to avoid the pericardium on the left. Costal cartilage can be harvested in large quantities and provides a thick piece of cartilage, which can be carved into shape to

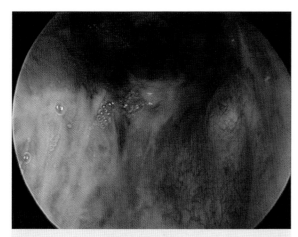

Fig. 22.16 A posterior graft.

fit the defect. Most surgeons try to preserve the perichondrium on the side of the graft used on the intraluminal surface as the perichondrium allows more rapid epithelialization than bare cartilage.

The anterior graft may be carved in a variety of shapes to fit securely into the laryngofissure. It is the authors' preference to carve a mortice cross-section (► Fig. 22.17), which stops the graft prolapsing into the lumen. The graft is secured with slow absorbing monofilament sutures (e.g., 4–0 PDS [Ethicon]) and an attempt is made to ensure the graft is airtight to improve wound healing and to reduce the risk of infection. As the wound is potentially not clean and the graft is not vascularized, the authors use prophylactic antibiotics.

The posterior graft is technically more challenging. The edges of the posterior cricoid split are harder to distract because of muscle attachment, and it is impossible to suture the graft into place without leaving suture ends in the lumen, which increases the risk of granulations and airway obstruction. It is possible to carve the graft with small flanges so that it can retain its position in the cricoid without suture, but the required dissection behind the cricoid plate can risk injury to the recurrent laryngeal nerves.

Two-Stage Laryngotracheal Reconstruction (Stenting)

In the two-stage approach, a stent is used to support the grafts until they heal into the surrounding tissue. The ideal stent needs to be the right size and shape to fit the airway, made of relatively inert material so that it does not promote granulations, and compatible with a tracheostomy tube. Commercial stents are available, but one can easily be fashioned from an ET tube.

Where the expansion and graft involves the glottis as well as subglottis, the stent will need to extend through the vocal cords, but if the expansion is limited to the subglottis, it is best to fix the stent below the level of the cords to avoid injury to the glottis.

Most stents are fixed in place with a suture that is removed at the second-stage procedure, although more specialized stents such as the Montgomery T-tube (► Fig. 22.18) may need to be removed quickly in the event of tube obstruction and are left unfixed. It is not uncommon to encounter significant granulations around the stent and they need to be removed or allowed to settle before decannulation.

Cricotracheal Resection

Decannulation rates after traditional LTR are much lower in severe stenosis (grades 3 and 4). When a very small (grade 3) or occluded (grade 4) lumen is expanded to the size of an age-appropriate subglottis, the graft takes up a

22

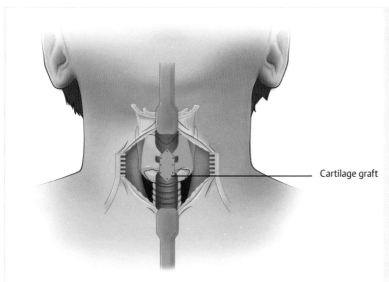

Fig. 22.17 Laryngotracheal reconstruction.

Cartilage graft

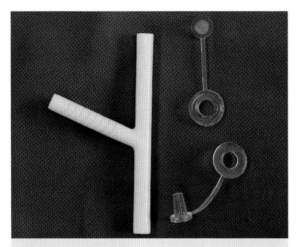

Fig. 22.18 Three-limbed Montgomery T-tube with washers and cap. The washer attaches to the ribbed limb of the tube preventing inward displacement and the cap can be used to close the lumen.

This approach may be considered in purely *subglottic* stenosis.

A major complication of cricotracheal resection (CTR) is the risk of anastomotic failure, with dehiscence of the tracheal segment from the thyroid cartilage. Some surgeons place sutures between the chin and sternum to prevent neck extension in in the early postoperative period to lessen this risk. CTR may be done as a two-stage procedure with a stent or as a single-stage procedure with postoperative intubation for 7 to 10 days.

CTR is technically challenging and is really only available in highly specialized centers (▶ Fig. 22.19).

large fraction of the lumen. The resulting slow healing and epithelialization creates a tendency for significant granulation and rescarring.

Monnier in Lausanne described and popularized a technique whereby the cricoid ring containing much of the stenosis is excised leaving only the posterior lamina of the cricoid with its overlying mucosa.[40,41] The free edge of the trachea is then anastomosed to the lower edge of the thyroid cartilage. To reduce tension on the anastomosis, the larynx needs to be mobilized from above by releasing the strap muscles superior to the hyoid (suprahyoid release) and below by dissecting the upper trachea away from the esophagus. There is a risk of injury to the esophagus and the recurrent laryngeal nerves.

22.4 Acquired Disorders of the Vocal Fold

22.4.1 Vocal Cord Palsy

Cord palsies in children may be congenital (see Chapter 21), but acquired cases, typically iatrogenic, are seen, especially after thoracotomy. The left recurrent laryngeal nerve is at greater risk, particularly with surgery around the aortic arch (e.g., closure of patent ductus arteriosus, correction of double aortic arch).

Presentation may be with airway obstruction or an abnormal cry. A temporary paresis due to transient

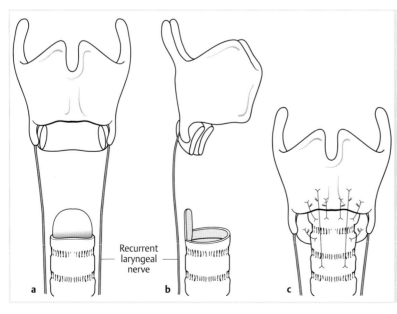

Recurrent laryngeal nerve

a   b   c

Fig. 22.19 Cricotracheal resection. **(a,b)** After resection of the narrowed tracheal segment, the pedicled membranous posterior flap of the trachea is identified. **(c)** Anterior thyrotracheal and lateral cricotracheal anastomosis. (Reproduced from Theissing J, Werner J, Rettinger G. ENT-Head and Neck Surgery: Essential Procedures. Thieme; 2011, with permission.)

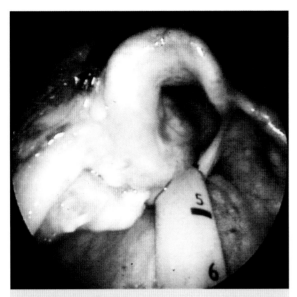

Fig. 22.20 B-cell lymphoma of the larynx in a child.

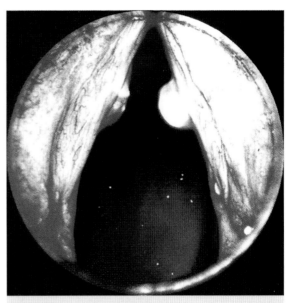

Fig. 22.21 Vocal cord nodules.

pressure on the nerve (neurapraxia), often for as long as 3 to 6 months, is far more common than the more serious transection of the nerve (neurotmesis), and in most cases, expectant treatment is appropriate. Aspiration may complicate the clinical picture.

The airway obstruction rarely warrants a tracheostomy, except in the very unusual case of a bilateral palsy. In older children with voice issues, speech and language therapy or injection of a bulking agent (calcium hydroxyl apatite) to the affected cord may be considered.

As in adults, a cord palsy can arise due to a lesion in or adjacent to the recurrent laryngeal nerve anywhere in its course from the brainstem through the skull base, the neck, and, in the case of the left nerve, the mediastinum, and the child will need to be investigated accordingly. Bilateral cord palsy is rare but can complicate some viral infections and may cause severe airway obstruction.

22.4.2 Mucosal Lesions of the Vocal Folds

These are often the result of endotracheal intubation trauma (see below), but cysts, polyps, and very rarely true neoplasms do occur in the pediatric larynx (▶ Fig. 22.20). Hoarseness needs to be thoroughly investigated, making sure you get a good view of the larynx even if this means general anesthesia. Vocal cord nodules are not uncommon in children (▶ Fig. 22.21). The etiology is similar to adults, and treatment is conservative.

22.5 Key Points

- Epiglottitis is now rare, but sporadic cases can occur. Stay vigilant.
- "Croup" or ALTB is common and usually responds to steroids.
- Bacterial tracheitis remains a serious condition with the potential to require PICU admission.
- RRP is caused by HPV and may require multiple surgical treatments.
- RRP may become very rare as the effects of HPV vaccination become apparent.
- Subglottic stenosis has reduced greatly in incidence as neonatal airway care has improved.
- Laryngotracheal injury and stenosis is now mainly iatrogenic.
- The management of laryngotracheal stenosis is now concentrated in specialist centers.
- LTR will in many cases avoid the need for tracheostomy.
- A small number of children are suitable for CTR.
- Acquired vocal cord palsy in children is often a complication of thoracotomy and is usually temporary.

References

[1] Wilson TG. Diseases of the Ear, Nose and Throat in Children. London: William Heinemann; 1955
[2] Carter P, Benjamin B. Ten-year review of pediatric tracheotomy. Ann Otol Rhinol Laryngol. 1983; 92(4 Pt 1):398–400
[3] Sobol SE, Zapata S. Epiglottitis and croup. Otolaryngol Clin North Am. 2008; 41(3):551–566, ix

[4] Tibballs J, Watson T. Symptoms and signs differentiating croup and epiglottitis. J Paediatr Child Health. 2011; 47(3):77–82

[5] McEwan J, Giridharan W, Clarke RW, Shears P. Paediatric acute epiglottitis: not a disappearing entity. Int J Pediatr Otorhinolaryngol. 2003; 67(4):317–321

[6] Acevedo JL, Lander L, Choi S, Shah RK. Airway management in pediatric epiglottitis: a national perspective. Otolaryngol Head Neck Surg. 2009; 140(4):548–551

[7] Fernandes RM, Oleszczuk M, Woods CR, Rowe BH, Cates CJ, Hartling L. The Cochrane Library and safety of systemic corticosteroids for acute respiratory conditions in children: an overview of reviews. Evid Based Child Health. 2014; 9(3):733–747

[8] Tebruegge M, Pantazidou A, Thorburn K, et al. Bacterial tracheitis: a multi-centre perspective. Scand J Infect Dis. 2009; 41(8):548–557

[9] Tan AK, Manoukian JJ. Hospitalized croup (bacterial and viral): the role of rigid endoscopy. J Otolaryngol. 1992; 21(1):48–53

[10] Hopkins A, Lahiri T, Salerno R, Heath B. Changing epidemiology of life-threatening upper airway infections: the reemergence of bacterial tracheitis. Pediatrics. 2006; 118(4):1418–1421

[11] Kuo CY, Parikh SR. Bacterial tracheitis. Pediatr Rev. 2014; 35(11):497–499

[12] Skjeldestad FE, Mehta V, Sings HL, et al. Seroprevalence and genital DNA prevalence of HPV types 6, 11, 16 and 18 in a cohort of young Norwegian women: study design and cohort characteristics. Acta Obstet Gynecol Scand. 2008; 87(1):81–88

[13] Tasca RA, Clarke RW. Recurrent respiratory papillomatosis. Arch Dis Child. 2006; 91(8):689–691

[14] Donne AJ, Clarke R. Recurrent respiratory papillomatosis: an uncommon but potentially devastating effect of human papillomavirus in children. Int J STD AIDS. 2010; 21(6):381–385

[15] Koutsky LA, Ault KA, Wheeler CM, et al. Proof of Principle Study Investigators. A controlled trial of a human papillomavirus type 16 vaccine. N Engl J Med. 2002; 347(21):1645–1651

[16] McMurray JS, Connor N, Ford CN. Cidofovir efficacy in recurrent respiratory papillomatosis: a randomized, double-blind, placebo-controlled study. Ann Otol Rhinol Laryngol. 2008; 117(7):477–483

[17] Peyton Shirley W, Wiatrak B. Is cidofovir a useful adjunctive therapy for recurrent respiratory papillomatosis in children? Int J Pediatr Otorhinolaryngol. 2004; 68(4):413–418

[18] Donne AJ, Rothera MP, Homer JJ. Scientific and clinical aspects of the use of cidofovir in recurrent respiratory papillomatosis. Int J Pediatr Otorhinolaryngol. 2008; 72(7):939–944

[19] San Giorgi MR, Tjon Pian Gi RE, Dikkers FG. The clinical course of recurrent respiratory papillomatosis after the use of cidofovir is influenced by multiple factors. Eur Arch Otorhinolaryngol. 2015; 272 (7):1819–1820

[20] Pawlita M, Gissmann L. Recurrent respiratory papillomatosis: indication for HPV vaccination? [in German]. Dtsch Med Wochenschr. 2009; 134 Suppl 2:S100–S102

[21] Young DL, Moore MM, Halstead LA. The use of the quadrivalent human papillomavirus vaccine (gardasil) as adjuvant therapy in the treatment of recurrent respiratory papilloma. J Voice. 2015; 29(2):223–229

[22] Silverberg MJ, Thorsen P, Lindeberg H, Ahdieh-Grant L, Shah KV. Clinical course of recurrent respiratory papillomatosis in Danish children. Arch Otolaryngol Head Neck Surg. 2004; 130(6):711–716

[23] Mullen S, Maney J, Casey C. Sweet on the outside but not on the inside -liquitab injuries in a tertiary paediatric emergency department (PED). Emerg Med J. 2015; 32:1009

[24] Wootten CT, Bromwich MA, Myer CM, III. Trends in blunt laryngotracheal trauma in children. Int J Pediatr Otorhinolaryngol. 2009; 73(8):1071–1075

[25] Fuhrman GM, Stieg FH, III, Buerk CA. Blunt laryngeal trauma: classification and management protocol. J Trauma. 1990; 30(1):87–92

[26] Merritt RM, Bent JP, Porubsky ES. Acute laryngeal trauma in the pediatric patient. Ann Otol Rhinol Laryngol. 1998; 107(2):104–106

[27] Schott SR. Laryngeal trauma. In: Myer CM, Cotton RT, Schott SR, eds. The Pediatric Airway. Philadelphia, PA: Lippincott Williams and Wilkins; 1994

[28] Schaefer SD. Management of acute blunt and penetrating external laryngeal trauma. Laryngoscope. 2014; 124(1):233–244

[29] Sittel C. Paediatric laryngotracheal stenosis [in German]. Laryngorhinootologie. 2012; 91(8):478–485

[30] Myer CM, III, O'Connor DM, Cotton RT. Proposed grading system for subglottic stenosis based on endotracheal tube sizes. Ann Otol Rhinol Laryngol. 1994; 103(4 Pt 1):319–323

[31] McCaffrey TV. Classification of laryngotracheal stenosis. Laryngoscope. 1992; 102(12 Pt 1):1335–1340

[32] Maronian NC, Azadeh H, Waugh P, Hillel A. Association of laryngopharyngeal reflux disease and subglottic stenosis. Ann Otol Rhinol Laryngol. 2001; 110(7 Pt 1):606–612

[33] Hartnick CJ, Hartley BE, Lacy PD, et al. Topical mitomycin application after laryngotracheal reconstruction: a randomized, double-blind, placebo-controlled trial. Arch Otolaryngol Head Neck Surg. 2001; 127 (10):1260–1264

[34] Warner D, Brietzke SE. Mitomycin C and airway surgery: how well does it work? Otolaryngol Head Neck Surg. 2008; 138(6):700–709

[35] Lang M, Brietzke SE. A systematic review and meta-analysis of endoscopic balloon dilation of pediatric subglottic stenosis. Otolaryngol Head Neck Surg. 2014; 150(2):174–179

[36] Wentzel JL, Ahmad SM, Discolo CM, Gillespie MB, Dobbie AM. White DR. Balloon laryngoplasty for pediatric laryngeal stenosis: case series and systematic review. Laryngoscope. 2014; 124(7):1707–1712

[37] Horn DL, Maguire RC, Simons JP, Mehta DK. Endoscopic anterior cricoid split with balloon dilation in infants with failed extubation. Laryngoscope. 2012; 122(1):216–219

[38] Cotton RT, Seid AB. Management of the extubation problem in the premature child. Anterior cricoid split as an alternative to tracheotomy. Ann Otol Rhinol Laryngol. 1980; 89(6 Pt 1):508–511

[39] Boardman SJ, Albert DM. Single-stage and multistage pediatric laryngotracheal reconstruction. Otolaryngol Clin North Am. 2008; 41 (5):947–958, ix

[40] Hartley BE, Cotton RT. Paediatric airway stenosis: laryngotracheal reconstruction or cricotracheal resection? Clin Otolaryngol Allied Sci. 2000; 25(5):342–349

[41] Yamamoto K, Jaquet Y, Ikonomidis C, Monnier P. Partial cricotracheal resection for paediatric subglottic stenosis: update of the Lausanne experience with 129 cases. Eur J Cardiothorac Surg. 2015; 47(5):876–882

23 Tracheostomy

R. W. Clarke

23.1 Introduction

Tracheotomy refers to an opening in the trachea to facilitate air entry. As the tracheal incision heals and becomes continuous with the surrounding tissues, it forms a stoma, *tracheostomy.* The operation has been in use throughout the history of medicine for the relief of airway obstruction by bypassing the upper airway. It is an important and often lifesaving measure in children.

Expertise in pediatric tracheostomy management now tends to be concentrated in specialist pediatric centers. Many children with tracheostomies are cared for at home by parents with the support of community health care professionals in the expectation that once the primary condition that necessitated a tracheostomy is resolved, the child's airway can be managed without a tracheostomy–*decannulation.*

As techniques for airway management have improved in recent decades, the need for tracheostomy has declined and the indications have changed.[1]

23.2 Indications

Tracheostomy is used to bypass an obstructed airway (▶ Fig. 23.1; ▶ Table 23.1 a). It reduces the respiratory "dead space" and permits easier instrumentation, including suctioning, of the tracheobronchial tree. It obviates the need for prolonged endotracheal (ET) intubation and facilitates respiratory ventilation (▶ Table 23.1 b) in ventilated patients. Home ventilation is now frequently used in children with conditions that in the past would not have been treated or would have meant long-term inpatient care (▶ Table 23.1 b,c) and is an increasingly common indication for tracheostomy.

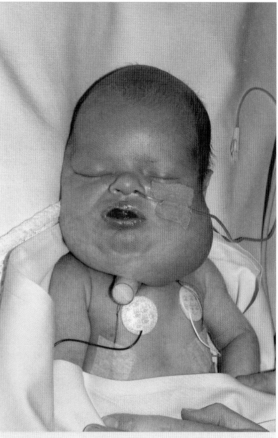

Fig. 23.1 Tracheostomy in a child with a large lymphangioma of the head and neck, extending into the tongue and obstructing the airway.

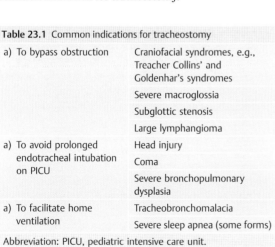

Table 23.1 Common indications for tracheostomy

a) To bypass obstruction	Craniofacial syndromes, e.g., Treacher Collins' and Goldenhar's syndromes
	Severe macroglossia
	Subglottic stenosis
	Large lymphangioma
a) To avoid prolonged endotracheal intubation on PICU	Head injury
	Coma
	Severe bronchopulmonary dysplasia
a) To facilitate home ventilation	Tracheobronchomalacia
	Severe sleep apnea (some forms)

Abbreviation: PICU, pediatric intensive care unit.

23.3 Emergency Tracheotomy

An emergency opening into the trachea can save a child who presents with complete or near-complete upper airway obstruction. This was a frequent occurrence in the preantibiotic era when diphtheria and epiglottitis were commonplace and steroids were not widely used in the management of acute laryngotracheobronchitis (ALTB) or "croup." Pediatricians and anesthesiologists were less skilled at managing ET intubation in the very young. A tracheotomy "in extremis" is now a very rare procedure, and a scheduled operation under optimum conditions with skilled pediatric anesthesia is much to be preferred.

23

> A child can nearly always be managed by airway supportive measures such as "bag and mask" or by ET intubation prior to a planned tracheostomy.

In a desperate situation, you can make an opening into the trachea using a large bore needle to puncture the cricothyroid membrane (cricothyroidotomy; see ▶ Fig. 20.3).

23.4 Preoperative Planning

Traditional advice has been that tracheostomy is preferable to "prolonged" intubation, that is, use of an ET tube for more than a few weeks. With modern-day ET tubes causing much less tissue trauma and with improved neonatal care and better overall management of very sick children, particularly premature neonates, ET intubation can now be prolonged often for several weeks before a tracheostomy is needed. Tracheostomy is typically considered when it becomes clear that a child who is being managed by ET intubation is unlikely to cope without some form of airway support. Often one or more attempts will have been made at extubation.

The parents or carers of a child needing a tracheostomy, and in the case of the older child the child him/herself, will need careful and detailed preoperative counseling.[2] In addition to an explanation of the condition and its natural history, with and without a tracheostomy, they should be aware of the possible complications and of the postoperative concerns as detailed in the next section. The child will initially be unable to vocalize, including crying, a prospect parents often find very distressing.[3,4] If home care of the child is planned, then the parents should be trained in how to change the tube, how to suction the trachea, how to ensure optimum humidification, and in basic resuscitation techniques. It can be useful to show them a variety of tracheostomy tubes, introducers and suction equipment using a teaching doll or mannequin (see below) prior to surgery.

23.5 Special Considerations in Children

The principles that govern tracheostomy apply to both adults and children, but there are some factors that make pediatric tracheostomy very different. The child has a short fat neck, and the surgical landmarks may be very close together. The trachea is much softer and less well anchored than in an adult and easily rolls away to one side when palpated. This, coupled with its small caliber and its proximity to surrounding structures such as the carotid sheath, can make the trachea difficult to identify, particularly if the surgeon is inexperienced or if there is

no ET tube in place. The small caliber of the trachea means that only a small diameter tube can be used. Pediatric tubes are typically single, that is, there is no "inner" and "outer" tube as in adults as this would reduce lumen of the tube. There is rarely room to accommodate a cuff, so pediatric tracheostomy tubes are generally uncuffed except for in the older child.

> Children are inclined to produce brisk inflammatory responses to foreign bodies (i.e., a tracheostomy tube). Peristomal granulations and granulation tissue at the site of the lower end of the tube where it abuts the tracheal wall are common and can give rise to bleeding and obstruction.

For this reason, fenestrated tubes are almost never used in children—the fenestra is liable to become blocked by inflammatory tissue.

Some technical issues of particular importance in children are discussed next, for example, the need to be extra cautious to avoid the possibility of tracheal stenosis by avoiding the removal of any cartilage and the need to ensure that there is a good gap between the end of the tube and the carina given the very short length of the trachea especially in the newborn.

23.6 Technique

The operation is almost invariably carried out under general anesthesia, often, but not always, with an ET tube in position.

- Position the child with the head stabilized in a rubber head ring and use a small shoulder roll to lift the upper chest. A standard sandbag is good for older children, but in babies, a rolled up draping towel placed under the shoulders is gentler. Be careful not to overextend the head or to use too bulky a shoulder support as otherwise the thoracic vessels, particularly the brachiocephalic vein, may be pulled into the neck where they are at risk during dissection. An adhesive tape under the child's chin and extending on either side to the head of the table helps to keep overhanging skin and soft tissue away and makes for an easier approach to the neck, particularly if the baby is a little "pudgy."
- Once the skin is prepared with a disinfectant and the child is draped, identify the landmarks: suprasternal notch, the trachea, the cricoid and thyroid cartilages, and the tracheal rings, and mark the site of incision halfway between the suprasternal notch and the cricoid.
- An injection of local anesthetic and a vasoconstrictor (the author uses "Lignospan" [Septodont] cartridges, which contain lidocaine and epinephrine) helps minimize bleeding.

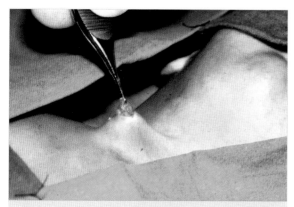

Fig. 23.2 Removing subcutaneous fat.

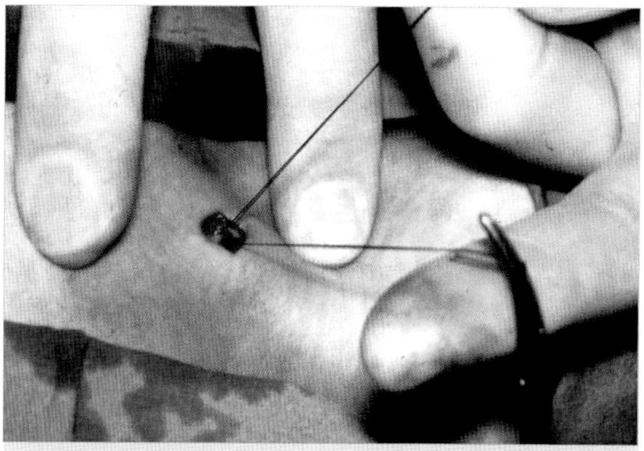

Fig. 23.3 Stay sutures help to open the trachea to facilitate insertion of the tube.

- Make a transverse skin incision and secure hemostasis with precise bipolar diathermy, tying the anterior jugular veins if they are bulky and get in the way. A little subcutaneous fat is inclined to prolapse through the skin wound and can be removed to facilitate access to the deeper structures (▶ Fig. 23.2).
- Incise the platysma. Separate and move the strap muscles laterally to expose the pretracheal fascia. If the thyroid isthmus is bulky and obscuring a good view of the trachea, it can be divided using monopolar diathermy but more often than not it can be left intact.
- Clean away the pretracheal fascia to expose the tracheal rings, making *absolutely certain* that you have identified the trachea to your own satisfaction and that of your assistant. There is rarely a need for extensive opening up of tissue planes, and if you confine your dissection as close as possible to the midline, the risk of trauma to adjacent structures, and the risk of troublesome bleeding, is minimized.
- If the child is intubated, you will feel the ET tube, which you can roll between finger and thumb. Count the tracheal rings up to the cricoid and prepare to incise the trachea vertically exactly in the midline between the second and fourth tracheal rings.
- Now place two stay sutures in the trachea, one on each side of the midline, and secure them with a knot well away from the trachea so they are easy to remove postoperatively. Make sure they are securely anchored in the tracheal cartilage as they can easily pull out if they are tentatively placed in the fascia.
- Liaise carefully with the anesthetist so that he/she knows you are about to open the airway.
- Check the tracheotomy tube. Make sure it is patent and that the introducer slides easily in and out as you can very occasionally get a poorly fitting introducer or a defective tube. A little lubricant jelly on the tip of the introducer helps to get it into position.
- Now ask your assistant to use the stay sutures to gently elevate the trachea and stabilize it as you incise it (▶ Fig. 23.3). Make your incision and extend it upward, staying well below the first tracheal ring.
- Now insert and position the tracheostomy tube as the anesthetist gradually withdraws the ET tube.
- The breathing circuit is now quickly attached to the tracheostomy tube and assuming the tube is correctly positioned, the anesthetist will soon detect carbon dioxide in the exhaled gases and both lungs will be easily ventilated.
- Many surgeons now recommend that the cut edges of the tracheal wall be sutured to the skin edge (maturation sutures) to make for easier tube replacement and to facilitate the development of a stoma.[5]
- Before securing the flanges, it is the author's practice to check the position of the lower end of the tube using a flexible endoscope, measuring first the distance from the upper opening of the tube to the carina and then withdrawing the endoscope to exactly the lower end of the tube and ensuring that this end is at least one centimeter above the carina, otherwise the tube is too long and may slip down into a bronchus, causing difficulty with ventilation of one lung in the postoperative period.
- Place the free ends of the stay sutures on the child's chest wall, taping them in place. Some units prefer to label them "right" and "left" to avoid the confusion that can arise in a fraught situation where the stay sutures need to be used to help open the stoma for rapid tube replacement.
- Now position the tapes around the child's neck so as to leave a good finger's width between the tape and the neck (▶ Fig. 23.4). Some units recommend suturing the flanges to the skin for extra security.

23

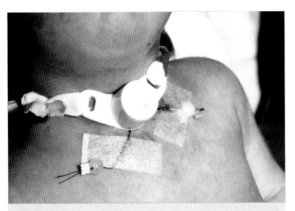

Fig. 23.4 Tracheostomy tube in position with tapes secured.

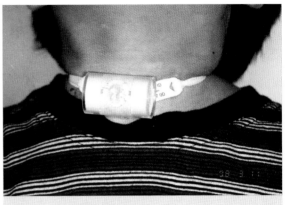

Fig. 23.5 A tracheal mask or a "Swedish nose."

23.7 Postoperative Care

> ℹ️
>
> Health care staff that look after a child in the early post-operative period need to be aware of the risk of the tube becoming obstructed or dislodged.

The tube can slip out of the airway or become blocked by secretions or clotted blood. It is important that the team handing over care from the operating room to the post-operative ward (typically the pediatric intensive care unit [PICU]) inform the staff clearly what was done.

> ℹ️
>
> Management protocols vary but the important thing is to have a routine and that staff become familiar with it.[6,7]

Point out that the stay sutures are anchored into the tracheal wall on either side and may be gently pulled to the sides to open the trachea and facilitate replacement of the tube. Some centers will do a routine chest X-ray to confirm the position of the tube and to check for a pneumothorax.

Regular gentle suction and humidification are essential, otherwise secretions will build up and may dry out forming a cast in the tube lumen. A nebulizer is a good way to administer humidification, as is a tracheal mask or a "Swedish nose" (▶ Fig. 23.5). This latter is an attachment containing a filter that becomes saturated, thus moistening inhaled air. A few drops of warm sterile saline applied directly into the stoma followed by gentle and controlled suction can help loosen secretions.

In our unit, the child is looked after on the PICU for the first 24 hours and then transferred to a ward where the staff have had specific training in tracheostomy care. It is especially important that front-line staff know what to do in the event of tube blockage or accidental decannulation. Some units have a bedside notice (▶ Fig. 23.6, ▶ Fig. 23.7). Arrangements for the first tube change vary; what is important is that an agreed protocol is established and agreed well in advance.[6,8] In the author's unit, the first tube change is planned for 5 days after surgery and is undertaken by a senior ear, nose, and throat surgeon with an anesthetist or a pediatric intensive care physician available. The stay sutures can now be removed.

23.8 Complications

Pediatric tracheostomy under controlled conditions with an appropriately trained surgeon, anesthetist, and nursing team is a safe operation, but is important to be aware of potential complications (▶ Table 23.2) and to know how to deal with them. Operative complications include profuse bleeding, acute airway obstruction, and trauma to adjacent structures, for example, a pneumothorax. A small pneumothorax can be managed expectantly but a large one may warrant a chest drain.

Airway obstruction is an ever-present risk during and after surgery. Vigilance in the early postoperative period is especially important when the risk of the tube slipping out of the trachea, or getting blocked by dried secretions or blood clot, is greatest. Air can enter the tissues of the neck or even the mediastinum (surgical emphysema or pneumomediastinum) especially if the wound is sutured tightly or dressings are too firmly applied, in which case they need to be loosened.

Persistent bleeding may be from the skin edges, the anterior jugular veins, or the parenchyma of the thyroid gland, and will usually settle. Occasionally, you may need to pack or reexplore the wound.

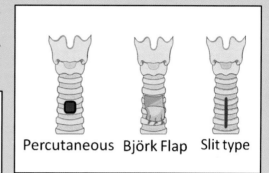

This patient has a

TRACHEOSTOMY

There is a potentially patent upper airway (Intubation may be difficult)

Surgical / Percutaneous

Performed on (date) ....

Tracheostomy tube size (if present) ....

Hospital / NHS number ....

Notes: Indicate tracheostomy type by circling the relevant figure.
Indicate location and function of any sutures.
Laryngoscopy grade and notes on upper airway management.
Any problems with this tracheostomy.

Percutaneous   Björk Flap   Slit type

| **Emergency Call:** | Anaesthesia | ICU | ENT | MaxFax | Emergency Team |

www.tracheostomy.org.uk

Fig. 23.6 Bedside notice for adult and pediatric tracheostomies. Please note that percutaneous and Björk flaps are not used in children. (Reproduced from McGrath BA, Bates L, Atkinson D, Moore JA. Multidisciplinary guidelines for the management of tracheostomy and laryngectomy airway emergencies. Anaesthesia. 2012;67(9):1025–1041, with permission from the Association of Anaesthetists of Great Britain & Ireland/Blackwell Publishing Ltd.)

> Erosion of the brachiocephalic vessels can cause a catastrophic bleed.

Torrential bleeding due to erosion of the brachiocephalic artery is a rare but catastrophic complication of tracheostomy.[9] The brachiocephalic (innominate) artery crosses the trachea, and if unusually high, it can lie very close to the tracheotomy site. If this situation is encountered at surgery, it is best to open the trachea a little higher than usual, accepting the slightly higher risk of tracheal stenosis, so that the tube is well away from the artery, reducing the potential for erosion of the vessel. A tracheal innominate fistula is rare but may be fatal.[9]

The skin around the stoma can become inflamed and excoriated, and good nursing care with close attention to the stoma will go a long way to alleviating conditions such as eczema and wound breakdown.

Stomal problems include granulations due to an inflammatory reaction to the tube. This can be made worse by a poorly fitting tube "chafing" the skin or by repeated traumatic tube changes. The child's tracheal mucosa is inclined to produce a brisk inflammatory response to a foreign body, such as a tracheostomy tube, and a mass of granulation tissue, often incorrectly called a "granuloma," can develop typically just above the tube (suprastomal granulation; ▶ Fig. 23.8) or at the lower end of the tube where the free end of the lumen is in contact with the anterior tracheal wall. Granulations sometimes need to be cauterized or removed. Cicatrization of the stoma can cause it to close down, often over a period of a few hours so that tube replacement can be very difficult.

Long-term complications include the ever-present risks of airway obstruction due to accidental decannulation or tubal blockage. The risk is difficult to quantify, but all of the large series that have followed children up for several years report a small but acknowledged fatality rate of the order of 2%.[1]

Some of the long-term complications only become apparent when the child is considered for decannulation. The tracheal wall above the stoma can become soft, prolapsing into the lumen (suprastomal collapse; ▶ Fig. 23.9).

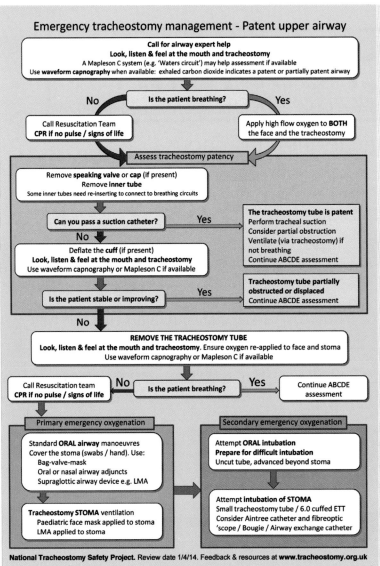

Fig. 23.7 Algorithm for managing a tracheostomy emergency. (Reproduced from McGrath BA, Bates L, Atkinson D, Moore JA. Multidisciplinary guidelines for the management of tracheostomy and laryngectomy airway emergencies. Anaesthesia. 2012;67(9):1025–1041, with permission from the Association of Anaesthetists of Great Britain & Ireland/ Blackwell Publishing Ltd.)

Table 23.2 Complications of tracheostomy

Immediate	Trauma to adjacent structures, e.g., pneumothorax
	Bleeding
	Injury to recurrent laryngeal nerves
Early	Accidental decannulation
	Blocked tube
	Surgical emphysema
	Bleeding
Late	Accidental decannulation
	Blocked tube
	Granulations: stomal, suprastomal, and tracheal
	Suprastomal collapse
	Tracheoinnominate fistula
	Tracheocutaneous fistula

Tracheal stenosis is rare nowadays. Surgeons are better trained to appreciate the importance of avoiding trauma to the cricoid cartilage and the first tracheal ring, and modern-day tubes are made of lighter and less irritant material (e.g., lightweight plastic or silicone rather than "red rubber") than was the case with older tubes.

> A persistent tracheocutaneous fistula is fairly common and may need surgical correction.

A tracheostomy inevitably disturbs the delicate mechanisms whereby the airway closes off during deglutition and some effect on swallowing and aspiration is common, although often the effects are surprisingly minor and of little clinical significance.

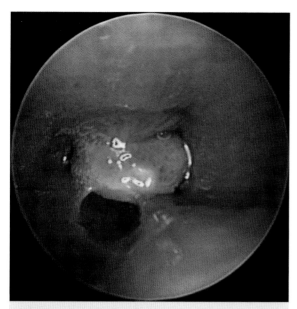

Fig. 23.8 Suprastomal granulation.

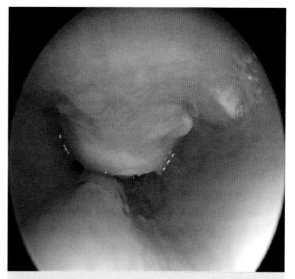

Fig. 23.9 Suprastomal collapse of the anterior tracheal wall obstructing the airway.

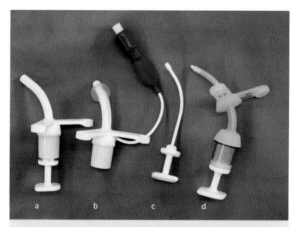

Fig. 23.10 A variety of tracheostomy tubes. **(a)** A standard "cuffless" tube with the introducer in position. **(b)** A cuffed tube, the cuff inflated. **(c)** The introducer for **(b)**. **(d)** An adjustable (flexible) flanged tube with introducer.

> A tracheostomy is a major life-changing event for a child and the family; the long-term psychosocial consequences, including the effect on voice, must not be forgotten.

23.9 Tracheostomy Tubes

The huge variety of tracheostomy tubes in the marketplace is a testimony to the fact that no tube is perfect.

The ideal tube should be light, flexible, easy to insert and remove, easy to clean, and made of material that neither harbors infection nor encourages a tissue foreign body reaction. Silicon and silastic are commonly used nowadays in preference to the older metal and rubber tubes. The material is light but strong, so a small thickness of the tube wall leaves room for a larger lumen, important in very small babies, and the flanges cause minimal chaffing to the skin of the neck. ▶ Fig. 23.10 shows a variety of tracheostomy tubes.

Consider both the diameter and the length when selecting a tube. In general, the wider the tube bore the better; a narrow tube is more likely to become blocked by secretions, but avoid a too snug fit as this may make tube change difficult and in extreme cases can cause mucosal ischemia. The child will need regular monitoring so the tube can be "upsized" as he/she grows.

> The tube should be long enough to sit well in the stoma so that it does not pop out, with the distal end a good 2 to 3 cm below the tracheotomy. It also needs to be 1 to 2 cm high of the carina so that it does not slip into a main stem bronchus, causing ventilation of just one lung.

This can be checked by a chest X-ray or by flexible tracheobronchoscopy.

Most manufacturers make tubes in "neonatal" or "pediatric" (longer) lengths. As a general rule, the "size" of the tube is the diameter in millimeters of the internal lumen, that is, a size 3.5 tube has an internal diameter of 3.5 mm, but this varies with manufacturers and tube types and is not absolute. Outer diameters and lengths also vary with different manufacturers and tube types. The measurements are usually clearly marked on the flanges (▶ Fig. 23.10). When inserting a first tracheostomy tube, the size of the ET tube is a good guide to what will be a best fit.

>
>
> There is no substitute for carefully selecting both the diameter and length based on the individual needs of the child.

Some children are especially difficult to "size," due to, for example, having a short or a fat neck or having a steep angle at the entrance to the trachea. An adjustable flange, or in some cases a customized tube "made to measure," may be needed.

Cuffed tubes are rarely needed in children but may be useful in the older child especially if the tracheostomy is for ventilation, when higher ventilatory pressures can be maintained with an inflated cuff. A cuff can also help reduce aspiration but needs careful management as an inflated cuff can cause mucosal ischemia.

A speaking valve allows air entry on inspiration but closes off on expiration, so air is forced into the glottis to permit phonation. Speaking valves are not often needed or well tolerated in children, and simply "downsizing" the tube so that air can be forced upward around the tube during expiration can bring about as good a result.

> Inner tubes are rarely used in children and fenestrated tubes almost never as they promote granulation.

23.10 Home Care

Unless the child has a chronic condition that warrants prolonged inpatient care, hospital stay after tracheostomy should be minimized and the parents or carers trained to look after the child at home, with suitable support from community health care professionals. Looking after a child with a tracheostomy is challenging both for parents and for those who come in contact with the child, for example, teachers. Many schools will not accept children with tracheostomies and some will insist the child has a dedicated "one-to-one" support worker. Every professional who comes in contact with the child will need to be made aware that the child has a tracheostomy and what that means in the particular circumstances. The child will not be able to participate fully in contact sports, and swimming or any water activities are prohibited. Training

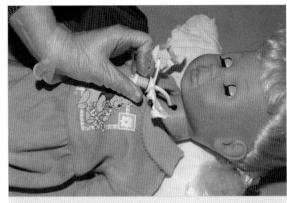

Fig. 23.11 A mannequin for teaching tracheostomy tube change to parents and carers.

commences as soon as practicable within the hospital setting and focuses on skills such as suction, provision of humidification, managing tube changes, resuscitation, and recognizing complications. Modern tubes have extended the interval between changes, and in a well-established tracheostomy, several weeks can go by between changes. A mannequin or teaching doll can be very useful (▶ Fig. 23.11).

Services and support vary greatly in different jurisdictions and between areas. Well-planned liaison between the hospital and the community teams is essential. Provision of suitable equipment, that is, suction apparatus, tubes, lubricants, tapes, dressings, and basic resuscitation equipment, is time-consuming and expensive, but not nearly as expensive as maintaining a child in hospital. There are support and advocacy groups for parents of children with tracheostomy (e.g., Association for Children with Tracheostomy in the United Kingdom) and they provide much useful information and a forum for contact between parents and carers. The equipment and support for home ventilation is even more complex, but is increasingly available.

23.11 Decannulation

A tracheostomy will be lifelong for some, but the aim for most children, as soon as the condition that necessitated tracheostomy is resolved or treated, is decannulation. Careful planning involves first a thorough assessment of the airway, including endoscopy, to confirm that the child is ready for an attempt at removing the tracheostomy tube. Suprastomal granulations (▶ Fig. 23.8) may need to be removed using laser or microdebrider. A degree of softening of the anterior tracheal wall above the stoma is inevitable in long-term tracheotomized children and will usually improve following decannulation. If it is severe, with prolapse of a segment into the lumen (suprastomal collapse; ▶ Fig. 23.9), it may warrant treatment before attempting decannulation. You may be able to excise the

V

segment, fix it to the skin of the stoma, or, in severe cases, support it with a cartilaginous graft.

Even if the child's airway is considered adequate to manage without a tube, he/she may struggle when the tube is blocked as it occupies a sizeable part of the lumen of the airway.

> ℹ A preliminary "downsize" or a series of incremental "downsizes" may help prepare for decannulation.

When the child is ready for decannulation, the parents and carers will need to be involved in a detailed discussion about the benefits and risks and are counseled carefully regarding the prospect of failure even after an initially apparent successful decannulation, with reestablishment of the tracheostomy. Many parents find the prospect of decannulation almost as alarming as they did the original operation; they are faced with the fear and worry of looking after a child whose airway has been compromised, but now without the safety of a tracheostomy tube. A specialist nurse visiting the home can support them by introducing short periods of "capping off" the tube under controlled conditions and with incremental increases in the time spent "capped." Decannulation needs to be undertaken in a safe setting, usually requiring the attention of an appropriately trained "one-to-one" nurse. Schedules and protocols vary from unit to unit and may need to be customized for the individual child and family.

Some children, for example, children with a head injury who have recovered well and needed a tracheostomy for temporary ventilation, may be best managed by immediate decannulation, that is, simply removing the tube ("cold turkey") and taping the wound in a situation where immediate resuscitation facilities are available and the tube can be speedily put back in.

23.12 Tracheocutaneous Fistula

In a long-standing tracheostomy, the track that runs from the skin to the trachea becomes lined with squamous epithelium and may remain patent after the tube is removed (▶ Fig. 23.12). This causes a troublesome mucus discharge sometimes with eczema of the skin and, of course, precludes activities such as swimming and immersion in the bathtub until the fistula is closed.

> ℹ A fistula that remains patent for 6 months following decannulation is unlikely to close spontaneously and will need surgical repair.

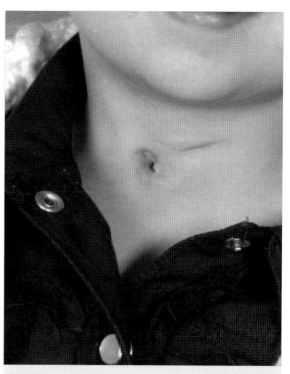

Fig. 23.12 Tracheocutaneous fistula.

It is the author's practice with persistent fistulas to check the airway endoscopically, reassess the caliber of the trachea to ensure that there is no stenosis and that there is sufficient lumen to withstand a surgical repair, deal with suprastomal granulations if need be, and then plan surgical closure.[10] The fistula is identified, dissected down to the tracheal wall, and resected with a cuff of tracheal cartilage before the cut edges are approximated and repaired. Very occasionally a cartilage graft may be needed to bolster the repair. The help of a skilled pediatric anesthesiologist is essential to ensure a smooth recovery without excessive coughing or straining as this may cause the repair to leak, giving rise to surgical emphysema. A single dose of dexamethasone helps to reduce postoperative mucosal swelling. The worst-case scenario is postoperative airway obstruction severe enough to warrant reinsertion of the tracheostomy tube, but this is happily very rare.

23.13 Key Points

- With appropriate training and support for parents and carers, most children who need a tracheostomy can be managed at home.
- Tracheostomies are now rarely needed for acute infection, for example, epiglottitis and ALTB.
- Most children can be safely intubated and ventilated for several weeks.

- Tracheostomy is very rarely needed as an emergency. Most children can be intubated, but in extreme circumstances, a cricothyroid puncture will buy time.
- Children's tracheostomy tubes are nearly always "single," that is, there is no inner tube.
- Children produce brisk inflammatory responses to tubes, causing "granulations."
- Stay in the midline when dissecting to expose the child's trachea.
- Make sure you identify the tracheal rings and stay well below the first ring when you incise the trachea.
- Beware the brachiocephalic vessels.
- Stay sutures, labeled and taped, make for safer postoperative care.
- Health care personnel looking after children with tracheostomies need appropriate training and support.
- Planned decannulation can be almost as traumatic for the parent and child as the original tracheostomy.
- Persistent tracheocutaneous fistula is common in children and may need surgical repair.

References

[1] Corbett HJ, Mann KS, Mitra I, Jesudason EC, Losty PD, Clarke RW. Tracheostomy—a 10-year experience from a UK pediatric surgical center. J Pediatr Surg. 2007; 42(7):1251–1254

[2] Callans KM, Bleiler C, Flanagan J, Carroll DL. The transitional experience of family caring for their child with a tracheostomy. J Pediatr Nurs. 2016; 31(4):397–403

[3] Flynn AP, Carter B, Bray L, Donne AJ. Parents' experiences and views of caring for a child with a tracheostomy: a literature review. Int J Pediatr Otorhinolaryngol. 2013; 77(10):1630–1634

[4] Brenner M, Larkin PJ, Hilliard C, Cawley D, Howlin F, Connolly M. Parents' perspectives of the transition to home when a child has complex technological health care needs. Int J Integr Care. 2015; 15: e035

[5] Craig MF, Bajaj Y, Hartley BE. Maturation sutures for the paediatric tracheostomy—an extra safety measure. J Laryngol Otol. 2005; 119 (12):985–987

[6] Lippert D, Hoffman MR, Dang P, McMurray JS, Heatley D, Kille T. Care of pediatric tracheostomy in the immediate postoperative period and timing of first tube change. Int J Pediatr Otorhinolaryngol. 2014; 78 (12):2281–2285

[7] eLearning for Healthcare. Tracheostomy Safety: Multidisciplinary resources for safer tracheostomy and laryngectomy care. Department of Health in association with Professional Bodies and the NHS. Available at http://www.e-lfh.org.uk/programmes/tracheostomy-safety/. Accessed February 11, 2016

[8] Website of the National Tracheostomy Safety Project. Available at http://tracheostomy.org.uk. Accessed February 11, 2016

[9] Wang XL, Xu ZG, Tang PZ, Yu Y. Tracheo-innominate artery fistula: diagnosis and surgical management. Head Neck. 2013; 35(12):1713–1718

[10] Tasca RA, Clarke RW. Tracheocutaneous fistula following paediatric tracheostomy—a 14-year experience at Alder Hey Children's Hospital. Int J Pediatr Otorhinolaryngol. 2010; 74(6):711–712

V

Part VI
Head and Neck

24 Neck Masses in Children: Congenital Neck Disease

Fiona B. MacGregor

24.1 Introduction

24.1.1 Development of the Pharyngeal Arches

In a developing embryo, the most typical features in the head and neck region are the external clefts that are part of the "branchial" or "pharyngeal" arches. The word *branchial* is derived from early observations of embryologists studying the development of the gills of fishes, and while "branchial" is still used to describe head and neck structures in humans, the terms *pharyngeal arches*, *pouches*, and *clefts* are preferred.

These rudimentary structures appear in the fourth and fifth weeks of development. Each pharyngeal arch consists of a core of mesenchyme, which is covered externally by ectoderm and internally by epithelium of endoderm origin (the primitive foregut). Each arch has its own muscular component and each of these components has their own cranial nerve supply.[1] They consist of bars of mesenchyme tissue separated by deep external clefts and internal pouches.

- The *first pharyngeal arch* includes the maxillary and mandibular processes and Meckel's cartilage, which will later form the incus and malleus. Musculature of the first arch includes the muscles of mastication, and the nerve supply is provided by the mandibular branch of the trigeminal nerve.
- The cartilage of the *second or hyoid arch* gives rise to the stapes, thyrohyoid process, and parts of the hyoid bone. The nerve of the second arch is the facial nerve.
- The *fourth and sixth pharyngeal arches* (the fifth is rudimentary) contribute to the formation of the laryngeal cartilages. The fourth arch musculature is supplied by the superior laryngeal branch, and the sixth arch by the recurrent laryngeal branch of the vagus.

> The ongoing development of the first pharyngeal pouch and cleft contributes much to the formation of the ear (▶ Fig. 24.1).

The first cleft penetrates the underlying mesenchyme and gives rise to the external auditory meatus with the lining at the bottom end of the meatus participating in the formation of the eardrum.

The mesenchyme of the second arch migrates inferiorly to overlap the third and fourth clefts. This forms a cavity

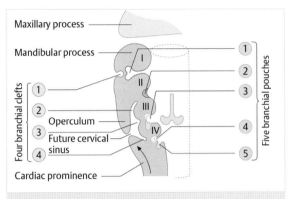

Fig. 24.1 Embryology of the pharyngeal arches.

lined with ectoderm epithelium, that is, the *cervical sinus*, which ultimately involutes.

> The second pharyngeal pouch contributes to the formation of the palatine tonsils.
>
> Epithelium from the third pouch differentiates into the inferior parathyroid gland and epithelium from the fourth pouch forms a superior parathyroid gland. Further cells from the fourth pharyngeal pouch become incorporated into the thyroid giving rise to the parafollicular or C cells that secrete calcitonin.

The thyroid gland develops at the level of the *foramen cecum* in the floor of the pharynx and subsequently descends in front of the primitive foregut as a bilobed diverticulum.

The gland reaches its final position in front of the trachea at the seventh week.

24.2 Congenital Neck Masses

Congenital neck masses in children may be apparent at birth (e.g., lymphangioma, fibromatosis colli) or may declare themselves later, for example, thyroglossal duct cysts.

24.2.1 Dermoid Cysts in the Neck

A dermoid cyst is thought to result from the inclusion of epithelial cells along the lines of embryonic closure. The resulting cyst contains ectodermal and mesodermal

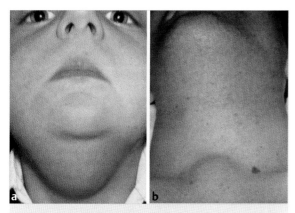

Fig. 24.2 Dermoid cyst. (Reproduced from Bull TR, Almeyda JS. Color Atlas of ENT Diagnosis (5th ed). Stuttgart, New York: Thieme; 2010, with permission.)

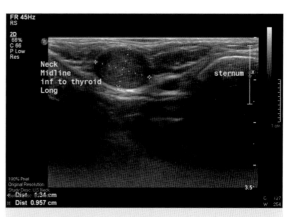

Fig. 24.3 Ultrasound of dermoid cyst.

elements and can result in the presence of hair follicles and sebaceous glands within the lesion.

Presentation

A dermoid cyst often presents in a similar fashion to a thyroglossal duct cyst with a small midline mobile smooth swelling. Infection is rare. It is often found in an inferior position in the neck to that of a thyroglossal duct cyst (▶ Fig. 24.2); it is usually more superficial and mobile and it does not move on protrusion of the tongue. In reality, it can be difficult to distinguish from a thyroglossal duct cyst.

An ultrasound scan is of limited benefit but will show the extent of the cyst and its position in relation to deeper structures (▶ Fig. 24.3). It is important to ask the radiologist to look for evidence of a connection to adjacent structures, for example, the presence of a track extending to the tongue base, as this would not be in keeping with a dermoid cyst but point to a thyroglossal duct cyst instead.

> i
>
> For aesthetic reasons, because these cysts can undergo troublesome recurrent infection and because of diagnostic uncertainty, excision is usually recommended.

Management

Surgery for a clinically obvious dermoid cyst is performed through a skin crease incision and then a simple cystectomy is carried out. If there is any doubt about the diagnosis, then it is best to assume that the lesion is a thyroglossal duct cyst and proceed accordingly (discussed next). A dermoid cyst typically contains a white cheesy material, whereas a thyroglossal duct cyst will usually yield a viscous gelatinous fluid.

24.2.2 Thyroglossal Duct Cyst

This is the most common congenital abnormality that presents in the head and neck region, making up approximately 70% of cases. Thyroglossal duct cysts occur because the duct fails to involute between the 8th week and the 10th week of gestation and a cyst can form anywhere along the duct's natural course from the foramen cecum to the thyroid gland. The majority of cysts are found in close proximity to the middle portion of the hyoid bone, and in approximately 30% of cases, a tract is found posterior to or adherent to the hyoid. Hence, resecting a segment of hyoid bone to ensure there are no cell rests left behind is important.

Presentation

A thyroglossal cyst most commonly presents in childhood with a midline lump in close proximity to the hyoid bone (▶ Fig. 24.4). It can occasionally become infected resulting in a red, painful swelling, which can discharge. Typically, the lump moves on swallowing and on protruding the tongue, but this is not always reliable.

Investigations

> i
>
> An ultrasound scan is the investigation of choice.

It is used to establish the presence of a cystic structure in the neck,[2] but also and more importantly to confirm that there is a separate and normal-looking thyroid gland present. This is important to prevent the rare possibility of inadvertent removal of an ectopic thyroid gland. In most cases, no further investigations are needed, but other imaging modalities may be helpful, depending on the ultrasound findings or in cases of recurrence.

24

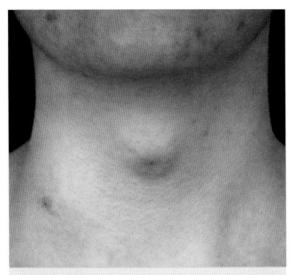

Fig. 24.4 Thyroglossal duct cyst in an adolescent.

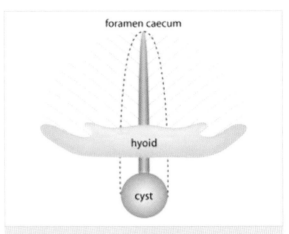

Fig. 24.5 Surgical excision of a thyroglossal duct cyst as described by Sistrunk. The middle portion of the hyoid bone, the cyst, and a core of tongue base muscle up to the foramen cecum are excised.

Treatment

> Surgical excision is the treatment of choice.

The operation is classically described by Sistrunk who appreciated the importance of excising the middle portion of the hyoid bone, the cyst, and a core of tongue base muscle up to the foramen cecum (▶ Fig. 24.5). Histological examination of the resected specimens has confirmed that the thyroglossal duct can have small branches extending laterally.

> A wide core of surrounding tissue should be excised en bloc with the specimen.

- The incision should be carried out through a horizontal skin crease. If the skin has been involved because of previous infection, then an ellipse should be taken and the edges undermined to permit a good aesthetic repair.
- The cyst is identified and the tissues dissected over a wide plane superiorly up toward the hyoid bone. It is important to identify the thyrohyoid membrane that will prevent inadvertent entry into the airway and will also guide the surgeon to the undersurface of the hyoid bone.
- The hyoid bone should be transected at the level of the lesser cornu bilaterally. In an older child, it may be well ossified and very hard, so a sharp bone-cutting forceps is needed.

- Cutting diathermy is useful to extend the dissection up to the tongue base taking a triangular core.

It is advisable to insert a drain for the first few hours postoperatively. There is often some oozing from the hyoid bone and there is also a significant dead space. Hematoma is therefore a distinct possibility.

Recurrence rates are very low if a wide local excision as described is performed, but simple cystectomy results in a 50% recurrence rate.

24.3 Pharyngeal Arch Disorders

> Anomalies in the developing arches may give rise to cysts, sinuses, or fistulas. They may become infected, or present as pits, masses, or discharging lesions in the head and neck.

24.3.1 First Pharyngeal Arch Anomalies

There are a number of classifications of this anomaly and the most frequently reported is that of Work, who described duplication anomalies of the first branchial groove, type I and type II.[3] Although these classifications may indicate the underlying embryological abnormality, they are not able to predict accurately the relationship of any abnormality to the facial nerve, which is, of course, of great importance in the surgical management of these patients.

VI

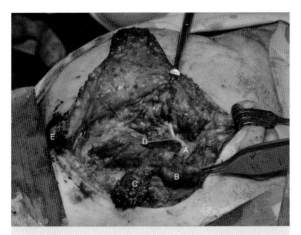

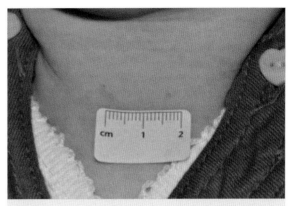

Fig. 24.7 Second pharyngeal arch sinuses.

Fig. 24.6 Left first pharyngeal cleft anomaly approached through superficial parotidectomy. The facial nerve trunk lies deep to the lesion at **(A)**. The lesion is a large cartilaginous tube **(B)** attached to the floor of the ear canal and extending forward to the skin punctum located at **(E)**. The superficial parotid lobe has been reflected inferiorly **(C)**. The mandibular branch of the facial nerve lies superficial to the lesion at **(D)**.

Presentation

First pharyngeal arch anomalies usually present as a cyst, sinus, or mass in the periauricular area (▶ Fig. 24.6) or they can present with a discharge from the ear in the presence of a normal tympanic membrane (due to a sinus in the external auditory canal). These abnormalities are rare and the presentations vary. Unfortunately, this often means that the diagnosis is made at a late stage following several episodes of infection in the same area. This can make excision more challenging.

It is important to distinguish a first pharyngeal arch anomaly from a simple preauricular sinus (see Chapter 6). Openings above the tragus are unlikely to be complex arch anomalies; they are more likely to arise from aberrant fusion of the developing aural tubercles.

Investigations

A magnetic resonance imaging (MRI) scan or a computed tomography (CT) scan may give some information about the deep extent of any sinus or swelling and its relationship to the facial nerve and middle ear. Ultrasound and sinograms are of limited benefit, although they might be appropriate in more complex cases. Imaging should ideally be discussed with a pediatric radiologist who has an interest in this area.

Management

Acute infections should be managed with antibiotics, and surgery should be considered once this has resolved.

Recurrence is more common if there is a history of multiple infections prior to surgery.[4]

> Because of the potential close anatomical relationship of any cyst or tract to the facial nerve, a parotidectomy incision is recommended with formal identification of the facial nerve and the use of a nerve monitor. Bear in mind the very superficial position of the nerve in children (see Chapter 26).

Complete excision of the lesion, including the entire tract, should take place and the operator must be prepared to follow any connections through or around the branches of the facial nerve, possibly running into the external ear canal and the middle ear.

The main and significant risk of surgery is damage to the facial nerve trunk or one of its branches, and a thorough preoperative work-up and fully informed consent should take place prior to surgical intervention.

24.3.2 Second Pharyngeal (Branchial) Arch Anomalies

These are usually blind-ended sinuses that extend from an external skin opening in the middle or lower neck along the anterior border of the sternomastoid (▶ Fig. 24.7). The sinus runs superiorly along the carotid sheath and up toward the tonsil fossa.

24

Occasionally, there is a true complete fistula opening into the tonsil fossa.

These lesions usually present in early childhood as the sinus is usually obvious within the neck and may discharge clear fluid. The discharging sinus may be associated with a more distal cyst, which may become infected.

The diagnosis is usually made clinically, but a sinogram can provide a good demonstration of the course of the tract. The ipsilateral tonsil should be examined.

If surgical intervention is indicated, then complete excision of the sinus or fistula is recommended.

- In a young child, this is usually performed through one elliptical skin incision around the external opening.
- The tract is then followed superiorly.
- Gentle insertion of a lacrimal probe can be useful as can instillation of methylene blue.

In young children, one skin incision is usually adequate, but in older children and adults or where the tract extends high into the neck, a second higher incision (step-ladder technique) may be required.

24.3.3 Third and Fourth Arch Anomalies

These are very uncommon and the diagnosis is often made only after several presentations with repeated infection in the neck.

Presentation

Most patients present in childhood or early adulthood with recurrent cervical abscess or recurrent thyroiditis. For reasons that remain unknown, the huge majority of these abnormalities occur on the left side and more often in females. These sinuses originate in the third and fourth internal pharyngeal pouches, and an opening may be seen in the apex of the pyriform sinus on flexible laryngoscopy (► Fig. 24.8).

Investigations

A barium swallow will confirm a tract extending down from the pyriform fossa toward the thyroid gland (► Fig. 24.9). It is important to treat any acute infection prior to performing this examination as edema may obliterate the sinus tract and prevent visualization. A CT scan can also be performed to determine the extent of the abnormalities.

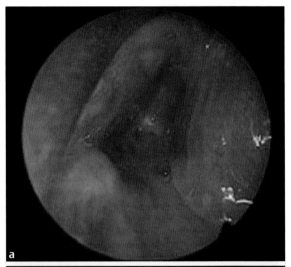

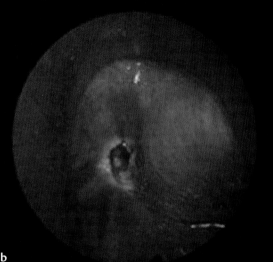

Fig. 24.8 Third or fourth arch anomaly. Rigid laryngoscopy showing sinus in left pyriform fossa before and after cautery.

Management

A preexisting infection should be treated with antibiotics and/or incision and drainage as appropriate.

Many of these abnormalities have now been treated conservatively with endoscopic cauterization of the sinus opening within the pyriform fossa.

This may require to be performed more than once, but current data has suggested that it is a safe and effective treatment in the majority of patients. If the problem recurs despite repeated cauterization, then surgical excision should be carried out. The tract should be removed

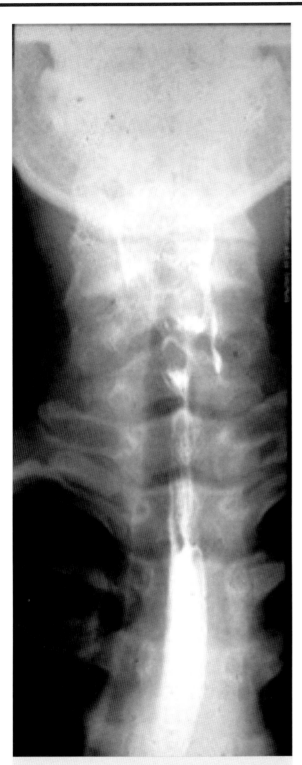

Fig. 24.9 Barium swallow showing fourth pharyngeal arch anomaly.

in its entirety excising the tract through the neck, suturing the pyriform sinus opening and occasionally taking the ipsilateral lobe of the thyroid gland if the patient has had significant problems with thyroiditis or a thyroid abscess.

Excision surgery is, of course, associated with a risk of damage to the neurovascular structures and in particular the superior and recurrent laryngeal nerves. Detailed preoperative counseling and informed consent are, of course, essential.

24.4 Vascular Malformations and Hemangiomas

There is a wide range of vascular pathologies that can present in the head and neck in children. They can be solid structures made up of a mass of endothelial tissue (hemangioma or birthmark) or more cystic structures composed of abnormal vessels including lymphatic cysts or dilated veins. They were classified by Mulliken and Glowacki into the following two main groups[5]:
1. Hemangiomas.
2. Vascular malformations.

The classification of these lesions is evolving,[6] and improved imaging techniques, particularly contrast-enhanced MRI, have made for ever more precise characterization, often without the need for histology.[7]

24.4.1 Hemangiomas

Often known as "birthmarks," these lesions exhibit rapid endothelial proliferation shortly after birth, growing in infancy and then resolving spontaneously in childhood.

Presentation

Lesions involving the skin tend to be red in appearance and grow rapidly from approximately 6 weeks of age. This growth phase lasts approximately 9 to 12 months and the lesion then slowly resolves over a period of several years. Deeper lesions such as these seen in the subglottis appear more bluish in color.

> **i**
>
> If the hemangioma becomes very large, cardiac failure can occur.

24

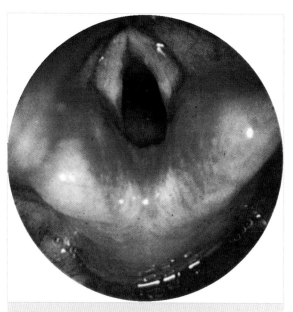

Fig. 24.10 Endoscopic view of subglottic hemangioma.

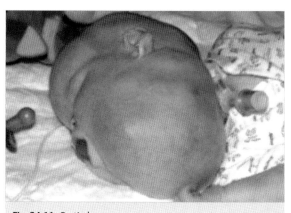

Fig. 24.11 Cystic hygroma.

The consequences of these abnormalities depend on the site involved. On the skin, the problem may simply be cosmetic, but if the lesion encroaches on the eye, for instance, then it can have serious functional consequences and intervention is required.

Hemangiomas can occur in the subglottic region and present with increasing stridor in the first few weeks of life (see Chapter 21).

Treatment

> ℹ
>
> The majority of hemangiomas require no treatment as they will regress spontaneously. The parents may need support and reassurance if the lesion is large and has an aesthetic impact.

Until recently, hemangiomas that had a functional impact on the child were treated with high-dose corticosteroids either orally or injected directly into the lesion. Interferon was a less popular alternative. However, in France in 2008, it was discovered by chance that oral propranolol can dramatically reduce the size of hemangiomas, and this medication has now been adopted as the treatment of choice in those hemangiomas that are large or are obstructing the airway or, in the case of facial and orbital lesions, are affecting vision.[8] Propranolol carries a risk of side effects such as hypotension, bradycardia, and syncope, and therefore patients undergoing this treatment must be closely monitored and cardiology assessment is advisable (see Chapter 21).

In those cases in which medical treatment has failed or where propranolol is contraindicated, surgery may be considered. Surgery for subglottic hemangiomas (▶ Fig. 24.10) is covered in Chapter 21.

24.4.2 Vascular Malformations

Lymphatic Malformations (Lymphangioma)

These have traditionally been known as *cystic hygromas*. They consist of a collection of thin-walled lymphatic cysts. These cysts can by very small and can infiltrate adjacent structures or can be macrocystic containing very large spaces that can compress, displace, and distort adjacent structures.

Presentation

> ℹ
>
> These lesions can, therefore, present with anything from minor cosmetic issues to a life-threatening obstruction (▶ Fig. 24.11).

Lymphatic malformations can present at birth or can become apparent throughout childhood. Very large malformations may be evident on prenatal scans and may prevent normal vaginal delivery and in this instance an ex utero intrapartum treatment (EXIT) procedure may be appropriate (see below) followed by tracheostomy to establish an airway.

VI

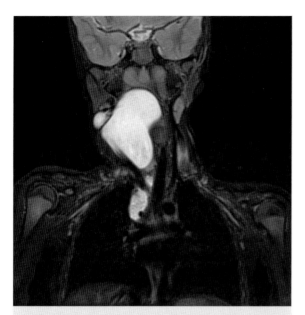

Fig. 24.12 T2-weighted coronal magnetic resonance imaging scan of a 3-year-old girl showing a large, right-sided, macro-cystic lymphatic malformation. It encases and displaces the carotid sheath laterally. It also displaces the trachea across to the left. The lesion extends down into the anterior mediastinum as far as the aortic arch.

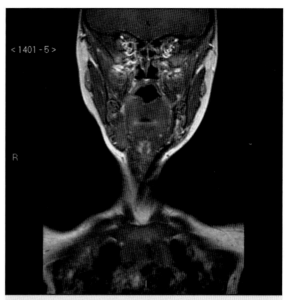

Fig. 24.13 magnetic resonance imaging showing a large, left-sided ectatic neck vein. This can present as a neck swelling, causing diagnostic confusion.

Lesions commonly involve the submandibular and parotid areas and can infiltrate the tongue and larynx. The tongue can protrude from the mouth, resulting in ulceration, bleeding and infection, and interference with feeding and development of speech.

Investigations

An MRI or a CT scan can aid in the diagnosis and display the extent of the pathology. Biopsy may be required where diagnosis remains uncertain or to characterize a particularly aggressive lesion, but high-quality MRI is usually definitive (▶ Fig. 24.12). Endoscopy may be useful to assess the airway and to establish the degree of infiltration of the supraglottic larynx.

Treatment

Treatment may be conservative when there are no functional sequelae and purely aesthetic issues may be addressed surgically as the child gets older. Where there are functional problems related to the airway, speech, and swallowing, intervention may be required at an early age.

- *Injection sclerotherapy* with substances such as OK432 have been shown to be effective, particularly in macrocystic disease.[9] It is ideally performed under ultrasound control by aspirating the individual cysts to dryness and then injecting the sclerosant. The neck can

then become quite inflamed and skin breakdown is a potential complication. In large lesions, there may be a very active inflammatory response with airway compromise occasionally needing endotracheal intubation. The resulting fibrosis may make surgical intervention at a later stage more challenging.

- *Surgery* can be fraught due to the intimate relationship of the cysts to surrounding structures and due to the difficulty of effecting complete excision, so recurrence is common. Major surgery is rarely performed to completely excise the lymphangioma and is often used as a debulking procedure. Some children with large lesions, especially involving the tongue base, may need a long-term tracheostomy. The aim is to improve function. This may involve a tongue reduction or partial removal of an obstructing neck mass. The cysts can infiltrate around important neurovascular structures, particularly the cranial nerves, and it is important to preserve these in managing this benign disease. When lesions are large, it can be very challenging to produce a good cosmetic result and these children are best looked after in specialist centers.

24.5 Venous Malformations

These are soft compressible bluish swellings that can occur in the head and neck region. They include ectatic veins (▶ Fig. 24.13) and can be misdiagnosed as solid

24

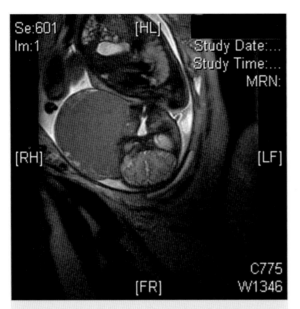

Fig. 24.14 Prenatal sonogram showing a large neck mass.

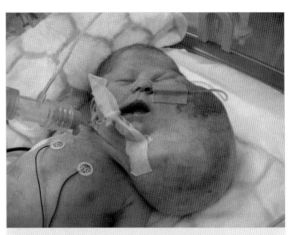

Fig. 24.15 The baby from ▶ Fig. 24.14 safely delivered through the ex utero intrapartum treatment (EXIT) procedure with an endotracheal tube securing her airway. Surgery for the neck mass was undertaken a few days after birth.

lumps. Injudicious attempts at surgical excision can cause torrential bleeding. Preoperative imaging is always wise with neck masses in children. These lesions can be challenging to resect and surgery should only be undertaken following careful preoperative assessment, in some cases including MRI scanning and/or angiography. Sclerotherapy and embolization are alternatives to surgical resection.

24.6 Teratomas

Teratomas arise from pluripotent cells and ectopic embryonic nongerm cells. They can present in the head and neck. They are usually mature in children and rarely malignant but may be locally aggressive.

24.6.1 Presentation

The tumor can result in a large neck mass or a nasopharyngeal or oropharyngeal swelling. It can present with airway obstruction and respiratory distress and require immediate excision.

Teratomas are often associated with polyhydramnios. Advances in prenatal scanning are such that diagnosis of these tumors is now often made at prenatal scanning while the child is in utero.

EXIT Procedure

In cases where severe upper airway obstruction is anticipated (▶ Fig. 24.14), a well-coordinated team including an obstetrician, an anesthetist, and an ear, nose, and throat surgeon may be able to secure the airway either by endotracheal intubation or by tracheotomy before the baby is separated from the placenta. The uteroplacental circulation can be prolonged for an extended period at delivery. This EXIT procedure can transform a potentially fatal neonatal emergency to a controlled intervention with a safe outcome for mother and baby (▶ Fig. 24.15). More definitive management can then proceed when the child is stable.[10] Specific indications and guidelines are likely to be refined as a consequence of ongoing advances in fetal intervention and antenatal imaging.

24.6.2 Investigations

Investigations may include a CT scan. Teratomas typically contain multiple calcified foci. Thyroid function should be assessed both pre- and postoperatively as the teratoma may include functioning thyroid tissue. Serum alpha fetoprotein can be used as a marker of malignancy, but this is rare in childhood teratomas.

VI

24.6.3 Management

Complete surgical excision is the treatment of choice. These tumors are usually well encapsulated and dissect out reasonably easily, although care must always be taken to avoid damage to adjacent structures.

24.7 Hamartomas

These are tumorlike malformations due to an anatomical error in the course of development. They are composed of tissue from a single specific germinal layer and differ in this way from teratomas and from dermoid cysts; lymphoid, vascular, and cartilaginous hamartomas have been described.

They are unusual in the head and neck region. They present with a swelling and treatment consists of surgical excision.

24.8 Fibromatosis Colli

This abnormality represents the most common neck mass in the immediate perinatal period and within the first 2 months of life. The older term for this condition is *sterno-cleidomastoid tumor of infancy*. The etiology is not well understood but it is thought to be related to an abnormal intrauterine position or birth injury that results in a fusiform swelling of the sternomastoid muscle. Fibrosis is found within the muscle and results in torticollis, which usually resolves within the first 6 months. In more severe and long-standing cases, the resulting torticollis can cause craniofacial asymmetry.

Babies present with a firm nontender lateral neck swelling or with head tilt. Examination reveals a hard spindle-shaped swelling within the sternomastoid muscle.

Diagnosis is usually clinical, but when doubt remains an ultrasound scan (► Fig. 24.16) will exclude other neck masses and confirm the intramuscular fusiform swelling.

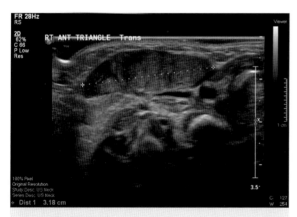

Fig. 24.16 Ultrasound showing large mass, fibromatosis colli, in the sternomastoid muscle in a newborn.

Conservative treatment consists of physical therapy and is effective in most cases. Those more severe cases may require surgery to divide the sternal and clavicular heads of the sternomastoid muscle and any tight deep cervical fascia. In more severe cases, division of the upper end of sternomastoid may be required.

Physical therapy must be employed postoperatively to avoid recurrence.

24.9 Key Points

- Understanding the embryological development within the head and neck region will aid in the diagnosis and treatment of congenital neck disease.
- Consider the diagnosis of a congenital anomaly in a child with recurrent head and neck abscesses.
- Beware the proximity of the facial nerve in first arch anomalies.
- Consider endoscopic cautery in the management of third and fourth pharyngeal arch sinuses.
- Ultrasound scanning followed by wide local excision is the management of choice in thyroglossal duct cysts.
- Many hemangiomas require no intervention as they will resolve with time but consider propranolol and/or surgical intervention when function affected.
- Consider the EXIT procedure when large lymphangiomas and head and neck teratomas are diagnosed in vitro.

References

[1] Sadler TW, ed. Head and neck. In: Langman's Medical Embryology. 11th ed. Philadelphia, PA: Lippincott, Williams and Wilkins; 2010:265–291

[2] Oyewumi M, Inarejos E, Greer ML, et al. Ultrasound to differentiate thyroglossal duct cysts and dermoid cysts in children. Laryngoscope. 2015; 125(4):998–1003

[3] Work WP. Newer concepts of first branchial cleft defects. Laryngoscope. 1972; 82(9):1581–1593

[4] Prosser JD, Myer CM, III. Branchial cleft anomalies and thymic cysts. Otolaryngol Clin North Am. 2015; 48(1):1–14

[5] Mulliken JB, Glowacki J. Hemangiomas and vascular malformations in infants and children: a classification based on endothelial characteristics. Plast Reconstr Surg. 1982; 69(3):412–422

[6] Wassef M, Blei F, Adams D, et al. ISSVA Board and Scientific Committee. Vascular anomalies classification: recommendations from the International Society for the Study of Vascular Anomalies. Pediatrics. 2015; 136(1):e203–e214

[7] Higgins LJ, Koshy J, Mitchell SE, et al. Time-resolved contrast-enhanced MRA (TWIST) with gadofosveset trisodium in the classification of soft-tissue vascular anomalies in the head and neck in children following updated 2014 ISSVA classification: first report on systematic evaluation of MRI and TWIST in a cohort of 47 children. Clin Radiol. 2016; 71(1):32–39

[8] Léauté-Labrèze C, Dumas de la Roque E, Hubiche T, Boralevi F, Thambo JB, Taïeb A. Propranolol for severe hemangiomas of infancy. N Engl J Med. 2008; 358(24):2649–2651

[9] Giguere CM, Bauman NM, Sato Y, et al. Treatment of lymphangiomas with OK432 (Picibanil) sclerotherapy: a prospective multi-institutional trial. Arch Otolaryngol Head Neck Surg. 2002; 128(10):1137–1144

[10] Taghavi K, Beasley S. The ex utero intrapartum treatment (EXIT) procedure: application of a new therapeutic paradigm. J Paediatr Child Health. 2013; 49(9):E420–E427

24

25 Neck Masses in Children: Acquired Neck Masses

Haytham Kubba

25.1 Introduction

Neck masses in children are very common but they can present significant diagnostic challenges. In adults, a new lump in the neck is assumed to be a malignancy and investigated accordingly. In children, however, the majority of new lumps in the neck are infectious or inflammatory in origin. The clinician is faced with the task of identifying without delay the small number of children who have serious pathology such as malignancy and at the same time avoiding unnecessary investigation and treatment of children with pathology that is benign and self-limiting.

Masses of congenital origin (such as thyroglossal duct cysts and lymphatic malformations) may only become clinically apparent sometime after birth and so must enter the differential diagnosis of neck lumps appearing in childhood. These congenital lesions have been discussed already in Chapter 24 and will not be mentioned further here.

Broadly speaking, children with neck masses present in one of the following two ways:

- In the acute or emergency presentation: the child has a short history of a neck mass in association with pain, fever, general malaise, and all the signs of an acute illness.
- In the nonacute presentation to the outpatient clinic: the child is typically systemically well and the neck mass is the only concern.

> **i**
>
> In the acutely unwell child, the cause is likely to be infection or an inflammatory disorder.
>
> In the systemically well child the main concern is to identify those with tumors from the majority with inflammatory cervical lymphadenopathy.

25.2 Neck Masses in Children Who Are Acutely Unwell

25.2.1 Clinical Assessment

> **i**
>
> In a child who presents acutely with pain, fever, malaise, and a neck mass, the most likely cause is infection, but the clinician should be aware of a few noninfective inflammatory conditions that require specific treatment.

We should also never forget that some malignancies (particularly lymphoma and neuroblastoma) and histiocytoses can present acutely with a neck mass and with symptoms such as weight loss and malaise, mimicking an infection.

For the child presenting as an emergency with a neck mass and fever, it is worth making an initial assessment of the child's general state. Deep neck-space infections may cause airway compression, while fever, septicemia, and poor oral intake may all lead to hypovolemia. These may need immediate attention regardless of the exact underlying diagnosis. The same is true for pain, and analgesia may allow for a more complete physical examination.

Once the situation is stabilized, focus on the duration of the illness, any preceding upper respiratory symptoms, symptoms associated with the mass itself, and systemic symptoms such as night sweats and weight loss. Any history of foreign travel or known conditions such as tuberculosis (TB) or human immunodeficiency virus (HIV) in the family is clearly important. The clinician should ask specifically if there was any preexisting lump or sinus opening to suggest an underlying branchial cleft or thyroglossal duct anomaly. Recurring neck abscesses around the left thyroid lobe may suggest a third/fourth pharyngeal pouch anomaly (see Chapter 24).

Evaluate the child's general health including temperature, state of hydration, and demeanor.

> **i**
>
> Note specific features of the mass such as size, site, consistency, fluctuance, tenderness, and discoloration of the overlying skin.

Examine the ears, nose, and oral cavity and consider awake transnasal fiberoptic laryngoscopy depending on the circumstances. Trismus, torticollis, palatal bulging, retropharyngeal swelling, and stertor are all worrying signs of deep neck-space infection. General examination may reveal diagnostic clues such as heart murmurs and swelling of the hands and feet in Kawasaki's disease; exudative tonsillitis and splenomegaly in Epstein–Barr virus (EBV) infection; and abdominal masses or lymphadenopathy in the axillae and groins in children with malignancy.

> **i**
>
> For the acutely unwell child with a neck mass, the most important initial investigation is ultrasound.

A full blood count and routine blood chemistry can give useful information, but ultrasound is the single test most likely to guide initial treatment. It will distinguish solid lesions from cysts and abscesses, as well as providing anatomical information. Cross-sectional imaging (such as computed tomography [CT]) is useful when deep neck-space infection is suspected.

25.2.2 Acute Lymphadenitis

Acute Viral Lymphadenitis

Acute viral lymphadenitis is extremely common in children and, it can be considered normal for a child with a viral upper respiratory tract infection to have palpable cervical lymph nodes for 3 or 4 weeks. A normal preschool child may get as many as eight upper respiratory tract infections a year, so fluctuating enlargement and regression of cervical lymph nodes is a normal physiological phenomenon as the lymphocytes in the lymph nodes do their job of processing and responding to foreign antigens. No specific investigation or management is required other than reassurance. More persistent lymphadenopathy can be associated with EBV or cytomegalovirus (CMV) infection and with the illness that accompanies the acquisition of HIV infection.

Acute Bacterial Lymphadenitis

Acute bacterial lymphadenitis most often occurs after an upper respiratory tract infection. *Streptococcus pneumoniae* and *Staphylococcus aureus* are common pathogens.
- In the initial stages, the child is feverish and unwell with a mass of swollen lymph nodes.
- These continue to enlarge and undergo central necrosis until a *superficial lymph node abscess* forms.
- At this stage, the lymph node mass will be large, fluctuant, red, hot, and tender.

Treatment is with systemic antibiotics, but if a fluctuant abscess has developed, incision and drainage under general anesthesia may be needed. Needle aspiration may be useful in selected cases. The child's general condition then improves quickly with fluid rehydration, intravenous if needed, analgesia, antipyretics, and continued antibiotics. This is a very common clinical situation with which every otolaryngologist is familiar.

Familiarity breeds complacency and there are several pitfalls in the management of acute cervical lymphadenopathy:
- First among these is the preschool age child presenting with a fluctuant subcutaneous abscess of a few weeks duration with reddish-purple skin discoloration and no fever or malaise. At first glance this looks like a typical bacterial abscess but it is in fact nontuberculous mycobacterial (NTM), sometimes called "atypical mycobacterial" (ATM), infection for which incision and drainage would be a poor choice of treatment (see section on Nontuberculous Mycobacterial Infection).
- The second pitfall is the child with a serious deep neck-space infection who is getting steadily sicker on the ward. This is often misdiagnosed as a superficial lymph node abscess. Thorough examination, including the oropharynx, with ultrasound scanning as needed should avoid this.
- The third is the occasional failure of radiologists and otolaryngologists to communicate effectively: the radiologist may report a small amount of early central necrosis in a lymph node as "liquefaction," which the otolaryngologist might interpret as meaning a collection large enough to justify drainage, only to find no pus at surgery. If surgery is being considered, it should go without saying that there is no substitute for a direct discussion with the radiologist about exactly what they have found and where.

25.2.3 Deep Neck-Space Infection

Peritonsillar Abscess

In older children and adolescents, management can usually proceed as for adults, with transoral needle drainage of the collection under local anesthetic, administration of antibiotics, and the expectation of rapid resolution. Diagnosis and treatment in younger children can be much more difficult as it may be almost impossible to see the oropharynx in an uncooperative, unhappy toddler with trismus.

Peritonsillar abscess (quinsy) occurs less often in children than in adults.
   Look carefully for airway compromise.

Investigation

Ultrasound scanning can sometimes give surprisingly good views of the tonsil capsule to make the diagnosis in a cooperative child, but in many cases, the diagnosis is presumptive. If there is any doubt, a CT scan will exclude any more serious deep neck-space infection, but the child will usually need a general anesthetic with endotracheal intubation to achieve good quality images and to ensure that the airway is secure throughout the procedure. This is no small undertaking as endotracheal intubation may be very difficult in the presence of trismus and oropharyngeal swelling.

25

Treatment

Assuming the child is stable, the best initial course of action is often simply to treat the child with intravenous rehydration, analgesia, antipyretics, and broad-spectrum antibiotics and then reassess after 12 to 24 hours.[1] Consider metronidazole, especially if there is not a rapid response as anaerobes are commonly implicated. The clinical condition usually improves quickly and physical examination becomes easier allowing the definitive diagnosis to be made. Many peritonsillar abscesses will settle in a few days with conservative treatment.

If the child is not stable or not improving rapidly with conservative management, then general anesthesia and a scan become inevitable. At this point, it is worth making a plan in advance to intervene under the same anesthetic once the diagnosis of peritonsillar abscess is confirmed. Needle aspiration under general anesthesia is often inadequate because of the high reaccumulation rate; it is much better to do something definitive at this stage to avoid the risk of having to repeat the general anesthetic. There is much variation in management strategies in different countries and health care systems, with immediate surgery the routine in Denmark.[2,3]

> "Hot" tonsillectomy drains the abscess and removes the focus of infection in one simple procedure.

Retropharyngeal Abscess

A retropharyngeal abscess most commonly occurs in children under the age of 5 years due to suppuration in lymph nodes secondary to upper respiratory tract infection.

Retropharyngeal abscess in an infant will often present in a similar manner to acute epiglottitis with a sick, feverish baby drooling saliva and breathing with a soft stertor. Such cases should be managed in the same way as epiglottitis until the diagnosis is established:
- Disturb the child as little as possible.
- Quickly assemble a team of experienced clinicians including an anesthetist and an otolaryngologist.
- Gently induce anesthesia with an inhalational agent to allow examination of the pharynx and larynx.
- Intubation can proceed at this point, along with transoral drainage of the abscess through a vertical incision in the posterior pharyngeal wall if the diagnosis is apparent.

> A sick baby with potential airway obstruction should never be sent to the radiology department for a lateral soft-tissue neck X-ray; to do so is potentially dangerous and a plain X-ray is too prone to artifact to be of much use.

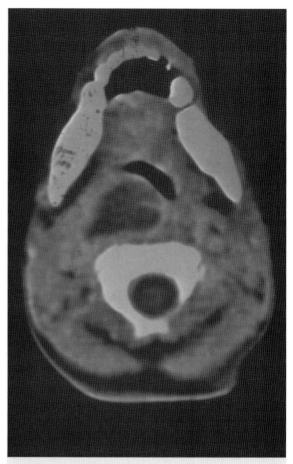

Fig. 25.1 Computed tomography of retropharyngeal abscess.

If a diagnosis of retropharyngeal abscess is being seriously considered, then the airway should be secured by endotracheal intubation and definitive imaging (a CT scan of the neck) arranged (▶ Fig. 25.1).

Parapharyngeal Abscess

Children may develop a *parapharyngeal abscess* secondary to lymph node suppuration, tonsillitis, or dental infection. The clinical presentation is very variable.[4]
- Some present with a rapidly progressive, fulminating illness and may even require admission to the intensive care unit.
- Others run a more insidious course with subtle signs such as neck stiffness, torticollis, low-grade pyrexia, and malaise.

The external swelling in the neck may be difficult to discern in the early stages, and oropharyngeal swelling may also be difficult to see in the early stage. The tonsil may be deviated if the parapharyngeal collection is large.

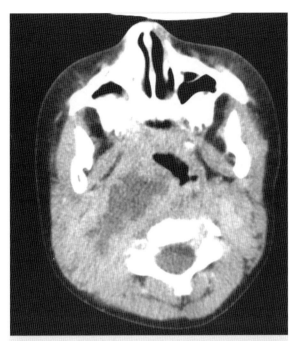

Fig. 25.2 Axial computed tomography scan with contrast of a child showing a large right parapharyngeal abscess displacing the tonsil medially and the carotid sheath laterally.

Ultrasound is an excellent first-line investigation, as it involves no ionizing radiation and the child does not need general anesthesia. Some radiologists may even attempt needle drainage of the abscess under the guidance of the ultrasound probe. Cross-sectional imaging such as CT gives much more useful anatomical information on the position of the abscess and its relationship to the carotid sheath and the pharynx (▶ Fig. 25.2)—information which is very useful for surgical planning. It allows estimation of the volume of pus present, which may support conservative management if the volume is small.

> **i**
>
> In most cases of parapharyngeal abscess, the treatment is formal incision and drainage under general anesthesia.

An external incision allows wide drainage and the placement of a drain to reduce the chance of reaccumulation, but in some cases, a transoral approach is quicker and easier. The tonsil is often the original site of suppuration, and once it has been removed, the abscess can be identified through the tonsil bed using a needle, followed by blunt dissection with forceps. This approach is best when the abscess has displaced the carotid sheath laterally. Preoperative imaging will identify the relationship of the abscess to the carotid sheath and aids surgical planning.

An external scar is avoided with a transoral approach, but the chance of reaccumulation of pus with the need for a second procedure is higher.

It is not uncommon to find that there is no pus at surgery despite the CT appearance of a collection. Early necrosis can be difficult to differentiate from liquid pus. magnetic resonance imaging (MRI) scanning tends to have even more false-positives for pus than CT. Ultimately, if there is doubt, then proceed with surgery.

25.2.4 Noninfective Inflammatory Conditions

There are a few nonsuppurative inflammatory causes of acute cervical lymph node swelling with fever of which the clinician should be aware. Some are serious in their own right, but some are important in that early diagnosis prevents the need for unnecessary further investigation and treatment. These diagnoses should be considered particularly for children whose fever does not respond rapidly to antipyretics and antibiotics.

Kawasaki's Disease

Kawasaki's disease (mucocutaneous lymph node syndrome) is an autoimmune vasculitis affecting children under the age of 5 years. It presents with fever, nontender cervical lymph node enlargement, edema of the hands and feet, and erythema of the conjunctiva, oral mucosa, and skin. Arthritis, aseptic meningitis, and myocarditis may also occur in the early stages. Skin desquamation on the hands and feet occurs later.

The most important feature is the potential for coronary artery aneurysms and the small but significant risk of death within the first few weeks after onset without treatment.

> **i**
>
> The fever is usually high and unresponsive to paracetamol, ibuprofen, or antibiotics. It lasts for a week or two in most cases, and the longer the duration of fever, the higher the risk of cardiac sequelae. Early diagnosis is essential but this can be difficult in practice as there is no single definitive test.

The diagnosis is based on clinical features, blood tests, and echocardiography. A full blood count will show a degree of anemia and thrombocytosis, and the erythrocyte sedimentation rate and C-reactive protein (CRP) will be elevated. Coronary artery aneurysms on echocardiogram are highly diagnostic in the right clinical setting. Temporal artery biopsy is rarely required. Diagnostic criteria[5] are set out in Box 25.1.[5]

25

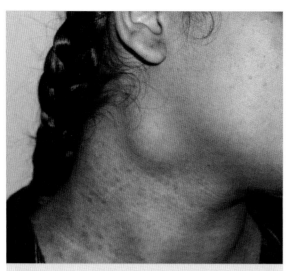

Fig. 25.3 Tuberculous lymph node in the neck of an adolescent girl.

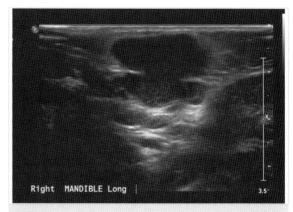

Fig. 25.4 Ultrasound showing "collar-stud" abscess typical of cervical tuberculosis.

Box 25.1 Diagnostic Criteria for Kawasaki's disease[5]

Fever of at least 5 days' duration with any four of the following five criteria:

- Erythema or cracking of the lips or oral mucosa.
- Rash on the trunk.
- Swelling or erythema of the hands or feet.
- Conjunctival injection.
- Enlarged cervical lymph node (15 mm or more).

Or, fever of at least 5 days' duration, coronary artery disease on echocardiography, and any three of the aforementioned criteria, when the features cannot be explained by any other known disease process.

The child needs to be admitted under the care of a pediatrician. Treatment should be prompt. This is one of the very few situations when aspirin is recommended for children. The fever responds rapidly to aspirin and intravenous immunoglobulin. The role of systemic steroids is uncertain.

Kikuchi–Fujimoto's Disease

Kikuchi–Fujimoto's disease (KFD or necrotizing lymphadenitis) is rare outside Japan but isolated cases have been reported in other parts of Asia, in Europe, and in North America. It usually occurs in people in their twenties, but cases have been reported in very young children.

The cause of the disease is unknown but it may be an excessive T-cell reaction to a nonspecific infectious trigger in a genetically susceptible individual.

Presentation is with tender cervical lymphadenopathy in association with headache, skin rash, weight loss, and fever. Ultrasound scanning of the neck shows enlarged coalescent nodes, with distortion of the normal hilar architecture. This is nonspecific but an important sign as a normal hilar architecture pattern virtually excludes significant lymph node disease. Blood tests are unhelpful.

> i
>
> KFD is a benign, self-limiting condition but may be misdiagnosed as more serious pathology such as TB (▶ Fig. 25.3, ▶ Fig. 25.4) or malignancy.[6] Diagnosis is by means of lymph node excision biopsy and histology. The histological pattern is characteristic and shows coagulative necrosis in the paracortical areas of the involved lymph nodes.
>
> The disease usually resolves spontaneously over a period of a few weeks or months. Treatment is supportive.

Periodic Fever, Aphthous Stomatitis, Pharyngitis, and Adenitis Syndrome

Periodic fever, aphthous stomatitis, pharyngitis, and adenitis (PFAPA) syndrome is of unknown etiology. It typically occurs in young children and is characterized by episodes of high fever with mouth ulcers, pharyngitis, and tender enlargement of cervical lymph nodes occurring every 3 to 5 weeks for at least 6 months. Throat cultures show no growth, but tonsillar fauna are now thought to play a role in some cases.[7] Blood tests may be useful to exclude cyclical neutropenia. In between episodes, the child is perfectly well.

Episodes often resolve quickly with steroids, but if the condition is disabling, then surgery may be considered. A review of 159 children in 13 observational studies and 2 randomized controlled trials suggested that a significant majority of children have complete resolution or improvement after adenotonsillectomy.[8] However, the condition usually regresses anyway as the child gets older, with one study showing 50 out of 59 children having resolution after a mean of 6.3 years,[9] suggesting that milder cases can be treated conservatively.

25.3 Neck Masses in Children Who Are Systemically Well

Cervical lymphadenopathy is one of the commoner presentations in pediatric otolaryngology practice. *Reactive lymphoid hyperplasia* is, of course, a physiological response to an infective or inflammatory stimulus. Children suffer from frequent upper respiratory infections, mostly viral in origin, so it should not be surprising that palpable lymph nodes are present in 62% of healthy children aged 3 weeks to 6 months, 52% of those aged 7 to 23 months, and up to 41% of those aged 2 to 5 years.[10]

> Persistent enlargement of cervical lymph nodes raises the concern that there may be serious underlying pathology (such as Hodgkin's disease), but the majority of children with persistently enlarged nodes have reactive hyperplasia and nothing else.

25.3.1 Clinical Assessment

In adults, enlarged cervical lymph nodes are assumed to be malignant until proven otherwise, and this can be quickly and reliably confirmed with fine needle aspiration cytology. The most common diagnosis is squamous carcinoma, which can spread to the skin if an excision biopsy is performed, but can be reliably detected cytologically due to the presence of keratin. In children, the situation is different. Rather than confirming malignancy, we are seeking to exclude it and this requires that tests have a very low false-negative rate.

Carcinoma is very rare in children, so seeding to the skin is not a concern. Most childhood tumors are difficult to diagnose on cytology, and fine needle aspiration can be difficult without anesthesia in young children. For these reasons, excision biopsy remains the "gold standard" investigation. However, this comes with a scar, wound discomfort, the risk of bleeding and infection, possible damage to the accessory, hypoglossal or marginal mandibular nerves, the risks of a general anesthetic, and the inconvenience of a hospital stay.

The challenge for the clinician is to identify the very small number of children who have a high suspicion of serious pathology and who therefore need to proceed without delay to excision biopsy under general anesthesia, and at the same time to find ways to reliably exclude anything serious for the vast majority, sparing them the risks of surgery. We do not do this well at present. Many children with malignant tumors of the head and neck suffer significant diagnostic delay, whereas the majority of children undergoing excision biopsy of cervical lymph nodes have only reactive hyperplasia. It is very common to see children being repeatedly reviewed in otolaryngology outpatient clinics over a period of many months until parents and clinicians finally proceed to excision biopsy out of sheer desperation at the lack of progress. In these circumstances, where the child has been reviewed for many months without any malignancy becoming apparent, it is almost certain that nothing serious will be found on histology of the excised nodes. It would be much better to make a decision on the child's first or second visit to the clinic, either to proceed to excision biopsy or to reassure and discharge.

In many cases, the child has a history of upper respiratory tract infections or skin conditions (particularly of the scalp) that are serving as an inflammatory stimulus to the lymph nodes. The nodes themselves are small (5 mm or less), mobile, bean-shaped, and soft. There is often a history that the nodes fluctuate in size, something that only really occurs in reactive hyperplasia. Systemic features such as night sweats and weight loss are absent. In these circumstances, it is perfectly reasonable to reassure and discharge the family with no further investigations as long as they are instructed to return if there is progressive enlargement of the node.

Some children have masses that are clearly worrying and they should proceed rapidly to excision (or incision) biopsy of the mass after cross-sectional imaging (usually MRI). Such worrying masses include anything bigger than 2 cm, rapidly growing masses, masses in children with a known history of malignancy, and any supraclavicular masses (Box 25.2).

Box 25.2 Neck Lumps: Red Flags for Pediatric Malignancy

- Size > 2 cm.
- Rapid growth.
- History of malignancy.
- Supraclavicular site.

When the diagnosis is less clear-cut, investigations have a role. A plain chest X-ray can be obtained from clinic and occasionally this reveals mediastinal lymphadenopathy suggestive of lymphoma or signs of TB. Ultrasound scanning is the most useful investigation, however. In the

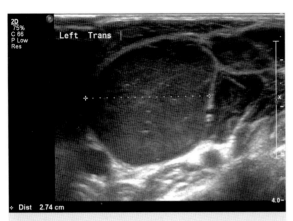

Fig. 25.5 Ultrasound of neck mass due to lymphoma.

hands of a skilled ultrasonographer, features such as round shape, loss of the normal hilum, and abnormal echogenicity can be highly predictive of lymphoma (▶ Fig. 25.5), whereas oval shape and normal lymph node architecture can be very reassuring of reactive hyperplasia.[11]

Blood should also be taken at this stage for serology. Positive serology for CMV, EBV, or *Bartonella henselae* (see section on Cat-Scratch Disease) provides a diagnosis and may therefore avoid the need for excision biopsy.

> **i**
>
> As many as 10% of children with cervical lymphadenopathy have positive serology, so the pickup rate is good and this is a worthwhile investigation.

The diagnostic role of full blood count and CRP testing is unclear, but if you are taking blood for serology, it is reasonable to order these tests as well.

Serology results can take a few weeks to appear, so a review appointment should be made for 4 to 6 weeks. During this period, a course of antibiotics may cause the nodes to shrink if the cause is chronic infection in the upper respiratory tract. At review, the serology and ultrasound results can be reviewed and the child reexamined to see if the nodes are getting larger or smaller. A clear decision to excise or discharge should then be possible and prolonged, repeated clinical review avoided.

25.3.2 Infective Causes

Cat-Scratch Disease

Cat-scratch disease (▶ Fig. 25.6) is caused by the gram-negative bacillus *Bartonella henselae*, which is transmitted to humans in the feces of cat fleas through small scratches or bites in the skin. It is usually asymptomatic in the early stages, although some individuals may have headache and fever a week or two after inoculation, fol-

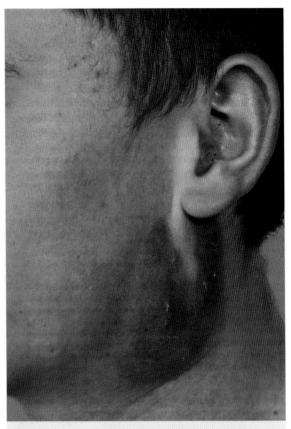

Fig. 25.6 Cat-scratch disease.

lowed by cervical lymphadenopathy lasting a few months. The condition is usually benign and self-limiting in immunocompetent individuals and its significance lies in the fact that serological diagnosis can lead to patient reassurance and the avoidance of excision biopsy of cervical lymph nodes. In the immunocompromised, more severe complications can occur, such as encephalitis, optic neuritis, blood-filled cysts of the liver and spleen, and vascular lesions in the skin.

Posttransplant Lymphoproliferative Disorder

In children who are immunosuppressed following a solid organ or bone marrow transplant, cervical lymphadenopathy with or without fever should raise suspicion of posttransplant lymphoproliferative disorder. Cervical lymph nodes and the tonsils are common sites for this condition, which is caused by B-cell proliferation due to EBV infection. Diagnosis is on histology of an excised node or other lymphoid tissue plus evidence of EBV infection. Treatment involves reducing immunosuppression whenever possible and use of antivirals. The condition is potentially serious as it can lead to non-Hodgkin's lymphoma in some cases.

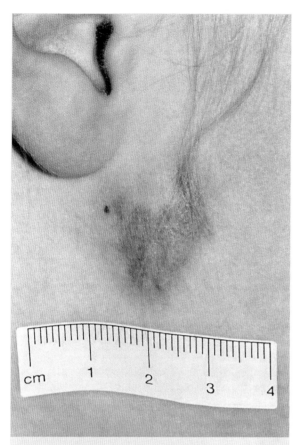

Fig. 25.7 Typical appearance of nontuberculous mycobacterial infection in the region of the right parotid tail.

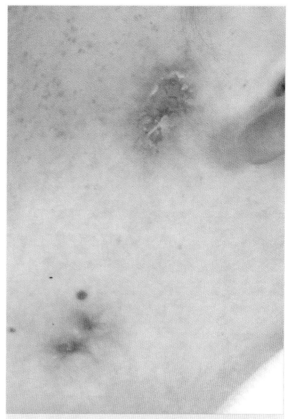

Fig. 25.8 Puckered scarring in the left parotid and submandibular regions 2 and a half years after presentation with nontuberculous mycobacterial infection. The parents declined any treatment.

HIV-Associated Lymphadenopathy

HIV-associated lymphadenopathy typically occurs soon after seroconversion in HIV infection. The lymphadenopathy is diffuse, generalized, and persistent for many months and may be associated with adenotonsillar hyperplasia. If stable, the lymphadenopathy can simply be observed, but a rapid change in the size of a node should raise the suspicion of non-Hodgkin's lymphoma, which is common in HIV infection.

Nontuberculous Mycobacterial Infection

NTM infection is surprisingly common and probably often misdiagnosed.[12] The organisms (*Mycobacterium bovis, M. scrofulaceum, M. avium intracellulare,* etc.) are widely present in the soil and in lime scale deposits in domestic plumbing. The condition is also known as ATM infection, something of a misnomer as it is far commoner than TB in western medical practice.

Although these organisms can cause serious disseminated infections in immunocompromised children (such as those with HIV), the vast majority of children with cer-

vical lymph node infection are immunocompetent. Toddlers are especially susceptible; the disease is very rare over 3 years of age, presumably because the child's immmune function has matured.

- The organisms enter through oral ingestion and pass to the regional lymph nodes, typically intraparotid and submandibular nodes.
- The child presents with a neck lump, and the overlying skin develops violet-red discoloration (▶ Fig. 25.7), with eventual skin breakdown in many cases.
- Some cases resolve without discharge, but in most, a sinus discharges for months before healing with a puckered scar (▶ Fig. 25.8).
- The whole process can take up to 3 years to complete.

The diagnosis is clinical on the basis of the characteristic skin appearance in a child who remains systemically well and apyrexial and whose history is longer than would be expected for a bacterial abscess (usually a few weeks). Aspiration should be avoided as it leads to skin breakdown and a discharging sinus. Incision and drainage should be avoided too for the same reason. In any event, even if a sample can be obtained for microbiology, culture

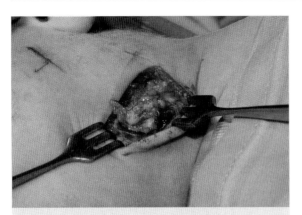

Fig. 25.9 Collar-stud abscess formation in nontuberculous mycobacterial infection. The abscess is formed from necrotic subcutaneous fat.

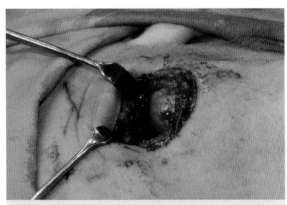

Fig. 25.10 Further dissection of the case shown in ▶ Fig. 25.5, deep to the deep fascia, reveals the underlying infected lymph node

takes 6 weeks and is only positive in a minority of cases. A chest X-ray is mandatory and ultrasound can be useful, although not specifically diagnostic. Tuberculin testing usually produces a weak positive response in individuals who have not been immunized with bacille Calmette–Guérin, and this can provide some partial support to the diagnosis.

> The organisms rapidly become resistant to monotherapy with either ciprofloxacin or clarithromycin, so in some centers, combined treatment with either of these drugs and antituberculous drugs is recommended.

Treatment of Nontuberculous Mycobacterial Infection

It is possible that some early infections with no (or minimal) skin changes may settle with antibiotic treatment, although there is one randomized trial suggesting that resolution occurs just as often by simply doing nothing.[13] The natural history of this condition is that it eventually resolves. The problem with antibiotics (or doing nothing) is that limited disease may progress and the ultimate cosmetic result may be worse (in about a third of cases). There is no real consensus at present on optimum treatment strategy, so it needs to be customized to the individual child and will vary with the experience and preference of the treating physician.[14]

For some infections, surgical excision is the treatment of choice if it is done early and the surgeon is sufficiently experienced in this sort of work to be sure that the risk of cranial nerve (especially facial nerve) damage is minimal. If surgery is planned, then a block dissection of lymph nodes suffices for limited disease, but a partial parotidectomy and supraomohyoid neck dissection are not uncom-

monly required for extensive disease. Discolored skin can usually be saved if it is in a cosmetically important site (such as the cheek) by curetting the subcutaneous abscess from the deep surface of the dermis—the skin color will eventually return to normal. Postoperative clarithromycin for 3 months is often prescribed but there is little evidence to support this. In cases where the skin has already broken down, skin must either be excised or the disease left alone to run its course.

> Prior to embarking on surgery, or prolonged medical therapy, parents need a detailed discussion regarding the natural history of the condition, the prospect of resolution without treatment, the likelihood of scarring, and the risk of facial nerve trauma. In skilled hands, good disease clearance can be achieved with a surgical scar that is less disfiguring than the result of untreated disease. This type of surgery is highly demanding (see Chapter 26) due to the very thin skin, the superficial position of the facial nerve, and the presence of a large mass of matted nodes often with overlying collar-stud abscesses in the subcutaneous plane (▶ Fig. 25.9, ▶ Fig. 25.10).

25.3.3 Noninfective Inflammatory Conditions

Rosai–Dorfman's Disease

Rosai–Dorfman's disease (sinus histiocytosis with massive lymphadenopathy) is an inflammatory condition of unknown etiology in which histiocytes (an old-fashioned term for macrophages and dendritic cells) accumulate in large numbers in lymph nodes and occasionally other

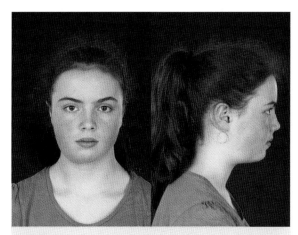

Fig. 25.11 Anteroposterior and lateral view of a mass in the submandibular region in a 14-year-old girl. At surgery, the submandibular gland was normal, and the mass was a group of matted nodes superficial to the gland. Histology confirmed Langerhans' cell histiocytosis.

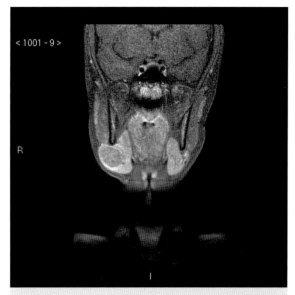

Fig. 25.12 Magnetic resonance imaging of the submandibular mass in ▶ Fig. 25.11. Langerhans' cell histiocytosis.

sites such as orbit, nose, oropharynx, and salivary glands. It typically causes massive bilateral cervical lymphadenopathy with fever and malaise in older children and young adults.[15] In most cases, it runs a prolonged but benign course with spontaneous regression. Excision biopsy of a lymph node is required to exclude lymphoma, and more extensive surgical debulking may be necessary for compression symptoms.

Langerhans' Cell Histiocytosis

Langerhans' cell histiocytosis (LCH) can also present with lymphadenopathy (▶ Fig. 25.11, ▶ Fig. 25.12). It tends to occur in the children under the age of 5 years and is characterized by clonal proliferation of Langerhans' cells and their accumulation in tissue. It is unclear whether this is a neoplastic or inflammatory process. LCH is a spectrum of disease from unifocal (previously known as *eosinophilic granuloma*), which presents as a solitary bone lesion, to multifocal multisystem disease (previously known as Letterer–Siwe's disease), which can involve bone lesions (often the mandible, causing jaw pain or loose teeth), skin eruptions (commonly on the scalp), pituitary gland lesions, chronic otitis media, and bone marrow involvement. Fever, lethargy, and weight loss may occur. LCH with cervical lymphadenopathy will usually be of the multifocal type. Diagnosis requires excision biopsy of an affected node for histological examination, together with radiology of the chest and any affected bones and MRI of the pituitary. Prognosis can be poor, especially in the under the age of 2 years, and aggressive treatment may be required with steroids and in severe cases cytotoxic chemotherapy. Mortality is approximately 10% overall, but 50% in multifocal disease in children under the age of 2 years.

Castleman's Disease

Castleman's disease presents as a mass of enlarged lymph nodes and its main importance is in the differential diagnosis of lymphoma. The diagnosis is histological. It is a B-cell lymphoproliferative disorder, and some cases are thought to have a viral cause. Children most often have the unicentric form, with nodes confined to one area of the neck. Surgical excision is all that is required. The multicentric condition is more common in adults and much more serious. It is associated with HIV infection in some cases and can run an aggressive course, requiring prolonged treatment with antivirals and monoclonal antibodies. For this reason, children with apparently unicentric disease should probably have imaging of the chest, abdomen, and pelvis, and HIV testing.

25.3.4 Tumors

Almost every child with a malignancy in the head and neck will have been falsely reassured that there is nothing serious going on by at least one doctor prior to the diagnosis being made. While malignancy in children is fortunately rare it does occur, and every clinician must remain vigilant to ensure prompt diagnosis.

> **i**
>
> Cancer remains the second commonest cause of death in childhood (the commonest being trauma), and 12% of all malignancies in childhood involve the head and neck.[16]

25

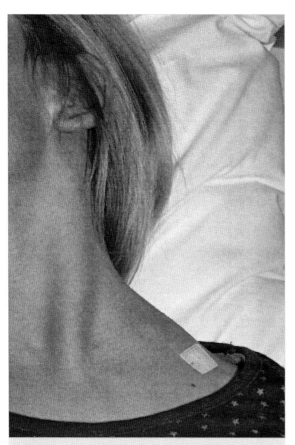

Fig. 25.13 Mass of rubbery lymph nodes in the left posterior triangle of a 10-year-old girl, typical of Hodgkin's disease.

Table 25.1 Ann Arbor staging system for Hodgkin's lymphoma

Stage	
I	One lymph node region or extralymphatic organ
II	Two or more lymph node regions on the same side of the diaphragm or one lymph node region and one extralymphatic organ on the same side of the diaphragm
III	Lymph node regions on both sides of the diaphragm plus an extralymphatic organ, the spleen or both
IV	Diffuse involvement of one or more extralymphatic organs with or without lymph node involvement
Suffixes	
A	No systemic symptoms
B	Weight loss, fever, or night sweats
E	Extralymphatic organ involvement
S	Splenic involvement

Hodgkin's Lymphoma

Hodgkin's lymphoma is the commonest type of lymphoma in children. It mostly occurs in teenagers and presents with painless firm lymphadenopathy (▶ Fig. 25.13). Previous EBV infection seems to be a risk factor. Splenic involvement, bone marrow infiltration, and superior vena cava obstruction can all occur. A staging system is shown in ▶ Table 25.1.

A good tissue sample (preferably a whole node) is required for diagnosis. Histologically, Hodgkin's is broadly divided into *classical* and *nonclassical*. The nonclassical form has a nodular lymphocyte predominant appearance, and the Reed-Sternberg's cells (which are the malignant cells in Hodgkin's lymphoma) express the B-cell marker CD20. It tends to run a less aggressive course.

Classical Hodgkin's is classified into the following subtypes:
* Lymphocyte depleted.
* Mixed cellularity.
* Nodular sclerosing.
* Lymphocyte predominant.

Treatment depends on subtype, stage, age and sex, but tends to include external beam radiotherapy and chemotherapy in some combination. Survival now exceeds 85% for advanced disease and well more than 95% for early disease with newer chemotherapy regimes and radiotherapy.[17]

Non-Hodgkin's Lymphomas

Non-Hodgkin's lymphomas make up a very diverse group of cancers that have little in common. In the latest World Health Organization classification system, the traditional Hodgkin's/non-Hodgkin's distinction has largely been

Large neck masses, rapidly growing masses, and supraclavicular masses are all particularly suspicious. In these circumstances, it is a matter of urgency to obtain good quality imaging (usually MRI) and a generous tissue biopsy. Most pediatric tumors appear as a densely packed mass of small, round, intensely staining cells on histology, so accurate diagnosis on cytology is difficult. For this reason, fine needle aspiration cytology is often unhelpful (with the exception of thyroid and salivary tumors where it can be very useful). A large piece of tissue, sent fresh to the laboratory, is often required for extensive immunohistochemistry studies. The oncology team should be involved as early as possible for children with suspicious lesions so that staging investigations (such as bone marrow aspiration) can be planned at the time of biopsy.

The commonest tumor types in children are as follows[16]:
* Lymphoma (27% of cases).
* Neural tumors (23%).
* Thyroid malignancies (21%).
* Soft-rissue sarcomas (12%).

Squamous cell carcinoma is very rare.

abandoned and 18 types of lymphoma are described, of which Hodgkin's is merely one. The remainder are classified largely according to the cell of origin (B cell, T cell, and NK cell) and surface markers such as CD5 and CD22.

While lymphadenopathy can occur, non-Hodgkin's lymphoma in children tends to be extranodal, presenting in sites such as the tonsil, larynx, or sinuses. It also tends to be of high grade, unlike the indolent disease often seen in adults. Progression can be very rapid in children, so prompt diagnosis and referral are essential. Treatment depends on histological type but will involve aggressive combination chemotherapy. Prognosis is generally very good, broadly comparable to that for Hodgkin's lymphoma.

Neurofibroma

A neurofibroma is a benign tumor of Schwann cells that most often occurs as part of *neurofibromatosis type 1* (NF1). NF1 is an autosomal dominant genetic condition, although 50% of cases are due to a new mutation rather than being inherited. The disease occurs due to a mutation in the tumor suppressor gene *NF1*. Diagnostic criteria for NF1 are listed in Box 25.3.

Box 25.3 Diagnostic Criteria for NF1

Any two of the following:
- Six or more café au lait spots > 5 mm (prepubertal) or > 15 mm (postpubertal).
- Two or more neurofibromas of any type or one of plexiform type.
- Specific osseous lesion with or without pseudoarthrosis.
- First-degree relative with NF1.
- Two or more Lisch nodules (iris hamartomas).
- Inguinal or axillary freckling.
- Optic glioma.

Neurofibromas occur in two types:
- Cutaneous.
- Plexiform.

The cutaneous ones form multiple unsightly lumps in the skin with no malignant potential, but in the context of the child presenting with a deep-seated neck mass, a plexiform neurofibroma is a more likely diagnosis. Plexiform lesions can arise from any nerve, but the vagus is common. In the early stages, they form discrete rounded masses but can go on to form huge, extensive, and widely infiltrating masses.

Surgical excision is the mainstay of treatment but recurrence is common. Extensive lesions are often better managed by observation unless surgical debulking is likely to improve cosmesis or function.

There is a 5% malignant transformation rate in plexiform lesions, forming a *malignant peripheral nerve sheath tumor*. These lesions are usually extensive and complete surgical excision difficult. Adjunctive radiotherapy and chemotherapy are required but recurrence and metastasis are common and prognosis is poor.

Neuroblastoma

Neuroblastoma is the most common malignancy of infancy with 40% occurring in the first year of life. The neck is an uncommon site, however. The tumor derives from neural crest cells in the sympathetic chain or adrenal medulla. Cervical lymph nodes may be involved in metastatic disease from a primary tumor in the abdomen or thorax, or the cervical sympathetic chain may be the primary site. Presentation is with a neck mass, Horner's syndrome, or compressive symptoms due to a retropharyngeal mass pressing on the upper aerodigestive tract. Diagnosis is based on histological examination, imaging, and urinary catecholamine metabolites. Surgery is ideal for localized lesions, but more advanced disease has a poor prognosis and combination therapy (usually chemotherapy) will be required.

Primitve Neuroectodermal Tumor

Primitive neuroectodermal tumor is a rare malignancy of neural crest origin that is biologically identical to *Ewing's sarcoma of bone*. It is very aggressive, and both chemotherapy and radiotherapy are used to control the disease.

Thyroid Nodules

Thyroid nodules are much less common in children than in adults, and a thyroid nodule in a child is much more likely to be malignant.

The most common cause of nodules in children is *follicular adenoma*, but the risk of malignancy in a nodule is at least 25%. *Papillary carcinoma* and *follicular carcinoma* are common (70 and 20% of malignant cases, respectively), but their behavior differs from that in adults. They are often more advanced at presentation (up to 90% have lymph node metastases, for example) but carry an excellent prognosis. Antecedent radiation exposure is a risk factor for thyroid tumors in children.

Diagnosis is based on history, examination, ultrasound, and fine needle aspiration cytology as in adults. Treatment is by means of total thyroidectomy, accompanied by a selective central and lateral neck dissection if nodes are involved. Well-differentiated thyroid malignancies in children are very sensitive to thyroid-stimulating hormone suppression with postoperative thyroid hormone, which may help to prevent recurrence.

Rhabdomyosarcoma

Rhabdomyosarcoma is a tumor of mesenchymal origin arising from primitive muscle progenitor cells. It is the most common soft-tissue sarcoma in children, and approximately 35% of cases occur in the head and neck. It is broadly grouped into embryonal and alveolar subtypes on histology: embryonal tumors are commoner, tend to occur at a younger age, and have a better prognosis. Presentation is usually as a mass, although metastases can occur through lymphatics to regional nodes or through blood to distant sites.

Head and neck primary sites are divided into the following:

- Orbital.
- Parameningeal (nasopharynx, middle ear, sinuses, and infratemporal fossa).
- Nonparameningeal (all other sites).

Parameningeal sites have the worse prognosis.

Treatment is with surgery whenever possible for localized disease, or more commonly chemoradiotherapy. Surgery also has a role for residual disease after chemoradiotherapy.

25.4 Key Points

- Cervical lymphadenopathy is very common and usually occurs due to reactive lymphoid hyperplasia. Tumors do occur, however, and the challenge is to diagnose them without delay and at the same time to avoid unnecessary excision biopsy for the majority of children with benign, self-limiting pathology.
- Large nodes (> 2 cm), supraclavicular nodes, rapidly growing nodes, and nodes with suspicious ultrasound features should be excised urgently for histology.
- Serology can be useful in diagnosing infectious causes such as EBV, *B. henselae*, and CMV, and thereby avoiding the need for excision biopsy.
- Fine needle aspiration cytology is most useful in thyroid and parotid masses, less so for cervical lymph node masses.
- The majority of cervical lymph nodes in children are small and fluctuate in size over time. They can be confidently diagnosed as reactive without the need for excision in most cases.
- Noninfective inflammatory causes of cervical lymphadenopathy include:
  - Kawasaki's disease—mainly affects children under the age of 5 years; characterized by cervical lymphadenopathy with high fever, erythema of mucosa, conjunctiva and skin, and swollen hands and feet; early treatment with immunoglobulin and aspirin is essential to minimize cardiac morbidity.
  - KFD—mainly affects adolescents; characterized by tender cervical lymphadenopathy, weight loss, skin rash, fever; benign, but needs biopsy to exclude other diagnoses.
  - PFAPA syndrome—mainly affects the young child; episodes of high fever occur every few weeks with aphthous ulcers and pharyngitis; management is supportive care with adenotonsillectomy if symptoms are especially disabling.

References

[1] Qureshi H, Ference E, Novis S, Pritchett CV, Smith SS, Schroeder JW. Trends in the management of pediatric peritonsillar abscess infections in the U.S., 2000–2009. Int J Pediatr Otorhinolaryngol. 2015; 79 (4):527–531

[2] Wikstén J, Blomgren K, Eriksson T, Guldfred L, Bratt M, Pitkäranta A. Variations in treatment of peritonsillar abscess in four Nordic countries. Acta Otolaryngol. 2014; 134(8):813–817

[3] Simon LM, Matijasec JW, Perry AP, Kakade A, Walvekar RR, Kluka EA. Pediatric peritonsillar abscess: quinsy ie versus interval tonsillectomy. Int J Pediatr Otorhinolaryngol. 2013; 77(8):1355–1358

[4] Grisaru-Soen G, Komisar O, Aizenstein O, Soudack M, Schwartz D, Paret G. Retropharyngeal and parapharyngeal abscess in children–epidemiology, clinical features and treatment. Int J Pediatr Otorhinolaryngol. 2010; 74(9):1016–1020

[5] Ozen S, Ruperto N, Dillon MJ, et al. EULAR/PReS endorsed consensus criteria for the classification of childhood vasculitides. Ann Rheum Dis. 2006; 65(7):936–941

[6] Kucukardali Y, Solmazgul E, Kunter E, Oncul O, Yildirim S, Kaplan M. Kikuchi-Fujimoto Disease: analysis of 244 cases. Clin Rheumatol. 2007; 26(1):50–54

[7] Tejesvi MV, Uhari M, Tapiainen T, et al. Tonsillar microbiota in children with PFAPA (periodic fever, aphthous stomatitis, pharyngitis, and adenitis) syndrome. Eur J Clin Microbiol Infect Dis. 2016; 35(6):963–970

[8] Garavello W, Pignataro L, Gaini L, Torretta S, Somigliana E, Gaini R. Tonsillectomy in children with periodic fever with aphthous stomatitis, pharyngitis, and adenitis syndrome. J Pediatr. 2011; 159(1):138–142

[9] Wurster VM, Carlucci JG, Feder HM, Jr, Edwards KM. Long-term follow-up of children with periodic fever, aphthous stomatitis, pharyngitis, and cervical adenitis syndrome. J Pediatr. 2011; 159(6):958–964

[10] Herzog LW. Prevalence of lymphadenopathy of the head and neck in infants and children. Clin Pediatr (Phila). 1983; 22(7):485–487

[11] Papakonstantinou O, Bakantaki A, Paspalaki P, Charoulakis N, Gourtsoyiannis N. High-resolution and color Doppler ultrasonography of cervical lymphadenopathy in children. Acta Radiol. 2001; 42(5):470–476

[12] Soni I, De Groote MA, Dasgupta A, Chopra S. Challenges facing the drug discovery pipeline for non-tuberculous mycobacteria. J Med Microbiol. 2016; 65(1):1–8

[13] Lindeboom JA. Conservative wait-and-see therapy versus antibiotic treatment for nontuberculous mycobacterial cervicofacial lymphadenitis in children. Clin Infect Dis. 2011; 52(2):180–184

[14] Mahadevan M, Neeff M, Van Der Meer G, Baguley C, Wong WK, Gruber M. Non-tuberculous mycobacterial head and neck infections in children: analysis of results and complications for various treatment modalities. Int J Pediatr Otorhinolaryngol. 2016; 82:102–106

[15] Pulsoni A, Anghel G, Falcucci P, et al. Treatment of sinus histiocytosis with massive lymphadenopathy (Rosai-Dorfman disease): report of a case and literature review. Am J Hematol. 2002; 69(1):67–71

[16] Albright JT, Topham AK, Reilly JS. Pediatric head and neck malignancies: US incidence and trends over 2 decades. Arch Otolaryngol Head Neck Surg. 2002; 128(6):655–659

[17] Fermé C, Eghbali H, Meerwaldt JH, et al. EORTC-GELA H8 Trial. Chemotherapy plus involved-field radiation in early-stage Hodgkin's disease. N Engl J Med. 2007; 357(19):1916–1927

VI

26 Salivary Gland Disorders in Childhood

Michael Gleeson

26.1 Introduction

In days gone by, almost every child would have experienced an acute salivary gland disorder before reaching adult life. Nowadays, as a result of widespread mumps vaccination, acute viral parotitis is extremely uncommon in the developed world. The presentation of a patient with acute unilateral parotid enlargement, now usually an adult, causes confusion and often results in a number of unwarranted investigations before the correct diagnosis is considered. It is humbling that any general practitioner living 50 years ago would have made the diagnosis immediately at a glance. The salivary diseases that prevail today in the pediatric age group are relatively uncommon. Some are extremely rare. Their management can be very difficult and, if surgery is involved, is better undertaken by a clinician with special training and a special interest.

26.2 Congenital Disorders

26.2.1 Anatomical Anomalies

Aplasia and Dysplasia

Congenital anomalies of the salivary glands are very uncommon. Aplasia of the major salivary glands and atresia of their ducts has been described, as has polycystic disease of the parotid glands. Polycystic disease may be unilateral or bilateral and presents with intermittent swelling of the parotid gland, particularly at meal times, only to subside shortly afterward. There is rarely any need for acute treatment of polycystic parotid disease and most cases have little impact on the child's life.

Ranula

The more common developmental salivary disorder is a mucous retention cyst of the floor of the mouth called a *ranula*. Occasionally, these cysts are found in the newborn but more typically in toddlers and preschool children.

They appear as a superficial translucent swelling in the floor of the mouth with a frog's belly appearance, hence their name. Ranulae usually lie just to one side of the midline. If sufficiently large, a ranula can extend well into the anterior triangle of the neck, displace the tongue upward, and interfere with swallowing (cervical or "plunging" ranula). Occasionally, these cysts rupture spontaneously or, as a result of unnoticed trauma, release thick viscid mucus. Recurrence is then common.

The diagnosis is clinical but imaging (ultrasound, magnetic resonance imaging [MRI], if needed) can demonstrate the limits of the swelling and help to plan treatment, particularly if there is extension into the neck. Surgical management was traditionally by simple generous marsupialization, opening the sac and suturing the edges to the adjacent normal mucosa, but recurrence was not uncommon and most surgeons now advocate a more thorough dissection with delivery and complete excision of the ranula. Many advise excision of the sublingual gland as well to further reduce the risk of recurrence.

26.2.2 Congenital Tumors and Hamartomas

Parotid Gland Hemangioma

Hemangiomas may be present at birth, in the first year of life, and certainly before the age of 10 years. Girls are affected more frequently than boys. The tumor presents as a diffuse soft swelling of the parotid gland and, if particularly large, appears bluish. Other salivary glands are hardly ever involved. Spontaneous regression sometimes with phlebolith formation is well recognized. These hemangiomas are partly or predominantly cavernous or are mixed hemangiomas. They follow the expected natural history of hemangiomas in that they grow to a peak in size and then regress, so the long-term prognosis is excellent.

Often these tumors progress rapidly in the first year of life and can cause extreme anxiety. Both parents and doctors may fear that the child has an aggressive malignancy. Imaging—ideally with MRI scanning under the supervision of an experienced pediatric radiologist—is essential and has greatly improved management and has reduced the need for biopsy as the diagnosis can usually be made with near certainty on MRI scanning. Parents can then be reassured that this is a benign condition with an excellent prognosis.

The discovery that childhood hemangiomas respond to propranolol has transformed the management of this condition (see Chapters 21 and 24). Children are now typically managed medically at least until the proliferative phase is over. Many will not require any further intervention, and if surgical treatment is needed at all, it should be delayed for as long as possible and certainly until the child is at least 5 years old.

26

Total excision of parotid hemangiomas is curative, but almost never needed nowadays. The surgeon who undertakes this type of work must have significant expertise. It is not difficult to imagine the difficulties that might be encountered operating on such a vascular tumor in close proximity to the facial nerve.

> ℹ️
>
> It is important not to confuse parotid hemangiomas with lymphangiomas as the management and expectations in terms of natural history are very different. Local sclerosants are not appropriate for hemangiomas. Systemic corticosteroids have been reported to control rapidly growing hemangiomas, but medical management with propranolol to reduce the proliferative phase of development of these lesions is now widely accepted as best practice.[1]

Propranolol is best given under the supervision of a pediatrician with careful monitoring of the cardiovascular effects, particularly in the early stages of treatment. In very aggressive hemangiomas, with particularly aggressive histology and if the lesion is encroaching on important structures (e.g., the orbit), a course of treatment with cytotoxic agents such as vincristine or methotrexate can be considered. This would be under the supervision of a pediatric oncologist.

Lymphangioma

Presentation and Management

These congenital, often multiloculated, lymphatic malformations (formerly known as cystic hygroma) are commonly found in the neck and frequently involve or infiltrate the parotid and submandibular salivary glands. Two main types, macrocystic and microcystic, are recognized, but mixed types are also seen. The cysts contain lymph and are now recognized as part of a spectrum of vascular malformations. They are not true neoplasms (see Chapter 24).

Lymphangiomas tend to increase in size over time and are subject to repeated episodes of infection that require antibiotic therapy and take a considerable time to respond. Management is discussed in Chapter 24. Essentially, it is either by expectant treatment, surgery, or sclerotherapy, often under the supervision of an interventional radiologist, or by a combination of any of these strategies. A number of injectable chemical agents, for example, biological products such as OK432 (see Giguere et al)[2] or alcohol, bleomycin, and doxycycline, have been used in attempts to cause sclerosis. They can be quite successful in macrocystic but less so in microcystic disease, presumably because they do not disperse evenly throughout the often multiple small cysts. Injection is best given

under the careful supervision of an interventional radiologist with good quality imaging and will usually require general anesthesia. For large lesions, a vigorous inflammatory reaction can ensue in the early postoperative period and the child may need to be managed in a high dependency unit or on occasion in a pediatric intensive care unit with endotracheal intubation. Surgery can be extremely challenging.

> ℹ️
>
> These lesions do not respect tissue planes and it is easy to inflict cranial nerve palsies (▶ Fig. 26.1).

Prenatal Diagnosis

Congenital anomalies of the head and neck, including lymphangiomas, are sometimes diagnosed by prenatal maternal ultrasonography, supplemented as needed by MRI scanning. They can be extremely large and may threaten the integrity of the airway.

> ℹ️
>
> Mothers of babies with large lymphangiomas detected at prenatal scanning are best delivered at major tertiary centers.

The newborn baby's airway can be secured while the placental circulation is still functioning, either by endotracheal intubation or, in extreme cases, by tracheotomy. This technique, ex utero intrapartum treatment (EXIT), can permit definitive treatment of babies who would otherwise not survive much beyond birth.[3]

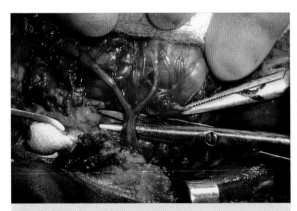

Fig. 26.1 An extensive macrocystic lymphangioma in the deep lobe of the right parotid gland. The facial nerve needed to be mobilized to remove the lesion.

26.2.3 Pharyngeal (Branchial) Arch Anomalies

First pharyngeal or "branchial" arch anomalies are uncommon and may present with a cutaneous sinus or fistula on the face or neck beneath the pinna overlying the parotid gland, usually between the tragus and the angle of the jaw. The superior opening, if present, may be either in front of the tragus or in the floor of the external auditory canal, usually at the junction of cartilaginous and bony part. While the superficial pits are noticeable at birth, they become more prominent and noticeable with each and every subsequent episode of infection. Aural discharge synchronous with purulent discharge from the cutaneous opening indicates that there is an opening within the external ear canal (see Chapter 24).

As recurrent infections become more frequent, surgical resection of the fistulous track or sinus becomes inevitable. A lazy "S" parotidectomy incision and approach may be used as the track runs a variable course often deep to the inferior division and branches of the facial nerve.

> **i**
>
> Frequent infections can make dissection from the nerve difficult and increase the likelihood of facial nerve morbidity. As with all parotid surgery, intraoperative facial nerve monitoring should be mandatory.

The internal opening of the fistula must be removed as well and occasionally is found to open into a duplicate cartilaginous canal lying inferior to the external auditory canal (▶ Fig. 26.2).

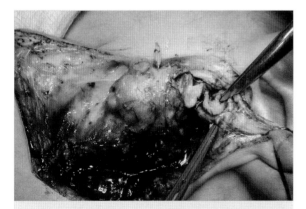

Fig. 26.2 Resection of first branchial arch anomalies. The fistulous external opening has been marked. The scissors point to the internal opening within the external auditory canal that has been excised in continuity with the anomaly. The lower division of the main trunk of the facial nerve can be seen running immediately posterior and deep to the track.

26.2.4 Parotitis in Cystic Fibrosis

Like other exocrine mucus-secreting glands, salivary glands are affected by this autosomal recessive disease. Abnormal mucus produced by the glands obstructs their ducts and causes progressive damage to the related parenchyma. The parotid gland, which mainly produces serous secretion, is less affected than the submandibular gland.

26.3 Acquired Salivary Gland Disorders

26.3.1 Salivary Gland Trauma

Mucous Extravasation Cysts

These mucoceles are relatively common and usually caused by trauma that tears the duct of a minor salivary gland allowing mucus to extravasate into the surrounding tissues. The commonest site is the lower lip, but these cysts are sometimes found in buccal mucosa or in the floor of the mouth. They present as soft, dome-shaped, swellings with a bluish hue. They are rarely more than a centimeter in diameter. Mucous extravasation cysts inevitably require excision as they do not resolve spontaneously.

Sialolithiasis (Salivary Gland Stones)

Though much more common in adults, particularly the elderly, salivary calculi may occasionally develop in children and be the cause of duct obstruction. The submandibular gland is the most frequently affected gland and this is thought to be due to its relatively mucoid secretion and the higher calcium concentration of its saliva.

The child may complain of intermittent pain that gets worse at mealtimes, making them reluctant to eat certain foods that provoke increased salivation. There may be a visible swelling in the submandibular triangle that slowly subsides. The gland will be tender to palpate and the calculus is often visible in the floor of the mouth close to the duct orifice. If the gland becomes infected, pus may exude from the duct, and a local lymphadenopathy may be apparent.

Salivary gland calculi are normally radiopaque and can be imaged using standard plain film techniques. If it is possible to milk the calculus toward the duct orifice, relief of obstruction can be achieved by a simple ductotomy or dilatation. In the young, this might necessitate a general aaesthetic, but older children could be amenable to this procedure under local anesthetic. In adults, calculi deeper in the gland can be retrieved using endoscopic techniques. At present, endoscopic techniques are being used to manage juvenile recurrent parotitis and this minimally invasive method is increasingly applied to calculus retrieval.[4,5,6]

26

26.3.2 Inflammatory Disorders

Viral Sialadenitis (Mumps)

A number of viruses may involve the salivary glands but the classical cause of viral sialadenitis is mumps caused by the mumps virus, a paramyxovirus, which can affect many glands other than the parotids and also the neural tissue. Infection is probably by droplet spread and is thus very contagious. The incubation period is typically 18 to 21 days. After a prodromal period of malaise and anorexia, there is characteristically swelling of one or both parotid glands and fever. The parotid swelling is tense and painful. Sometimes, the submandibular glands may also be affected.

The diagnosis is not difficult and can be made on the basis of clinical signs only, especially when there has been a recent outbreak of the disease.

> With widespread immunity as a result of measles, mumps, and rubella (MMR) vaccination, mumps is nowadays sometimes not considered in the differential and it may take days to make the diagnosis on the basis of exclusion of other conditions. Simple blood tests will fail to show the characteristic neutrophil leukocytosis that is present with other forms of parotitis, and the precise diagnosis can be confirmed by serology using enzyme-linked immunosorbent assay (ELISA).

Mumps is usually a mild, self-limiting disease. If contracted after puberty, approximately 20% of males with mumps develop orchitis, but sterility rarely results. Other possibilities include oophoritis or pancreatitis. Serious complications include aseptic meningitis, encephalitis, and permanent, usually unilateral, profound sensorineural hearing loss.

There is no specific treatment, and vaccination against mumps is therefore important for children over 1 year of age to avoid the risk of deafness. In Britain, the recommended preparation is MMR triple vaccine, which is more than 95% effective.

Cat-Scratch Disease

Cat-scratch disease is common in the United States and less commonly seen in Europe. The infection follows a scratch or bite from a cat and is caused by the gram-negative bacterium *Bartonella henselae* or *Bartonella quintana*. The event that introduced the infection is often not remembered but usually takes place 2 to 4 weeks previously. A small papule or pustule forms at the site and is associated with a regional lymphadenopathy in the neck. The child may develop parotid swelling and it has been known for a facial palsy to develop which can confuse the situation. There is normally mild pyrexia, malaise, muscular aches and pains, decreased appetite, and sometimes conjunctivitis. The infection is usually mild and self-limiting and does not require any specific treatment. Much more serious complications can very rarely include encephalopathy and endocarditis.

The diagnosis is made on clinical signs and on the histological appearances of biopsied tissue. More recent tests using the polymerase chain reaction are extremely sensitive.

Granulomatous Disease

Tuberculous Parotitis

Tuberculosis is a rare cause of sialadenitis that is seen from time to time. The parotid glands are the most commonly affected site. The infection may involve the intraglandular lymph nodes or the gland parenchyma. It is far less common than nontuberculous mycobacteria but needs to be considered, particularly in children at high risk. These include especially those with immune system compromise, and human immunodeficiency virus (HIV) and those from a background of extreme poverty and deprivation. *Mycobacterium tuberculosis* is the cause of tuberculous sialadenitis.

Nontuberculous Mycobacteria

The incidence of this condition is increasing greatly in Europe. The child will present with a tumor-like swelling of the neck, often in the region of the parotid or the submandibular gland. The parotid gland in children has a much higher content of lymphoid tissue, as distinct from salivary parenchymal tissue, than in the adult, hence the tendency for cervical lymphadenopathy in this area. Affected children are generally 18 months to 3 years old. The skin may develop a characteristic violet hue and may break down. Children are usually well with no fever and no pain.

Diagnosis is largely clinical but can be confirmed histologically when the characteristic granulomas are seen. Aspiration cytology usually produces a thin green fluid that often shows no more than lymphocytes on cytological examination. Culture is often unhelpful.

> The condition is entirely benign and self-limiting with inevitable regression of the lesions over a period of a year or so.

Management is discussed in Chapter 25.

Human Immunodeficiency Virus Associated Parotitis

Generalized enlargement of the parotid glands, persistent lymphadenopathy of the parotid nodes, or the development of cysts with benign lymphoepithelial lesions is seen in HIV-positive children. The other major salivary glands may also be affected. Some children may also have a dry mouth. The diagnosis can be confirmed by ultrasound, computed tomography (CT), or MRI combined with fine needle aspiration biopsy to exclude other causes.

These children are best managed with antiretroviral medication and close observation with supportive care to prevent or minimize the effects of a dry mouth on the developing dentition. In some children, aspiration of enlarging cysts can be helpful and lessen the aesthetic impact. Fortunately, more radical therapies such as radiotherapy and surgery are rarely indicated.[7]

Recurrent Parotitis

This disorder is of unknown etiology even though it is considered to be infective, possibly caused by the Epstein–Barr virus. The main clinical features are recurrent, tender swellings of one or both parotid glands. The interval between attacks may be six or more months and individual attacks typically last for days to weeks. Ultrasonic examination shows duct dilatation. There may be considerable adverse effects on parotid function.[8]

In children, the disease has usually been reported to resolve spontaneously at or near puberty. Management is expectant unless the symptoms are extremely disabling. It can present in younger children, but typically they are over 10 years of age.

Antibiotics appear to shorten the duration of attacks and are the usual first line of treatment. They are repeated as necessary until there is spontaneous resolution. Salivary gland endoscopy with dilatation of developing ductal strictures together with lavage, with or without hydrocortisone, shows promise and may prevent more severe glandular damage.[4] Very occasionally and in severe cases, widespread parenchymal destruction will happen with fistula formation through the skin, and resection of the affected parotid gland may have to be considered. If so, a total conservative parotidectomy would be necessary and with it increased potential facial nerve morbidity.

26.3.3 Pediatric Salivary Gland Tumors

The most common salivary gland tumors of early infancy or the neonatal period are hemangiomas. In older children, those over 10 years of age, the most common type of epithelial tumor is the benign pleomorphic adenoma, but approximately 50% of salivary tumors in children prove to be malignant. This is a much higher relative proportion of malignant tumors than is seen in the adult population. Of the malignant tumors, mucoepidermoid carcinomas and acinic cell carcinomas are the most frequent. As in adults, there is a female preponderance, and tumors in the parotid gland outnumber those in the submandibular and minor glands by a factor of nearly 2:1 (▶ Table 26.1).

In probably the largest series reported, Shikhani and Johns[9] analyzed the relative incidence of different histological tumor types among 472 previously reported cases and among their own cases of childhood salivary gland tumors. No fewer than 50% were malignant, and they confirmed that malignant salivary gland tumors were proportionately more frequent than in adults. These malignant tumors were mainly in older children and presented more frequently in the parotid glands. Of the 229 benign tumors, pleomorphic adenomas formed 86.6%,

26

Table 26.1 Distribution of juvenile salivary gland tumors by site and type

Tumor type	Site					
	Parotid (%)	Submandibular (%)	Sublingual (%)	Intraoral (%)	Lip (%)	Unknown (%)
Pleomorphic	26 (55)	14 (29.8)	0	4 (8.5)	0	3 (6.4)
Warthin's	1 (100)					
Monomorphic	1 (100)					
Mucoepidermoid	3 (50)	2 (33)		1 (17)		
Acinic cell	1 (100)					
Adenoid cystic	1 (100)					
Adenocarcinoma				1 (50)	1 (50)	
Undifferentiated	1 (33)				2 (67)	
Unclassified	1 (100)					
Others	9 (90)	1 (10)				
Total number	44 (61)	17 (24)		6 (8)	3 (3.5)	3 (3.5)

Source: British Salivary Gland Tumor Panel data, 1986.

whereas of the 243 malignant tumors, mucoepidermoid carcinomas comprised 49.6%, acinic cell carcinomas 12.2%, undifferentiated carcinomas 8.9%, and adenoid cystic carcinomas 6.5%. They also summarized the treatment and outcome of 272 cases where sufficient data were available and noted that the recurrence rate of pleomorphic adenomas after enucleation was more than 39% but much less, 19.5%, after superficial parotidectomy. These exceptionally high recurrence rates were probably a reflection of the difficulties of operating on small glands by inexperienced surgeons unfamiliar with the surgical anatomy of the facial nerve. Two of these recurrent tumors underwent transition to highly aggressive carcinomas. Overall, 32 patients (11.4%) including one who had had a pleomorphic adenoma died from their tumors—a very salutary lesson.

> **i**
>
> The diagnosis of salivary gland tumors in children should be made in exactly the same way as for an adult patient.

In other words, take a good clinical history, examine the neck carefully, and perform fine needle aspiration cytology if there are good local facilities for this. Arrange appropriate imaging with CT, MRI, and ultrasound. Sadly, these tumors are so uncommon that there is often a delay in diagnosis, the parents being inappropriately and incorrectly reassured that their child merely has an enlarged lymph node. Rarely periparotid tumors that have developed from the overlying hair matrix of the skin may be encountered. These may be indistinguishable from parotid tumors on clinical examination and only diagnosable prior to surgery by aspiration cytology and imaging (▶ Fig. 26.3). More unfortunately, some children with

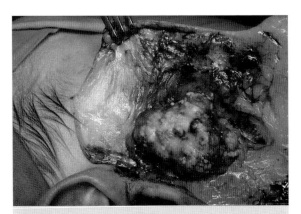

Fig. 26.3 This pilomatrixoma had developed slowly over a period of 3 months and was indistinguishable on clinical examination from a suppurating lymph node. The child had received several courses of antibiotic therapy before the diagnosis was made on the basis of an aspiration biopsy.

parotid tumors will already have undergone inadequate surgery by the time definitive treatment is started, often an open biopsy that might lead to increased subsequent morbidity caused by seeding into the surrounding tissues.

> **i**
>
> Once the diagnosis has been confirmed, the tumor should be excised in exactly the same way as one would manage an adult.

- For benign tumors, a superficial parotidectomy will suffice.
- When a malignant tumor is present, a total conservative parotidectomy is necessary.
- In the very rare situation where a malignant tumor has already caused a facial palsy, a radical parotidectomy would be required with adjuvant radiotherapy.

26.4 Pediatric Parotidectomy

While resection of the parotid gland in children has already been mentioned for developmental disorders, for example, first pharyngeal (branchial) arch anomalies, lymphangioma, and vascular abnormalities, the consequences of poorly performed surgery are so great that further discussion is warranted. Parotid surgery is slightly more difficult in children than in adults for the following reasons:

- The facial nerve is smaller and courses more superficially within the parotid in children than in adults. This is partly due to incomplete development of the mastoid process, which leaves the stylomastoid foramen and its contents, the facial nerve, relatively unprotected at the base of the skull. As a result, the nerve may be encountered at a very early stage in the surgical procedure and can be inadvertently damaged (▶ Fig. 26.4).
- The parotid tissue may have been subject to recurrent or chronic infection as with pharyngeal (branchial) arch anomalies, vascular malformations, recurrent parotitis, and granulomatous infection. Over time, the gland will have become densely scarred and the plane of dissection around the facial nerve almost nonexistent. In this situation, iatrogenic facial weakness or paralysis is a very significant risk and is a complication about which parents should be very clearly forewarned.
- Lesions such as vascular malformations are either so diffuse or bleed so easily that surgical landmarks can be lost and accidental heat damage to the facial nerve from bipolar coagulation is an ever-present risk.

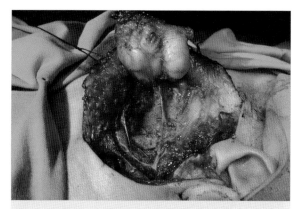

Fig. 26.4 This congenital mass in the parotid gland had been identified at birth and grew rapidly such that it doubled in size during the first 3 months of life. An aspiration biopsy proved difficult to interpret and there was concern that the tumor might be malignant. There was no facial weakness. The tumor, a sialolipoma, was removed completely and without complication in this neonate. The facial nerve trunk was extremely superficial as the mastoid process had yet to develop.

> ℹ
>
> The use of intraoperative facial nerve monitoring for this type of surgery cannot be recommended too strongly and should be a standard of care. Not only does it help predict the impending proximity of the facial nerve trunk, but it also helps minimize trauma to its finer branches, which can be irrevocably damaged all too easily. It hardly needs repeating that facial palsy is a devastating handicap to carry through life for the child, the parents, and the surgeon.

26.5 Sialorrhea (Drooling)

> ℹ
>
> Sialorrhea (drooling) is a distressing complaint most often seen in children with neurologic dysfunction, typically cerebral palsy. The fundamental disorder is that of neuromuscular incoordination, children being unable to swallow or control their saliva rather than producing too much.

It is easy to underestimate the social impact of this condition. Parents of severely affected children may need to change their child's clothing many times every day or submit their child to long-term hospitalization. In severe cases, aspiration is an added risk.

26.5.1 Multidisciplinary Management

A multidisciplinary approach to assessment and management is essential. Speech and language therapists (SALTs), physical therapists, dental surgeons, and otolaryngologists can all make valuable contributions. Surgery should only be contemplated after a period of intense conservative therapy and prolonged observation. Some children may improve spontaneously with further development, and surgical intervention at an early age cannot be justified. Close attention should be paid to the correction of abnormal body posture, dental malocclusion, and nasal obstruction. All of these worsen drooling but are easily correctable. Such capacity as there is to initiate and complete swallowing should be maximized by appropriate sensory training.

In some patients, behavioral modification by auditory evoked conditioned reflexes using commercially available devices was found to be helpful. The so-called dribbling boxes consisted of a collecting box containing a sensor. The box was placed beneath the child's chin and bleeped each time saliva dripped into it. These devices are less frequently used nowadays and postural and behavioral modification is much more often managed under the supervision of a SALT with a special interest in this type of work (see Chapter 5).

26.5.2 Pharmacotherapy

Pharmacotherapy with anticholinergic drugs, for example, hyoscine, may be useful particularly when administered by a transdermal skin "patch," but the side effects of these drugs (constipation, urinary retention, impaired visual accommodation and often, agitation) often compound the patient's troubles.

In recent years, the use of botulinum toxin A injected into the salivary glands has been found to be effective. Two to three nonoverlapping points on the parotid and submandibular glands are injected taking great care not to administer too much toxin and to ensure that the toxin is injected into the gland and not the superficial tissues.

> ℹ
>
> Ultrasound guidance is advocated particularly for the submandibular gland as it almost eliminates the risk of temporary facial weakness.

It must be remembered that botulinum toxin A preparations vary in their strength and that Botox (Allergan) or Xeomin (Merz Pharma GmbH & Co) is three times stronger

26

than Dysport (Biophar, Ltd). A total dose of 22.5 units of Botox/Xeomin is considered appropriate for the parotid gland and 15 units for the submandibular gland.

26.5.3 Surgical Management

Surgical approaches to the control of drooling that have been proposed range from excision of the major glands and denervation procedures to relocation or ligation of the salivary ducts. The submandibular salivary glands, as the major contributors to resting salivary flow, have received most attention in this respect.

> Naturally all operations have to be undertaken bilaterally. This is therefore a serious consideration in treatment planning. These procedures are major undertakings even in typically developing children, let alone those with neurologic disabilities.

Surgical Approaches to Sialorrhea

A number of different surgical strategies have been tried. These include the following:
- Denervation by chorda tympani section.
- Tympanic plexus interruption through a tympanotomy approach.

This provided a satisfactory outcome in only approximately 50% of patients and left children with temporary hearing loss and permanent loss of taste on the anterior two-thirds of the tongue. Bilateral resection of the salivary glands was far too drastic and had significant potential facial nerve morbidity, but in extreme cases, bilateral submandibular gland excision may still be considered.

Nowadays, good results can be obtained by relocation (transposition) of the submandibular salivary gland ducts (▶ Fig. 26.5). The ducts are dissected out through a transoral approach and repositioned in the tonsillar fossa. This procedure can be undertaken bilaterally and simultaneously. It avoids an external scar and any facial nerve morbidity.
- Under general anesthesia with a nasal endotracheal tube and with the surgeon seated at the head of the table, an elliptical island of mucosa is incised around the submandibular papillae.
- Using blunt dissection, the individual ducts and lingual nerves are identified.
- The island is then divided and a submucosal tunnel created on each side of the floor of the mouth to open at the base of each tonsillar fossa approximately 1 cm behind the anterior tonsillar pillar.
- The mucosal cuff surrounding each duct orifice is passed through this tunnel and sutured in the tonsillar fossa.

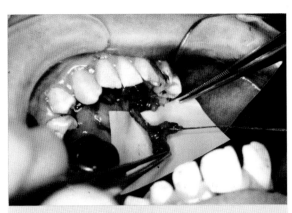

Fig. 26.5 Transposition of submandibular salivary ducts for sialorrhea. The duct, together with a triangle of surrounding mucosa, has been dissected and mobilized ready for relocation/transposition posteriorly.

Most patients develop swelling of the floor of the mouth that normally subsides within 2 to 3 days. Intravenous access for fluid replacement and drug administration is frequently necessary postoperatively until a normal diet is established and patients can take drugs by mouth. This is rarely necessary for more than 24 to 48 hours as the majority of patients are fit for discharge home by the second or third postoperative day. These children will often be under the care of a pediatrician and many will need appropriate perioperative medical management, including drug control of epilepsy.

Complications of Surgical Management of Sialorrhea

Complications are not common, but early ranula formation and submandibular duct obstruction have been reported. Many surgeons feel that simultaneous excision of the sublingual glands at the time of the original surgery reduces this risk. Late obstruction of relocated submandibular ducts may be associated with extremely large tonsils, especially in children with recurrent tonsillitis. Surgical removal of these glands can be difficult because of adhesions.

Outcomes of Surgical Management of Sialorrhea

Reduction in the severity of drooling should be achieved in at least 80% of patients, but that is not synonymous with the cessation of sialorrhea. Saliva is still present on the chins of up to 70% of those cases deemed by the surgeon to be successful. Success is therefore very difficult to assess and greatly depends on the expectations of the patient or parents. At one extreme, a patient may be happy with a minor improvement in drooling despite persistence of saliva on the chin; at the other extreme, the patient may cease drooling as a result of removal of the major glands but be made unhappy by the discomfort of a dry mouth.

Surgical treatment should be tailored for each particular patient and not undertaken until all other potential strategies have been properly addressed and tried. There is always much to commend a single surgical intervention customized for the individual child. Patients with incessant, drenching sialorrhea should therefore be considered for more radical therapy than those less severely affected. Whatever the procedure adopted, it is important, first, to counsel patients or parents that it may be a major undertaking and, second, to caution them against any excessive hopes of total cure.

26.6 Key Points

- A confident diagnosis of parotid hemangioma can be made on the basis of imaging characteristics alone. Few need to be resected as they tend regress over time and most of those that do not can be managed medically with propranolol. Some aggressive hemangiomas will require cytotoxic therapy.
- Surgical intervention for pharyngeal arch anomalies has to be carefully timed. Anomalies that have been subject to frequent infections are difficult to remove completely and there is an increased risk of inadvertently damaging adjacent structures, for example, the facial nerve.
- Consider mumps as the cause of unilateral parotid enlargement in an unwell child. Undertake serological tests early in the illness.

- Tuberculous parotitis is likely to become more common as migration increases from poorer countries and war-stricken zones. Some of those infected may have immune system compromise.
- Pediatric parotidectomy should be undertaken by specialist surgeons and not by the occasional operator. Facial nerve monitoring is essential.
- The drooling child needs a multidisciplinary approach using the expertise of a large number of different clinicians.

References

[1] Marsciani A, Pericoli R, Alaggio R, Brisigotti M, Vergine G. Massive response of severe infantile hepatic hemangioma to propanolol. Pediatr Blood Cancer. 2010; 54(1):176

[2] Giguere CM, Bauman NM, Sato Y, et al. Treatment of lymphangiomas with OK432 (Picabanil) sclerotherapy:a prospective multi-institutional trial. Arch Otolaryngol Head Neck Surg. 2002; 128(10):1137–1144

[3] Lazar DA, Olutoye OO, Moise KJ, Jr, et al. Ex-utero intrapartum treatment procedure for giant neck masses—fetal and maternal outcomes. J Pediatr Surg. 2011; 46(5):817–822

[4] Nahlieli O, Shacham R, Shlesinger M, Eliav E. Juvenile recurrent parotitis: a new method of diagnosis and treatment. Pediatrics. 2004; 114 (1):9–12

[5] Rosbe KW, Milev D, Chang JL. Effectiveness and costs of sialendoscopy in pediatric patients with salivary gland disorders. Laryngoscope. 2015; 125(12):2805–2809

[6] Ramakrishna J, Strychowsky J, Gupta M, Sommer DD. Sialendoscopy for the management of juvenile recurrent parotitis: a systematic review and meta-analysis. Laryngoscope. 2015; 125(6):1472–1479

[7] Dave SP, Pernas FG, Roy S. The benign lymphoepithelial cyst and a classification system for lymphocytic parotid gland enlargement in the pediatric HIV population. Laryngoscope. 2007; 117(1):106–113

[8] Xie LS, Pu YP, Zheng LY, Yu CQ, Wang ZJ, Shi H. Function of the parotid gland in juvenile recurrent parotitis: a case series. Br J Oral Maxillofac Surg. 2016; 54(3):270–274

[9] Shikhani AH, Johns ME. Tumors of the major salivary glands in children. Head Neck Surg. 1988; 10(4):257–263

26

27 Ear, Nose, and Throat Problems in Cleft Lip and Palate

Ravi K. Sharma and Simon van Eeden

27.1 Introduction

Children with cleft palate will present to ear, nose, and throat (ENT) surgeons in two ways. First, the incidence of otitis media with effusion (OME) is higher in children with cleft palate resulting from Eustachian tube dysfunction. For similar reasons, they may have more persistent problems with retraction pockets and cholesteatomas. Second, these children may present with challenging airways (Pierre Robin [PR] sequence). The nasal deformity arising from poor septal support may lead to both cosmetic and functional problems.

This chapter discusses the different types of cleft palate and goes on to describe the common syndromes associated with cleft palate. The ENT manifestations in such syndromes and their treatments are also discussed.

27.2 Incidence

Clefts of the lip and/or palate are the commonest facial anomaly, occurring in approximately in 1:700 live births. Cleft lip (with or without cleft palate) and clefts of the palate are two distinct conditions. Clefts of the lip may occur in isolation or may be associated with clefts of the palate.

Clefts of the lip range from incomplete clefts to complete unilateral or bilateral clefts of the lip, alveolus, and palate. Cleft lips make up approximately 55% of referrals to a regional cleft lip and palate (CLP) service. These can be divided into:
- Cleft lip (CL) alone (unilateral or bilateral): 23%.
- Unilateral CLP (UCLP): 22%.
- Bilateral CLP (BCLP): 10%.

In clefting of the lip and/or palate, there is racial variation in incidence. In Chinese children, clefting occurs in approximately 1 in 500 live births as against an incidence of approximately 1 in 2,000 African children. Approximately 15 to 30% of affected babies will have a cleft as part of a syndrome (▶ Table 27.1).

27.3 Etiology

Both genetic and environmental factors are implicated. The environmental factors include the following:
- Maternal use of anticonvulsants such as phenobarbital and phenytoin (tenfold increase).
- Alcohol.
- Cigarette smoking (twofold increase).
- Corticosteroids (threefold increase).

Maternal folic acid deficiency may also contribute to clefting.

Clefting is also associated with chromosomal abnormalities—abnormalities of chromosomes 1, 2, 4, 6, 11, 14, 17, and 19 have been reported. Genetic and environmental interaction may increase the risk of clefting, for example, clefting risk is increased six times if the mother smokes and has a defect in chromosome 2; a defect on chromosome 4 increases the risk for mothers who drink alcohol or smoke cigarettes.

27.4 Diagnosis

Clefts may be diagnosed antenatally or at birth. The diagnosis may be delayed if the cleft is missed at the baby's birth check.

27.4.1 Antenatal Diagnosis

It is now possible to diagnose clefting as early as 12 weeks of gestation by transvaginal ultrasound. Ultrasound is more accurate in diagnosing isolated CL and CLP (67–93%) but is limited in making the diagnosis of isolated cleft palate (7–22%). Detection rates improve markedly after 20 weeks of gestation.

> **i**
>
> Expectant mothers with a normal early ultrasound but with known risk factors for having a baby with a cleft should have a repeat scan at 20 weeks' gestation.

Clefts may be classified ultrasonically into the following five types:
- Type 1: isolated CL.
- Type 2: UCLP.
- Type 3: BCLP.
- Type 4: median CL.
- Type 5: clefts associated with amniotic banding of limb–body–wall complex.

> **i**
>
> The type of the cleft has been correlated with chromosomal abnormalities, structural anomalies, and fetal death. The more severe the cleft, the greater the risk of associated chromosomal abnormalities, structural anomalies, and fetal death.

Table 27.1 ENT manifestation in syndromes commonly associated with cleft palate

Syndrome/sequence	Incidence	Genetic transmission	Primary defect (if any)	ENT manifestation	Other important manifestations
PR sequence	1:8,500		Micrognathia with relative macroglossia	Airway problems, feeding, obstructive sleep apnea, recurrent otitis media, conductive HL	Associated with other syndromes such as Stickler's syndrome
Stickler's syndrome	1:7,500	Autosomal dominant	Affecting collagen	Recurrent acute otitis media, possibly SN HL, flat nasal bridge and facies, bifid uvula, associated PR sequence (30%)	Myopia, retinal detachments, cataracts, bone abnormalities
Velocardiofacial syndrome	1:2,000	Deletion of chromosome 22q11	Abnormal pharyngeal arch development	Hypernasal speech, ear infection	Cardiac anomalies in 75%, parathyroid and immune deficiency
Otopalatal digital syndrome		X-linked with expression in males		HL, cleft palate	Skeletal abnormalities, growth deficiency, Arnold–Chiari malformation
Branchio-otorenal syndrome	1:40,000	Autosomal dominant	Deficiency in first and second branchial arches	Preauricular pits (80%) and external ear deformities; conductive (80%), SN, or mixed HL; branchial fistula; high arch/cleft palate	Renal dysplasia (60%)
Treacher Collins' syndrome	1:50,000	Autosomal dominant (treacle gene mapped on 5q32-q33.1)	First branchial arch abnormality	Low set ears, microtia, stapes abnormalities, deafness usually conductive, retrognathia	Coloboma of the eyes (70%), antimongoloid slant of eyes, craniofacial clefts
Apert's syndrome	1:70,000	Autosomal dominant	FGFR 2 gene abnormality	Midfacial hypoplasia, wide cochlear aqueduct, recurrent acute otitis media, conductive HL, cleft palate (30%)	Craniosynostosis with syndactyly of the hand and feet

Abbreviations: ENT, ear, nose, and throat; HL, hearing loss; PR, Pierre Robin; SN, sensorineural.

Once the diagnosis has been made antenatally, the parents should immediately be referred to the local cleft team for appropriate counseling and support. Counseling will include feeding advice with information about breast-feeding, explanation of the surgical protocol, sharing of pre- and postoperative photographs, and details of local and national support groups.

27.4.2 Diagnosis and Counseling at Birth

> **i**
>
> In those cases where an antenatal diagnosis has not been made, the aim is to diagnose all clefts at birth and for parents to be contacted by a member of the local cleft team within 24 hours of delivery.

Specialist feeding and nursing advice should be provided at the time of birth. Soon after diagnosis, the designated cleft nurse specialist should be available to give further counseling and support to the family where necessary, including advice by telephone and home visits where needed.

> **i**
>
> Feeding advice is particularly important, as neonates with clefts of the palate are unable to either compress the breast against the palate or to develop the vacuum necessary for feeding.

They therefore need to be positioned in a semi-upright position and fed with special soft teats and soft "squeezy" bottles. It is possible to breast-feed neonates with isolated CLs. Mothers can be encouraged to express breast milk where breast-feeding is not possible.

The discussion about the surgery may include pre- and postoperative photographs. It is important to emphasize that the child's appearance will change after lip surgery and that there will be a period of adjustment.

27

At the multidisciplinary clinic, the parents should also be given information about the following:

- Dental development and the need for alveolar bone grafting where indicated.
- The effect of clefting on speech and the possible need for speech therapy (10–15% of patients with palatal clefts) and speech surgery (in 5–20% of cases).
- OME.

Parents should be made aware of the need to monitor hearing and should also be offered psychological support and genetic counseling. Genetic advice is especially important if a syndromic diagnosis is suspected.

27.5 Surgical Management of Cleft Lip and Palate

Clefts of the lip may result in both cosmetic and functional problems. Functional problems include impairment in the production of bilabial sounds (pa, pi) and impairment of maxillary growth secondary to scar constriction. Babies with isolated CL can usually feed normally although they may have difficulty creating an adequate lip seal.

The main anatomical defects in UCLP and in BCLP are shown in ▶ Table 27.2 and ▶ Table 27.3 and in ▶ Fig. 27.1 and ▶ Fig. 27.2.

Lip repair is usually carried out between 3 and 5 months in the United Kingdom.

- The lip, nose, and hard palate are repaired at the first surgery at 3 to 5 months of age in healthy children.
- The hard palate is repaired with an unlined, superiorly pedicled turnover flap from the vomer.
- Apart from closure of the cleft lip and nose, repair should aim to give a functional and symmetrical lip of equal vertical height with a naturally appearing "cupid's bow" with minimal scarring and a symmetrical and functional nose.

Table 27.2 Anatomical defects in unilateral cleft lip and palate

Lips	Discontinuity of the skin, muscle, and oral mucosa of the upper lip on cleft side
	Vertical soft-tissue deficiency on the medial aspect of the cleft
	Abnormal muscle insertions into the nasal spine and alar base
Nose	Rotation of the septum, columella, and nasal spine away from the cleft
	Separation of the domes of the alar cartilages at the nasal tip and kinking of the lateral crus on the cleft side
	Dislocation of the lower and upper lateral cartilages on the cleft side
	Displacement of the alar base in all three planes of space, inferiorly or superiorly, depending on the cleft, posteriorly and laterally
	Displacement and flattening of the nasal bone on the cleft side
Alveolus	An alveolar cleft in the region of the lateral incisor tooth on the cleft side
	Missing, malformed, or supernumerary teeth in the line of the cleft
Palate	Defect in primary palate anterior to the incisive foramen
	Complete cleft of the hard palate
	Vomer inserted into the hard palate on the noncleft side
	Complete cleft of the soft palate
	Abnormal palatal muscle insertions: tensor veli palatini inserted into the back of the hard palate and palatopharyngeus inserted into the cleft of the soft palate and into the back of the hard palate
	Levator veli palatini inserted into the margin of the cleft in the soft palate
	Palatoglossus inserted into the cleft of the soft palate

Table 27.3 Anatomical defects in bilateral cleft lip and palate

Lip	Discontinuity of the skin, muscle, and oral mucosa of the upper lip bilaterally
	Central segment consisting of prolabium and premaxilla with short columella
	No labial sulcus
	Lack of orbicularis oris continuity with fibers terminating in the lateral lip elements
Nose	Lack of columella height
	Alar domes and middle crura are splayed, caudally rotated like a bucket handle, and subluxed from their normal anatomical position overlying the upper lateral cartilages
Alveolus	Bilateral defect of alveolus and anterior palate
	Missing, malformed, or supernumerary teeth in the line of the cleft
	Collapse of lateral palatal segments behind premaxilla
Palate	Bilateral cleft of the hard palate
	Vomer attached to premaxilla in the center line
	Complete cleft of the soft palate with similar muscle insertions to the soft palate in UCLP

Abbreviation: UCLP, unilateral cleft lip and palate.

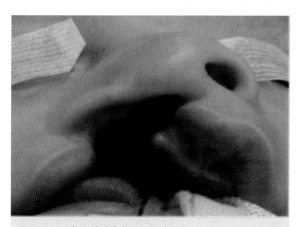

Fig. 27.1 Unilateral cleft lip and palate.

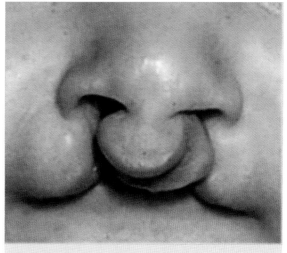

Fig. 27.2 Bilateral cleft lip and palate.

There is wide variation in the techniques, timing, and protocols for the repair of BCLP. To maintain symmetry, it is easier to repair both sides simultaneously.

The timing of palatal repair is controversial. A balance has to be struck between the beneficial effect of early palatal repair (before 1 year of age) on speech and delaying hard palate closure to improve growth.

Asynchronous bilateral lip repair (repairing one side and then the other side on a separate occasion) is practiced by some surgeons. It is important to establish primary muscle continuity (unless there is undue muscle tension at the time of primary repair, when the final muscle repair is deferred for 9 months to a year). The labial sulcus is reconstructed using mucosa from the prolabium and from the lateral lip elements. Some surgeons rely on muscle action to create a labial sulcus and do not formally reconstruct the sulcus.

Repair of the hard palate varies widely from complete closure with a vomer flap on both sides, to complete closure on one side and partial repair of the opposite side, to complete closure on one side only leaving the contralateral side open for repair a few months later on a separate occasion. Surgeons vary in their approach to hard palate repair as many fear that raising a full bilateral vomerine flap may compromise the blood supply to the premaxilla, but by raising the flap up to the prevomerine suture on one side, the blood supply to the premaxilla is maintained.

27.5.1 Palate Repair

Functional palatal repair is important for speech and may be important for Eustachian tube function.

It has been shown that improved growth only consistently occurs when hard palate closure is delayed until adolescence. This results in unacceptably poor speech. Common practice in the United Kingdom is to close the soft palate in patients with CLP and the entire palate in isolated cleft palates between 6 and 9 months.

The hard palate in patients with complete CLP is widely repaired in the United Kingdom using a vomer flap as shown in ▶ Fig. 27.3. Several earlier techniques have been

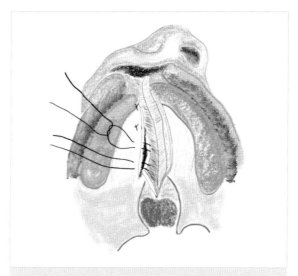

Fig. 27.3 Cleft palate repair using a vomer flap.

largely abandoned in the United Kingdom because of unfavorable midfacial growth, compromised dental arch formation, difficult fistulas, excessive palatal scarring, and poor speech outcomes.

27.5.2 Alveolar Bone Grafting

i
Some children will need alveolar bone grafts (Box 27.1).

Assessment for alveolar bone graft surgery is normally undertaken by the cleft surgeon and orthodontist together. It is important to time the procedure so that tooth eruption occurs into the graft soon after the bone graft is placed. If it is done too early, the bone placed into the cleft will be lost, and if too late, the bony and periodontal support for the tooth will be compromised. The timing of surgery is determined from panoramic and occlusal radiographs (and now more recently cone-beam computed tomography) taken during the mixed dentition. The ideal time to graft is when the root of the tooth erupting into the cleft is between half and two-thirds formed. Several autogenous donor sites have been used for alveolar bone grafting including iliac crest, rib, calvarium, tibia, and mandibular symphysis. In the United Kingdom, the iliac crest is regarded as the gold standard for alveolar bone grafting as it is rich in osteogenic cells, is rapidly transformed into alveolar bone, substantial amounts of cancellous bone can be easily obtained, and excellent long-term outcomes have been reported.

Box 27.1 Aims of Alveolar Bone Grafting

- Stabilize the alveolar arch.
- Restore arch integrity.
- Allow teeth to erupt into optimal position.
- Permit orthodontic alignment of arch.
- Repair oronasal fistula.
- Create a platform for prosthetic replacement, for example, implants.
- Optimize maxillary surgery.
- Create support for the nose (alar base) and lip.

27.6 ENT Problems in Cleft Lip and Palate

- The otorhinological problems encountered in patients with cleft palate can be categorized into the following:

- Otologic disorders.
- Nasal deformity.
- Airway disorders.

27.6.1 Otitis Media with Effusion

i
Conductive hearing loss is almost universal in children with cleft palate, with a reported incidence rates of 94 to 100%. Sensorineural or mixed hearing loss is present in 5% of cases.

OME in children with CLP is due to the poor function of the tensor veli palatini and levator palatini muscles. This results from the cleft in the palatine raphe, causing increased compliance in the Eustachian tube due to its inability to open during swallowing.[1] Persistent OME frequently causes hearing loss in otherwise healthy (i.e., without cleft palate) children aged 2 to 4 years with a quoted incidence of 21%. The spontaneous resolution rate is 65%, hence the rationale for the 3-month waiting period. OME with persistent hearing loss of worse than 25 dB in the better hearing ear is usually considered a surgical indication for inserting ventilation tubes.[2] As the child gets older, this functional loss has less effect with improved hearing and tubal function in adolescents.[3]

Management

Ongoing otological and audiological surveillance is an important part of the multidisciplinary care of children with cleft palate. Routine use of tympanostomy tubes in all cases is now discouraged and a customized approach to the individual child is preferred.[4,5]

The protocol used in our unit is outlined in ▶ Fig. 27.4.[6] Pediatric hearing assessment in children with cleft palate up to the age of 3 months is done objectively using otoacoustic emissions, auditory brainstem recording, and high-frequency tympanometry.[2] Beyond the age of 7 months, behavioral tests are employed (distraction tests, performance tests, visual reinforced audiometry; see Chapter 13). Pure-tone audiograms are reliably performed beyond the age of 4 years in most children. Normal speech intensity varies between 50 and 60 dB. A significant hearing impairment above 50 dB in the better hearing ear is likely to affect speech perception and language development.

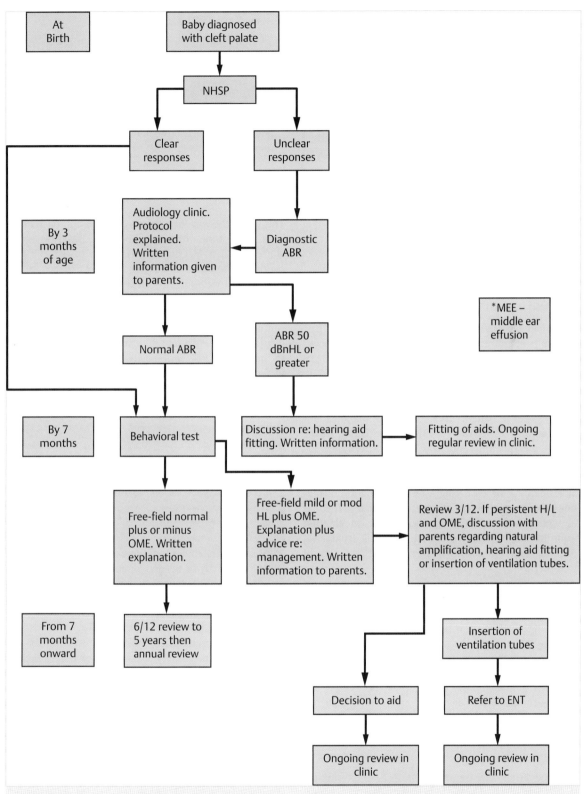

Fig. 27.4 Audiological care pathway for cleft palate children. ABR, auditory brainstem response; NHSP, neonatal hearing screening program.

27

Tips and Tricks

Hearing management[7]:

- Insertion of ventilation tubes at *primary closure* of the cleft palate should be performed only after careful otological and audiological assessment.
- Children with CLP need ongoing ontological and audiological surveillance into adult life.
- Persistent hearing loss ≥ 25 dB beyond 3 months needs intervention.
- Intervention: hearing aids or ventilation tubes.
- If considering ventilation tubes, use only short-term ones.
- Ventilation tubes may generate more complications in children with CLP.

27.6.2 Tympanic Membrane Retraction and Cholesteatoma

Eustachian tube dysfunction in children with cleft palate results in an increased incidence of retraction pockets with potential for cholesteatoma. In a study of 116 patients who underwent cleft palate repair, followed up for 72 months, the incidence of cholesteatoma has been quoted to be approximately 15%. The incidence was slightly lower in patients treated with ventilation tubes (14%) compared to those without ventilation tubes (16.7%), but this difference was not statistically significant. In adults with submucosal cleft, it rises to 26%.[8] Other studies have reported an incidence of 5.9% for cholesteatoma, necessitating a recommendation of life-long otological follow-up for these patients.[1,9] There is an eightfold, statistically significant, rise in children requiring surgery for chronic otitis media (tympano-mastoidectomy) following insertion of three sets of grommets.[3,10]

A retraction pocket with no keratin collection or hearing loss needs to be monitored, with consideration of grommet insertion if it is felt that the retraction is worsening. Keratin collection with migration of squamous epithelium into the middle ear makes it a cholesteatoma, and the child then needs a formal mastoid exploration. In children, performing a combined-approach tympanoplasty (CAT) may be reasonable, keeping the posterior canal wall intact. Echoplanar diffusion-weighted magnetic resonance imaging scanning is effective in diagnosing a recurrence greater than 5 mm and may enable the surgeon to defer second look surgery for longer.[11]

For persistent disease, extensive disease or multiple recurrences, a canal wall down mastoidectomy is preferred. Tympanomastoid surgery is more fully discussed in Chapters 9 and 10.

27.6.3 Nasal Deformity

The nasal deformities in UCLP and BCLP are described earlier.

Primary nose repair is performed at the time of the primary lip repair. Long-term outcomes of a consecutive series of patients with UCLP and BCLP showed that primary rhinoplasty does not compromise nasal growth.[12,13]

This paved the way for a more aggressive approach to the nose at the time of primary lip repair. Nasal dissection started with a McComb dissection releasing the skin overlying the lower and upper lateral cartilages on the cleft side carried out through the lip incisions and then progressed to open approaches to the lower and upper lateral cartilages through rim incisions. Work on the septum followed with dissection of the septum from the displaced nasal crest into the midline. Various techniques to maintain cartilage repositioning following surgery include external and internal suspensory sutures, temporary tie-over splints, and longer-term internal and external silicone splints.[14,15]

Secondary surgery of the nose is still often indicated despite improved results following primary rhinoplasty at the time of lip repair, and adjustment may be needed on more than one occasion.

Early secondary rhinoplasty between 3 years of age and adolescence, may be needed for aesthetic reasons, specifically to address obvious deformities of the tip, the lower lateral cartilage and alar base in patients with UCLP, and the shortened columella and widened alar bases in patients with BCLP.

Formal septorhinoplasty (including osteotomies and grafting where necessary) is usually delayed until skeletal maturation is complete. It should only be carried out after orthognathic surgery, where indicated, has been undertaken. The cleft nose deformity is complex and patients have usually been operated on more than once, thus increasing the difficulty of the surgery. Unless only very minor adjustments are indicated, complete cleft septorhinoplasties are best carried out as open or external approach procedures. It is important to try to address the patient's concerns and wishes as long as these are realistic and these patients often benefit from at least one session with the team psychologist.

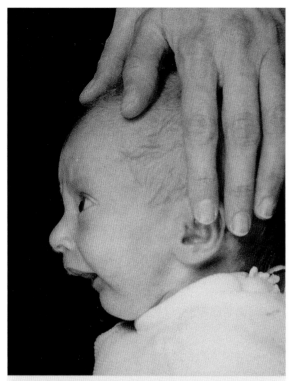

Fig. 27.5 Child with Pierre Robin sequence. Note the micrognathia and retrognathia with low set ears. (Reproduced from Entezami M, Albig M, Gasiorek-Wiens A, Becker R. Ultrasound Diagnosis of Fetal Anomalies. Stuttgart/New York: Thieme; 2004, with permission.)

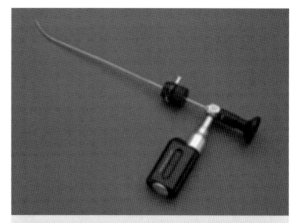

Fig. 27.6 Bonfils intubation endoscope. An age-appropriate endotracheal tube (ETT) is mounted on the rigid telescope that has a fixed-angle bend anteriorly. This is guided into the laryngeal inlet and the ETT is slipped into the trachea. An ETT can also be railroaded into the larynx using a flexible bronchoscope.

27.6.4 Airway Disorders

Pierre Robin Sequence

This is the most common congenital disorder associated with cleft palate with an incidence of 12%.[16] The primary defect is a small jaw (micrognathia; ▶ Fig. 27.5), which results in the normal-sized tongue being pushed cranially, preventing the fusion of the palatine plates in intrauterine life and resulting in the cleft palate. The relative reduction in the oral cavity results in the tongue prolapsing into the oropharynx (glossoptosis), which contributes to upper airway obstruction. The child will have stertorous breathing, often with feeding difficulties, and will require assistance with breathing in the early neonatal period.

There is increased mandibular growth in the first year of life that reduces the need for assisted breathing beyond 6 to 9 months of age in the majority of children.

Management

Airway assessment includes confirming the patency of the nasal airway to exclude choanal atresia and performing a direct laryngotracheoscopy. Access at endoscopy is challenging due to the typically anteriorly placed larynx in children with PR sequence. An anteriorly placed larynx can be a challenge to intubate and for the introduction of a rigid endoscope. Using a McCoy hinged tongue blade is helpful in improving the visibility of the larynx. Lately, Bonfils (Karl Storz) rigid intubation endoscopes have proved useful to gain access in a difficult airway (▶ Fig. 27.6).

Pulse oximetry is best done overnight and ideally at home and will indicate the number and severity of desaturations.

These babies are best nursed in the prone position, despite current advice to get healthy babies to sleep on their backs ("back to sleep"). The treatment options include insertion of a nasopharyngeal airway (NPA), noninvasive ventilation (continuous positive airway pressure, bilevel positive airway pressure), or, as a very last resort, a tracheostomy. An obstruction above the larynx, for example, tongue collapse in PR sequence, can be treated with an NPA inserted at birth for period of 3 to 6 months. A well-placed NPA will project just below the free edge of the soft palate in the nasopharynx. The NPA is customized for each child, and the length is measured from nasal ala to the angle of mandible or tragus of the ear (▶ Fig. 27.7). The NPA secures the airway and allows a period for mandibular development.

Mandibular advancement surgery may need to be considered in children with persistent retrognathia, usually in association with severe craniofacial deformity.

27

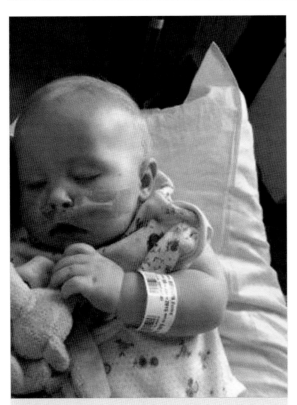

Fig. 27.7 A baby with a nasopharyngeal airway.

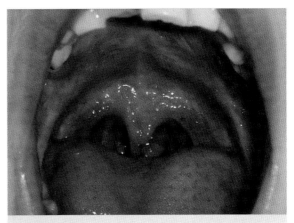

Fig. 27.8 Calnan's triad of signs of submucosal cleft palate.

Tips and Tricks

Airway management:
- Assess nasal patency bilaterally.
- Differentiate between stridor and stertor.
- Beware of the anteriorly placed larynx.
- In retrognathic patients (PR sequence, Treacher Collins' syndrome): insert an NPA.
- Sizing of NPA: nasal ala to the angle of the mandible.
- Avoid adenoidectomy in patients with submucosal cleft palate.

27.7 Submucosal Cleft Palate

Submucosal cleft palate is defined as the presence of a muscular or bony defect underlying a normal appearing mucosal surface in the roof of the oral cavity. It is usually characterized by the presence of a "Calnan's triad" of signs—bifid uvula, furrow along the midline of the soft palate (may appear bluish or white), and notch or a dented feel along the hard cleft palate (▶ Fig. 27.8)—but it may have a variable expression. The incidence of bifid uvula[17] in the normal population, without a submucosal cleft palate, is 1 to 7.5%. A submucosal cleft palate may

occur in 1 to 10% of the population without speech dysfunction.[18]

An ENT surgeon must be aware of the condition, feeling for the palate when confronted with a bifid uvula in a child admitted for adenotonsillectomy. If a submucosal cleft is suspected, it is advisable to avoid performing an adenoidectomy, as the adenoid pad may be the only supporting tissue against which the palate may close during swallowing, thus preventing velopharyngeal incompetence and nasal regurgitation. The child should be referred to the local cleft palate department.

The modern techniques for adenoidal surgery (coblation or suction diathermy adenoidectomy; see Chapter 18) allow for controlled removal of tissue under the surgeon's vision either using a nasendoscope or a postnasal mirror. The technique involves a controlled ablation of the obstructing choanal tissues and creating lateral channels through the adenoidal tissue, keeping a central core intact for supporting the palate. This has been performed by the first author on a number of cases with bifid uvula as a compromise to improve the sleeping pattern of the child (by improving the nasal breathing) while maintaining functional support for the soft palate. It must be stressed that this is attempted only in a center offering cleft palate services.

27.8 Key Points

- Children with cleft palate need to be assessed in a multidisciplinary setup.
- Incidence of OME is higher in children with cleft palate. This requires close surveillance and intervention with hearing aids or ventilation tube insertion, if required.
- Management of retraction pockets and cholesteatomas may prove challenging.
- Children with small jaw (PR sequence) have a difficult access airway. They may require flexible intubation.

- NPA in newborns with PR sequence provides a safe airway bypassing the obstruction caused by a prolapsing tongue. Further surgery in form of tracheostomy or mandibular advancement may be considered for difficult airway.
- ENT surgeons should check for submucosal cleft in children with bifid uvula.

References

[1] Coutinho MB, Magalhães A, Matos C. Bone anchored hearing aids in children with cleft palate. J Int Advanced Otol. 2009; 5(2):261–264

[2] Andrew PJ, Chorbachi R, Sirimanna T, Sommerlad B, Hartley BEJ. Evaluation of hearing thresholds in 3-month-old children with a cleft palate: the basis for a selective policy for ventilation tube insertion at time of palate repair. Clin Otolaryngol. 2004; 29:10–17

[3] Sheahan P, Miller I, Sheahan JN, Earley MJ, Blayney AW. Incidence and outcome of middle ear disease in cleft lip and/or cleft palate. Int J Pediatr Otorhinolaryngol. 2003; 67(7):785–793

[4] Kuşcu O, Günaydın RÖ, İcen M, et al. The effect of early routine grommet insertion on management of otitis media with effusion in children with cleft palate. J Craniomaxillofac Surg. 2015; 43(10):2112–2115

[5] Smallridge J, Hall AJ, Chorbachi R, et al. Functional outcomes in the Cleft Care UK study—part 3: oral health and audiology. Orthod Craniofac Res. 2015; 18 Suppl 2:25–35

[6] Gani B, Kinshuck AJ, Sharma R. A review of hearing loss in cleft palate patients. Int J Otolaryngol. 2012; 2012:548698

[7] National Institute for Health and Care Excellence. Clinical Guideline 60: Surgical management of children with otitis media with effusion. NICE 2008. Available at http://www.nice.org.uk. Accessed June 2012

[8] Reiter R, Haase S, Brosch S. Repaired cleft palate and ventilation tubes and their associations with cholesteatoma in children and adults. Cleft Palate Craniofac J. 2009; 46(6):598–602

[9] Goudy S, Lott D, Canady J, Smith RJH. Conductive hearing loss and otopathology in cleft palate patients. Otolaryngol Head Neck Surg. 2006; 134(6):946–948

[10] Phua YS, Salkeld LJ, de Chalain TMB. Middle ear disease in children with cleft palate: protocols for management. Int J Pediatr Otorhinolaryngol. 2009; 73(2):307–313

[11] Aikele P, Kittner T, Offergeld C, Kaftan H, Hüttenbrink KB, Laniado M. Diffusion-weighted MR imaging of cholesteatoma in pediatric and adult patients who have undergone middle ear surgery. AJR Am J Roentgenol. 2003; 181(1):261–265

[12] McComb HK. Primary repair of the bilateral cleft lip nose: a long-term follow-up. Plast Reconstr Surg. 2009; 124(5):1610–1615

[13] McComb HK, Coghlan BA. Primary repair of the unilateral cleft lip nose: completion of a longitudinal study. Cleft Palate Craniofac J. 1996; 33(1):23–30, discussion 30–31

[14] Morselli PG, Pinto V, Negosanti L, Firinu A, Fabbri E. Early correction of septum JJ deformity in unilateral cleft lip-cleft palate. Plast Reconstr Surg. 2012; 130(3):434e–441e

[15] Lu TC, Lam WL, Chang CS, Kuo-Ting Chen P. Primary correction of nasal deformity in unilateral incomplete cleft lip: a comparative study between three techniques. J Plast Reconstr Aesthet Surg. 2012; 65(4):456–463

[16] Kay DJ, Nelson M, Rosenfeld RM. Meta-analysis of tympanostomy tube sequelae. Otolaryngol Head Neck Surg. 2001; 124(4):374–380

[17] Oji T, Sakamoto Y, Ogata H, Tamada I, Kishi K. A 25-year review of cases with submucous cleft palate. Int J Pediatr Otorhinolaryngol. 2013; 77(7):1183–1185

[18] Shapiro BL, Meskin LH, Cervanka J, Pruzansky P. Cleft uvula: a microform of facial clefts and it genetic basis. Birth Defects Orig Artic Ser 1971;7(7):80–82

27

28 Disorders of the Esophagus and Gastroesophageal Reflux

Marcus K. H. Auth and Balaji Krishnamurthy

28.1 Introduction

Disorders of the esophagus are usually the province of the general pediatrician, the pediatric gastroenterologist, and the general pediatric surgeon. Some conditions present to otolaryngologists, and gastroesophageal reflux disease (GERD) may be important in the pathogenesis of many pediatric ear, nose, and throat (ENT) disorders, including laryngomalacia, laryngotracheal stenosis, rhinosinusitis, and otitis media. This chapter considers the principal disorders of the esophagus that may come to the attention of an otolaryngologist.

28.2 Congenital Disorders

28.2.1 Tracheoesophageal Fistula

Anatomy, Prevalence, and Associations

Tracheoesophageal fistula (TEF) describes an abnormal communication between the trachea and the esophagus. The prevalence is approximately 1 in 1,400 live births. In approximately 85% of cases, the esophageal lumen ends in a blind pit, *esophageal atresia*, and the fistula connects this lumen with the anterior tracheal wall (▶ Fig. 28.1 a).

If a TEF occurs without esophageal atresia, the fistula connects obliquely from the trachea in a caudal direction toward the esophagus. The fistula enables air to pass from the trachea to the esophagus, and esophageal contents (saliva, milk, and gastric juices) into the trachea, as in the far less common *H-type fistula* (▶ Fig. 28.1 b).

> **i**
> The baby with an *H-type fistula* can have a normal or near-normal swallow but will aspirate some of the contents of the esophagus into the airway. Diagnosis can be delayed as the baby may continue to feed.[1]

Additional major congenital anomalies are present in approximately 50% of babies with a TEF. These include the VATER or VACTERL (*v*ertebral defects, *a*norectal anomalies, *c*ardiac anomalies, *t*racheoesophageal disorders, cardiac defects, *r*enal defects, and *l*imb disorders), and the CHARGE (*c*oloboma, congenital *h*eart disease, choanal *a*tresia, *r*enal and *g*enital anomalies, and *e*ar abnormality) complexes of disorders.

Presentation and Diagnosis

Maternal polyhydramnios can be one sign of esophageal atresia, particularly if there is a *TEF with esophageal atresia*; there may be suspicion based on prenatal ultrasound scanning.

After birth, the child is reported to be mucus-ridden, with saliva drooling from the mouth. Feeding results in choking, respiratory distress, cyanotic attacks, aspiration into the lungs and pneumonia, or unexplained abdominal distensions. Symptoms are relieved by nasogastric tube feeding unless the baby has esophageal atresia.

Suspect esophageal atresia if a 10-gauge catheter (preferably relatively stiff) passed through the mouth becomes arrested approximately 9 to 13 cm from the gums. To determine if the secretion aspirated from the catheter is neutral or near-neutral (usually pH 4 and higher), pH paper should be used. Normal stomach pH is 3.5 and lower.

Investigations

> **i**
> A plain X-ray of the abdomen and thorax helps differentiate the different forms of TEF: if it shows a gasless abdomen, the child probably has no distal TEF, but may have a proximal TEF or esophageal atresia alone. In a distal TEF, there is air in the abdomen below the diaphragm.

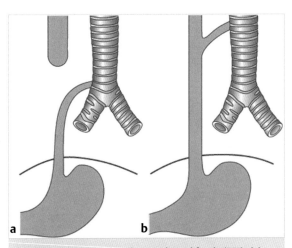

Fig. 28.1 Illustration of tracheoesophageal fistula (TEF). **(a)** Esophageal atresia with distal TEF (common type). **(b)** H-type fistula (rare). (Reproduced from Tytgat GNJ, Tytgat SHAJ. Grading and Staging in Gastroenterology. Stuttgart/New York: Thieme; 2009, with permission.)

rings are thin, fragile structures that partially or completely obstruct the esophageal lumen. An *esophageal web* is a thin mucosal fold protruding into the lumen, most commonly located anteriorly in the cervical esophagus, causing focal narrowing in the postcricoid area.

Schatzki "B" rings are smooth, thin mucosal structures at the gastroesophageal junction. They may cause dysphagia. Muscular rings are very rare, typically located within 2 cm of the squamocolumnar junction.[1]

Symptoms and Treatment

Most esophageal rings are asymptomatic, are found incidentally, and do not require treatment. If symptomatic, esophageal dilatation is the best treatment. Esophageal strictures, webs, and rings have not been associated with globus pharyngeus.[2]

28.3 Acquired Esophageal Disorders

28.3.1 Esophageal Strictures

Etiology

A stricture is a fixed narrowing within the lumen. It may be caused by inflammation, fibrosis, or intraluminal neoplasia. Extraluminal causes include direct invasion by a neoplasm or mediastinal lymph node enlargement. More often a stricture is benign, secondary to the following:
- Severe GERD;
- Caustic ingestion;
- Previous surgery; or
- Infection (candida, herpes virus, meningococcus).

Other causes include inflammation (epidermolysis bullosa, chronic granulomatous disease), chemotherapy, or radiotherapy. Some children develop iatrogenic esophageal stricture secondary to sclerotherapy of varices.

Presentation

Infants and children may present with recurrent vomiting, coughing, choking, cyanosis with feeds, and irritability during or after feeds. Older children may present with dysphagia, odynophagia, frequent regurgitation of swallowed food bolus, vomiting, and weight loss.

Investigation and Diagnosis

Diagnosis is by endoscopy (esophagogastroduodenoscopy [EGD]), possibly combined with barium swallow/meal. Computed tomography may be helpful in selected cases (► Fig. 28.3, ► Fig. 28.4).

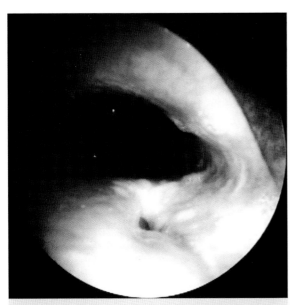

Fig. 28.2 Tracheoesophageal fistula evident at bronchoscopy. An H-type fistula can be especially difficult to detect as the baby often feeds normally.

Tracheobronchoscopy can demonstrate an upper pouch fistula or identify the point at which the distal fistula enters the airways (► Fig. 28.2). Moderate-to-severe tracheomalacia is a common accompaniment to a TEF and will need the attention of a pediatric otolaryngologist. Upper esophagoscopy (rigid or flexible) will not always detect an H-type TEF, but if performed, it will demonstrate the blind-ending esophageal pouch in esophageal atresia.

An upper pouch fistula or the subtle signs of an H-type TEF can be demonstrated by contrast introduced by a catheter placed in the midesophagus under continuous video fluoroscopy (tube esophagoscopy).

Management

The infant should be stabilized and kept warm with minimal handling and adequate oxygenation. Place the infant in the right lateral position, allowing draining of saliva and preventing gastric contents from coming up. The child will need frequent gentle suctioning and should be transferred as soon as is practicable to a specialist pediatric center for surgery under the care of a suitably trained pediatric surgical team.

28.2.2 Esophageal Strictures, Web, and Rings

Etiology and Presentation

In contrast to acquired strictures (see Chapter 28.3.1), congenital esophageal strictures are very rare. *Esophageal*

28

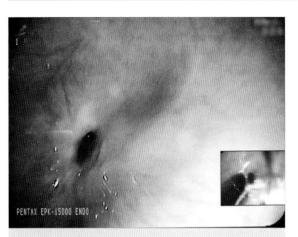

Fig. 28.3 Filiforme fibrotic stricture secondary to chronic gastroesophageal reflux.

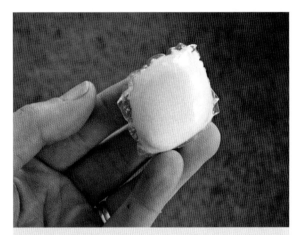

Fig. 28.5 Bleach crystal pack.

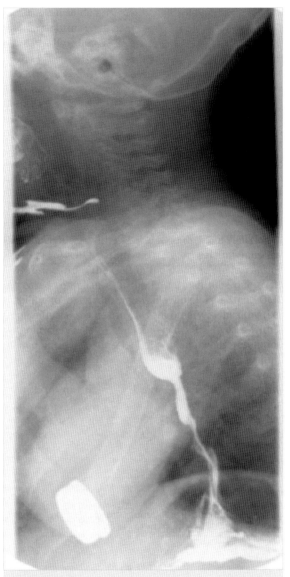

Fig. 28.4 Irregular extensive stenosis in severe gastroesophageal reflux disease.

Management

Children with minimal symptoms may require no treatment. It may be helpful to counsel parents regarding smaller meals and antireflux medications as needed. Balloon dilatation under fluoroscopic guidance may be helpful if symptoms are more severe, and in extreme cases, surgery (stricturoplasty) can be considered. There is a small risk of perforation and recurrence with these techniques.[2]

28.3.2 Caustic Esophageal Damage

This is caused by mucosal and mural ulceration brought about by ingestion of chemicals. It has become relatively rare in western communities due to improved safety, awareness, and labeling of household cleaner containers, for example, caustic soda, and increased parental awareness of the dangers of chemical ingestion by children. Caustic strictures are still a major health problem in the developing world (see Chapters 4 and 22).

Very significant damage can be caused to the oropharynx, the esophagus, stomach, and the larynx by alkaline liquid agents (e.g., dishwasher fluid) or crystalline drain cleaners, which adhere to the oropharynx, become lodged in the upper esophagus, and cause tissue injury by liquefactive necrosis. Household bleach (▶ Fig. 28.5, ▶ Fig. 28.6) may induce severe mucosal burns and edema.[3] "Liquitabs" containing dishwasher fluid or detergent are a particular modern hazard (see ▶ Fig. 20.5).

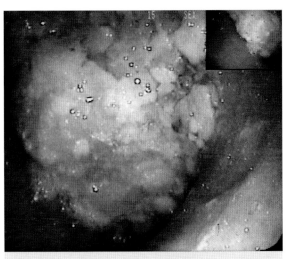

Fig. 28.6 Soluble bleach crystals in esophagus and stomach (depicted here) following accidental ingestion. Note the large amounts that in this case required surgical retrieval through laparotomy, following joint assessment from ear, nose, and throat, gastroenterology, anesthetics, general surgery, and respiratory medicine.

Symptoms

In the acute situation, there may be burns of the hands, face, and oral cavity. The child may present with vomiting, dysphagia, drooling, epigastric and abdominal pain, and refusal to drink. Shock and severe respiratory distress may occur if there is mediastinal penetration.

In long-standing cases, there may be mucosal erythema and edema. Noncircumferential superficial mucosal ulcerations do not always cause long-term complications. Sequelae of esophageal caustic injuries are as follows:
- Stricture formation.
- Development of achalasia.
- "Brachyesophagus."
- Gastroesophageal reflux (GER).
- The development of malignancy (a late complication).

Diagnosis

A chest radiograph can detect air in the mediastinum if there is perforation and mediastinitis.

A joint approach by ENT, gastroenterology, surgery, anesthetics, and respiratory physicians should be planned and coordinated to determine the type of injury and to remove toxic material adhering to the mucosa before it causes further tissue damage.

For ingested liquids, flexible endoscopy may be performed *with great care* within 12 to 36 hours after ingestion to assess the extent of damage.[3] A contrast swallow can be performed 2 to 3 weeks after ingestion.

Treatment

In the emergency situation, make no attempt to induce vomiting or to neutralize the caustic agent due to the risk of exothermic reaction and additional injury.[3]

Admit the child to hospital even for an apparently minor injury and commence resuscitation. Early treatment with H_2 blocker or proton pump inhibitors (PPIs) is indicated. Nasogastric tubes should not be placed blindly. Usually, parenteral fluids are required until after endoscopic assessment when, depending on the findings, patients may be considered safe to swallow liquids. Children are at ongoing risk of additional complications and need to be monitored for respiratory symptoms on a ward with surveillance facilities (e.g., a high dependency unit).

If "liquitabs" or granules are swallowed, they should be removed either by safe endoscopy (e.g., wrapped in a net and ideally sealed, if the equipment is available), or following diagnostic endoscopy, a laparoscopic surgical removal may be needed to retrieve larger amounts of the substance.

If nasogastric tube placement is considered (e.g., difficult venous access), the placement requires endoscopic guidance (laryngoscopy and flexible esophagoscopy) to avoid a perforation. Depending on the type or amount of ingested chemical, the extent of epidermal or mucosal damage, the presence of respiratory symptoms and signs of systemic inflammation or infection, and the perceived risks of aspiration, admission and treatment on a pediatric intensive care unit may be indicated. This is to facilitate airway protection by intubation and ventilation.

In severe cases and if there is evidence of incipient shock, an intravenous fluid bolus, continued intravenous fluid therapy, or even total parenteral nutrition may be needed.

There is some evidence that early high-dose steroids (1-g methylprednisolone/1.73 m^2/day for 3 days) reduces secondary stricture formation.[4] Antibiotics may be used if there is any suspicion of perforation.

In the long term, repeated esophageal dilatation or reconstructive surgery may be needed.

28

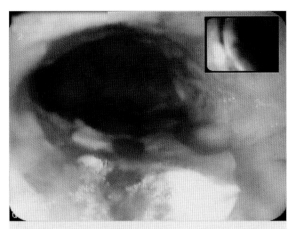

Fig. 28.7 Grade III gastroesophageal reflux disease with fresh bleeding and fibrinous ulcerations.

28.3.3 Gastroesophageal Reflux

Introduction

Some reflux of gastric contents into the esophagus above the gastroesophageal junction is physiological, especially in infancy. Reflux as a developmental variation of gastrointestinal (GI) motility resolves as the infant matures. The distinction between this "physiological" and "pathological" GER in infancy and childhood is determined not merely by the number and severity of reflux episodes but also, and most importantly, by the presence of reflux-related complications. These can include failure to thrive, erosive esophagitis, esophageal stricture formation, and chronic respiratory disease (▶ Fig. 28.7).[5]

> Pathological GER warrants appropriate diagnostic testing and medical or surgical management.

When GER causes such complications, it is often referred to as GERD.

Pathophysiology

A low resting tone of the lower esophageal sphincter (LOS) is associated with GER in a subgroup of infants and children with neurologic impairment. LOS pressure is, however, normal in most children with GER. Transient relaxation of LOS is now considered the most important factor in GER. This can be triggered by obesity, food allergies, liquid diet (infants), and other causes including high intrathoracic pressures associated with airway obstruction. GERD is for this reason an important accompaniment of many pediatric ENT disorders.

Clinical Features

GER can present as effortless vomiting after feeds. There can be regurgitation immediately or some hours after feeding. Crying, irritability, poor appetite, weight loss and poor growth (failure to thrive), heartburn, dysphagia, halitosis, and poor dentition can be pointers. Atypical symptoms include chronic cough, sore throat, wheezing, recurrent pneumonitis, stridor, hoarseness, apnea, bradycardia, and "apparent life-threatening events."

Investigations

The diagnosis of GERD is based largely on history and examination.

- *Endoscopy* is useful to assess complications such as esophagitis and stricture formation and to screen for underlying conditions such as *Helicobacter pylori* infection, eosinophilic esophagitis (EoE), or Barrett's esophagus (BE).
- *Twenty-four-hour esophageal pH/impedance-pH monitoring* is useful for assessing and quantitating GER.
- A *barium swallow* is used to rule out anatomical abnormalities but is a poor tool in diagnosing GERD.
- *Radionuclide scans* (milk scan), adding radioisotope to feeds, is useful in measuring gastric emptying and subsequent scanning of pulmonary fields is useful for demonstrating aspiration.
- Esophageal manometry can measure LOS pressure and esophageal motility.

Treatment

Many children need little or no active treatment. Conservative therapy such as thickening of infant feeds and the use of lower volume and lower osmolality feeds reduces regurgitation, can decrease crying, and increases sleep time. In older children, elevation of the head of bed can be helpful. In milk protein intolerance, protein hydrolysate feeds may be tried.

With significant symptoms, medications are indicated and include antacids, ranitidine, omeprazole, and esomeprazole, ideally under the supervision of a pediatrician. Prokinetic agents (domperidone, metoclopramide, low-dose erythromycin) have some empirical benefit but the evidence base for their use is poor.

In very severe cases, the baby may need to be fed slowly through a nasogastric tube. Reflux is occasionally severe enough to warrant the fashioning of a percutaneous gastrostomy for continued feeding.

> The indications for surgery in refractory GERD should be carefully evaluated by joint assessment by a pediatric gastroenterologist and a pediatric surgeon.

A Nissen fundoplication, sometimes in combination with vagotomy and pyloroplasty, may be considered. Surgical jejunostomy may be indicated, or in very severe cases, usually children with intractable neurodisability, total gastroesophageal dissociation (Bianchi's procedure) has been undertaken.[6]

28.3.4 Barrett's Esophagus

> **i**
>
> BE is defined by the presence of intestinal mucosa above the gastroesophageal junction.

The diagnosis is endoscopic, with histological confirmation as required. Endoscopic features include velvety red "tongues" of a villiform surface appearance extending up the esophagus from the proximal gastric fold at the gastroesophageal junction, with islands of residual white squamous mucosa along with other endoscopic changes including ulceration and nodularity or friability.[7] Chronic GERD is an accepted risk factor, particularly in severe neurologic disease or in autism.[7]

The child needs to be referred to a gastroenterologist as BE is a risk factor for malignancy.[8]

> **i**
>
> While for adults, the treatment is endomucosal resection, children are usually only monitored by regular upper GI endoscopies, with treatment of GER using ranitidine, omeprazole, or lansoprazole. It is essential that these patients are handed over to an adult gastroenterology service for ongoing surveillance because of the high cancer risk.

Long-term treatment involves prevention of acid reflux by PPIs or H_2 blockers.

28.3.5 Eosinophilic Esophagitis

Etiology

EoE is a chronic immune/antigen-mediated eosinophilic inflammation leading to esophageal dysfunction in the absence of GER.[9]

Triggers identified are the potent eosinophilic chemokines interleukin 5 and eotaxin. Prevalence is increasing, reaching 9 to 10 per 100,000, and cows' milk protein intolerance is considered an etiological factor.

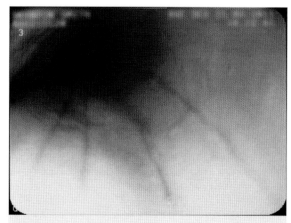

Fig. 28.8 Linear vertical furrowing of the mucosa in eosinophilic esophagitis.

The condition can spare the lower esophagus, and therefore multiple biopsies should always be taken from the proximal in addition to the distal esophagus.

Symptoms

Onset of symptoms is in the first or second decade, with a male predominance.[9]

In infants and toddlers, typical symptoms are feeding problems, vomiting, regurgitation, excessive crying or irritability, and food refusal. In the younger child, they include vomiting and retrosternal pain, whereas the older child may present with dysphagia and food impaction. The diagnosis should be considered if there is lack of response to high-dose PPIs in the absence of GER.

Nongastroenterological features include wheeze, eczema, and allergic rhinitis.

Diagnosis

Diagnosis is endoscopic, with histological confirmation. There are characteristic concentric indentations in the esophagus (concentric rings), white exudates or plaques (eosinophilic microabscesses), and longitudinal furrows (▶ Fig. 28.8).

The diagnosis is based on histological evidence of dense esophageal tissue eosinophilia in both upper and lower esophagus of more than 15 eosinophils per high power field, often associated with eosinophilic microabscesses and basal zone hyperplasia.

Complications

If unrecognized, the condition can lead to impaction of a food bolus in the esophagus, which can present as an emergency requiring rigid or flexible endoscopy for foreign body removal.

28

Treatment

> Currently, the cornerstone of treatment is dietary intervention or the use of swallowed or inhaled corticosteroids if dietetic changes are either not feasible or unsuccessful.[9]

If the history is strongly suggestive of dietetic triggers or if allergy testing shows conclusive evidence of food-related causes, different dietetic restrictions are indicated:

- "Targeted" diet is tried if specific food allergies are confirmed by symptoms, such as dysphagia triggered by specific foods, or by allergy tests (radioallergosorbent test [RAST] or skin-prick test).
- "Six-food elimination" (elimination of dairy, soya, wheat, egg, nut, fish/shellfish) is recommended if no specific food triggers are detectable, but compliance can be difficult in younger children. The rationale is to exclude the main nutritional allergy sources.
- Elemental diet with an amino-based formula milk is indicated for severe forms of EoE to reverse the inflammatory cascade.

If allergy exclusions are not feasible, medical options provide an alternative. After exploring the effect of omeprazole over 4 weeks (which may be combined with domperidone, but restrictions apply to the use of domperidone due to potential severe side effects[10,11]), medical options include the following:

- Off-label topical swallowed steroids (see Box 28.1).
- Systemic oral steroids.
- Azathioprine.

Box 28.1 Topical Steroids for EoE

Budesonide can be prepared in an oral viscous form by dissolving 1 mg (in younger children < 30 kg) or 2 mg (> 30 kg) in a viscous sweetener solution (e.g., Splenda). When swallowed, this exerts its effect locally on the esophageal mucosa. Alternatively, Fluticasone 880 µg/day divided in two doses can be used as a spray to administer topical steroids to the esophagus. Evaluation of treatment by endoscopic biopsies is recommended after 1 month. In refractory disease, systemic steroids (e.g., prednisolone 1 up to 40 mg/kg) and azathioprine (2 mg/kg) can be used.

28.3.6 Esophageal Foreign Body

> Foreign body aspirations and ingestions are common in children (see also Chapter 4).[12]
>
> - Button battery: these are potentially life-threatening in children. When the battery becomes lodged in the esophagus, battery-induced damage can extend to the mediastinum, causing potentially fatal injury to the trachea or aorta. Battery retention in the esophagus requires urgent endoscopic removal, esophageal assessment, prevention of acid reflux, and occasionally parenteral nutrition (see Chapter 4).
> - Coins should be promptly removed from the esophagus if there is any evidence of stridor, cough, drooling, pain, or inability to swallow or drink. Both flexible and rigid endoscopy may be suitable, depending on local skills. If asymptomatic, an observation period of 8 to 16 hours is considered safe to enable spontaneous passage of the coin, which occurs in approximately 25 to 30% of children.

28.3.7 Infections

Infections of the esophagus are rare in healthy children, but can occur in immunosuppression, for example, in children receiving cancer chemotherapy. In infants, candida colonization is associated with typical white plaques present in the mouth, tongue, and pharynx. Viral infections include papilloma (human papillomavirus [HPV]), or aphthous ulcerations by cytomegalovirus (CMV). Aphthous ulcerations in the esophagus can occasionally be found in Crohn's disease.

28.3.8 Dysphagia and Regurgitation

School children frequently present with effortless regurgitation, bringing up saliva, gastric secretion, or food components (usually undigested) into the esophagus, larynx, or pharynx. These children, typically adolescents, are usually asymptomatic with no heartburn, chest pain, epigastric pain, or loss of appetite. The family history often reveals that the symptoms have been described in a parent or grandparent in their childhood.

Barium study and EGD with histology (to exclude EoE and GERD) are usually normal apart from signs of mild reflux. Unfortunately, there is no specific treatment and neither prokinetics nor antacids are particularly helpful. The prognosis appears benign, although evidence-based studies are lacking.

28.3.9 Esophageal Motility Disorders in Children

This is a group of disorders caused by disrupted peristalsis, involving smooth muscles and its innervation.

Achalasia

Achalasia is a disorder of esophageal motility presenting as a functional obstruction at the esophagogastric junction characterized by a lack of esophageal peristalsis, increased LOS pressure, and partial or incomplete LOS relaxation.[8] It presents in children older than 5 years as dysphagia for both solids and liquids, and regurgitation of undigested food.

Theories have been postulated suggesting that the defect is genetic, neurogenic, myogenic, hormonal, or infectious. Incomplete relaxation of the LOS is believed to be secondary to the fact that the postganglionic inhibitory nerves are absent, reduced in number, functionally impaired, or lacking in central connections.[13] Ganglion cell degeneration appears to be prominent in the early years of the disorder, with progressive loss of neurons detected after a decade or more. Achalasia has been associated with adrenocorticotropic hormone insensitivity and alacrima (triple-A or Allgrove's syndrome).

Investigations

A chest radiograph may show a widened mediastinum with an air–fluid level and a lack of air in the stomach.

Barium swallow usually shows a widened tortuous esophagus with a narrowed distal "beak" (▶ Fig. 28.9).

Endoscopy is used to exclude other causes but esophageal manometry is the diagnostic gold standard.

Treatment

Experience with medical therapy is still limited and efficacy is poor. Surgical treatment, for example, disruption of the LOS by pneumatic dilatation or "Heller's myotomy," is usually required.

Globus Pharyngeus

Globus pharyngeus describes a persistent or intermittent nonpainful sensation of a lump or foreign body in the throat. It is a common condition in ENT clinics of adulthood, whereas the incidence in childhood or adolescence is not defined. Persistence of symptoms over several years has been reported for the majority of adult patients. GER has been described as one potentially major cause

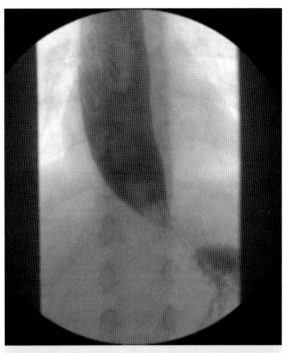

Fig. 28.9 Barium meal fluoroscopy of achalasia: distal esophageal stenosis of neuromuscular origin with typical proximal dilatation.

perhaps due to acid reflux by direct irritation and inflammation or by vagovagal reflex hypertonicity. Other potential causes include abnormal upper esophageal sphincter function, pharyngeal inflammatory disorders, hypertrophy of the base of the tongue, thyroid diseases, cervical heterotopic gastric mucosa, psychological factors and stress, and very rarely childhood tumors.

Since globus is considered an essentially benign disorder, focus should be on a detailed patient history, evaluation of high-risk symptoms, assessment of associated reflux, and attention to psychological problems. Physical examination of the neck and a flexible endoscopic nasolaryngeal examination are usually sufficient, with no need for more extensive or invasive investigations. PPIs taken 30 to 60 minutes before meals for up to 3 months often bring about a response in the presence of reflux symptoms. Flexible upper GI endoscopy may be helpful if there is no improvement, with pH or impedance monitoring as needed.

Barium swallow and video fluoroscopy are useful in ruling out esophageal causes or identifying rare pharyngeal dysfunction in a small subgroup of patients. Manometry is rarely indicated.

Dietetic and lifestyle regulations are helpful. A speech and language therapy referral can be beneficial. Relaxation techniques and cognitive behavioral therapy should be considered, particularly in situations where there is a significant psychological component.[2]

28

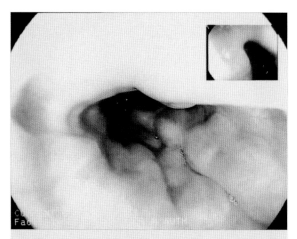

Fig. 28.10 Grade III esophageal varices near gastroesophageal junction.

28.3.10 Upper Gastrointestinal Bleeding

The etiology of upper GI bleeds in children differs substantially from that in adults.

Some of the conditions discussed previously can cause fresh bleeding and include severe GERD, which can also cause vomiting of hematin. Children with diaphragmatic or hiatal hernia can bleed from erosions that can occasionally be seen in the lower esophagus.

Infants may swallow maternal blood when breast-fed, or bleeding can be a sign of a cow's milk protein intolerance. In infants, major fresh upper GI bleeding and melena can result from esophageal varices, usually following a history of prolonged jaundice. EGD shows typical longitudinal venous dilatation in one to three strings (▶ Fig. 28.10). Clearly biopsies from the esophagus are then contraindicated.

ℹ

Emergency treatment of bleeding esophageal varices comprises resuscitation with an intravenous fluid bolus and continued infusion, sometimes blood transfusion, and intravenous octreotide perfusion. Octreotide is a somatostatin analog that reduces portal venous pressure. Sclerotherapy treatment or rubber band ligature may need to be performed by an experienced gastroenterologist.

28.4 Key Points

- Neonates and infants may have severe anatomical problems including TEF.
- Some GER is normal. It only becomes problematic if it causes symptoms or signs (GERD).
- Choking, coughing, and vomiting are often symptoms of gastroesophageal disorders, but regurgitation is common and may not require treatment.
- Consider ingestion of foreign bodies and be alert to the dangers of button batteries.
- School-aged children often have EoE.
- In conditions with desaturations or aspirations, joint assessment by ENT and gastroenterology (and respiratory medicine in some cases) is advisable.

References

[1] Beasley SW. Oesophageal atresia and trachea-oesophageal fistula. In: David M Burge, D Mervyn Griffiths, Henrik A Steinbrecher, Wheeler RA, eds. Paediatric Surgery. 2nd ed. London: Hodder Arnold; 2006:120–133

[2] Lee BE, Kim GH. Globus pharyngeus: a review of its etiology, diagnosis and treatment. World J Gastroenterol. 2012; 18(20):2462–2471

[3] Wasserman RL, Ginsburg CM. Caustic substance injuries. J Pediatr. 1985; 107(2):169–174

[4] Usta M, Erkan T, Cokugras FC, et al. High doses of methylprednisolone in the management of caustic esophageal burns. Pediatrics. 2014; 133(6):E1518–E1524

[5] Rudolph CD, Mazur LJ, Liptak GS, et al. North American Society for Pediatric Gastroenterology and Nutrition. Guidelines for evaluation and treatment of gastroesophageal reflux in infants and children: recommendations of the North American Society for Pediatric Gastroenterology and Nutrition. J Pediatr Gastroenterol Nutr. 2001; 32 Suppl 2:S1–S31

[6] de Lagausie P, Bonnard A, Schultz A, et al. Reflux in esophageal atresia, tracheoesophageal cleft, and esophagocoloplasty: Bianchi's procedure as an alternative approach. J Pediatr Surg. 2005; 40(4):666–669

[7] Spechler SJ, Goyal RK. Barrett's esophagus. N Engl J Med. 1986; 315 (6):362–371

[8] Podas T, Eaden J, Mayberry M, Mayberry J. Achalasia: a critical review of epidemiological studies. Am J Gastroenterol. 1998; 93(12):2345–2347

[9] Papadopoulou A, Koletzko S, Heuschkel R, et al. Management guideline of eosinophilic esophagitis (EoE) in childhood. J Pediatr Gastroenterol Nutr. 2014; 58(1):107–118

[10] European Medicines Agency. Restrictions on the use of domperidone-containing medicines. London: EMA; September 2014. Available at http://www.ema.europa.eu/ema/index.jsp?curl=pages/medicines/human/referrals/Domperidone-containing_medicines/human_referral_prac_000021.jsp&mid=WC0b01ac05805c516fEuropean. Accessed January 27, 2016

[11] National Institute for Health and Care Excellence. Gastro-oesophageal reflux disease in children and young people: diagnosis and management. NICE guidelines [NG1]. London: NICE; 2015

[12] Brumbaugh DE, Colson SB, Sandoval JA, et al. Management of button battery-induced hemorrhage in children. J Pediatr Gastroenterol Nutr. 2011; 52(5):585–589

[13] Seelig MH, DeVault KR, Seelig SK, et al. Treatment of achalasia: recent advances in surgery. J Clin Gastroenterol. 1999; 28(3):202–207

Appendix: Strength of Clinical Evidence

Table 1 Category of evidence

Ia	Evidence from meta-analysis of randomized controlled trials
Ib	Evidence from at least one randomized controlled trial
IIa	Evidence from at least one controlled study without randomization
IIb	Evidence from at least one other type of quasiexperimental study
III	Evidence from nonexperimental descriptive studies, such as comparative studies, correlation studies, and case–control studies
IV	Evidence from expert committee reports or opinions or clinical experience of respected authorities, or both

Table 2 Strength of recommendation

A	Directly based on category I evidence
B	Directly based on category II evidence or extrapolated recommendation from category I evidence
C	Directly based on category III evidence or extrapolated recommendation from category I or II evidence
D	Directly based on category IV evidence or extrapolated recommendation from category I, II, or III evidence

Index

Note: Page numbers set **bold** or *italic* indicate headings or figures, respectively.